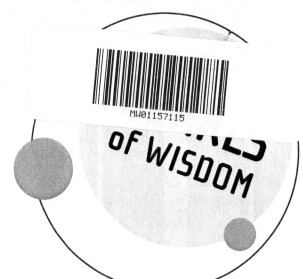

of WISDOM

Urology
BOARD REVIEW

Third Edition

Stephen W. Leslie, M.D., F.A.C.S.

Lorain Surgical Specialties, Inc.
Assistant Clinical Professor of Urology
Medical College of Ohio School of Medicine
Amherst, Ohio

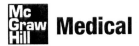 **Medical**

New York Chicago San Francisco Lisbon London Madrid Mexico City Milan
New Delhi San Juan Seoul Singapore Sydney Toronto

34567890 IBT/IBT 14 13 12

ISBN 978-0-07-160583-0
MHID 0-07-160583-5

Notice

Medicine is an ever-changing science. As new research and clinical experience broaden our knowledge, changes in treatment and drug therapy are required. The author and the publisher of this work have checked with sources believed to be reliable in their efforts to provide information that is complete and generally in accord with the standards accepted at the time of publication. However, in view of the possibility of human error or changes in medical sciences, neither the author nor the publisher nor any other party who has been involved in the preparation or publication of this work warrants that the information contained herein is in every respect accurate or complete, and they disclaim all responsibility for any errors or omissions or for the results obtained from use of the information contained in this work. Readers are encouraged to confirm the information contained herein with other sources. For example, and in particular, readers are advised to check the product information sheet included in the package of each drug they plan to administer to be certain that the information contained in this work is accurate and that changes have not been made in the recommended dose or in the contraindications for administration. This recommendation is of particular importance in connection with new or infrequently used drugs.

This book was set in Adobe Garamond by Aptara®, Inc.
The editor was Kirsten Funk.
The production supervisor was Sherri Souffrance.
Project management was provided by Satvinder Kaur.
The cover designer was Handel Low.
IBT Global was printer and binder.

This book is printed on acid-free paper.

Library of Congress Cataloging-in-Publication Data

Urology board review / [edited by] Stephen W. Leslie. – 3rd ed.
    p. ; cm. – (Pearls of wisdom)
  Includes bibliographical references.
  ISBN-13: 978-0-07-160583-0 (pbk. : alk. paper)
  ISBN-10: 0-07-160583-5
  1. Urology–Examinations, questions, etc.   I. Leslie, Stephen W.
II. Series: Pearls of wisdom.
  [DNLM: 1. Urologic Diseases–Examination Questions.
2. Urology–Examination Questions. WJ 18.2 U771 2009]
  RC871.U764 2009
  616.60076–dc22
                                      2009011874

DEDICATION

"To David A. Levy MD who skillfully edited the First Edition, to Scott Plantz MD who decided at the last minute to give me this unique editorial opportunity, and especially to my wife Rosemary, my parents and family for their sacrifices which helped me achieve my professional goals; and to all of my teachers who took their time to educate and instruct me so I could learn how to provide care for others."

Stephen

CONTENTS

CONTRIBUTORS

Tamer Aboushwareb, MD
Research Instructor
Wake Forest Institute for Regenerative Medicine
Wake Forest University Baptist Medical Center
Winston-Salem, North Carolina
Congenital Disorders of the Lower Urinary Tract

Madhu Alagiri, MA, FAAP
Associate Professor of Surgery
Director of Pediatric Urology
University of California, San Diego
San Diego, California
Megaureter

David M. Albala, MD, FACS
Professor of Urology
Director of Minimally Invasive and Robotic
    Urologic Surgery
Duke University Medical Center
Durham, North Carolina
Radionuclide
Upper Urinary Tract Obstruction
Adult Urinary Tract Infections

Sultan Saud Alkhateeb, MD
Fellow, Urologic Oncology
Department of Surgical Oncology
University Health Network
University of Toronto
Toronto, Ontario
Canada
Intestinal Segments in Urology

Anthony Atala, MD
Professor and Chair
Department of Urology
Director, Wake Forest Institute for Regenerative
    Medicine
Wake Forest University School of Medicine
Medical Center Boulevard
Winston-Salem, North Carolina
Congenital Disorders of the Lower Urinary Tract

Daniel A. Barocas, MD
Instructor
Department of Urologic Surgery
Vanderbilt University Medical Center
Nashville, Tennessee
Adrenal Physiology

Mark F. Bellinger, MD
University of Pittsburgh
Children's Hospital of Pittsburgh
Pediatric Urology Associates
Pittsburgh, Pennsylvania
Embryology of the Genitourinary Tract

Jay Laurence Bloch, MD
Chief
Urological Specialists of Southern New Jersey
Voorhees, New Jersey
Renovascular Hypertension

Benjamin N. Breyer, MD
Chief Resident
University of California, San Francisco
Department of Urology
San Francisco, California
Urethral Lesions

Venu Chalasani, MBBS, FRACS
Divisions of Urology & Surgical Oncology
University of Western Ontario
London, Ontario
Canada
Surgical Anatomy of the Pelvis

Bilal Chughtai, MD
Resident Physician
Division of Urology
Albany Medical Center
Albany, New York
*Treatment of Locally Advanced or Recurrent
    Prostate Cancer*

Christopher L. Coogan, MD
Associate Professor
Department of Urology
Rush University Medical Center
Chicago, Illinois
Urinary Diversion and Undiversion

Paul L. Crispen, MD
Fellow, Urologic Oncology
Department of Urology
Mayo Clinic
Rochester, Minnesota
Adrenal Tumors
Renal Tumors, Adults

James M. Cummings, MD
Professor
Department of Surgery
Division of Urology
St. Louis University School of Medicine
St. Louis, Missouri
Genitourinary Trauma

Cole Davis, MD
Fellow, Urologic Oncology
Clinical Instructor in Urology
University of California, San Francisco
San Francisco, California
Uroradiology

John W. Davis, MD
Assistant Professor of Urology
The University of Texas
The M.D. Anderson Cancer Center
Houston, Texas
Penile Cancer

David A. Diamond, MD
Associate Professor of Surgery (Urology)
Harvard Medical School
Boston, Massachusetts
Disorders of Sexual Development

Damon Dyche, MD
Resident Physician
Department of Urology
William Beaumont Hospital
Royal Oak, Michigan
TCC of the Bladder

Ernie L. Esquivel, MD
Assistant Professor of Clinical Medicine
Renal-Electrolyte and Hypertension Division
University of Pennsylvania School of Medicine
Philadelphia, Pennsylvania
Renal Section
Department of Medicine
Philadelphia Veterans Affairs Medical Center
Philadelphia, Pennsylvania
Renal Physiology

Kevin M. Feber, MD
Division of Pediatric Urology
William Beaumont Hospital
Royal Oak, Michigan
Congenital Disorders of the Upper Urinary Tract

Fernando Ferrer, MD, FAAP, FACS
Vice-Chairman
Department of Surgery
Associate Professor of Surgery (Urology) and
    Pediatrics (Oncology)
University of Connecticut School of Medicine
Farmington, Connecticut
Surgeon-in-Chief
Director Division of Pediatric Urology
Connecticut Children's Medical Center
Hartford, Connecticut
Urological Emergencies in the Newborn
Pediatric Oncology

Andrew I. Fishman, MD
Department of Urology
Saint Vincent Catholic Medical Center
New York Medical College
New York, New York
Renal/Ureteral Stone Surgery

Matthew T. Gettman, MD
Associate Professor
Department of Urology
Mayo Clinic
Rochester, Minnesota
Adrenal Tumors
Renal Tumors, Adults
Renal Tumors, Children

Reza Ghavamian, MD
Associate Professor of Urology
Director Urologic Oncology
Montefiore Medical Center
Albert Einstein College of Medicine
Bronx, New York
*Squamous Cell Carcinoma and Adenocarcinoma
of the Bladder*

Gamal M. Ghoniem, MD, FACS
Head, Section of Female Urology,
    Voiding Dysfunction
    & Reconstructive Surgery
Cleveland Clinic Florida
Weston, Florida
Urodynamics

Marc Goldstein, MD, DSc (hon), FACS
Professor of Reproductive Medicine, and Urology
Senior Scientist, Population Council
Surgeon-in-Chief, Mail Reproductive Medicine
    and Surgery
Cornell Institute for Reproductive Medicine
    and Surgery
Weill Cornell Medical College
New York, New York
Male Infertility

Michael Grasso III, MD
Chairman
Department of Urology
Saint Vincent Medical Center
New York, New York
Professor and Vice Chairman
New York Medical College
Valhala, New York
Renal/Ureteral Stone Surgery

Graham F. Greene MD, FACS
Associate Professor of Urology
Chair in Urologic Oncology
University of Arkansas for Medical Sciences
Little Rock, Arkansas
Retroperitoneal Anatomy

A. Ari Hakimi, MD
Resident Physician
Department of Urology
Montefiore Medical Center
Albert Einstein College of Medicine
Bronx, New York
*Squamous Cell Carcinoma and Adenocarcinoma
of the Bladder*

Stephen B. Haltom, MD
Radiology Resident Physician
University of New Mexico School of
    Medicine
Albuquerque, New Mexico
Radiology: CT/Ultrasound

J. Nathaniel Hamilton, MD
Resident Physician
Department of Urology
Medical University of South Carolina
Charleston, South Carolina
*Interstitial Cystitis and Other Inflammatory
    Conditions of the Lower Urinary Tract*

Sang Won Han, MD
Department of Urology
Yonsei University
Seoul, Korea
Enuresis

Daniel M. Hoffman, MD, FACS
Genito-Urinary Surgery & Pediatric
    Urology
Urology Associates of Fredericksburg
Fredericksburg, Virginia
Surgical Therapy for Prostate Cancer

Daniel S. Hoyt, MD
Resident Physician
Division of Urology
University of Missouri School of Medicine
Columbia, Missouri
Prostatitis

Jonathan I. Izawa, MD, FRCSC
Assistant Professor
Departments of Surgery & Oncology
Divisions of Surgical Oncology & Urology
Schulich School of Medicine & Dentistry
University of Western Ontario
London Health Sciences Centre - Victoria
    Hospital
London, Ontario
Canada
Surgical Anatomy of the Pelvis

Joseph E. Jamal, MD
Staff Physician
Department of Surgery
Division of Urology
Lenox Hill Hospital
New York, New York
Neurogenic Voiding Dysfunction

Thomas W. Jarrett, MD
Professor and Chairman
Department of Urology
Medical Faculty Associates
George Washington University
Washington, DC
TCC of the Upper Urinary Tracts

Evan J. Kass, MD
Division of Pediatric Urology
William Beaumont Hospital
Royal Oak, Michigan
*Congenital Disorders of the Upper
    Urinary Tract*

Howard H. Kim, MD
Fellow
Male Reproductive Medicine and
    Microsurgery
Department of Urology
Cornell Institute for Reproductive Medicine
    and Surgery
Weill Cornell Medical College
New York, New York
Male Infertility

Ja-Hong Kim, MD
Fellow
Female Urology, Urodynamics, and Pelvic
    Reconstruction
Department of Urology
David Geffen School of Medicine
University of California, Los Angeles
Los Angeles, California
Female Incontinence and Vesicovaginal Fistula

Laurence Klotz, MD
Professor of Surgery
University of Toronto
Chief of Urology
Sunnybrook Health Science Centre
Toronto, Ontario
Canada
Intestinal Segments in Urology

Badrinath Konety, MD, MBA, FACS
Department of Urology
University of California, San Francisco
San Francisco, California
Urethral Lesions

Harry P. Koo, MD, FAAP, FACS
Professor and Chairman
Division of Urology
Virginia Commonwealth University School of
    Medicine
Richmond, Virginia
Cryptorchidism: Diagnosis and Management

Howard J. Korman, MD, FACS
Attending Physician
William Beaumont Hospital
Department of Urology
Comprehensive Urology PLLC
Royal Oak, Michigan
TCC of the Bladder

Brian F. Kowal, MD
Urology Resident Physician
Dartmouth Medical School
Dartmouth Hitchcock Medical Center
Lebanon, New Hampshire
Testicular and Para Testicular Tumors

Gregory J. Kubicek, MD
Department of Radiation Oncology
Thomas Jefferson University Hospital
Philadelphia, Pennsylvania
Radiation Therapy for Prostate Cancer

Christian S. Kuhr, MD, FACS
Director of Transplanation
Section of Urology
Department of Surgery
Virginia Mason Medical Center
Seattle, Washington
Renal Transplantation

Udaya Kumar, MD
Professor of Urology
University of Arkansas for Medical Sciences
Chief of Urology
McClellan's Memorial Veterans Affairs Hospital
Little Rock, Arkansas
Radionuclide
Upper Urinary Tract Obstruction
Adult Urinary Tract Infections

Peter Langenstroer, MD, MS
Associate Professor of Urology
Medical College of Wisconsin
Milwaukee, Wisconsin
Genitourinary Tuberculosis

Hye Young Lee, MD, MS
Clinical Research Assistant Professor
Department of Urology
Yonsei University College of Medicine
Seoul, Korea
Enuresis

David A. Levy, MD
Department of Urology
Case Medical Center
University Hospitals of Cleveland
Cleveland, Ohio
Diagnosis and Staging of Prostate Cancer

Mary Ann Lim, MD
Renal-Electrolyte and Hypertension Division
University of Pennsylvania School of Medicine
Philadelphia, Pennsylvania
Renal Physiology

Tom F. Lue, MD
Professor and Vice-Chair
Department of Urology
University of California, San Francisco
San Francisco, California
Urethral Strictures
Male Sexual Function and Dysfunction

Donald F. Lynch, Jr., MD, FACS
Professor and Chairman
Department of Urology
Eastern Virginia School of Medicine
Norfolk, Virginia
Penile Cancer

John H. Makari, MD, MHA, MA
Assistant Professor of Surgery
Division of Urology
University of Connecticut School of Medicine
Farmington, Connecticut
Attending Surgeon
Department of Pediatric Urology
Connecticut Children's Medical Center
Hartford, Connecticut
Urological Emergencies in the Newborn

James Mandell, MD
Professor of Surgery (Urology)
Harvard Medical School
President and CEO
Children's Hospital Boston
Boston, Massachusetts
Disorders of Sexual Development

Patrick H. McKenna, MD
Professor and Chair
Department of Surgery
Division of Urology
Southern Illinois University School of Medicine
Springfield, Illinois
Urological Emergencies in the Newborn

Badar M. Mian, MD, FACS
Associate Professor of Surgery
Division of Urology
Albany Medical College
Albany, New York
Treatment of Locally Advanced or Recurrent
  Prostate Cancer

Manoj Monga, MD
Department of Urology
University of Minnesota
Minneapolis, Minnesota
Medical Aspects of Urolithiasis

Jeremy B. Myers, MD
Fellow
University of California, San Francisco
San Francisco General Hospital
San Francisco, California
Urethral Strictures

Durwood E. Neal, Jr. MD
Professor and Chairman
Division of Urology
University of Missouri
Columbia, Missouri
Prostatitis

Elizabeth Phillips, MD
Department of Urology
University of Minnesota
Minneapolis, Minnesota
Medical Aspects of Urolithiasis

Shlomo Raz, MD
Professor of Urology
Chief, Pelvic Medicine and Reconstruction
Department of Urology
David Geffen School of Medicine
University of California, Los Angeles
Los Angeles, California
*Female Incontinence and Vesicovaginal
    Fistula*

Pramod Reddy, MD
Associate Professor of Surgery
University of Cincinnati
Director of Pediatric Urology Fellowship
Cincinnati Children's Hospital Medical
    Center
Cincinnati, Ohio
Radionuclide

Koon H. Rha, MD, FACS, PhD
Associate Professor
Department of Urology
Director, Robotic & MIS Training Center
Yonsei University College of Medicine
Seoul, Korea
Enuresis

Julie M. Riley, MD
Resident Physician
Division of Urology
University of Missouri
Columbia, Missouri
Prune Belly Syndrome

Jonathan C. Routh, MD
Department of Urology
Mayo Clinic
Rochester, Minnesota
Renal Tumors, Children

Eric S. Rovner, MD
Professor
Department of Urology
Medical University of South Carolina
Charleston, South Carolina
*Interstitial Cystitis and Other Inflammatory Conditions
    of the Lower Urinary Tract*

John D. Seigne, MB
Associate Professor of Surgery (Urology)
Dartmouth Medical School
Dartmouth Hitchcock Medical Center
Lebanon, New Hampshire
Testicular and Para Testicular Tumors

Alan W. Shindel, MD
Clinical Instructor
Department of Urology
University of California, San Francisco
San Francisco, California
Male Sexual Function and Dysfunction

W. Bruce Shingleton, MD
Division of Urology
University of North Carolina School of Medicine
Chapel Hill, North Carolina
Prostatic Hyperplasia

Anthony Y. Smith, MD
Professor and Chief
Division of Urology
University of New Mexico School of Medicine
Albuquerque, New Mexico
Uroradiology
Radiology: CT/Ultrasound

Frederick L. Taylor, MD
Resident in Urology
Rush University Medical Center
Chicago, Illinois
Urinary Diversion and Undiversion

Richard K. Valicenti, MD, MA
Associate Professor and Chief
Department of Radiation Oncology
Thomas Jefferson University Hospital
Philadelphia, Pennsylvania
Radiation Therapy for Prostate Cancer

Mark R. Wakefield, MD, FACS
Director, Renal Transplantation
Assistant Professor of Surgery/Urology
University of Missouri School of Medicine
Columbia, Missouri
Prune Belly Syndrome

John Chandler Williams, MD
Beaches Urology
Jacksonville Beach, FL
Benign Renal Cystic Disease

Michael B. Williams, MD, MS
Fellow
Department of Urologic Oncology
MD Anderson Cancer Center
Houston, Texas
Clinical Instructor
Department of Urology
Eastern Virginia Medical School
Norfolk, Virginia
Penile Cancer

Michael R. Williamson, MD
Professor
Department of Radiology
University of New Mexico
Albuquerque, New Mexico
Uroradiology

Jeffrey P. Wolters, MD, MPH
Resident Physician
Division of Urology
Virginia Commonwealth University School of
    Medicine
Richmond, Virginia
Cryptorchidism: Diagnosis and Management

Timothy R. Yoost, MD
Resident Physician
Department of Urology
Medical University of South Carolina
Charleston, South Carolina
*Interstitial Cystitis and Other Inflammatory Conditions
    of the Lower Urinary Tract*

George P. H. Young, MD, FACS
Attending Urologist
Lenox Hill Hospital
New York, New York
Neurogenic Voiding Dysfunction

Richard N. Yu, MD, PhD
Clinical Fellow in Urology
Children's Hospital Boston
Boston, Massachusetts
Disorders of Sexual Development

INTRODUCTION

Congratulations! *Urology Board Review: Pearls of Wisdom* will help you pass urology and improve your board scores. *Urology Board Review*'s unique format differs from all other review and test preparation texts. Let us begin, then, with a few words on purpose, format, and use.

The primary intent of *Urology Board Review* is to serve as a rapid review of urology principles and serve as a study aid to improve performance on urology written and practical examinations. With this goal in mind, the text is written in rapid-fire, question/answer format. The reader receives immediate gratification with a correct answer. Questions themselves often contain a "pearl" reinforced in association with the question/answer.

Additional hooks are often attached to the answer in various forms, including mnemonics, evoked visual imagery, repetition and humor. Additional information not requested in the question may be included in the answer. The same information is often sought in several different questions. Emphasis has been placed on evoking both trivia and key facts that are easily overlooked, are quickly forgotten, and yet somehow always seem to appear on urology exams.

Many questions have answers without explanations. This is done to enhance ease of reading and rate of learning. Explanations often occur in a later question/answer. It may happen that upon reading an answer the reader may think—"Hmm, why is that?" or, "Are you sure?" If this happens to you, GO CHECK! Truly assimilating these disparate facts into a framework of knowledge absolutely requires further reading in the surrounding concepts. Information learned, as a response to seeking an answer to a particular question is much better retained than that passively read. Take advantage of this. Use this book with your urology text handy and open, or, if you are reviewing on train, plane, or camelback, mark questions for further investigation.

Urology Board Review risks accuracy by aggressively pruning complex concepts down to the simplest kernel. The dynamic knowledge base and clinical practice of medicine is not like that! This text is designed to maximize your score on a test. Refer to your mentors for direction on current practice.

Urology Board Review is designed to be used, not just read. It is an interactive text. Use a 3×5 card and cover the answers; attempt all questions. A study method we strongly recommend is oral, group study, preferably over an extended meal or pitchers. The mechanics of this method are simple and no one ever appears stupid. One person holds the book, with answers covered, and reads the question. Each person, including the reader, says "Check!" when he or she has an answer in mind. After everyone has "checked" in, someone states his or her answer. If this answer is correct, on to the next one. If not, another person states his or her answer, or the answer can be read. Usually, the person who "checks" in first gets the first shot at stating the answer. If this person is being a smarty-pants answer-hog, then others can take turns. Try it—it's almost fun!

Urology Board Review is also designed to be re-used several times to allow, dare we use the word, memorization. I suggest putting a check mark every time a question is missed. A hollow bullet has been arbitrarily provided. Another suggestion is to place a check mark when the question is answered correctly once; skip all questions with check marks thereafter. Utilize whatever scheme of using the check boxes you prefer.

We welcome your comments, suggestions and criticism. Great effort has been made to verify these questions and answers. There will be answers we have provided that are at variance with the answer you would prefer. Most often this is attributable to the variance between original source. Please make us aware of any errata you find. We hope to make continuous improvements in a subsequent edition and would greatly appreciate any input with regard to format, organization, content, presentation, or about specific questions. Please write to Stephen W. Leslie, M.D. at swleslie@pol.com. We look forward to hearing from you.

Study hard and good luck!

S. W. L.

TEST-TAKING TIPS

BEFORE THE TEST

Review old tests to become familiar with the format and type of questions. Prepare all the materials you're allowed to bring and make sure they work. Bring extra pens, pencils, and erasers. Bring a watch so that you can pace yourself.

Make a quick study sheet or flash cards of all the material, from *Urology Board Review*, that you have trouble remembering or keep getting wrong. Go over the flash cards or study sheet repeatedly until the material becomes familiar. Review the study sheet/flash card material just before bed and first thing in the morning. This will help reinforce the information.

THE DAY BEFORE

Trying to cram the night before won't help, so get a good night's sleep. Set your alarm and have a backup. Avoid any sleeping pills that can have side effects the next morning.

Make sure you know exactly where the test is being given and how to get there. Have a backup plan for transportation just in case.

Bring or wear a sweater. If the room is too warm, you can always take it off. A slightly cool room is ideal. Have a good meal before the test. Having food in your stomach will help, but avoid having too many heavy foods that can make you groggy. Carry a protein bar in case you get hungry. Use the bathroom before the test. You don't need any bodily distractions.

TAKING THE TEST

Try to pick a comfortable spot in the room with plenty of space. Scan the entire test before actually starting. Read the directions and rules carefully and make sure you understand them. It's amazing how often mistakes are made because the rules and directions weren't followed exactly.

Read the entire question carefully, even if you think you know the question type and the answer right away. Be certain you've answered all parts of the question and didn't leave anything out.

Answer the easiest questions first. Mark the questions you're passing in the test booklet, if allowed, so you can quickly find them later. When you reach the end of the test, go back and finish the skipped questions. With multiple-choice questions, try to determine the correct answer before you read the possible solutions. Don't get worried or anxious if others finish before you do. It's not a race.

DEALING WITH TOUGH QUESTIONS

When dealing with a tough question, start by eliminating the answers that are clearly wrong, are probably wrong, or just don't seem to fit. Go back and read the entire question again. Test preparers don't usually add unnecessary words and details to their questions; every word is important. Look for a keyword or phrase that might be the key to the solution and circle it.

XX   Test-Taking Tips   ● ● ●

If two answers are virtually identical, chances are both are incorrect. Work on a problem question until you get stuck. Think about it for a minute or two, but if nothing else comes, go on to the next question. If allowed, place a mark by that question so that you can find it easily later. Sometimes there will be clues in later questions—these can help you with an earlier problem.

Look for grammatical clues. For example, the word "an" before a blank indicates that the answer starts with a vowel. Go with your first impulse as it's usually right. If you try to overthink the question, you'll probably get it wrong. If you really can't decide between two or more answers, the longer and more detailed answer is usually correct more often. If all else fails and there's no penalty for guessing, go for it!

Don't panic. You are probably not going to get every question right, but getting anxious over it won't help. If you feel yourself hyperventilating, getting anxious, or sweating, just do the following: Put down the pencil, close your eyes, take a few deep breaths, and consciously relax any muscle groups that you're clenching (jaw, neck, stomach). When you've calmed down, go back to the examination.

THE BIG FINISH

Use all of your time. Even if you finish early, check for silly mistakes and make sure all your marks are clear, legible, and in the correct space. Don't go back and change an answer unless you misread or misinterpreted the question. Make sure there are no stray marks on the answer sheet and that each answer completely fills in the little bubble.

Every few pages, make sure the test numbers and the answer numbers match. It's very easy to put an answer in the wrong place, especially if you skipped a question but forgot to skip marking the answer sheet, and then all the subsequent answers will be mismatched and incorrect. Make absolutely sure that your name and identification numbers are correct.

Good luck!

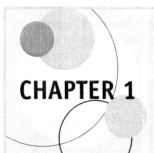

CHAPTER 1 Uroradiology

Cole Davis, MD, Anthony Y. Smith, MD, and Michael Williamson, MD

○ **A 23-year-old man has a history of microscopic hematuria and an intravenous urogram (IVU) is planned for evaluation. The patient reports a history of an allergy to shellfish. He has not previously received IV contrast. The next step should be?**

Patients with a history of asthma, drug allergy, or allergy to shellfish have approximately a twofold greater risk of a contrast reaction. Minor reactions include hot flushes, nausea, vomiting, or urticaria while major reactions include bronchospasm, hypotension, laryngeal edema, and cardiac arrest. The overall incidence of contrast reactions is estimated to be 13% with high-osmolality agents and only 3% with low-osmolality agents. The alternatives to consider in this patient include substitution of a different study (particularly had there been a severe prior reaction), the use of lower osmolality contrast agents, and pretreatment with steroids and antihistamines. A reasonable pretreatment regimen for adults consists of 50-mg prednisone at 13, 7, and 1 hour prior to the study, and 50 mg of diphenhydramine 1 hour before the examination. H1 and H2 blockers can also be used.

Another option would be to use either ultrasound and/or noncontrasted CT scan to examine the kidneys in a case of microscopic hematuria, particularly when the patient is only 23 years old.

Contraindications to IVP include previous anaphylactic reactions to IV contrast, positive azotemia (creatinine >2.0), relative contraindications include dehydration, diabetes, multiple myeloma, and pregnancy.

○   **A 30-year-old female is undergoing a workup for microhematuria. Her serum pregnancy test is negative. The 15-minute film from the IVU is shown. The next step should be?**

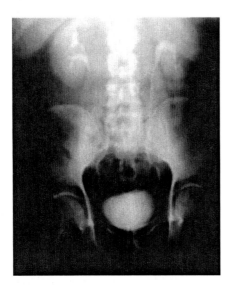

The patient should have a cystoscopy to complete the workup. The IVU is normal. (It is not uncommon to have a normal study appear on a board examination.) While the film as shown is normal, it is important to point out that the top of the left kidney is "cropped." The entire kidney should be visible on an IVU. If not, additional films should be taken.

○   **Describe the proper technique for performing and reviewing an IVU.**

In a normal IVU, a KUB or scout film is obtained following which approximately 1 cm^3/kg of intravenous contrast is administered. On the KUB, careful attention should be paid to any and all unusual calcifications, organs outside the urinary tract, and bony abnormalities as well as any technical flaws. A 30-second film shows the nephrogram phase of the IVU and is regarded as the best film to assess renal masses and renal contour. During the excretion phase, 5-, 10-, and 15-minute films are generally taken. There should be symmetric excretion. The left kidney should be no more than 2-cm longer than the right kidney. Kidneys should be approximately 3 to 5 vertebral bodies in length. Forniceal angles should be sharp. Blunting of the forniceal angles is said to be the earliest radiographic sign of hydronephrosis on IVU. Three major infundibula should be visualized along with roughly 13 to 14 calyces for each kidney. The angle, orientation, outlines, shape, and position of the kidneys should be reviewed and tomograms should be taken if there is any doubt about the integrity of the kidneys. The ureter should not show a standing column (columnization) of contrast and the bladder contour, best seen on the 15-minute film, should be smooth. A postvoid film should also be done. Posterior oblique films can be performed to better visualize the distal ureters.

○ **A 70-year-old man presents with microhematuria and a portion of the initial KUB done for the IVU is shown. Prior to cystoscopy, what should be the next step?**

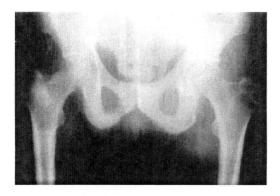

Four things to look for on the scout film are "masses, gasses, bones, and stones." Each time you look at a scout film review those four things and comment about whether they are normal or abnormal. Symmetry is also important. In this case, there is asymmetry on either side of the pubic symphysis with sclerosis evident on the left. There is a somewhat moth-eaten appearance to the periosteum on the left superior and inferior pubic rami as well. Sclerotic bone lesions are found in patients with breast and prostate cancer. On plain films, a 50% change in cortical density is required to visualize metastatic disease. In this elderly man, the next step should be a prostate specific antigen and a prostate examination.

○ **A child with multiple birth defects had a renal ultrasound suggestive of duplication and hydronephrosis. An IVU was performed to further evaluate the finding. The KUB obtained prior to the study is shown. What is the radiographic finding demonstrated?**

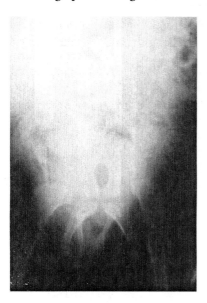

The radiograph is a classic picture of complete sacral agenesis. The sacrum is absent causing the pelvic ring to look like an inverted teardrop. Incomplete agenesis may be more difficult to diagnose. The diagnosis may be delayed until failed attempts at toilet training prompt urological evaluation for neurogenic bladder. Sacral agenesis may be one component of the VACTERL syndrome (V = **V**ertebral anomalies, A = imperforate **A**nus, C = **C**ardiac anomalies, TE = **T**rach**E**oesophageal fistula, R = **R**enal anomalies, and L = **L**imb anomalies).

○   **This KUB accompanied the IVU done for evaluation of congenital urological problems in a child. What is the radiographic finding demonstrated?**

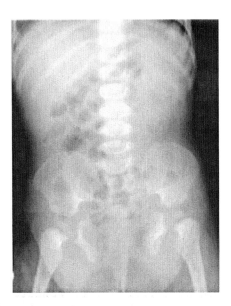

The three conditions that are associated with widening of the symphysis pubis include pregnancy, trauma, and the congenital condition of exstrophy/epispadias, of which this is an example. The femurs are rotated laterally. There is no separation of the SI joint to suggest trauma. This abnormality is thought to occur as a result of failed mesodermal ingrowth and consequent failure of descent of the cloacal membrane that produces eventration of the bladder onto the abdominal wall. The spectrum ranges from pure epispadias with a dorsal penile meatus and urethra to cloacal exstrophy with eventration of both bowel and bladder.

○   **A 35-year-old female presents many years after a sterility procedure in which silicone was injected into the fallopian tubes. She has had significant microscopic hematuria. The likely diagnosis is?**

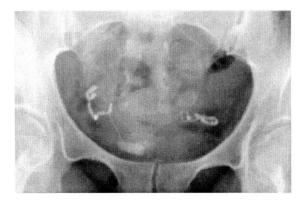

The diagnosis is a bladder stone secondary to foreign body, which in this case was the silicone that eroded through the bladder wall producing a nidus for stone formation. It is important to consider the possibility of outlet obstruction or foreign body when treating a patient with a bladder stone.

○   **This plain film was obtained in a patient undergoing a workup for microhematuria and pyuria. A routine urine specimen submitted for culture was negative. What is the likely diagnosis?**

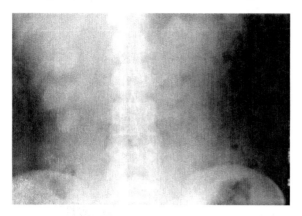

This film shows the classic "paste" stones of genitourinary tuberculosis. The stones are faint on plain film and represent dystrophic calcification of the caseating granulomas that infiltrate the parenchyma of the kidney. The tissue sloughs into the collecting system giving rise to these stones.

○   **A 20-year-old diabetic female presents to the emergency department with fever to 104°C and a white count of 33,000 associated with a left shift. The scout film from an IVU is shown. What is the most likely diagnosis?**

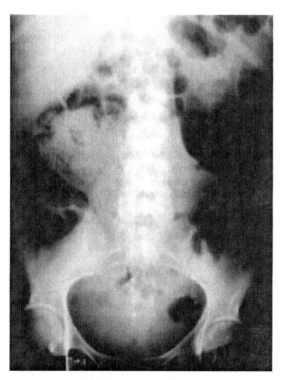

There is gas essentially replacing the left renal outline in a classic case of emphysematous pyelonephritis. The treatment is broad-spectrum antibiotics and nephrectomy. A CT scan, if the patient is stable enough to tolerate the procedure, may help to distinguish a perinephric abscess caused by a gas-forming organism. Gas may outline the kidney in cases of duodenal or colon (retroperitoneal) trauma as well.

○   **An elderly man presents with obstructive voiding symptoms, microhematuria, and a palpable abdominal mass. A KUB was obtained prior to the IVU. The next step should be?**

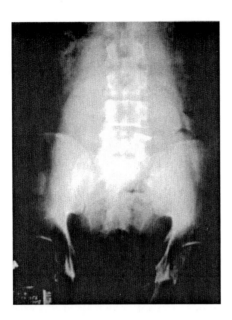

The plain film while overpenetrated shows a midline abdominal mass extending from the pelvis to well above the presumed umbilicus. The next step should be to place a Foley catheter, which in this case resulted in resolution of the mass. This is a bad case of urinary retention.

○   **A patient undergoing a workup for microhematuria has the following KUB obtained prior to the IVU. What is the radiologic finding and what are the top three possible diagnoses associated with this radiographic finding?**

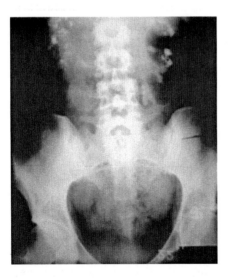

The film shows medullary nephrocalcinosis. This finding is seen most commonly with medullary sponge kidney, type I renal tubular acidosis, and hyperparathyroidism. Cortical nephrocalcinosis is rarely seen in the present era. In the past, it typically was seen as a consequence of postpartum hypotension and renal infarction that produced atrophic kidneys with calcified cortices.

○ **This scout film was obtained to evaluate left flank pain and fever. The urinalysis shows a pH is >7.2 and many gram-negative rods. What are the significant findings on the film? What is the most likely organism cultured from the urine? In addition to antibiotics, what immediate procedure is probably necessary?**

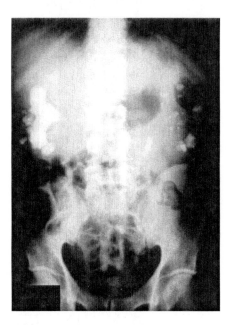

This film shows a large staghorn calculus on the right and multiple stones in both the kidneys. To be classified as a staghorn calculus, the stone should fill and outline at least one calyx and infundibulum. In addition, there appears to be a large calcification medial to the left kidney which could represent ureterolithiasis. These are likely magnesium ammonium phosphate (struvite or triple phosphate) stones associated with urea splitting organisms such as a *proteus* species accounting for the alkaline urinary pH. Subsequent films confirmed obstruction on the left and a left nephrostomy was placed. *In a septic patient with obstruction, a percutaneous nephrostomy is safer than a double J stent.*

○   **A 50-year-old homeless woman presents with gross hematuria and severe dysuria. This KUB was obtained as part of the initial workup. What is the significant radiographic finding?**

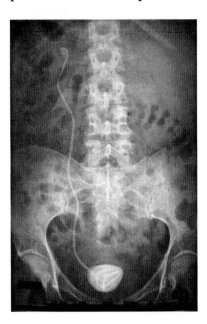

This KUB shows a retained ureteral stent with a large bladder calculus incorporated into the distal coil. Further questioning this patient revealed a history of ureterolithiasis and ureteral stent placement at an outside facility 18 months ago. *It is imperative to secure follow-up in all patients with ureteral stents.* The management should be based on functional findings on the right kidney with a study such as a diuretic renogram.

○   **A 30-year-old female involved in a motor vehicle accident presents with gross hematuria and underwent an IVU. What is the significant finding on the IVU?**

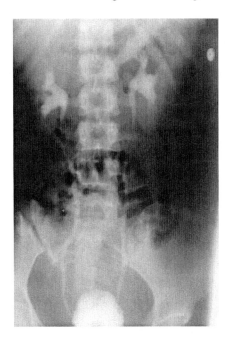

The IVU shows a pelvic fracture with obvious displacement of the SI joint on the right. *It is important on any film presented to look at surrounding structures.* Be especially careful if you are given only one film from a series to review. In this case, the Foley catheter has already been successfully placed. A cystogram and drainage film did not show any evidence of bladder rupture.

○ **A 75-year-old female is evaluated for an episode of gross painless hematuria. The IVU obtained is significant for two abnormalities. Identify these problems.**

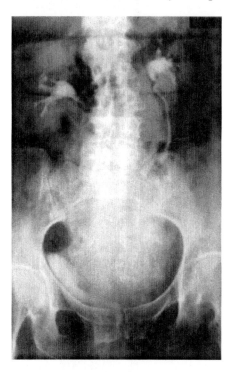

In elderly patients, it is especially important to look for associated findings. In this film, the left ureter deviates laterally in the upper third. There is a fine rim of calcification and a suggestion of a midline mass. On the left side, these findings are suspicious for an aortic aneurysm, which this proved to be. In addition, there is a large calcified pelvic mass displacing the bladder, which ultimately proved to be a Brenner tumor of the ovary. Not well seen is the invasive transitional cell carcinoma of the bladder, which was diagnosed by cystoscopy. *Always remember that finding renal pathology does not exclude bladder and lower urinary tract pathology.*

○   **A 40-year-old man undergoes an IVU to evaluate microhematuria. The 15-minute film is shown. What is the abnormality shown?**

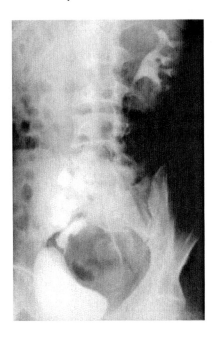

Close inspection of the IVU shows a portion of a calyceal system just below the right pelvic brim and overlying the sacrum. This is an example of an ectopic kidney. The plain film in this case demonstrated a stone in the pelvic kidney. Up to 50% of pelvic kidneys will have hydronephrosis or reflux.

○   **A 42-year-old man who presented with a history of a febrile UTI was evaluated with an IVU. What is the likely diagnosis?**

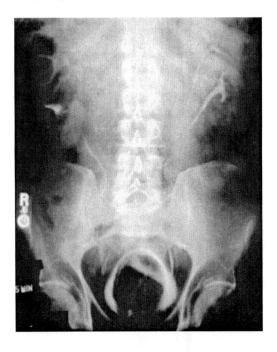

This is an IVU that we do not often see in adults. There is duplication of the collecting system on the left. **Duplication of one collecting system should immediately raise suspicion about duplication in the other kidney.** The right collecting system is notable for only two major infundibula and tilts to the right, a finding labeled as the "drooping lily" sign. The collecting system is missing the upper pole calyx, which often bears close resemblance to a "ball peen hammer." Additionally, there is a large lucent smooth filling defect in the bladder, which could be confused with a tumor or BPH. However, putting the whole picture together, it is likely that this is an ectopic ureterocele with obstruction of an upper pole ureter in a complete duplication on the right. Ectopic refers to the location of the ureteral orifice, which is likely to be outside the trigone. The Meyer–Weigert rule governing the configuration of duplicate orifices is "the upper pole drains lower and lower pole drains lateral." The lower pole orifice is located more laterally on the trigone and is therefore more prone to reflux, while the upper pole orifice enters more medially and is more often obstructed, ectopic, or associated with a ureterocele.

○   **A 27-year-old man presents with right flank pain. His urinalysis shows 0 RBCs/hpf, 2–4 WBCs/hpf, and no bacteria. An IVU is ordered. A delayed film of the IVU is shown. The left kidney was normal on the earlier films. Also a film from a later retrograde ureteropyelography is shown. What radiographic diagnosis is most likely?**

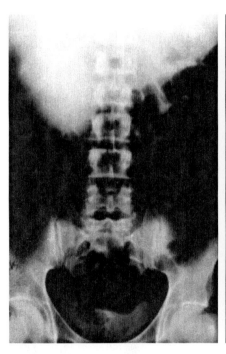
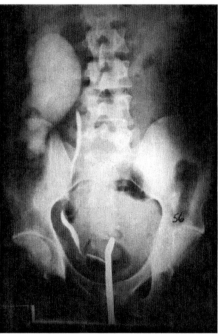

The IVU shows massive hydronephrosis on the right side with no hydroureter, an appearance consistent with a ureteropelvic junction obstruction. A Lasix renogram may give a better estimate of relative function and degree of obstruction but, more importantly, may give a more sensitive test to use to assess outcome after repair. Retrograde ureteropyelography confirms the diagnosis. Many times the formal repair is done in the same setting as the cystoscopy with retrogrades.

○   **A retrograde pyelogram was attempted in a 10-year-old male with intermittent flank pain and hydronephrosis on ultrasound. The ureter is incompletely filled. What is the diagnosis?**

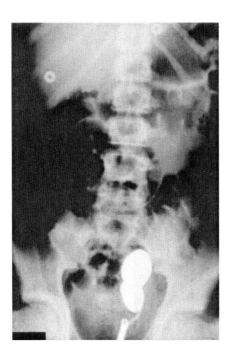

This film shows the classic appearance for a distal adynamic segment associated with a primary obstructed megaureter. The pathology is believed to be due to disordered smooth muscle in the distal segment of the ureter associated with increased collagen deposition. This segment fails to conduct the peristaltic wave and creates a functional obstruction. A similar mechanism is postulated for the majority of UPJ obstructions.

○   **A 30-year-old man presented with right-sided flank pain. His urinalysis showed 0 RBCs/hpf. An IVU was obtained. A 10-minute film is shown. What are the two likely diagnoses?**

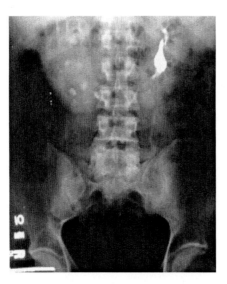

The lower pole of the left kidney has a medially based calyx, which is suggestive of a horseshoe kidney. In addition, the renal axis is shifted laterally. Approximately one-third of horseshoe kidneys may have a contralateral ureteropelvic junction obstruction. The renal pelves are oriented anteriorly, so the pyeloplasty is performed transabdominally. Ureterolithiasis with hydronephrosis is a possibility but no stone is seen and the patient had no significant hematuria making this diagnosis less likely. A retrograde pyelogram at the time of surgery would confirm the diagnosis and rule out a stone or distal adynamic segment.

○ **An IVU was obtained to evaluate microhematuria in a young man. The radiographic diagnosis is?**

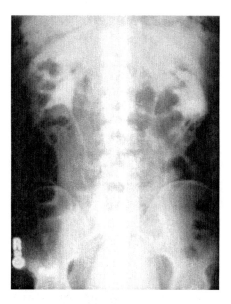

While a medially based calyx is suggestive of a horseshoe kidney, here is the exception. The left kidney has medial calyces but the right does not. This is a malrotated left kidney. The renal pelvis is oriented anteriorly during renal ascent and the kidney then rotates medially. Most malrotated kidneys rotate laterally instead so the vessels cross anteriorly.

○   **A retrograde pyelogram was obtained to evaluate an abnormality seen on IVU for microhematuria. A representative film is shown. What is the abnormality?**

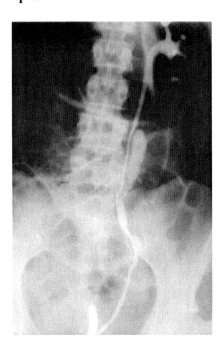

The abnormality is a blind-ending ureter on the left associated with an aborted partial duplication. Blind-ending ureters commonly have a 2:1 length-to-width ratio. They are histologically identical to normal ureters. Ureteral diverticula fail to meet these criteria. The management is individualized but may include excision where either symptoms or infection supervene.

○   **A 19-year-old male had an IVU performed for intermittent right flank pain. He has had a prior left nephrectomy. The IVU suggested obstruction of the upper one-third of the ureter. A representative film from a retrograde pyelogram is shown. What is the diagnosis?**

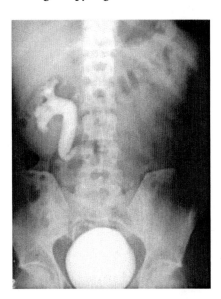

The film is classic for retrocaval ureter with medial deviation of the upper third of the right ureter. The embryologic derivation of the condition is best remembered by referring to the condition as persistent subcardinal vein. The first description of a dismembered pyeloplasty performed for this condition was by Andersen and Hynes.

○   **A 45-year-old man presented with left flank pain and gross hematuria. A representative film from the IVU is shown. What is the likely diagnosis?**

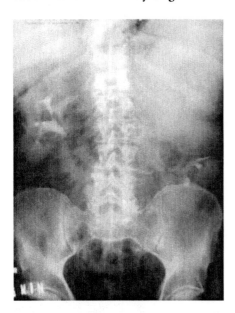

This film shows a different kind of "drooping lily" on the left. There appear to be three major infundibula suggesting normal collecting system architecture and arguing against a duplication. However, the "ball peen hammer" appearance has been modified by what appears to be compression due to a large mass. There are several densities seen in the middle of the mass and while those could represent pooling of contrast, a more likely explanation would be the presence of parenchymal calcification, which of course implies cancer. The differential would include renal cell carcinoma versus adrenal tumor but statistics favor the former. One must consider the possibility of adrenal disease when the kidney is displaced in this fashion.

○   **An IVU is obtained on a 50-year-old man that presents with gross hematuria. What is the most likely diagnosis?**

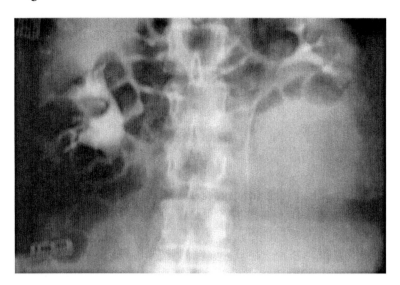

This film illustrates the principle that masses frequently stretch and distort portions of the urinary tract. The left kidney is displaced cephalad and the ureter is stretched and bowed medially. These findings suggest a lower pole renal mass, which is suspicious for renal cell carcinoma. An ultrasound or CT scan would confirm that it is solid and not a simple cyst.

○   **A 28-year-old man presents with a history of gross hematuria. A retrograde pyelogram is undertaken because of the findings on an IVU showing delayed function and hydronephrosis of the right kidney. What is the radiographic sign demonstrated? What is the likely diagnosis?**

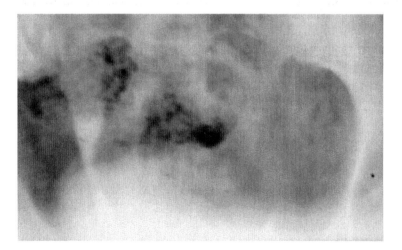

This is Bergman's sign or the "goblet sign". There is dilation of the ureter distal to a ureteral mass. The cause of this phenomenon is not well known but it may be caused by "to and fro" peristalsis of the mass. This leads to a radiographic appearance resembling a chalice or goblet on retrograde pyelogram. The likely diagnosis is transitional cell carcinoma of the ureter.

○   **A 70-year-old man who has a long smoking history presents with painless gross hematuria. A retrograde pyelogram has been done to evaluate the right ureter for hydronephrosis seen on the IVU. The most likely explanation for the findings is?**

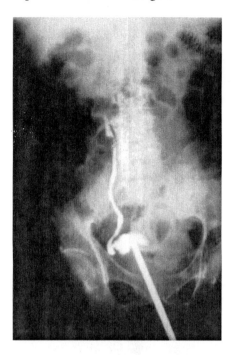

We like to apply the "rat bite" guideline of film interpretation in this case. **If the film looks like a rat has been at work, it is cancer until proven otherwise.** The retrograde pyelogram demonstrates a filling defect in the upper third of the ureter. The initial decision is to determine whether the defect is an intraluminal or extraluminal process. Extraluminal processes tend to displace and compress the ureter. In this case, a portion of the ureter appears to be "eaten" away and the diagnosis is most likely transitional cell carcinoma of the ureter. Other causes of lucent filling defects would be a lucent stone, sloughed papilla, polyp, blood clot, fungus ball, or malakoplakia/cystitis cystica. However, the classic "rat bite" appearance points to malignancy as the likely cause in this case. Ureteroscopy will confirm the diagnosis.

○   **A 70-year-old man with a long smoking history presents with painless gross hematuria. An IVU is performed as part of the diagnostic evaluation. What is the likely diagnosis?**

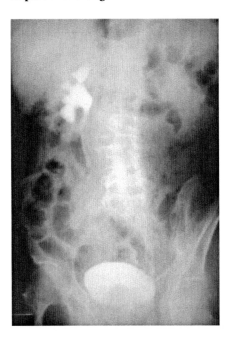

This IVU is notable for nonvisualization of the left kidney. There is a filling defect in the bladder, which could be mistaken for BPH except that it is somewhat irregular. In addition, the right kidney has a standing column of contrast to the middle third of the ureter and early hydronephrosis evidenced by blunting of the forniceal angles. Given the history, the likely diagnosis is muscle invasive transitional cell carcinoma of the bladder, with obstruction of the left ureter causing nonfunction of the left kidney. In addition, the findings on the right are suspicious for transitional cell cancer of the ureter, which proved to be the case as the retrograde showed. This film makes the point that **transitional cell carcinoma can be a bilateral process and the contralateral kidney must be evaluated carefully.** Ureteral obstruction signals invasive cancer up to 90% of the time.

○   **Shown is a representative film from the IVU of a patient who presented with painless gross hematuria. The patient has a long smoking history. What are the two significant findings on this study?**

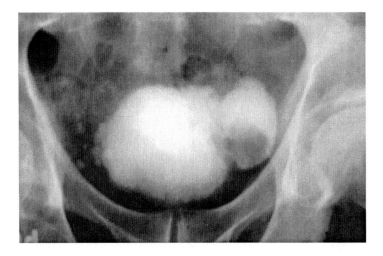

The IVU shows a bladder diverticulum with a filling defect present in the diverticulum. The filling defect is slightly irregular and given the history, the mass most likely represents a transitional cell cancer in a diverticulum. This usually carries a more ominous prognosis.

○   **An IVU is performed for gross hematuria and the collecting system is not well visualized. A retrograde pyelogram is performed. What is the likely diagnosis?**

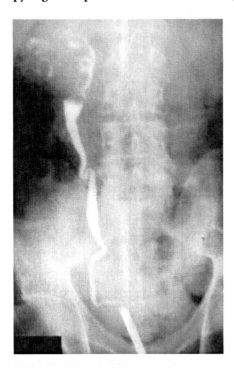

There is a nice goblet sign in the upper ureter, and the collecting system architecture has been destroyed. A "rat" has been at work here and the diagnosis is most likely transitional cell carcinoma. However, the differential should also include xantho granulomatous pyelonephritis and tuberculosis.

○   **This IVU was performed on a 65-year-old male presenting with gross hematuria and a serum creatinine of 1.8. What are the radiographic findings?**

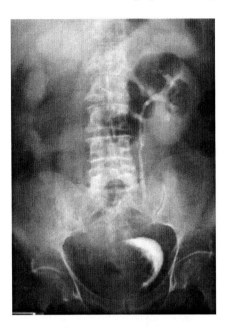

The IVU shows no right nephrogram and a large filling defect in the bladder, which appears to originate from the right bladder wall. This likely represents a bladder tumor and the right kidney is completely obstructed. Upper tract obstruction is worrisome for ureteral involvement of the tumor. A CT scan of the abdomen would be helpful in this setting in addition to transurethral resection of the bladder tumor for therapy and staging.

○   **A 15-year-old nonsmoker presents with an episode of gross hematuria. An IVU shows delayed function of the left kidney. The CT scan findings suggest a soft tissue mass in the ureter. A retrograde pyelogram was performed. What are the significant findings on the study? What are the two most likely diagnoses?**

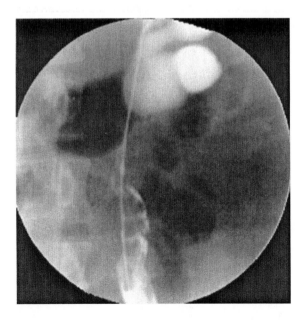

The retrograde pyelogram shows a somewhat lobulated filling defect in the upper ureter. Transitional cell carcinoma is always a possibility, but in a younger patient, the differential would include a fibroepithelial polyp which, in fact, this turned out to be. The CT scan is useful to rule out a radiolucent stone. Ureteroscopy will confirm the diagnosis.

○   **A middle-aged man referred for microhematuria has 10 RBCs/hpf and 20 WBCs/hpf. A urine culture is negative. Urine cytology is negative. A representative film from the IVU is shown for the right kidney. What is the most likely diagnosis?**

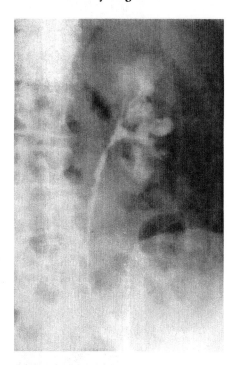

The diagnosis is tuberculosis. Most of the features of tuberculosis are illustrated in this film. Tuberculous strictures occur classically in the infundibula, ureteropelvic junction, and ureterovesical junction. In this film, there are strictures of the upper pole infundibulum and UPJ with some degree of "beading" of the upper ureter. There is evidence of papillary necrosis and actual tissue slough in the film. Damage to parenchyma may progress to calyceal amputation or frank autonephrectomy. Faint amorphous calcifications were evident on the plain film.

○   **This patient has a history of pyuria and vague right flank pain. Routine urine cultures have been negative. This film is the 15-minute film from an IVU. What is the most likely diagnosis?**

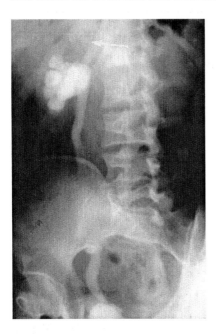

The diagnosis is again tuberculosis. The film illustrates something that both tuberculosis and transitional cell carcinoma do and that is to amputate calyces. The upper pole calyx of the right kidney is seen as just a whisp of irregular contrast (arrow). There is a distal ureteral stricture, which is not well demonstrated on the film. The bladder is contracted and the left kidney is not working and has undergone a functional autonephrectomy.

○   **This film shows bilateral retrograde pyelograms obtained in a patient who had a chronic indwelling stent on the right, which had recently been removed. What diagnosis is suggested by the radiographic finding shown?**

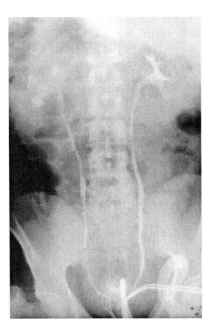

The retrograde pyelogram on the right shows extensive notching of the ureter with smooth, small round filling defects. The history and radiographic findings are most consistent with ureteritis cystica. Other possibilities in the differential would be tuberculosis, malakoplakia, persistent fetal ureter, or transitional cell carcinoma.

○ **This patient underwent an evaluation for microhematuria and pyuria. Past history was remarkable for an extensive travel history including trips to Africa and China. An IVU was obtained and shown are a portion of the scout and 5-minute films. What is the most likely diagnosis?**

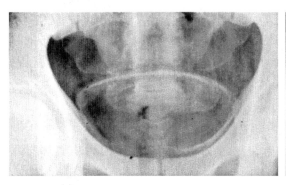 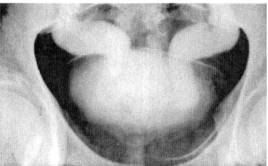

There are few things that will calcify the bladder wall and the first one that should come to mind in this clinical scenario is *Schistosoma*. Schistosomiasis is found in rivers in Africa and other parts of the world. Once in the host, the *Schistosoma hematobium* reside in the perivesical venous plexus and lay their eggs in the bladder wall and venous tributaries of the bladder. The eggs are then shed in the urine completing its life cycle. The result of this process is an intense inflammatory reaction in the bladder. Schistosomiasis can acutely present with hematuria and inflammatory changes in the bladder wall on IVU. Late findings include calcification of the bladder and ureteral walls. Similar to tuberculosis, there may be extensive ureteral strictures. Nonfunction, stones, polypoid masses, and hydronephrosis are also seen. The risk of bladder cancer is high in these patients. Consistent with the intense inflammatory reaction, there is a higher risk of squamous cell cancer and adenocarcinoma. **When there is a suspicion of an inflammatory condition involving the urinary tract, ask about the travel history.**

○   **A 45-year-old female presented with a history of recurrent urinary tract infection. A catheterized urine specimen grew multiple gram-negative organisms. An IVU was obtained. The significant findings on the film are? The most likely diagnosis to explain the film is?**

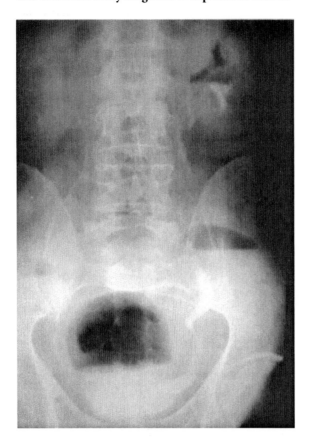

The IVU shows a large amount of gas in the bladder and outlining of the left upper pole calyx. Gas can occur in the urinary tract in association with infection caused by a gas-forming organism. Gas in the amounts seen on this film should raise suspicion for a vesicoenteric fistula, particularly given the history of a polymicrobial infection. Sometimes gas will appear in the wall of the bladder in association with a urinary tract infection known as emphysematous cystitis. Gas outlining the collecting system with no parenchymal gas occurring in the presence of a urinary tract infection is because of emphysematous pyelitis, which responds to antibiotics more favorably than emphysematous pyelonephritis. Renal pelvic gas can also be caused by reflux of air associated with instrumentation. The most likely diagnosis in this case is colovesical fistula caused by diverticulitis. Crohn's disease, colon cancer, and other pelvic malignancies can also cause fistulas.

○   **A 50-year-old female presented with a history of malaise, left-sided flank pain, and a low-grade fever. On physical examination, a hard mass was palpable in the left upper quadrant. A urine culture grew *Proteus*. The IVU suggested a left renal mass associated with several calcifications, which appeared to be stones, and the kidney was essentially nonfunctional. A representative film from the retrograde pyelogram is shown. What is the likely diagnosis?**

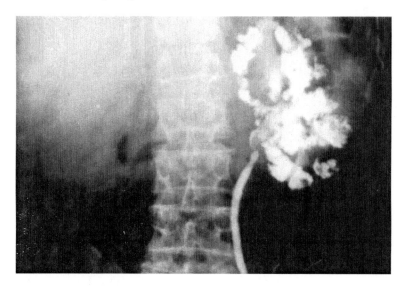

The constellation of renal mass and stones raises the differential of xanthogranulomatous pyelonephritis versus squamous cell carcinoma of the kidney. The presence of the proteus infection makes the former more likely. Renal calculi are seen in one-third of cases and a mass is found in two-thirds. *Proteus* is the most common organism but *E. coli* is also common. The retrograde pyelogram shows destruction of parenchyma and collecting system with multiple abscess cavities. There is a suggestion of a filling defect in the renal pelvis corresponding to the stone seen on plain film.

○   **A middle-aged female presented with a history of recurrent urinary tract infection. The infections have all been characterized by dysuria and frequency but without fever. A postvoid film from the IVU is seen. The likely diagnosis is?**

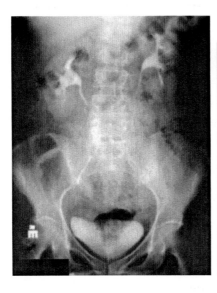 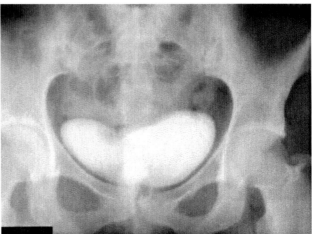

The film shows a relatively smooth double-contrast density at or just distal to the bladder neck. In a female, the likely diagnosis is a urethral diverticulum. Urethral diverticula may be a cause of recurrent UTI. They may be difficult to diagnose. The diagnosis should begin with a good physical examination that includes palpation of the urethra. An IVU and particularly the postvoid bladder film may identify the diverticulum. A voiding cystogram, "double bubble" urethrogram using a special double balloon urethral catheter, and cystoscopy may also be useful.

○   **A 25-year-old female presented with a history of intermittent right flank pain and hematuria. A faint stone was seen overlying the right bladder shadow on plain film. Hexagonal crystals were present in the urine. What is the significant radiographic sign demonstrated in this IVU and what is the most likely diagnosis?**

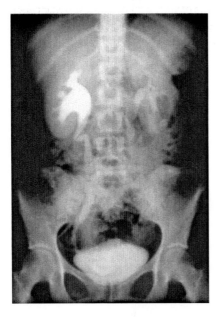

The IVU shows a "cobra head" deformity of the distal right ureter consistent with a simple orthotopic ureterocele. The orifice is likely to be on the trigone. The faint lucency seen in the middle of the ureterocele is likely to be a "relatively" radiolucent stone composed of cystine. The crystalluria confirms this and a sodium nitroprusside test on the urine would be positive. Unlike uric acid stones, which are not seen on a plain film, cystine stones are faintly seen on the plain film but appear lucent versus contrast on the IVU. Cystine and uric acid stones are both visible on noncontrast CT scans. Only medication stones (indinivir) are invisible on both noncontrast CT scans and plain films. IVU should be used for diagnosis of possible stones in patients on indinivir and similar medications.

○   **This patient had an IVU performed for hematuria. A urinalysis showed numerous RBCs, no WBCs or bacteria, and a pH of 5.0. The plain film did not show a stone. What are the significant findings and what is the most likely diagnosis? What test should be performed next to confirm the diagnosis?**

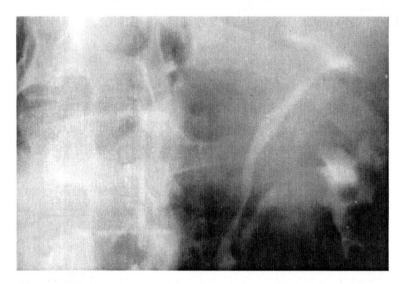

This film shows a smooth lucent filling defect in the lower pole system of a partial duplication. The surface of the defect is smooth. While the usual differential of tumor, stone, clot, papilla, and fungus ball applies, the findings are most consistent with a radiolucent uric acid stone. This could be confirmed with a noncontrast (renal colic) spiral CT scan since uric acid stones appear bright white, while the other possibilities would show only soft tissue. An ultrasound would show a solid stone if the calculus is large enough.

○   **This man presented with gross hematuria. The scout film from the IVU and a set of retrograde pyelograms are shown. A urine culture is sterile. What is the diagnosis and what is the stone composition likely to be?**

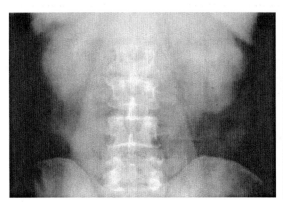 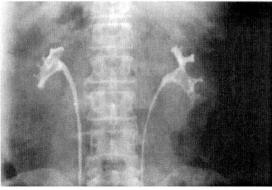

This patient has bilateral staghorn calculi. The stones are relatively radiolucent. Staghorn calculi are most often composed of struvite or magnesium ammonium phosphate and are accompanied by infection with urea-splitting organisms such as *Proteus*. Struvite has a relative density of 0.20, while cystine is slightly lower at 0.15 compared to bone which has a relative radiographic density of 1. These stones are relatively radiolucent and the diagnosis in this patient was staghorn calculi composed of cystine.

○   **A 35-year-old man presented with a history of hypertension, gross hematuria, and abdominal masses. A representative film from the IVU and a retrograde pyelogram are shown. The diagnosis is most likely?**

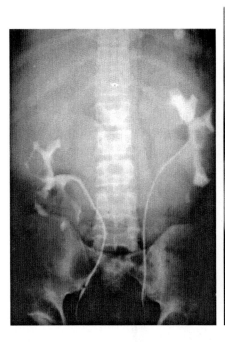 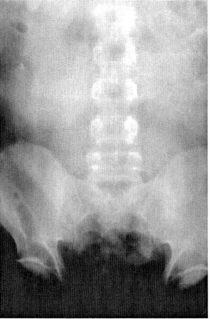

This is a set of films we do not see too often in the era of CT scanning. A normal kidney should be roughly three vertebral bodies in length. The IVU shows large kidneys bilaterally with diffuse splaying of both collecting systems due in this case to multiple cysts. The retrograde pyelogram confirms the IVU findings but also shows some degree of ureteral displacement because of the large kidneys. The diagnosis is autosomal dominant polycystic kidney disease. The patient may have a strong family history. Because of the risk of infecting cysts, the decision to perform retrograde pyelograms in these patients is a serious one and prophylactic antibiotics should be given. The differential diagnosis for large kidneys is long and includes bilateral hydronephrosis, bilateral duplication, bilateral renal tumors, acute bilateral renal vein thrombosis, renal lymphoma, leukemic infiltrates, acute tubular necrosis, diuretic or contrast administration, preeclampsia, lupus, Wegener's, Goodpasture's syndrome, and myeloma with amyloidosis.

○   **This patient with an ileal conduit and a history of transitional cell carcinoma of the bladder had an IVU performed as part of a routine follow-up evaluation. The serum creatinine was elevated to 1.7 mg/dL. The likely diagnosis is?**

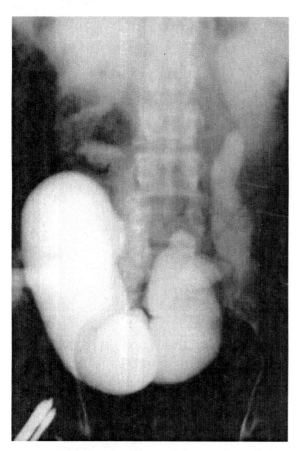

This is a classic film demonstrating stomal stenosis. The presence of bilateral hydronephrosis and a large dilated ileal loop is the conduit equivalent of bladder outlet obstruction confirming the diagnosis of stomal stenosis. A gentle digital examination of the stoma would confirm this.

○   **This young man sustained a gunshot wound to the abdomen and underwent a laparotomy with closure of several small bowel perforations. Two weeks later, he presented with a history of fever to 104°C and flank pain. An ultrasound revealed left hydronephrosis. A representative film of the IVU is shown. What is the likely diagnosis and how should it be managed?**

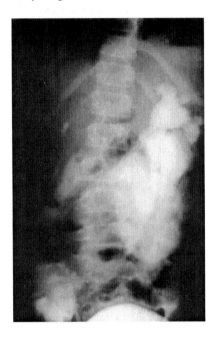

The IVU shows marked extravasation of contrast into a large urinoma. The likely diagnosis is a missed ureteral injury with an infected urinoma. Management in this case consisted of percutaneous drainage of the kidney and urinoma, antibiotics, and delayed repair. **As a general radiologic principle of trauma, whether blunt or penetrating, medial extravasation of contrast should raise suspicion for a ureteral injury.**

○   **This 20-year-old male was involved in a motor vehicle accident. He had multiple long bone fractures. His blood pressure in the field was 70 mm Hg but he responded quickly to fluids. He had no hematuria. A trauma IVU was performed in the trauma suite. What is the likely diagnosis?**

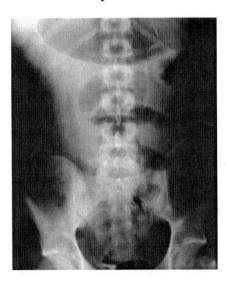

The film shows the left kidney to be functioning normally but there is absence of a nephrogram and function of the right kidney. In addition, there is a fracture of the right L1 transverse process. **Fractures of transverse processes in the region of the renal hilum raise concern for a right renovascular injury.** An expeditious angiogram or contrasted CT scan would confirm the diagnosis. The presence of shock, hematuria, or high suspicion as with major decelerating trauma in the absence of hematuria should prompt urological evaluation. The advent of high-speed CT scanning has largely supplanted the use of IVU in the evaluation of the trauma patient. The two-shot trauma IVU consists of a scout film followed by an injection of 1 mL/kg of IV contrast. A second film is taken at 10 minutes postcontrast injection.

○   **This 50-year-old man presented with poorly localized abdominal pain and was found by ultrasound to have bilateral hydronephrosis and a serum creatinine of 6.0 mg/dL. Past history is significant for migraine headaches. The prostate examination is normal and a trial of catheter drainage does not improve things. Bilateral retrograde pyelograms were obtained and the film for the right side is shown and the film on the left was nearly identical. A stent was passed easily on both sides and the creatinine responded and decreased to 2.0 mg/dL. What is the most likely diagnosis?**

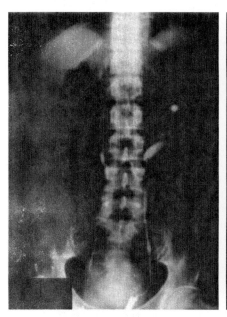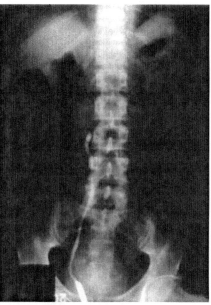

The retrograde pyelograms show medial deviation of the ureter over the spine. The fact that a stent passed easily makes the diagnosis of a stricture less likely and with medial deviation, the diagnosis is most likely retroperitoneal fibrosis. Migraine headaches provide an additional clue to the possible use of methysergide which has been used to treat migraines and has been associated with retroperitoneal fibrosis. A CT scan may be useful to confirm the presence of a fibrous mass encircling the aorta and vena cava and encasing the ureters as well. **Remember that on examinations, the examiners usually don't usually give you any information that isn't relevant to the case in some way, such as travel, medications, allergies, or surgical history.**

○   **The prenatal ultrasound of a newborn male showed bilateral hydronephrosis. A follow-up study confirmed the presence of bilateral hydronephrosis. A serum creatinine was 1.7 mg/dL 3 days postpartum. A representative film of the voiding cystourethrogram is shown. What is the likely diagnosis?**

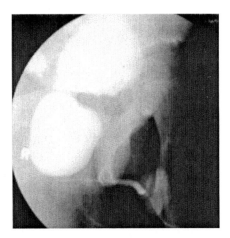

Any history of bilateral hydronephrosis should prompt a look at the bladder outlet. A normal bladder outlet should be funneled and nondilated. This film shows the three-key radiographic characteristics of posterior urethral valves, which are dilation and elongation of the posterior urethra and indentation of the bladder neck. The voiding film also shows high-grade vesicoureteral reflux, which is frequently seen with posterior urethral valves. The differential would include membranous uretheral stricture or external sphincter dyssynergia, neither of which fit the history.

○   **This KUB and voiding cystourethrogram were obtained in a male infant with undescended testes and bilateral hydronephrosis on ultrasound. What is the likely diagnosis?**

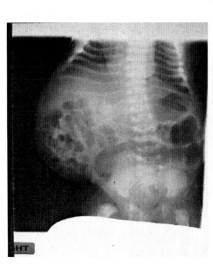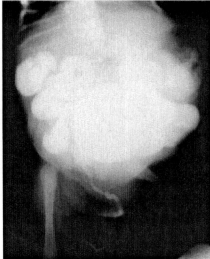

This classic film which needs little history is a case of the Eagle-Barrett or "prune-belly" syndrome. The classic triad consists of a male with absent abdominal wall musculature, bilateral undescended testes, and urological anomalies. The rib cage is flared and the flanks are bulging. There is massive reflux bilaterally into tortuous and dilated ureters. In this patient, the posterior urethra is nondilated making the diagnosis of posterior urethral valves unlikely. However, the prostate may be hypoplastic in these patients causing the posterior urethra to appear dilated. The bladder is usually large but smooth walled as obstruction is not generally present.

○ **Here is another voiding cystourethrogram performed in a male infant with hydronephrosis on antenatal ultrasound confirmed in the postnatal period by repeat ultrasound. What is the diagnosis?**

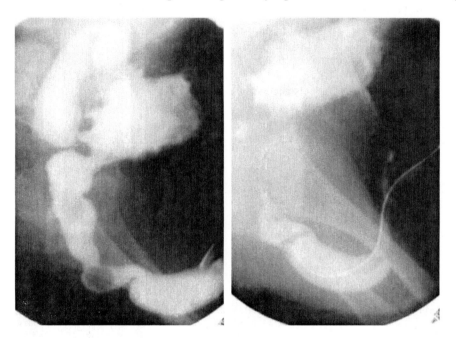

'n this case, both the posterior and anterior urethra are dilated and the catheter identifies a "flap" of tissue at the distal end of a diverticulum. There is a heavily trabeculated bladder and at least unilateral massive reflux. The film demonstrates an anterior urethral diverticulum or anterior urethral valves. This is a very rare cause of outlet obstruction in newborn males.

○   **This cystogram was obtained in a young male with recurrent febrile urinary tract infections. His physical examination is normal. What is unusual about the film and what is the diagnosis?**

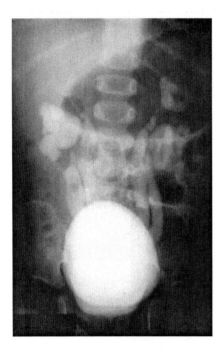

The diagnosis is bilateral vesicoureteral reflux. The cystogram shows high-grade vesicoureteral reflux into duplicate collecting systems on either side. The unusual finding on the film is the presence of reflux into both collecting systems. In association with the Meyer–Weigert rule, the upper-pole ectopic orifice more commonly obstructs and is located more inferomedially while the lower-pole system refluxes. However, reflux can occur into both segments. An alternative explanation for this film might be a low-lying, incomplete duplication with reflux into the solitary orifice on each side.

○   **This cystogram was obtained in a child who had a febrile urinary tract infection. What is the most likely diagnosis?**

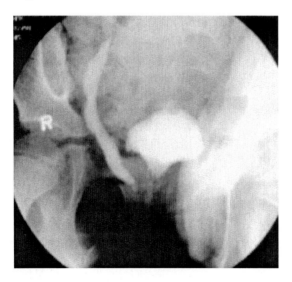

The right ureter is opacified due to reflux, and it inserts into the urinary tract at a site distal to the bladder neck. The diagnosis is a refluxing ectopic ureter. In females, ectopic ureters are more often associated with the upper pole segment of duplication while in males, the ureter more commonly drains a nonduplicated system. In females, the ureter may insert into the uterus, vagina, cervix, bladder neck, vestibule, or urethra while in males, insertion is most commonly in the bladder neck, prostatic urethra, seminal vesicles, vas deferens, or ejaculatory duct.

○ **This child presented with umbilical discharge. A voiding cystogram was obtained. What is the diagnosis?**

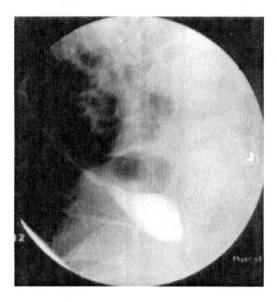

The cystogram shows a patent urachus. While persistence of the urachus has been attributed to intrauterine bladder outlet obstruction, the majority of patients with a patent urachus do not have obstruction.

○ **This is a voiding cystourethrogram obtained in a child who presented with a history of voiding with two streams. What is the diagnosis?**

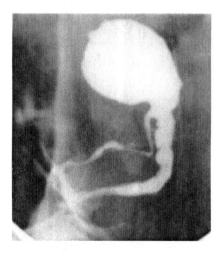

The cystogram shows a sagittal or epispadiac complete urethral duplication. Collateral or side-by-side duplications also exist and are more often associated with other pelvic anomalies such as imperforate anus or penile duplication.

○   **In the previous case, which urethra is the normal one?**

In the overwhelming majority of cases, the ventral urethra is the normal variant.

○   **This cystogram lateral view was obtained in a young male who had obstructive urinary symptoms. What is the likely diagnosis?**

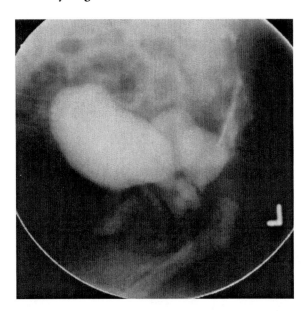

The study shows bilateral congenital bladder diverticula. While bladder diverticula may be associated with posterior urethral valves or neurogenic bladder, they may occur as an isolated entity. In this case, the posterior urethra is nondilated and the bladder is relatively smooth making these two diagnoses less likely. Diverticula may be associated with infection but also may cause outlet obstructive symptoms. In this case, simple resection of only diverticula relieved the symptoms.

○ **This 3-year-old female had an episode of gross hematuria. A cystogram was obtained. What is the likely diagnosis?**

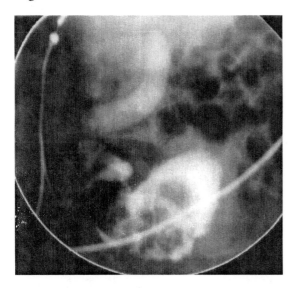

The classic cystographic appearance of a botryoid rhabdomyosarcoma of the bladder is that of a **"cluster of grapes,"** which the filling defect in this cystogram certainly resembles. Sarcoma botryoides is a variant of embryonal type rhabdomyosarcoma which forms polypoid tumor masses.

○ **This patient was involved in a motor vehicle trauma and had gross hematuria. The patient initially had abdominal CT scanning which was unremarkable. A cystogram was then obtained. What is the likely diagnosis?**

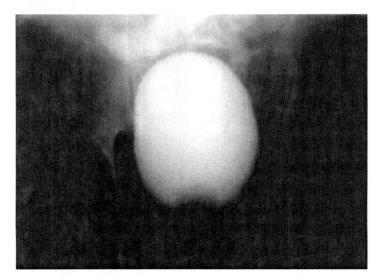

This film illustrates the importance of obtaining a scout film prior to the introduction of bladder contrast. In this case, the diagnosis is suspicious for an intraperitoneal bladder rupture. However, the contour of the bladder is smooth and appears to be intact. In fact, it was subsequently proven that the contrast seen was actually oral contrast, which had been given to the patient at the time of CT scanning. **Drainage films are also important since extravasation can hide behind the opacified bladder.** Oblique views should also be obtained.

○   **This older male had just undergone a transurethral resection of the prostate. A cystogram was obtained at the conclusion of the procedure because of a concern about a possible bladder perforation. What is the most likely diagnosis and how should it be treated?**

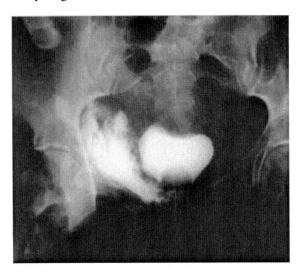

This film shows a classic extraperitoneal bladder rupture. The pattern of contrast extravasation is **"flame shaped"** and "whispy" in appearance and extends from the base of the bladder cephalad. Treatment is with catheter drainage. A repeat cystogram should be done in 7 to 10 days. Eighty-five percent of patients will be healed by that time. Virtually, all will be healed by 3 weeks after the injury.

○   **This patient was involved in a motor vehicle accident and sustained a pelvic fracture. A retrograde urethrogram was normal and a cystogram was performed. What is the likely diagnosis and how should it be treated?**

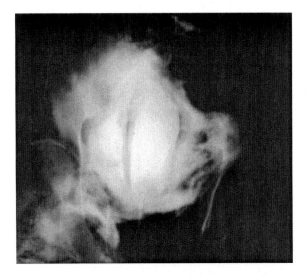

The cystogram shows a classic **"teardrop"** shape caused by compression by the pelvic hematoma. There is "flame-shaped" extravasation extending in a whispy fashion from the base of the bladder. The picture is typical for an extraperitoneal bladder rupture. Some concern for intraperitoneal rupture might be raised because of contrast-located cephalad to the bladder, but there is no obvious contrast outlining loops of bowel. While only 10%

of pelvic fractures manifest bladder rupture, virtually 100% of traumatic extraperitoneal bladder ruptures are associated with pelvic fracture. Roughly 10% are combined intra- and extraperitoneal injuries. **In adults, at least 300 mL of a water-soluble iodinated contrast should be instilled into the bladder by gravity pressure for a cystogram in order to exclude bladder rupture. A retrograde urethrogram should always be done first.**

○ **What is the formula used to calculate the estimated bladder capacity in children?**

Bladder capacity equals 60 mL + (30 mL × age in years).

○ **This patient presented following a motor vehicle accident. The patient had been drinking at the local bar prior to the accident. On presentation, he had suprapubic tenderness and a urinalysis showed gross hematuria. He did not have a pelvic fracture by plain film. An abdominal CT scan with a passive "CT cystogram" was normal. In spite of this, a standard trauma cystogram was performed. What does the study show and what is the diagnosis?**

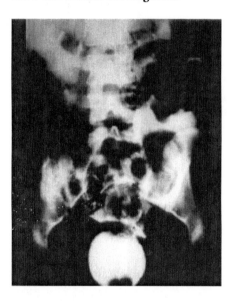

The study shows a classic intraperitoneal bladder rupture. As opposed to extraperitoneal ruptures, the contrast outlines loops of bowel and the direction of extravasation is cephalad. **Bladder ruptures in which there is significant contrast-located cephalad to the bladder should raise suspicion for intraperitoneal rupture.** A diagnostic maneuver that may help in equivocal cases is placing the patient in Trendelenburg position and repeating the film. Contrast may be seen over the liver or spleen. An active CT cystogram is usually a very sensitive test, but it should be done with the standard 300 mL contrast instillation into the bladder rather than using just the passive filling by the IV contrast used with CT. **Cystograms are best done before any oral, rectal, or IV contrast.**

○   **This 20-year-old male presents to the ER after a motor vehicle accident with blood at the urethral meatus. The patient is hemodynamically stable and undergoes a retrograde urethrogram after a failed single passage of a Foley catheter. What are the significant radiographic findings?**

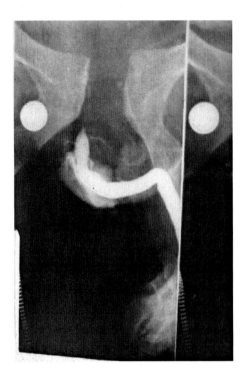

This retrograde urethrogram film shows significant pubic diastasis and urethral extravasation of contrast material consistent with urethral disruption. With this mechanism of injury, the most common place for a urethral injury is at the membranous urethra; however, this particular patient has sustained a bulbar urethral injury. No contrast material can be seen within the bladder. The patient will likely require a suprapubic cystostomy. Careful flexible urethroscopy and subsequent Foley catheter placement over a guidewire could be considered as a primary therapy.

○   **This retrograde urethrogram was obtained on a 35-year-old male presenting with a history of perineal trauma 2 years ago. What is the significant radiographic finding and how should it be treated?**

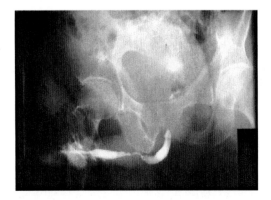

This urethral stricture extends from the distal bulbar urethra to the proximal pendulous urethra. Its length is estimated at 3.5 cm. **Remember that length of a urethral stricture must be measured from the point where tapering begins.** Options for repair include excision and primary anastomosis, augmented anastomotic repair, graft repair, and flap repair. Primary anastomosis can be attempted, but is usually reserved for strictures 2.5 cm or less. Augmented anastomotic repair would be a good choice for this length of stricture and the buccal mucosa would be an ideal graft material.

○ **This 40-year-old male with diabetes presented with fever, chills, and severe scrotal pain. What is the significant finding on KUB and what is the next step?**

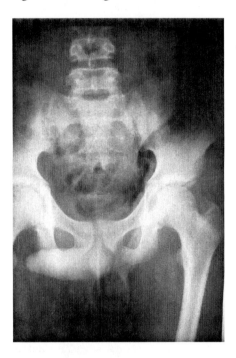

This film shows a likely left scrotal abscess. Air is seen but appears to be confined to the tunica vaginalis. Air on KUB in a diabetic, febrile patient should be considered a surgical emergency because of the possibility of Fournier's gangrene. Physical examination findings of subcutaneous crepitus and a rapidly expanding erythema would be worrisome. Wide excision and debridement is mandatory and potentially lifesaving along with antibiotics.

○ **Which common medication is specifically contraindicated and must be stopped prior to intravenous contrast administration; how long should it be held and why?**

Metformin (Glucophage) needs to be stopped before intravenous contrast studies and not resumed for at least 48 hours. A renal function test should be done to verify normal renal function before resuming the medication. Lactic acidosis is associated with the concomitant use of metformin and intravenous contrast. If it develops, severe lactic acidosis is associated with a 50% mortality rate.

○   **What prophylactic treatments can be used to prevent IV contrast-induced nephropathy?**

The most effective appears to be acetyl cysteine and sodium chloride hydration. Sodium bicarbonate may be more effective than plain saline hydration, but reports are conflicting. Other possible preventive therapies include theophylline and fenoldopam (a selective dopamine-receptor agonist), but their roles are still unclear with conflicting reports on their efficacy. Lasix, steroids, and mannitol have not shown any benefit.

○   **Gadolinium can cause what potentially serious complication when used in patients with renal failure?**

Nephrogenic systemic fibrosis.

CHAPTER 2 Radionuclide Studies

David M. Albala, MD, Udaya Kumar, MD, and Pramod Reddy, MD

○ **What are the half-lives of ^{99m}Tc, ^{123}I, and ^{131}I?**

The half-lives are 6 hours, 13.2 hours, and 8 days, respectively.

○ **What exactly is a rad?**

The amount of radiation energy absorbed by a patient's tissue is expressed in rad. The rad is defined as 100 ergs absorbed per gram of tissue.

○ **What is the difference between a roentgen and rad?**

A roentgen is a measure of ionization of the air by x-rays or gamma rays. Although the terms roentgen and rad are often used interchangeably, it should be remembered that roentgen is a measure of exposure, whereas the rad is a measure of energy absorbed by tissue.

○ **What are the most common instruments used to clinically detect ionizing radiation?**

Although gas detectors such as Geiger-Muller counters are used in nuclear medicine laboratories, solid crystal detectors are most commonly employed to detect ionizing radiation. The Anger camera used in most departments uses a sodium iodide crystal.

○ **What isotopes are used to measure the glomerular filtration rate (GFR)?**

Although ^{14}C inulin would give an accurate measurement of GFR, it is impractical to use. ^{51}Cr EDTA and ^{99}Tc DTPA are alternatives. In practice, ^{99m}Tc DTPA is usually used, as it also provides excellent renal images.

○ **Which isotopes are useful in measuring renal blood flow (RBF)?**

^{131}Hippuran, ^{123}I-Hippuran, and ^{99m}Tc-MAG3 are useful. ^{99}Tc-MAG3 is most commonly used in the United States for these purposes.

○   **How is ^{99m}Tc DTPA processed in the kidney?**

^{99}Tc DTPA is filtered and concentrated in the tubules and is then excreted through the collecting system. In a normal kidney, activity in the renal pelvis and ureter decrease after 5 to 10 minutes making it a useful test to detect obstruction.

○   **What does a DMSA scan demonstrate?**

^{99m}Tc DMSA accumulates progressively in the kidneys over several hours and images the renal cortex well. It is useful to detect renal scarring, early stages of renal damage from infection, and to differentiate functioning from nonfunctioning renal masses.

○   **What are the common uses of radionuclide studies after renal transplantation?**

They are useful in evaluating complications such as complete renal artery occlusion, urinary obstruction, or leakage. Acute tubular necrosis and rejection cause reduced perfusion and prolonged parenchymal transit times.

○   **What isotopes are useful in investigating occult suppuration in the abdomen or pelvis?**

Gallium-67 citrate–labeled or Indium-111–labeled leukocytes is used.

○   **What is the advantage of scanning with Indium-111 labeled leukocyte over Gallium-67 citrate in localizing infection?**

Studies with Indium-labeled leukocytes often can be completed in 24 hours, whereas those using Gallium-67 may take 48 to 72 hours to complete. In addition, the latter may be taken up by certain tumors such as lymphomas and hepatomas and is taken up by kidneys, which may confuse the diagnosis.

○   **How is MAG3 (mercaptoacetylglycine) cleared by the kidney?**

MAG3 is cleared by the kidneys primarily by tubular secretion and to a lesser extent by glomerular filtration. Therefore, it is an excellent agent for estimating the effective renal plasma flow. It is used to define UPJ obstruction and differential renal function.

○   **What is nuclear cystography and what is its value in ureteral reflux?**

It is the scintigraphic equivalent of conventional cystography. It is an accurate method for detecting and following reflux, although it does not provide the anatomic detail of fluoroscopic studies.

○   **True or False: In screening siblings for reflux, the nuclear scan is preferable to a standard voiding cystography.**

True. The radiation exposure in a nuclear scan is lower than a cystogram and when anatomic detail of VCUG is not essential, the nuclear scan is preferable.

○   **What are the nuclear scan findings in testicular torsion?**

The testicle appears avascular. In cases of epididymitis hypervascularity is noted. However, in cases of intermittent torsion and late torsion, hypervascularity may result from an inflammatory response. Occasional false-positive and false-negative results and limited availability of the nuclear scan 24 hours a day limit its usefulness in the diagnosis of torsion.

○ **What is the "doughnut sign" on the nuclear scan in testicular torsion?**

In a missed torsion (i.e., one that is several days old), there is often an area of hyperemia surrounding the central ischemic region of the testis. The central area appears photopenic surrounded by a rim of increased activity (doughnut).

○ **What factors affect the drainage curve of the nuclear scan in patients with UPJ obstruction?**

In addition to the severity of obstruction, the size and compliance of the collecting system, the hydration of the patient, the timing of diuretic and bladder drainage influences the drainage curve. A poorly functioning kidney may not respond adequately to the diuretic.

○ **True or False: The advantages of the ^{99m}Tc DMSA scan over IVU in the evaluation of renal damage from pyelonephritis include (a) lack of study impairment by bowel gas, (b) earlier detection of renal damage, (c) clear visualization of kidneys despite overlying bony structures, (d) improved ability to image the kidneys in various positions to delineate specific lesions, and (e) the collecting system is visualized more clearly.**

False. All are true except that the visualization of the collecting system in the DMSA scan is not nearly as good as with an IVU.

○ **True or False: Captopril is used to improve the accuracy of nuclear scan findings of renovascular hypertension.**

True. Captopril exaggerates the differences between the perfused and nonperfused areas of the kidney in patients with renovascular hypertension.

○ **What is the rationale behind the performance of a captopril renogram in the diagnosis of obstructive uropathy?**

Renin is secreted by the juxtaglomerular apparatus in renovascular hypertension and/or obstructive uropathy as a result of poor tissue perfusion. The local vascular regulatory mechanisms of the kidney:

- release thromboxane, causing vasoconstriction of the afferent arteriole, causing a further decrease of renal blood flow
- activate the renin–angiotensin system (RAS) that results in the formation of angiotensin II, which in turn increases the efferent arteriolar tone and is primarily responsible for restoring and maintaining glomerular filtration pressure.

Use of an angiotensin-converting enzyme inhibitor such as captopril can block this mechanism by preventing the vasoconstriction of the efferent arteriole, thereby causing a drop in GFR and relative renal function. This decrease is demonstrable with captopril renography.

○ **What is the correct dose of captopril administered for a captopril renogram?**

0.3 mg/kg is administered orally 1 hour prior to the radioisotope injection. A change of at least 5% (baseline scan vs. captopril scan) is considered significant when interpreting the results.

○ **What is an MIBG scan and what is it used for?**

Metaiodobezylguanidine (MIBG) is taken up by adrenal neurons. It is labeled with iodine and used to image the adrenal medulla and other active adrenergic tissues such as pheochromocytomas and neuroblastomas.

○ **How are nuclear scans helpful in carcinoma of the prostate?**

Bone scans with ^{99m}Tc methylenediphosphonate (MDP) are most useful in the staging of prostate cancer. They are more than 95% sensitive in detecting bony metastases from carcinoma of the prostate.

○ **What is a "superscan" in a patient with prostate cancer?**

When there is extensive involvement of the bony skeleton with metastasis in a patient with prostate cancer, the isotope is extensively taken up by the bone and the kidneys are not visualized.

○ **Bone scans typically are almost always negative and therefore not particularly useful until the PSA level reaches what point?**

A PSA level of 20 or more is usually necessary before a bone scan will be positive.

○ **Can nuclear scans be used in renal failure?**

Yes. ^{123}I and ^{131}I-hippurate and MAG3 can be concentrated even in kidneys with minimal renal function. They are of immense value in patients with renal failure or renal transplantation.

○ **What are the features of renal obstruction in a patient with hydronephrosis on a nuclear scan?**

During the excretory phase of the scan, the renogram demonstrates increasing activity over time, even after administration of furosemide, but the test may be unreliable in patients with poorly functioning kidneys or massively dilated collecting systems.

○ **How accurate is the MIBG scan in localizing pheochromocytomas and neuroblastomas?**

^{123}I MIBG scan is 85% to 90% sensitive and nearly 100% specific for localizing pheochromocytomas. It is almost 100% specific and 100% sensitive for neuroblastomas.

○ **What constitutes a "Well-Tempered Renogram" and how is it done?**

The Society for Fetal Urology and the Pediatric Nuclear Medicine Council of the Society of Nuclear Medicine published guidelines for the "Well-Tempered Diuresis Renogram" in 1992:

• Small field of view gamma camera is used for pediatric studies.
• If the child is younger than 4 months, MAG-3 should be the radioisotope used for the study.
• In children older than 4 months, MAG-3 is still the preferred radioisotope, however, DTPA may be substituted instead.
• The patient is well hydrated. A normal saline IV (15 mL/kg) given over 30 minutes is begun 15 minutes prior to the administration of the radioisotope. For the remainder of the study, a maintenance IV at 200 mL/kg/24 h is administered. The child's bladder should be catheterized to prevent any lower urinary tract dysfunction from influencing the results of the study.

○ **What is the recommended dose of diuretic (Lasix) for a "Well-Tempered Diuresis Renogram"?**

The dose of diuretic (Lasix) used should be 1 to 2 mg/kg IV.

○ **What is an indirect radionuclide cystogram (IRC)?**

The IRC is a diagnostic test to detect vesicoureteral reflux (VUR). It employs ^{99m}Tc DTPA as the radionuclide tracer. It provides information about the emptying phase of the bladder and can demonstrate VUR. Since it does not provide any information about the filling phase, it will miss the 3% of VUR known to occur during this phase of the bladder cycle. The high sensitivity of the IRC combined with the advantages of lower radiation and avoidance of bladder catheterization make it a valuable alternative to the VCUG.

○ **Match the following radionuclide tracers with method of action tracers**

1. DTPA	A. 80% tubular secretion
2. OIH	B. Both GFR-dependent and tubular secretion for clearance
3. MAG3	C. Localizes to the proximal convoluted tubules (PCT)
4. DMSA	D. Mostly tubular secretion
5. GH	E. GFR-dependent for clearance

1–E; 2–A; 3–D; 4–C; 5–B.

○ **What advantages does radionuclide cystography (RNC) have over a standard VCUG?**

The RNC is more sensitive and specific for the detection of vesicoureteral reflux than a VCUG. It also has a significantly lower gonadal radiation dose (RNC = 0.001–0.005 rads vs. VCUG = 0.208 rads).

○ **What are the disadvantages of radionuclide cystography (RNC)?**

- Limited ability to grade reflux.
- It does not provide additional radiographic data, i.e., the presence of constipation or bony abnormalities, etc.

○ **In a child presenting with flank pain, high fever, and dysuria, which radionuclide study would be appropriate to order?**

The child has features suggesting an acute pyelonephritis. DMSA renal imaging has been shown to demonstrate areas of decreased perfusion (inflammation vs. scar) in the kidneys. In order to differentiate between scar and inflammation, a renal ultrasound could be used or one could repeat the DMSA scan in 6 months. Persistent cortical defects represent parenchymal scars.

○ **What is the role of radionuclide imaging in the management of a duplex collecting system with an obstructed upper pole moiety?**

Radionuclide scanning (with a cortical agent) can provide information about the degree of function and amount of functioning renal tissue in each moiety of the duplex kidney. In the case of an obstructed upper pole moiety, it will also serve as a diagnostic test to determine efficacy of surgical intervention.

○ **Are there any potential complications to keep in mind or to counsel the parents about, while ordering a radionuclide study?**

For the most part, nuclear medicine studies are quite safe and the radiation dose involved is minimal. There is a small risk of a nosocomial UTI from urethral catheterization in radionuclide cystography. Some children may experience significant abdominal discomfort during a Lasix renogram, especially if they have intermittent obstruction and the study reproduces an obstructive episode.

○ **What are the contraindications to performing a radionuclide study on a patient?**

There are no absolute contraindications to the use of radionuclides for diagnostic purposes. A relative contraindication is pregnancy; therefore, nuclear medicine scanning should not be performed on patients in the reproductive age group without first performing a pregnancy test.

○ **Is there a role for radionuclide scanning in the acute evaluation of a trauma patient?**

The advent of ultrafast spiral CT scanners has changed the imaging algorithm for the evaluation of the trauma patient, so there is little need for radionuclide scanning in these cases. In certain select cases, radionuclide scanning with a renal cortical agent might be indicated to evaluate the degree of function and amount of functioning renal tissue.

○ **What is the best radionuclide agent to use in a 1-month-old infant with severe hydronephrosis, suggestive of bilateral ureteropelvic junction obstruction?**

Normally, it is not recommended to perform a Lasix scan on children younger than 3 months because of the relative functional immaturity of the kidneys, which limits the reliability of the results. However, there are instances where the physician has to perform the test sooner, as in the above clinical case. In such instances, MAG3 is the agent of choice, as it has lower uptake in the liver and spleen and higher renal extraction providing a better target to background ratio.

○ **In what clinical setting is "static" radionuclide imaging utilized?**

Static radionuclide imaging is used to evaluate vesicoureteral reflux, urinary tract infections, hypertension, and cystic diseases of the kidney. It can document renal scarring, acute pyelonephritis, and differential renal function.

○ **In what clinical settings is "dynamic" radionuclide imaging utilized?**

Dynamic renal functional imaging is useful for evaluating a suspected obstruction in cases of possible ureteropelvic junction obstruction and megaureters (although the $t_{1/2}$ values are of limited clinical relevance in light of the compliance of the dilated ureter). It is also useful in evaluating renal function in cystic kidney diseases, hypertension, as well as after a renal transplant or pyeloplasty.

○ **What is "SPECT" radionuclide scanning?**

"SPECT" (single photon emission computed tomography) is an imaging technique associated with single gamma ray emitting radiopharmaceuticals. The images are obtained using a scintillation camera which moves around the patient to capture images from multiple angles for tomographic image reconstruction. It results in better image quality and improves the sensitivity of the test.

○ **What is the agent used for a positron emission tomographic scan (PET)?**

The PET scan uses a radioactive glucose molecule as the radiotracer to identify metabolically active tissues. The radiotracer is a glucose analog called FDG ([18F]-2-fluoro-2-deoxy-D-glucose).

○ **What is the mechanism/physiologic principle that a PET scan is based on?**

During a PET scan, the patient is injected with a radiotracer; a glucose analog called FDG ([18F]-2-fluoro-2-deoxy-D-glucose). FDG is preferentially taken up by tumor cells and phosphorylated by the enzyme hexokinase to FDG-6-PO4. Unlike Glucose-6-PO4, PDG-6-PO4 cannot enter into the glycolytic pathway and be further broken down; it therefore remains trapped intracellularly. This allows the hypermetabolic tissue of a tumor to be distinguished from the surrounding normal tissue.

○ **What GU malignancy is best suited for imaging with a PET scan?**

PET scanning is best suited for radiographic staging in testis cancer. Testis cancer and its metastatic lesions have a high glycolytic rate, and therefore accumulate a high concentration of the radiotracer FDG.

○ **What is the role of PET scanning in the management of prostate cancer?**

PET scanning does not currently have a significant role in the diagnosis and imaging of prostate cancer as the cancerous prostatic tissue has a relatively low glycolytic rate, and therefore does not accumulate high concentrations of the radiotracer FDG.

○ **In testicular cancer, which modality has the higher diagnostic accuracy in detecting metastases: PET or CT scanning?**

PET scanning has a higher diagnostic accuracy than a CT scan for both initial staging of testis cancer and restaging after surgical and chemotherapeutic interventions.

○ **What is Fanolesomab and what is its utility in nuclear medicine imaging?**

Fanolesomab (FNB) is a 99 ^{m}technetium-labeled murine anti-CD15 IGM monoclonal antibody that specifically targets neutrophils. It is a radiopharmaceutical agent that has been designed to specifically target and localize acute infections. It is much more sensitive than an indium-111–tagged or gallium-tagged white blood cell scan that is the current gold standard.

○ **What factors can limit the utility of the Lasix renogram?**

The following are the factors that can significantly alter the results of a Lasix scan being performed to detect an obstructive lesion at the ureteropelvic junction (UPJ):

- The volume of the collecting system. (A very large pelvis is compliant and can hold a lot of tracer, falsely affecting the drainage time.)
- Renal insufficiency.
- The hydration status of the patient.
- Renal tubular disorders, i.e., acute tubular necrosis, Fanconi's syndrome.

○ **What are some of the pitfalls and limitations of the angiotensin-converting enzyme inhibitor (ACEI) renogram?**

The rationale of the ACEI renogram is that the ACEI blocks the vasoconstriction of the efferent arteriole and causes a decrease in the glomerular filtration pressure and a demonstrable decrease in the GFR:

- Patient hydration—overhydration can cause a false-negative result and underhydration can cause a false-positive result.
- Selection of the radiotracer—DTPA is better than MAG-3.
- Choice of the ACEI—captopril versus enalapril.
- Asymmetric small kidney with poor function often is unresponsive to the effects of ACEI.
- Renal insufficiency results in a nondiagnostic ACEI renogram.
- Bilateral disease limits the diagnostic ability of the test.

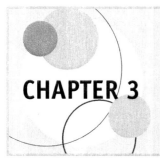

CHAPTER 3   Retroperitoneal Anatomy

Graham F. Greene, MD, FACS

○ **When closing a flank incision, which muscle layer has an obvious free border?**

The external oblique muscle has a free border laterally that extends from the lower border of the 12th rib to its aponeurotic insertion along the iliac crest.

○ **Between which two muscle layers do the intercostal nerves and vessels course?**

They course between the transversus abdominis and the internal oblique muscles. This is important when closing incisions to avoid entrapment of these structures.

○ **What is another name for Gerota's fascia?**

Perirenal fascia. It is a specialized condensation within the intermediate stratum of the retroperitoneal connective tissue. It forms a barrier to benign and malignant processes.

○ **Does Gerota's fascia form a tight seal around each kidney?**

No. Gerota's fascia is weakest at its caudal aspect along the course of the gonadal vessels and ureter.

○ **When resecting a large left upper pole renal mass from an anterior approach, what medial attachments need to be divided to allow reflection of the spleen, pancreas, and stomach?**

Division of the phrenicocolic, splenorenal, the gastrosplenic, and the gastrophrenic ligaments will allow reflection of the spleen, pancreas, and stomach from the craniolateral aspect of the retroperitoneum exposing the upper pole of the left kidney and adrenal gland.

○ **What surgical maneuver will allow access to the intra- and suprahepatic vena cava?**

Division of the right and left triangular ligaments and continuing the incision along the cranial and caudal coronary ligaments will allow reflection of the right lobe of the liver, providing dramatic exposure to the inferior vena cava as it receives the hepatic veins and perforates the diaphragm.

○ **What nerve is commonly seen coursing anterolaterally in the inguinal canal?**

The ilioinguinal nerve (L1) courses through the inguinal canal on the cord to exit the external ring and provide sensation to the pubic area.

○ **What other nerve besides the ilioinguinal nerve follows the cord through the inguinal canal?**

The genital branch of the genitofemoral nerve (L1, L2). It is less conspicuous than the ilioinguinal nerve and has a dual function supplying motor innervation to the cremasteric muscle and sensation to the anterior scrotum or labia majora.

○ **What nerve is clearly visualized coursing along the ventrum of the psoas muscle and proves useful in defining the lateral border for a complete pelvic lymph node dissection?**

The genitofemoral nerve (L1, L2) serves a dual purpose in supplying motor function to the cremasteric muscle and sensation to the perineum and anterior thigh.

○ **Define the arterial blood supply of the right adrenal gland.**

The right adrenal receives its blood supply from three main sources. The two obvious ones include branches from the inferior phrenic artery as well as branches from the right renal artery. A branch that is often forgotten that passes behind the inferior vena cava is the middle adrenal artery. This can lead to significant bleeding if unrecognized and cut during a right adrenalectomy.

○ **Into what structures do the gonadal vessels on either side drain?**

The right gonadal vein enters the inferior vena cava on its ventral lateral aspect at an oblique angle. The left gonadal vein empties into the left renal vein.

○ **What is the significance of a varicocele that does not diminish when examined in the supine position?**

Suspect a retroperitoneal mass or process that is impairing venous drainage such as lymphoma, testicular cancer, renal cell carcinoma, or retroperitoneal fibrosis.

○ **What are the primary sites of lymphatic drainage from the left testis?**

The most common site on the left side is the left para-aortic lymph nodes followed by the preaortic, interaortocaval, left common iliac, and left suprarenal lymph nodes in decreasing order. Left-to-right lymphatic drainage tends not to occur unless there is lymphatic obstruction.

○ **What are the primary sites of lymphatic drainage from the right testis?**

The most common site on the right side is the interaortocaval lymph nodes followed by precaval, preaortic, right paracaval, right common iliac, and left para-aortic lymph nodes in decreasing order. Lymphatic drainage proceeds from the right to left side of the retroperitoneum. Alternative routes can occur when there is lymphatic obstruction.

○ **Which division of the renal artery supplies the majority of the kidney?**

The anterior division supplies more than 75% of the kidney, including apical, upper, middle, and lower vascular segments of the kidney. The posterior renal artery supplies the majority of the dorsal aspect of the kidney.

○ **How often can a surgeon anticipate accessory renal arteries?**

In 25% to 40% of cases, there is more than one renal artery arising from the lateral aorta at the level of the second lumbar vertebra. Accessory renal arteries to the right lower pole will often cross anterior to the vena cava. It becomes important to recognize such branches so that they are not divided when exposing the right renal hilum.

○ **Where do the renal pelvis and the upper ureter receive their arterial blood supply?**

There are three anastomosing arteries providing the upper ureter and renal pelvis with blood supply. They include the renal artery, aorta, and gonadal artery.

○ **Which adrenal gland is more intimate with the cranial aspect of the kidney?**

The left adrenal gland is most intimate with the cranial aspect of the left kidney. It often will drape over the ventral aspect of the upper pole. The right adrenal gland is decidedly cranial to the right kidney, and care must be given when removing it because of its short adrenal vein entering dorsolaterally into the inferior vena cava.

○ **What is an alternate route for venous drainage of the left adrenal gland?**

The left inferior phrenic vein. The adrenal gland vein drains into the left renal vein. Close to where it enters, it is joined by the inferior phrenic vein which cranially also empties into the inferior vena cava above the level of the hepatic veins. This means that you can divide the adrenal vein at the level of the renal vein without compromising its venous drainage.

○ **Does ligation of the gonadal arteries at the level of the aorta compromise the gonads?**

No. The rich collateral circulation provided by the artery to the vas deferens and external spermatic artery in the male and the uterine artery in the female provide collateral blood supply to the gonad.

○ **What are the first branches of the intra-abdominal aorta?**

The paired inferior phrenic arteries are the first branches of the intra-abdominal aorta. They give origin to the superior supra-adrenal arteries.

○ **What are the three main arterial blood supplies to the small bowel and colon?**

They include the superior mesenteric artery, inferior mesenteric artery, and the inferior and middle hemorrhoidal arteries, which are branches from the internal iliac artery.

○ **When is it possible to completely resect the infrahepatic vena cava for renal cell carcinoma and an IVC thrombus?**

't is possible to resect the infrahepatic vena cava when removing a large right renal mass and associated renal vein thrombus. This is due to the rich collateral venous drainage of the left kidney through the lumbar (azygos) system. The right kidney is not afforded a similar venous drainage.

○ **Other than the gonadal vein, what other vein drains into the caudal aspect of the left renal vein?**

A left lumbar vein. This large lumbar vein provides collateral venous drainage as well as a potential source of bleeding when ligating the left renal vein.

○ **If the inferior mesenteric artery is ligated during a retroperitoneal lymph node dissection, what artery insures blood supply to the upper rectum, sigmoid colon, descending colon, and part of the left transverse colon?**

The marginal artery of Drummond. This artery provides collateral circulation between the superior mesenteric artery and the inferior and middle hemorrhoidal vessels.

○ **When assessing left para-aortic lymphadenopathy on CT scan, what clue helps you distinguish retroperitoneal structures from mesenteric structures?**

At the level of the L3 vertebra (or inferior pole of the kidneys), the inferior mesenteric artery and inferior mesenteric vein run in a craniocaudal direction. The ureter can be seen posterolateral to these distinct vessels. Any structures dorsomedial are in the retroperitoneal space as compared to ventrolateral structures that are in the mesentery or coelomic space.

○ **In what direction does most lateral lumbar lymphatic flow proceed?**

Right to left. The lymphatics coalesce posterior to the aorta to form a localized dilation of lymphatic chain known as the cisterna chyli. This structure lies in a retrocrural position, just anterior to the first or second lumbar vertebra, and empties into the thoracic duct through the aortic hiatus of the diaphragm.

○ **What is Kocher's maneuver?**

The Kocher's maneuver refers to the surgical reflection of the second and third part of the duodenum craniomedially, to provide access to the right renal vessels and inferior vena cava. When combined with mobilization of the small bowel mesentery, this maneuver exposes the great vessels in anticipation of retroperitoneal dissection. It is important to recognize that the Kocher's maneuver also mobilizes the head or uncinate process of the pancreas. Carefully placed retraction in this area will help prevent pancreatic injury.

○ **What happens to the ipsilateral adrenal gland in cases of renal ectopia or agenesis?**

They will present in their normal anticipated location within the retroperitoneum. The adrenal glands are embryologically and functionally distinct from the kidneys. Physically they are separated from the kidneys by connective tissue septa that are in continuity with Gerota's fascia as well as varying amounts of perinephric fat.

○ **During embryologic development the adrenal medulla has received what specialized cells and from where?**

The adrenal medulla consists of chromaffin cells, which are derived from the neural crest and are intimately associated with the sympathetic nervous system. Chromaffin cells belong to the family of APUD (amine precursor uptake decarboxylase) cells and produce neuroactive catecholamines that are released directly into the blood stream.

○ **What zone of the adrenal cortex produces glucocorticoids?**

The zona fasciculata. The adrenal gland consists of three zones or strata. The outermost layer of cells makes up the zona glomerulosa that produces aldosterone (mineralocorticoids). The next layer is the zona fasciculata that produces glucocorticoids, and in the normal adrenal gland is usually the thickest of the three layers. The innermost zona reticularis is responsible for producing sex steroids.

○ **Which layer of the adrenal cortex is not regulated by pituitary release of adrenocorticotropic hormone (ACTH)?**

The zona glomerulosa is not under direct pituitary regulation by ACTH. The zona glomerulosa, which is the outermost layer of the adrenal cortex, produces aldosterone in response to stimulation by the renin–angiotensin system.

○ **On which kidney can you find a dromedary hump?**

Both. This normal variation of renal contour is found much more commonly on the left than the right side. It is seen as a focal bulge on the midlateral border of the kidney.

○ **Between which two layers is the pararenal (paranephric) fat located?**

Between the transversalis fascia and Gerota's fascia. Within Gerota's fascia, the kidney is suspended in the perirenal fat. Depending upon the body habitus of the patient, varying amounts of pararenal fat can be found external to Gerota's fascia. When surgically approaching the kidney, the transversalis fascia can sometimes be mistaken for Gerota's fascia due to the underlying pararenal fat. Failure to incise transversalis fascia impends access to the retroperitoneum.

○ **Which segmental branch of the main renal artery is most constant?**

The posterior segmental artery is most constant. Prior to entering the renal hilum, the main renal artery divides into an anterior and posterior division. The posterior segmental artery supplies the majority of the dorsum of the kidney, whereas the anterior division gives rise to four anterior segmental arteries (apical, upper, middle, and lower) supplying the rest of the kidney. During nephron sparing surgery, mistaking the often long posterior segmental artery for the main renal artery can lead to incomplete arterial occlusion and blood loss.

○ **Describe intrarenal arterial anatomy.**

The renal artery divides into four or five segmental branches including the posterior, apical, upper, middle, and lower segmental renal arteries. The segmental arteries travel through the renal sinus and branch to give rise to lobar arteries. These lobar arteries divide again and enter the renal parenchyma as interlobar arteries and traverse the renal parenchyma through the renal columns of Bertin. At the base of the renal pyramids, the interlobar arteries branch into the arcuate arteries. In turn, the arcuate arteries branch to give rise to multiple interlobular arteries. These interlobular arteries branch within the renal cortex giving rise to the afferent arterioles of the glomerular capsule and contributing small branches to the renal capsular plexus. Blood leaves the glomerulus via the efferent arteriole and meets the venous system at the vasa recta within the renal medulla or through a capillary network within the cortex.

○ **What is implied when renal arteries are referred to as end arteries?**

The renal artery and its successive branches do not have anastomosis or collateral circulation. Therefore, occlusion of any of these vessels will result in ischemia and infarction of the renal parenchyma that it supplies.

○ **Describe renal venous drainage.**

The capillary bed within the cortex and the vas recta drain into interlobular veins, and then into arcuate, interlobar, lobar, and segmental veins, respectively. There are usually three to five segmental veins that empty into a main renal vein. Unlike renal arteries, renal parenchymal veins anastomose freely, especially in the arcuate vessels.

○ **Within the kidney where would the stellate veins be located?**

The stellate veins form a subcapsular venous plexus that form a communication between the interlobular veins and veins within the perinephric fat.

○ **How can renal vasculature obstruct the urinary collecting system?**

Accessory lower pole arteries may cross anterior to the urinary collecting system. In that orientation, they can become an extrinsic cause of ureteral pelvic junction obstruction.

○ **What is the significance of the anatomic landmark along the convex border of the kidney called "Brodel's white line"?**

It is often mistaken for the relative avascular plane of the kidney used to gain access to the renal collecting system during an anatrophic nephrolithotomy. The white line of Brodel is a longitudinal crease 1 to 2 cm ventral to the convex border of the kidney. The actual location of the avascular longitudinal plane lies 1 to 2 cm dorsal to the convex border of the kidney between the posterior segmental circulation and the anterior.

○ **Within the nephron of the kidney, describe the location and function of the juxtaglomerular apparatus.**

The juxtaglomerular apparatus is a specialized association between the proximal aspect of the distal convoluted tubule and the afferent renal arteriole. Specialized macula densa cells within the renal tubule detect changes with intratubular sodium concentration. They communicate with juxtaglomerular cells of the afferent arteriole that are responsible for secreting renin into the afferent arteriole and renal lymph. The juxtaglomerular cells will respond to changes in wall tension and receive input from renal nerves that can stimulate renin secretion.

○ **Within the renal collecting system, what is the significance of compound papillae?**

When two renal pyramids fuse during their development, they form a "compound" papillae. They usually occur at the renal poles. Their physiologic significance lies in the fact that the configuration of the collecting ducts (of Bellini) allows for reflux of urine and potentially bacteria into the kidney. Renal parenchymal scarring secondary to infection is typically most severe, overlying these compound papillae.

○ **Describe the anatomy of a major calyx.**

There are usually two to three major calyces within a kidney. Each major calyx receives two or more infundibula, each of which drain two or more minor calyces.

○ **Describe the muscle layers of the ureter.**

The smooth muscle layers of the ureter orient themselves in two layers: the inner longitudinal layer and an outer layer of circular and oblique muscle. The ureter's muscle wall is thickest in its pelvic portion. The circular and oblique fibers become integrated into the smooth muscle of the bladder and Waldeyer's ring. The inner longitudinal muscle fibers traverse the intramural ureter toward the ureteral orifice and trigone.

○ **What are the three distinct narrowings normally present along the course of the ureter?**

The first of these is the ureteropelvic junction, the second is the crossing of the iliac vessels, and the third is the ureterovesical junction within the bladder.

○ **Which of these is the smallest?**

The ureterovesical junction is usually the most narrow.

○ **What is the nomenclature used to describe ureteral segments intraoperatively and for radiologic purposes?**

The ureter can be divided into an abdominal and pelvic portion. The abdominal ureter extends from the renal pelvis to the iliac vessels. The pelvic portion extends from the iliac vessels down to the bladder. For radiologic purposes, the ureter can be divided into proximal, middle, and distal segments. The proximal segment extends from the renal pelvis to the upper border of the sacrum. The mid ureter lies between the upper and lower borders of the sacrum. The distal ureteral segment extends from the lower border of the sacrum to the bladder.

○ **Describe the innervation of the kidney.**

The kidney receives preganglionic sympathetic fibers from T8 (thoracic) through L1 (lumbar) spinal segments. Postganglionic fibers arise from celiac and periaortic ganglia. Parasympathetic innervation arises from the lesser and lower splanchnic nerves as well as the vagus nerve.

○ **Describe the innervation of the ureter.**

The ureter receives preganglionic sympathetic fibers from T10 through L2 spinal segments. Postganglionic fibers arise from ganglia in the aortorenal, superior, and inferior hypogastric plexus. Parasympathetic input arises from the second through fourth sacral spinal segments.

○ **Does the ureter require autonomic innervation to maintain peristalsis?**

Intrinsic pacemaker sites located in the minor calices of the collecting system initiate the contraction, which is then propagated down the ureter.

○ **What is necessary for any abdominal hernia (including inguinal hernias) to occur?**

A defect (weakness) in the transversalis fascia, which is the outer stratum of the retroperitoneal connective tissue, is essential for a hernia to occur.

○ **When performing laparoscopic port placement in the lower abdomen, what vessels of the anterior abdominal wall can be injured leading to significant, often unrecognized bleeding?**

Inferior epigastric vessels; these vessels originate from the external iliac arteries and traverse in a cranial direction posterior to the body of the rectus muscle and anterior to the posterior rectus sheath. Laparoscopic ports will often tamponade (mask) injury to these vessels only later to be recognized at the time of port removal or postoperatively as a posterior rectus hematoma. The surgical principle of checking all port sites prior to proceeding will identify this injury early, which is amenable to either open or laparoscopic suture ligation.

○ **What perforating vessels of the anterior abdominal wall help identify the midline of the fascia?**

The musculocutaneous perforators from the superior and inferior epigastric arteries that perforate the anterior rectus fascia providing circulation to the dermis and skin. They emerge at regular intervals, approximately 2 to 4 cm cranial caudally and 2 cm off midline. Encountering these vessels can help the surgeon correct their midline approach. Ligation or cautery of these vessels can lead to fat necrosis and devascularization of the skin.

○ **What is the lymphatic drainage of the left kidney and the right kidney?**

Left kidney drains into the left para-aortic nodes; right kidney drains into the right paracaval lymph nodes. In either case, the lymph nodes can lie anterior, lateral, or posterior to the aorta and vena cava, respectively. Infrequently, lymph nodes may be classified as hilar lymph nodes based on their association with renal hilum instead of regional lymph nodes. To insure adequate lymph node sampling during radical nephrectomy, a staging lymphadenectomy may be required.

○ **What is the Pringle maneuver?**

It is the compression of the portal triad in order to arrest hepatic blood flow during complicated inferior vena cava thrombectomy. Care is taken not to injure the structures of the portal triad, including the hepatic artery, portal vein, and common bile duct as well as minimizing the warm ischemia time during clamping.

○ **What vessel associated with the posterior lateral border of Gerota's fascia can lead to persistent annoying bleeding during radical nephrectomy?**

The renal capsular vein that connects the renal capsular plexus with the venous drainage of the posterior abdominal wall exiting at the intersection of the transversus abdominis and quadratus lumborum muscles with the iliac crest. This vessel is one of many that can get quite large if parasitized by a renal tumor.

○ **What fascia layer is often mistaken for Gerota's (perirenal fascia) during an open-flank approach to the kidney?**

Transversalis fascia, lying deep to the thoracolumbar fascia and covering the pararenal fat, together mimicking the perirenal fascia and perirenal fat which surrounds the kidney.

○ **What are the most ventral renal structures coursing over the isthmus of a Horseshoe kidney?**

The ureters.

○ **What is the Cisterna chyli and where is it located?**

The cisterna chili is located posterior medial to the aorta. It drains into the thoracic duct that enters the chest medial to the right crus of the diaphragm. The cisterna chyli is the confluence of the left and right lymphatic trunks, each with anterior and posterior branches to the renal vessels. Injury to the lymphatics at this level can result in chylous ascites.

○ **Do the lumbar sympathetic nerves travel anterior or posterior to the vena cava?**

Posterior, often located cranial to the junction of the lumbar veins and the posterior vena cava.

○ **What structures lie anterior to the hilum of the left kidney?**

The tail of the pancreas, the splenic artery, and the splenic vein.

○ **What are the various orientations of the right ureter to the vena cava?**

Paracaval (normal) and retrocaval (circumcaval).

○ **Where do the gonadal arteries originate?**

From the ventral abdominal aorta, cranial to the inferior mesenteric artery and caudal to the renal arteries.

○ **What nerve is seen exciting behind the psoas major muscle at the L2 level, traveling on top of the quadratus lumborum muscle in a lateral direction over the iliacus muscle?**

The lateral femoral cutaneous nerve of the thigh. Other obvious nerves in this area include the genitofemoral nerve, which is more medial and runs on top of the psoas muscle, and the ilioinguinal and iliohypogastric nerves, which lie lateral and more cranial to the lateral femoral cutaneous nerve.

○ **Describe the association of the pleura to the 11th and 12th ribs.**

The majority of the 11th rib and the dorsal–lateral half of the 12th rib. The 11th and 12th ribs are free-floating ribs that help the surgeon plan percutaneous, laparoscopic, and open surgical approaches to the kidneys. The pleura lie on the inner surface of the rib, medial to the insertion of the intercostal muscles, and superior to the diaphragmatic insertion.

○ **The most important lumbar nerves for preserving antegrade ejaculation arise from which sympathetic ganglia?**

L3 and L4 sympathetic ganglia.

○ **Parasympathetic fibers reach the inferior mesenteric plexus via what nerves?**

Pelvic splanchnic nerves via the superior hypogastric plexus.

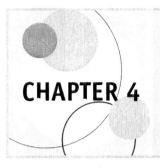

CHAPTER 4

Surgical Anatomy of the Pelvis

Venu Chalasani, MBBS, FRACS, and Jonathan I. Izawa, MD, FRCSC

○ **What is the thinnest of the pelvic bones?**

The pubic bones, which are often fractured in blunt pelvic trauma. Their fragments may injure the bladder, urethra, and vagina.

○ **True or False: The sacroiliac (SI) joint is often fractured in pelvic trauma.**

False. The synovial SI joint gains additional strength from anterior and posterior ligaments and fractures rarely involve this joint.

○ **What is the origin of the muscles of the pelvic diaphragm?**

The origin of the pubococcygeus and iliococcygeus muscles is the tendinous arch of the levator ani.

○ **What types of muscle fibers make up the pelvic diaphragm?**

Type I (slow-twitch fibres) and type II (fast-twitch) fibers. These provide tonic support of the pelvic contents and allow for sudden increases in intra-abdominal pressure, respectively.

○ **What organs does the inner stratum cover in the pelvis and what is its clinical importance?**

The inner stratum covers the rectum and the dome of the bladder. It also forms Denonvilliers' fascia, which acts as a barrier between the rectum and prostate, which contributes to the low rate of local extension of prostate cancer into the rectum.

○ **The endopelvic fascia is continuous with which layer of the abdominal wall?**

The transversalis fascia.

○ **What fascial structure extends medially from the arcus tendineus fascia in the female pelvis and what is its clinical significance?**

This structure is referred to as the periurethral, pubovesical, or urethropelvic ligament and it provides support to the urethra and anterior vaginal wall. Compromise to this fascia may contribute to stress urinary incontinence, bladder neck hypermobility, cystocele or urethrocele formation.

○ **True or False: As the dorsal vein of the penis passes within the pelvis under the pubic arch it forms a venous complex and part of this complex runs within the anterior and lateral walls of the striated urinary sphincter.**

True. One must be cautious during ligation and division of the dorsal venous complex, as damage to the striated sphincter can occur.

○ **What anatomic reason may account for the relatively higher incidence of axial skeletal and pelvic bone metastases in patients with metastatic prostate cancer, as opposed to lung metastases for example?**

There are numerous interconnections between the pelvic venous plexuses and the emissary veins of the pelvic bones and vertebral venous plexuses, which may be routes of dissemination of infection or tumor from the diseased prostate.

○ **What artery has its origin off the inferior epigastric artery and can be identified medial to the femoral vein during pelvic surgery?**

The accessory obturator artery arises from the inferior epigastric artery in 25% of patients and continues on through the obturator canal.

○ **What is the most common origin of the superior vesical artery?**

The proximal portion of the obliterated umbilical artery.

○ **What structures besides the rectum does the middle rectal artery supply?**

The middle rectal artery anastomoses with the superior and inferior rectal arteries to supply the rectum. It also gives small branches to provide additional arterial supply to the seminal vesicles and prostate.

○ **What accessory vein drains into the inferior surface of the external iliac vein in at least 50% of patients?**

The accessory obturator vein. Care must be taken to not tear this vein at the time of pelvic lymph node dissection.

○ **During a psoas hitch procedure, in which direction should the sutures be placed and why?**

The sutures should be placed in the direction of the muscle fibers and femoral nerve to avoid femoral nerve entrapment or damage. Caution must also be taken with retractor blades on the psoas muscle for prolonged periods, as this may also cause a femoral nerve palsy.

○ **What nerve is located lateral to the psoas muscle in the iliacus fascia?**

The lateral femoral cutaneous nerve.

○ **During a radical cystectomy in a 65-year-old male patient for clinical T3a transitional cell carcinoma of the bladder, you notice a nerve visible on the surface of the right psoas major muscle has been damaged by an electrosurgical injury. What sensory loss do you anticipate this patient may experience if the nerve function cannot be salvaged?**

The right genitofemoral nerve has been injured. Sensory loss to the anterior right thigh below the inguinal ligament and the anterior right hemiscrotum may occur.

○ **A 67-year-old male patient, 3 months postradical retropubic prostatectomy, but otherwise healthy, describes difficulty in moving his left leg into the car when he is on the driver's side. He has noticed this only in the postoperative period. What nerve injury likely occurred during his surgery?**

The patient likely sustained a left obturator nerve injury. The obturator nerve supplies the adductor muscles of the thigh.

○ **Where is the obturator nerve located in relation to the obturator artery and vein?**

The obturator nerve lies lateral and superior to the obturator vessels.

○ **During a sacrospinous colposuspension, what nerve or nerve plexus is at relatively high risk of injury?**

The sacral plexus, as it leaves the pelvis via the greater sciatic foramen and is immediately posterior to the sacrospinous ligament. If injured, there may be sensory and motor nerve supply compromise to the posterior thigh and lower leg.

○ **Where is the sacral plexus located?**

The sacral plexus is located on the surface of the piriformis muscle, deep to the endopelvic fascia and posterior to the internal iliac vessels.

○ **What nerve passes through the greater sciatic foramen and supplies sensory branches to the perineum and posterior aspect of the scrotum?**

The posterior femoral cutaneous nerve.

○ **Where is the location and anatomic orientation of the pelvic plexus?**

The pelvic plexus is rectangular, 4 to 5 cm in length, oriented in the sagittal plane and is located at its midpoint at the tip of the seminal vesicles.

○ **What are the anatomic relations of the communicating nerve fibers of the left and right components of the pelvic plexus?**

These fibers communicate posterior to the rectum, as well as anterior and posterior to the bladder neck.

○ **True or False: There is no pelvic parasympathetic efferent innervation to the descending and sigmoid colon.**

False. Some pelvic parasympathetic efferent fibers travel up the hypogastric nerves to the inferior mesenteric plexus, where they will subsequently provide innervation to the descending and sigmoid colon.

○ **True or False: Longitudinal smooth muscle fibers from the rectum join Denonvilliers' fascia.**

True. The fibers are located anteriorly at the inferior portion of the rectal ampulla.

○ **True or False: Intramural longitudinal vessels run the length of the ureter in 75% of patients.**

True. These vessels are formed by anastomoses of segmental ureteral vessels. In the other 25% of patients, the intramural ureteral vessels form a fine interconnecting mesh with less collateral flow and render the ureter more prone to ischemic insult. This intramural, interconnecting meshlike vascular pattern is often found in the pelvic ureter and therefore this portion of the ureter is less suited for ureteroureterostomy.

○ **True or False: The pelvic ureter has rich adrenergic and cholinergic autonomic nerve supply and will lose its peristaltic activity if it is denervated.**

False. The ureter will continue to have peristaltic activity despite its pelvic denervation and this is driven from pacemakers in the upper urinary tract.

○ **In a normal adult male, at what anatomic location are the ureters closest to each other?**

The ureters are closest and are located within 5 cm of each other as they cross the iliac vessels.

○ **What arteries usually supply the ureter with its largest pelvic branches?**

The inferior vesical and uterine arteries.

○ **Where does the ureteral smooth muscle terminate distally?**

The verumontanum. The muscle of the trigone is made up of three distinct layers; the superficial layer, derived from the longitudinal smooth muscle of the ureter, extends down to the verumontanum.

○ **Where does the bulk of the lymphatic fluid from the bladder drain?**

The external iliac lymph nodes. Some drainage may go to the obturator, internal iliac, and common iliac lymph nodes.

○ **During a radical cystectomy/anterior exenteration in a 65-year-old female patient with clinical T3a transitional cell carcinoma of the bladder, what ligaments are part of the lateral and posterior bladder pedicles that will be divided?**

The cardinal and uterosacral ligaments.

○ **True or False: The bladder wall has many postganglionic cell bodies.**

True. The vast majority of these synapse with parasympathetic cholinergic nerve endings.

○ **True or False: Presacral neurectomies are reasonably effective in relieving bladder pain.**

False. Afferent innervation from the bladder travels with the parasympathetic nerves as well as the sympathetic nerves, which travel via the hypogastric nerves.

○ **During a radical retropubic prostatectomy, the endopelvic fascia is divided lateral to the arcus tendineus fascia pelvis and is mobilized off the levator ani medially with the prostate. Is this endopelvic fascia visceral or parietal?**

It's the parietal endopelvic fascia.

○ **True or False: Normal prostatic glands may be within the striated urethral sphincter.**

True. There is no fibromuscular stroma or prostate capsule with these glands.

○ **What is the principal arterial supply to prostatic adenomas in benign prostatic hyperplasia?**

The inferior vesical arteries have urethral artery branches that enter the prostate posterolaterally at its junction with the bladder and these branches are the principal arterial supply to the adenomas.

○ **Can a local anesthetic alone achieve a complete prostatic block?**

Yes. It must be instilled into the pelvic plexus to block all afferent neurons.

○ **True or False: Bilateral pudendal nerve injury will cause loss of striated external sphincter function at the level of the membranous urethra.**

False. The striated sphincter has additional somatic nerve supply from a branch off the sacral plexus and it is located on the levator ani. Autonomic innervation from the cavernous nerves is also present, but this may not be significant for urinary continence.

○ **To what nodal locations do the lymphatics of the vas deferens and seminal vesicles drain?**

The external and internal iliac lymph nodes.

○ **What structures do the uterine arteries supply?**

The proximal vagina, uterus, and medial two-thirds of the fallopian tubes.

○ **What course do the nerves from the pelvic plexus travel to reach the female pelvic viscera?**

The nerves from the pelvic plexus travel through the cardinal and uterosacral ligaments. During a hysterectomy, these ligaments are divided and therefore may result in a neurogenic bladder.

○ **Which nerve crosses the distal end of the external iliac artery?**

The genital branch of the genitofemoral nerve.

○ **What two branches of the external iliac artery are within the pelvis?**

The inferior epigastric and the deep circumflex iliac arteries.

○ **At what anatomic site does the internal iliac artery branch into its anterior and posterior trunks?**

The greater sciatic foramen.

○ **Where is the obturator artery origin?**

The obturator artery has a variable origin. It can arise from the anterior trunk of the internal iliac artery, the inferior epigastric artery, or the inferior gluteal artery.

○ **The middle sacral vein is usually a tributary of which vein?**

The left common iliac vein.

○ **True or False: The external iliac lymph nodes can be further separated anatomically and functionally into three chains.**

True. The external, middle, and internal chains. For example, the external chain does not receive any lymphatic drainage from organs within the pelvis and these lymph nodes are located lateral to the external iliac vessels.

○ **What is unique about the Cherney incision?**

This incision involves access to the pelvic cavity and detaches the rectus muscles from the symphysis.

○ **What forms the arcus tendineus fascia pelvis?**

Fusion of the visceral and parietal components of the pelvic fascia forms the arcus tendineus fascia pelvis. It appears as a white line of condensation within the pelvis that runs in a sulcus lateral to the prostate from the puboprostatic ligaments to the ischial spine.

○ **Is smooth muscle present within the puboprostatic ligaments?**

Yes. There are smooth muscle fibers within the puboprostatic ligaments derived from the outer layer of detrusor musculature. Once the puboprostatic ligaments are divided during a radical retropubic prostatectomy, the ligaments contract due to their smooth muscle components and are no longer apparent.

○ **In what percentage of patients undergoing radical retropubic prostatectomy does the superficial dorsal vein of the penis appear to be absent?**

Approximately 10%.

○ **What areas of a normal bladder may be more prone to diverticular formation?**

The dome of the bladder where the urachus anchors the apex of the bladder to the anterior abdominal wall due to a paucity of detrusor muscle at this site. The hiatus in the detrusor, where the intramural ureter passes is also more prone to diverticular formation.

○ **During cystoscopic examination of a normal bladder, the urothelium over the trigone appears relatively smooth compared to the surrounding urothelium. How is this explained?**

The urothelium over the trigone is usually three cells thick and the lamina propria is dense here with strongly adherent epithelial cells. Therefore, during changes in bladder volume, the trigonal epithelium remains smooth in appearance endoscopically.

○ **True or False: The entire prostate is enclosed by a capsule composed of collagen, elastin, and abundant smooth muscle.**

False. The prostate is devoid of a capsule at the apex and base; therefore, no true capsule separates the prostate from the striated urethral sphincter or the bladder. The capsule is composed of collagen, elastin, and abundant smooth muscle and is continuous with the prostatic stroma.

○ **When an accessory pudendal artery is present and is supplementing or replacing penile arterial supply by the common penile artery, what is its origin and anatomic course in relation to the prostate gland?**

An accessory pudendal artery is present in approximately 4% of patients undergoing a radical retropubic prostatectomy and arises from the inferior vesical artery or obturator artery. It runs anterolateral to or within the prostate to reach the penis.

○ **What three muscles combine to make up the pubococcygeus muscle in the female?**

The pubococcygeus muscle is a thick "V-shaped" muscle band comprising three sections—the pubovaginalis muscle anteriorly, the puborectalis muscle, and the puboanalis muscle. These muscles pull the rectum, vagina, and urethra anteriorly against the pubic bone to compress the lumen of each.

○ **What is the primary muscular component of urethral support in the female?**

The pubovaginalis muscle, which is the most anterior part of the levator ani.

○ **While performing the incision for a radical retropubic prostatectomy, the pyramidalis muscle is observed to be present. What is the innervation of this muscle?**

The 12th thoracic nerve. Contraction of this muscle tenses the linea alba.

○ **During a radical cystectomy and pelvic lymph node dissection, care should be taken to avoid dissection below the presacral fascia. Why?**

This dissection may disturb the presacral veins and cause unnecessary blood loss.

○ **What is the lymph node of Cloquet's anatomic location?**

The lymph node of Cloquet lies within the femoral canal, medial to the external iliac vein, and beneath the inguinal ligament.

○ **What structure is often described as the inferolateral limit of a pelvic lymph node dissection in a radical cystectomy?**

The genitofemoral nerves. The fibroareolar tissue is divided medial to this structure in a pelvic lymph node dissection during a radical cystectomy.

○ **True or False: In a nerve sparing cystoprostatectomy, the unilateral internal iliac artery should be ligated and divided to improve hemostasis and facilitate the nerve sparing procedure, thereby possibly maintaining erectile function.**

False. The internal iliac artery should be preserved and the superior vesical artery should be ligated and divided proximally in order to maintain the integrity of the internal pudendal artery and to prevent vasculogenic erectile dysfunction.

○ **If the right internal iliac artery was ligated, what principal vessels might contribute to collateral circulation?**

The anastomoses of the following would possibly allow collateral circulation:

- The ovarian artery from the aorta with the uterine artery.
- The vesical arteries of the contralateral side with the same vessels on the ligated side.
- The middle rectal artery branches of the internal iliac artery with the superior rectal artery from the inferior mesenteric artery.
- The obturator artery with the inferior epigastric artery and the medial femoral circumflex artery, and by means of the pubic branch of the obturator artery, with the same vessels from the contralateral side.
- The circumflex artery with perforating branches of the deep femoral artery and the inferior gluteal artery.
- The superior gluteal artery with the posterior branches of the lateral sacral arteries.
- The iliolumbar artery with the last lumbar artery.
- The lateral sacral artery with the middle sacral artery.
- The iliac circumflex artery with the iliolumbar and the superior gluteal arteries.

○ **What artery arises posteriorly at the level of the aortic bifurcation and what does it supply?**

It is the middle sacral artery and it supplies the sacral foramina and the rectum.

○ **Name the muscles of the true pelvis.**

Piriformis, coccygeus, obturator internus, and the Levator ani.

○   **What muscles comprise the Levator ani?**

Puborectalis, pubococcygeus, and iliococcygeus.

○   **During a radical cystectomy (anterior exenteration) and an ileal conduit in a 65-year-old female, the vagina is observed to have very good vascular supply when the anterior wall is resected en bloc with the specimen. What is the main arterial supply to the vagina?**

The vaginal arteries, which can be represented by one, two, or three arterial vessels. These include arterial branches that can arise from the uterine artery, inferior vesical artery, or separate arterial branches directly from the anterior trunk of the internal iliac artery.

○   **What are the branches of the obturator artery within the pelvis?**

The iliac, vesical, and pubic arterial branches. The iliac branches ascend in the iliac fossa and supply the iliacus muscle and ilium, while anastomosing with branches of the iliolumbar artery. The vesical branch courses medially and posteriorly to help supply the bladder. The pubic branch arises from the obturator artery just before it leaves the pelvis and ascends inside the pelvis to communicate with the same vessel on the contralateral side and with the inferior epigastric vessels.

○   **What are the anatomic relations of the internal pudendal artery in the male?**

The internal pudendal artery in the male lies anterior to the piriformis muscle, sacral plexus of nerves, and the inferior gluteal artery. As it crosses the ischial spine, it is covered by the gluteus maximus muscle and overlapped by the sacrotuberous ligament. The pudendal nerve is medial to the artery and the nerve to the obturator internus muscle is lateral to the internal pudendal artery.

○   **What is the venous drainage of the vagina?**

The venous drainage occurs by means of the vaginal plexus of veins along the lateral aspect of the vagina. These are in continuity with the uterine, vesical, and rectal venous plexuses. The vaginal plexuses are drained by one or two vaginal veins on each side that flow into the internal iliac veins either directly or through the connections with the internal pudendal veins.

○   **How many external iliac lymph nodes are usually present in the normal adult and what is their anatomic arrangement?**

There are usually eight to ten external iliac lymph nodes that lie along the external iliac vessels. They are arranged in three groups. One group is on the lateral aspect, another on the medial aspect, and a third group on the anterior aspect of the external iliac vessels. The third group of lymph nodes on the anterior aspect of the vessels is sometimes absent.

○   **What are the origins of the arteries that supply the seminal vesicles?**

These arteries are derived from the middle vesical, inferior vesical, and middle rectal arteries.

○   **How does the ureteral smooth muscle change as the ureter approaches the bladder?**

The spirally oriented mural smooth muscle fibers become longitudinal. The fine longitudinal smooth muscle fibers from the ureter pass to either side of their respective orifices to join the lateral and posterior ureteral wall fibers and fan out over the base of the bladder. The fibers form the triangular and superficial muscle of the trigone.

○   **What is the origin and insertion of the pyramidalis muscle?**

It arises from the pubic crest and inserts into the linea alba.

○   **What blood vessels run in Campers fascia ?**

The superficial circumflex iliac, external pudendal, and superficial inferior epigastric vessels. They are branches of the femoral vessels.

○   **Describe the medial and inferior limits of Scarpa's fascia.**

Inferiorly, it fuses with the deep fascia of the thigh 1 cm below the inguinal ligament along a line from the anterior superior iliac spine to the pubic tubercle. Medially, it is continuous with Colles fascia of the perineum.

○   **What is the anatomical basis for a butterfly hematoma in the perineum?**

Colles fascia attaches to the ischiopubic rami laterally and to the posterior edge of the perineal membrane, hence limiting the spread of blood and urine following injury. Colles fascia is continuous with the dartos fascia of the penis and scrotum.

○   **Where is the arcuate line and what is its significance?**

The arcuate line is located two-thirds of the distance from the pubis to the umbilicus, and is the point at which all aponeurotic layers abruptly pass anterior to the rectus abdominis leaving this muscle clothed only by transversalis fascia and peritoneum posteriorly.

○   **What structures can be injured by paramedian incisions lateral to the rectus and what problems ensue?**

The last six thoracic segmental nerves enter the rectus abdominis laterally to supply it; division of these nerves can cause atrophy of the rectus and may predispose to ventral hernia. The inferior epigastric vessels may also be injured.

○   **At the start of a robotic transperitoneal radical prostatectomy, what folds are visible on the internal surface of the anterior abdominal wall and what do they contain?**

Approached laparoscopically, three elevations of the peritoneum, referred to as the median, medial, and lateral folds, are visible below the umbilicus. The median fold overlies the urachus; the medial fold the obliterated umbilical artery; and the lateral fold the inferior epigastric vessels.

○   **Why is the medial umbilical fold an important landmark for the surgeon?**

It contains the obliterated umbilical artery, which may be traced to its origin from the internal iliac artery to locate the ureter, which lies on its medial side.

○   **Is the configuration of the pelvic diaphragm flat, bowl-shaped, or near vertical?**

At the urogenital and anal hiatus, the muscles lie in a near-vertical configuration.

○   **What are the branches of the internal iliac artery?**

The posterior trunk gives rise to three parietal branches: the superior gluteal, the ascending lumbar, and the lateral sacral branches. The anterior trunk gives rise to seven branches: the superior vesical, the middle rectal, the inferior vesical, the uterine, the internal pudendal, the obturator, and the inferior gluteal branches.

○ **What nerve may be injured by retractor blades resting on the psoas muscle and what does it innervate?**

The femoral nerve that originates at L2-4 can be easily injured in this way. Other areas of potential femoral nerve injury or compression include the iliopsoas groove and at the inguinal ligament. An injury to the femoral nerve is most noticeable as a weakness in the quadriceps which causes difficulty with ambulation.

○ **During a radical retropubic prostatectomy, where are the cavernosal nerves most vulnerable?**

At the apex of the prostate, where they closely approach the prostatic capsule at the 5- and 7-o'clock positions.

○ **Describe the course of the cavernosal nerves in the pelvis.**

They originate from the most caudal portion of the pelvic plexus, then pass the tips of the seminal vesicles and lie within leaves of the lateral endopelvic fascia near its juncture with, but outside, Denonvilliers' fascia. They travel at the posterolateral border of the prostate on the surface of the rectum and are lateral to the prostatic capsular vessels.

○ **Does the blood supply to the pelvic ureter enter laterally or medially?**

Laterally. The pelvic peritoneum should be incised only medial to the ureter.

○ **When completely filled, what is the approximate maximum capacity of the normal bladder?**

450 to 500 mL.

○ **What are the layers of the bladder?**

- Transitional epithelium.
- Lamina propria.
- Detrusor.
  - Inner longitudinal.
  - Middle circular.
  - Outer longitudinal.

○ **What are the distinct muscle layers of the trigone of the bladder?**

There are three layers:

1. A superficial layer, derived from the longitudinal muscle of the ureter.

2. A deep layer, which continues from Waldeyer's sheath.

3. A detrusor layer, formed by the longitudinal and middle circular smooth muscle layers of the bladder wall.

○ **Is the bladder more richly supplied with sympathetic or parasympathetic nerves?**

Parasympathetic cholinergic nerve endings predominate.

○ **In what areas of the prostate is the capsule deficient and why is this important?**

At the apex and at the base. Normal prostatic glands can be found to extend into the striated urethral sphincter with no intervening "capsule." At the base of the prostate, outer longitudinal fibers of the detrusor fuse and blend with the fibromuscular tissue of the capsule. As with the apex, no true capsule separates the prostate from the bladder. This makes assessment of margins somewhat difficult in radical prostatectomy specimens.

○ **Which nerves carry sympathetic and parasympathetic innervation to the prostate?**

The cavernosal nerves.

○ **What is the lining of the female urethra?**

Its lining changes gradually from transitional to nonkeratinized stratified squamous epithelium.

○ **What layers of the abdominal wall are encountered during a Gibson incision?**

- The aponeurosis of the external oblique.
- The internal oblique muscle.
- The transversus abdominis muscle.

○ **What is the thickest part of the bladder?**

The bladder base.

○ **What does the verumontanum contain?**

It contains the prostatic utricle and the ejaculatory ducts.

○ **How is the venous drainage of the bladder different from normal venous drainage?**

Instead of following the arteries, the veins of the bladder drain into the lateral plexuses about the ureter and into the prostatovesical plexus along with the deep dorsal vein of the penis and the cavernous vein. From the plexus, the veins run in the lateral prostatic ligaments to empty into the internal iliac veins.

○ **Does the urachus reach the umbilicus?**

The urachus does not usually reach the umbilicus in the adult; rather, it may terminate adjacent to one of the obliterated hypogastric arteries, or it may join both arteries, or it may be short and partially degenerate into the subumbilical fibrous plexus of Luschka.

○ **Describe the course of the right ureter in the female pelvis.**

Passing medially at the level of the ischial spine, it lies behind the ovary in close association with the suspensory ligament of the ovary and forms the posterior limit of the ovarian fossa. The ovarian vessels make an oblique crossing over the ureter. Entering the parametrium of the broad ligament, it runs successively through the uterosacral ligament, the cardinal ligament, and the vesicouterine ligament. In its course, the ureter runs for a short distance with the uterine artery, which originating from the internal iliac artery lies lateral and anterior to it.

○ **Where is Bogros space, what does it represent, and what are its anatomical limits?**

Bogros space is located at the pelvic opening of the spermatic cord. It is lateral and superior to Retzius space. It represents the retroinguinal preperitoneium. Its limits are:

- Medially, the epigastric vessels, spermatic cord, iliac vessels, and space of Retzius.
- Anteriorly, the transversalis muscle.
- Laterally, the psoas muscle and lateral cutaneous nerve.

○ **What spinal nerve root or roots supply the cremasteric muscle?**

Spinal nerve root S-4.

○   **What abdominal muscle layer is in continuity with the cremasteric muscle?**

The internal oblique muscle.

○   **Lymphatics from the pelvis and testes cross the midline at what level?**

At the level of the renal hilum.

○   **What are the zones of the prostate?**

- Anterior fibromuscular stroma.
- Transition zone.
- Central zone.
- Peripheral zone.

CHAPTER 5

Embryology of the Genitourinary Tract

Mark F. Bellinger, MD

○ **A female infant is found to have unilateral renal agenesis. Ultrasound examination of the contralateral kidney and bladder and pelvis are normal. What concern should lead the urologist to recommend long-term monitoring of this child?**

Females with unilateral renal agenesis have a significant incidence of ipsilateral mullerian anomalies, and may present in early adolescence with a pelvic mass indicative of hydrometrocolpos due to any of a spectrum of uterine or vaginal anomalies, commonly uterus didelphys with an obstructed uterine horn.

○ **Ectopic and fused kidneys often have anomalous collecting systems. What is the orientation of the renal pelvis in most anomalous kidneys?**

The renal pelvis begins development in an anterior position and the kidneys rotate during ascent so that the pelves come to lie in a medial position. Most kidneys that are anomalous in location display incomplete rotation. The pelves are likely to be located in an anterior position.

○ **A 1-month-old female has a duplex left kidney with hydroureteronephrosis of the lower pole segment, which has a thin cortex. What is the most likely explanation for the hydronephrosis?**

In a completely duplicated collecting system, the upper pole is most likely to be hydronephrotic because of ureteral obstruction (ectopic ureter, ureterocele), while hydronephrosis of the lower pole system is most likely caused by vesicoureteric reflux.

○ **A 2-month-old male is found to have a right ureteral duplication with upper pole hydroureteronephrosis and a cystic mass in the bladder. What is the first logical therapeutic intervention to consider?**

The child's most likely diagnosis is ureteral duplication with a ureterocele subtending the upper pole ureter. In most cases, transurethral incision of the ureterocele is an appropriate first therapeutic intervention.

○ **A 7-year-old boy is found to have a complete right ureteral duplication with hydroureteronephrosis of the upper pole system during evaluation for nocturnal enuresis. Is this anomaly likely to be a cause of his incontinence?**

No. Ectopic ureters in males insert into the lower genitourinary tract above the external sphincter, including insertion into the Wolffian duct system (vas, seminal vesicle).

○ **An infant is found to have a right multicystic dysplastic kidney. What studies should be done to evaluate the left kidney?**

An ultrasound should be done to rule out hydronephrosis, and a voiding cystourethrogram should be performed since there is greater than 30% incidence of contralateral vesicoureteric reflux.

○ **An infant has drainage of clear fluid from the umbilicus. A small catheter is placed into the umbilical sinus and contrast injected is seen to pass into the gastrointestinal tract. What is the diagnosis?**

The child has persistence of the omphalomesenteric (vitelline) duct that connects with the terminal ileum at the site at which a Meckel's diverticulum would be found.

○ **Early rupture of the cloacal membrane may result in a spectrum of urological anomalies. List them.**

Cloacal exstrophy, exstrophy of the bladder, and epispadias.

○ **Horseshoe kidneys have an incidence of hydronephrosis that in some cases is caused by anomalous renal vasculature. Why is the incidence of this type of ureteral obstruction so high?**

Horseshoe kidneys take their vascular supply from a ladder of vessels that alternately appear and involute as the kidneys ascend toward the flank. Persistence of such "anomalous" vessels may result in ureteral obstruction, most commonly at the ureteropelvic junction obstruction.

○ **In cases of unilateral renal agenesis, is ipsilateral adrenal agenesis likely to occur?**

No. Ipsilateral adrenal agenesis occurs in less than 10% of cases.

○ **In crossed renal ectopia, are the kidneys more likely to be fused or nonfused?**

Fused renal ectopia is more common.

○ **In cross-fused renal ectopia, where does the ureter of the crossed kidney usually enter the bladder?**

The ureter draining the ectopic kidney usually crosses the midline to enter the contralateral trigone.

○ **Explain the Meyer–Weigert law in relation to ureteral duplication.**

The law states that in complete ureteral duplication, the orifice to the lower pole ureter inserts into the bladder in a more lateral and cranial position, while the ureter to the upper pole inserts in a more caudal and medial position.

○ **A 14-year-old male is found to have right ureteral obstruction secondary to retrocaval ureter. What is the embryologic explanation for this anomaly?**

Retrocaval ureter is a result of persistence of (failure of involution of) the right subcardinal vein.

○ **The fetal testis produces two hormones that are essential for the development of the internal genitalia. Name these hormones and indicate what effect they have on the developing genital structures.**

Testosterone supports the development of the Wolffian duct structures (seminal vesicles, vas, etc.). Mullerian-inhibiting substance acts ipsilaterally to suppress the development of the mullerian structures (fallopian tube, uterus, upper vagina).

○ **A 1-month-old male is found to have a left flank mass. What are the two most likely diagnoses and what would be your first imaging study in this case.**

The most likely diagnoses are hydronephrosis and multicystic renal dysplasia. The primary imaging technique for infants with abdominal masses should be ultrasound.

○ **A female neonate has a midline pelvic abdominal mass and a bulging interlabial mass. What is the most likely diagnosis?**

The most likely diagnosis is hydrometrocolpos secondary to imperforate hymen.

○ **A 12-year-old male presents with terminal hematuria and is found to have a polyp in his posterior urethra arising from the verumontanum. What is the cause of this polyp and the most likely pathologic diagnosis? Where else in the urinary tract are similar lesions occasionally found?**

The polyp is most likely a benign fibroepitheliomatous polyp of congenital origin. Similar polyps may be found in the ureter and renal pelvis.

○ **A 15-year-old male with dysuria is found to have a cystic lesion in the bulbous urethra. What is its most likely embryologic origin?**

This is most likely a Cowper's duct cyst.

○ **A 12-year-old boy with dysuria and bloody urethral spotting is found to have a small diverticulum on the roof of the distal urethra in the fossa navicularis. What is the correct term for this diverticulum?**

This lesion is known as a lacuna magna.

○ **A 1-month-old female is found to have a cystic mass prolapsing through the urethral meatus, and ultrasound of the abdomen shows hydronephrosis of the upper pole of the left kidney. What is the most likely diagnosis?**

The mass is a prolapsed ureterocele, which subtends the upper ureter of a completely duplicated left collecting system.

○ **A 3-year-old girl is found to have grade 3 left vesicoureteric reflux. What is the most likely anatomic location of the left ureteral orifice as seen at cystoscopy, and what is the embryologic explanation for its position?**

The ureter will likely be positioned in the bladder in a position lateral to the normal trigonal position. This is thought to be the result of a ureteral bud arising from the mesonephric duct in a position more caudal than usual. As a result, as the caudal mesonephric duct becomes absorbed into the trigonal structure, the ureteral orifice will migrate into a dorsolateral position in the bladder base.

○ **A 3-year-old boy is found to have a small, hydronephrotic left kidney and ureter. At cystoscopy, no left ureteral orifice can be identified. Where does the ureter most likely insert?**

The ureter most likely is inserted into the Wolffian system (seminal vesicle, vas). This anomaly represents failure of the ureteral bud to separate from its Wolffian duct origin.

○ **An infant being evaluated after urinary tract infection has an intravenous urogram performed. The study shows small folds in the upper portion of the left ureter without significant hydronephrosis. What is the nature and significance of these ureteral findings?**

The IVP has demonstrated "fetal folds" in the upper ureter. These persistent fetal infoldings generally are insignificant and disappear with time.

○ **What is the embryologic explanation for bifid ureters?**

Bifid ureters are thought to be the result of bifurcation of the ureteral bud during its ascent toward the renal mesenchyme.

○ **What is the most proximal extent of the ureteral bud in the renal collecting system?**

The ureteral bud ascends to join the metanephric blastema and unite with the glomerular structures. The collecting ducts of the kidney are the most proximal extent of the ureteral bud.

○ **Explain the differences in embryogenesis between multicystic renal dysplasia and autosomal dominant polycystic disease.**

The cysts in multicystic renal dysplasia are a reflection of failure of normal organogenesis; immature renal parenchyma and cystic dysplasia are found. In polycystic disease, the normal architecture of the nephron is destroyed by the obstruction of the nephron and resulting cystic deformation.

○ **At what stage of fetal development does the kidney begin to produce urine?**

At approximately 9 to 12 weeks.

○ **Congenital spinal anomalies may be associated with what urinary tract anomaly?**

Congenital spinal anomalies may be found in association with renal anomalies, in particular unilateral renal agenesis.

○ **Describe the syndrome in which urethral valves may be associated with unilateral renal dysplasia.**

In the VURD syndrome (vesicoureteric reflux, renal dysplasia), a dysplastic kidney may be found to be associated with massive unilateral vesicoureteric reflux.

○ **What ureteral anomaly is found in conjunction with multicystic renal dysplasia?**

Ureteral atresia.

○ **Explain the anomalies found in the Triad syndrome.**

The Triad, or Prune-Belly syndrome is a constellation of abnormal abdominal musculature, intra-abdominal undescended testes, and an abnormal (dysmorphic) urinary tract.

○ **What embryologic explanations have been proposed to explain the Prune-Belly syndrome?**

The explanations offered have been primarily those of anomalous development of the mesenchyme and a transient infravesical obstruction during early embryogenesis.

○ **What is the state of the prostate in boys with Prune-Belly syndrome?**

The prostate is hypoplastic.

○ **It is very difficult to pass a urethral catheter into the bladder of a boy with hypospadias. What is the likely explanation for this?**

The child most likely has an enlarged prostatic utricle.

○ **A 1-year-old male has a nonpalpable right testis. At the time of exploration, the inguinal canal is empty. Where should the surgeon look to be sure that the testis is absent?**

The testis descends from a position above the internal inguinal ring. Testes above the ring are located in the abdominal cavity if they are not congenitally absent. In most cases, a testis or blind-ending vas and vessels can be found in the abdomen by laparoscopy or open exploration. Retroperitoneal dissection, as practiced in the past, may allow the surgeon to miss an abdominal testis.

○ **At the time of exploration, an undescended testis is found outside of the external inguinal ring. The cord structures are long enough to reach the scrotum easily. Should the tunica vaginalis overlying the testis be opened?**

Yes. Since most undescended testes have a persistently patent processus vaginalis that does not close after the testis descends into the inguinal canal. This processus should be ligated at the internal inguinal ring.

○ **At exploration for an undescended testis, a blind-ending vascular structure is noted in the inguinal canal. Is exploration complete?**

No. To be sure that a testis is not present, the vas deferens should be identified. The vas and vessels may, in a small number of cases, be separate.

○ **At the time of inguinal herniorrhaphy in a 2-year-old boy, a bright yellow circular nodule approximately 3 mm in diameter is noted in the inguinal canal attached to the cord structures. What does this represent?**

This is an adrenal rest. No therapy is necessary. It represents the common precursor of the genitourinary ridge in early development.

○ **A 30-week-gestation neonate is noted to have bilateral canalicular testes. Is there any chance that descent will occur after birth?**

Yes. The incidence of cryptorchidism in premature infants is approximately 30%, while it is approximately 3% in full-term neonates and less than 1% at 1 year of age.

○ **In the classical literature of urology, what is the embryologic importance of epididymitis in a prepubescent male?**

The worry is that the boy may have an ectopic ureter draining into the vas deferens or seminal vesicle. Renal ultrasound examination is warranted in these cases.

○ **Describe the anatomy of the exstrophic tissue seen in cloacal exstrophy.**

The exstrophic tissue classically consists of a midline segment of hindgut, frequently with a prolapsed ileum and one or more openings to at least one appendix. The bladder is split into two hemibladders by the hind gut. Widely separated genital tubercles are seen as a hemiscrotum and hemipenis on each side, or a hemiclitoris on each side. The anus is imperforate. Most children also have a myelomeningocele and an omphalocele.

○ **Primary obstructive megaureter is most commonly caused by what anatomic entity?**

Obstructive megaureter is thought in most cases to be due to an adynamic distal ureteral segment.

○ **Vaginal atresia may be associated with anomalies of the urinary tract. What is the most commonly recognized urinary tract anomaly seen?**

Unilateral renal agenesis.

○ **What is the embryologic origin of the vagina?**

The upper portion of the vagina originates from the mullerian duct. The lower portion (distal to the hymen) originates from the urogenital sinus.

○ **The appendix testis is an embryologic remnant of what structure?**

The mullerian duct.

○ **A neonate with imperforate anus is seen to pass meconium per urethra. What is the most likely site of the connection between the urinary and gastrointestinal tracts?**

Embryologically, the most likely site of the fistula is the posterior urethra, although fistulization may occur at the base of the bladder.

○ **List at least three mechanisms that have been proposed to explain why testicles descend from the abdomen into the scrotum.**

The first is the abdominal pressure theory, which proposes that intra-abdominal pressure forces the testis out of the abdomen. The second is that the process is entirely controlled by hormonal influence. Another theory is that the gubernaculum pulls the testis into the scrotum.

○ **What is the embryologic origin of the appendix epididymis?**

The Wolffian duct.

○ **What is the embryologic explanation for uterus didelphys?**

The mullerian ducts are paired structures that fuse distally to form the upper portion of the vagina and the uterus, the cranial unfused portions forming the fallopian tubes. Failure of fusion may result in one of several anomalies of the uterus, including uterus didelphys and bicornuate uterus.

○ **Explain the embryologic cause of midshaft hypospadias.**

Hypospadias is a result of incomplete formation of the urethra. If the urethral folds fail to fuse in the midline, hypospadias may result.

○ **In cloacal exstrophy, how can an anomaly such as hemiscrotum with hemiphallus come to exist?**

If the cloacal membrane ruptures early, this acts as a wedge to keep the genital tubercles and genital folds widely separate, so each component of the hemiscrotum and hemiphallus develops widely separate from its contralateral mate.

○ **At what stage in gestation is nephron formation completed?**

Nephron formation is usually complete by approximately 36 weeks.

○ **What is the embryologic explanation for communicating hydrocele?**

The explanation is that the processus vaginalis fails to obliterate (persistence of a patent processus vaginalis).

○ **Glomerular filtration rate progressively increases during fetal development. At what postnatal age does GFR reach its peak?**

At approximately 4 months.

○ **A male neonate is found to have bilateral hydroureteronephrosis, echogenic renal parenchyma, and bilateral pneumothorax. What is the most likely diagnosis?**

This child is likely to have urethral obstruction secondary to posterior urethral valves.

○ **What is the mechanism of neonatal testicular torsion?**

The mechanism of this type of torsion, i.e., extravaginal torsion, is thought to be different from intravaginal torsion seen in adolescents and adults. In extravaginal torsion, the entire spermatic cord and its coverings appears to twist.

○ **In Potter's syndrome (bilateral renal agenesis), are the adrenal glands usually absent?**

No. The adrenals are usually normal.

○ **What is the renal anatomic defect found in association with megacalycosis?**

Underdevelopment of the renal medulla.

○ **What is the likely location of a ureter that originates from a higher than normal site on the mesonephric duct?**

According to Mackie and Stephens, the ureter will come to lie more caudal and medial in the bladder than a normal ureteral orifice.

○ **What is the importance of the mesonephric kidney to normal embryonic development of the genitourinary tract?**

The mesonephric kidney never functions in the human, but the mesonephric (Wolffian) duct is key to the genital ducts in the male and to the development of the ureteral bud, and thus the kidney.

○ **Explain one theory for the development of ureteroceles.**

Failure of normal perforation of Chawalla's membrane, which separates the ureter from the bladder, is thought to result in the formation of ureteroceles.

○   **What are the anatomic correlates of the mullerian tubercle in both male and female?**

The verumontanum and the hymen, respectively.

○   **In patients with a thoracic kidney, is a diaphragmatic hernia necessarily present?**

No.

○   **What is a proposed etiology for the formation of calyceal diverticula?**

It is proposed that failure of involution of third- and fourth-order branches of the ureteral bud may result in formation of calyceal diverticula.

○   **Infundibulopelvic stenosis may represent an embryologic midpoint between which two congenital renal anomalies?**

Ureteropelvic junction obstruction and multicystic renal dysplasia.

○   **What is the embryologic origin of the seminal vesicle?**

The Wolffian duct.

○   **What is the mechanism by which the cloaca becomes divided into the urogenital sinus and rectum?**

The urorectal septum grows to meet the cloacal membrane, forming the perineal body as it fuses with the cloacal membrane. This divides the cloacal membrane into an anterior urogenital membrane and a posterior anal membrane.

○   **Which portions of the male urethra have their embryologic origin from the urogenital sinus?**

The prostatic and membranous urethra.

○   **As a horseshoe kidney ascends from the pelvis, which vessel may prevent its ascent into the flank?**

The inferior mesenteric artery.

○   **Which embryonic structure, extending from the bladder to the umbilicus, may remain patent and result in urinary drainage?**

The allantois.

○   **For normal gonadal development, the primary germ cells must migrate from the wall of the yolk sac to paired structures along the dorsal portion of the embryo between the dorsal mesentery and the mesonephros. What are these paired structures that will develop into the primitive gonad?**

They are the genital ridges.

○   **There have been two general theories to explain the formation of the glanular urethra. Explain each theory.**

The first is that the urethral folds, which fuse to form the pendulous urethra, fuse all the way to the glans. The second theory holds that the pendulous urethra is formed in this manner, while a solid core of ectoderm burrows into the glans to unite with the proximal urethra and then canalize.

○ **Explain the embryologic origins of the labia minora and labia majora.**

The labia minora are formed from the urethral folds, while the labia majora are derived from the genital swellings.

○ **Explain the proposed etiology for exstrophy of the urinary bladder.**

Exstrophy occurs when early rupture of the cloacal membrane causes failure of mesenchymal migration into the area.

○ **Explain the embryogenesis of vasoureteral fusion.**

The ureter forms as a branch (ureteral bud) off of the Wolffian duct. In normal male embryogenesis, as the distal Wolffian duct is assimilated into the trigone during bladder formation, the ureteral bud (ureter) and the Wolffian duct (now the vas deferens) separate. Failure of this distal assimilation and separation may result in vasoureteral fusion, or more precisely, a failure of separation of the two structures.

○ **Define Potter syndrome. List its common etiologies and phenotypic (clinical) findings.**

Potter syndrome is the result of oligohydramnios secondary to prenatal kidney disease and renal failure. Bilateral renal agenesis is a common cause of the most severe and fatal form of this disease. Early rupture of membranes, renal cystic disease, and posterior urethral valves are other causes. Pulmonary hypoplasia, sacral agenesis, and various cardiovascular anomalies may also be present.

The common facial characteristics of the syndrome (Potter's facies) include low-set ears, prominent inner canthal folds, a flattened or blunted nose, a prominent depression between the lower lip and the chin. In addition, the babies appear prematurely senile and often have bowed legs and clubbed feet. Most of these findings are thought to be deformations resulting from the severe oligohydramnios.

○ **What anomalies of the male internal genital structures may be found in association with unilateral renal agenesis?**

Ipsilateral absence of the vas deferens and hypoplasia or cystic deformation of the seminal vesicle are found most often.

○ **Are congenital anomalies of the urinary tract more likely to occur on the right side or on the left side of the body?**

Left-sided anomalies predominate.

○ **What other congenital anomalies may be found in patients with renal ectopia?**

Genital anomalies are not uncommon: primarily uterine and vaginal anomalies in females and cryptorchidism, hypospadias, or other urethral anomalies in males.

○ **What is one proposed embryologic explanation for the development of megacalycosis?**

A proposed mechanism is nonobstructive enlargement of the calyx caused by hypoplasia or malformation of the renal papilla.

○ **List some of the common histologic findings of renal dysplasia.**

Distorted renal architecture with immature glomeruli, cartilage, and primitive ducts, lined with columnar epithelium and surrounded by fibromuscular collars.

○   **There are two predominant theories that aim to explain the development of renal dysplasia. List them.**

The first theory is that dysplasia results from obstruction of the developing nephron. The second, or "bud" theory, proposed by Mackie and Stephens, proposes that abnormal ureteral bud development causes the ureter to join the metanephric blastema abnormally, such that abnormal renal parenchyma results.

○   **What is an Ask-Upmark kidney, what is its clinical significance, and what other urological abnormality is it often associated with?**

An Ask-Upmark kidney is a small kidney with areas of segmental hypoplasia and sometimes dysplasia. Although originally thought to be an embryologic error, there is concern that the histologic changes might be in part because of renal scarring. Ask-Upmark kidneys can be a cause of severe hypertension. Most are associated with vesicoureteric reflux.

○   **What is the most common congenital anomaly of the contralateral kidney in a child with a congenital ureteropelvic junction (UPJ) obstruction?**

The most common finding is another UPJ obstruction.

○   **List the components of the VATER syndrome.**

They are **V**ertebral defects, imperforate **A**nus, **T**racheoesophageal fistula, and **R**enal and **R**adial dysplasia.

○   **What structures in male and female are formed from the genital swellings?**

Male: the scrotum. Female: the labia majora.

○   **What anatomic structure often herniates into the groin in female inguinal hernia.**

The ovary.

○   **Which specific Y chromosome gene is felt to be responsible for male sex differentiation and where is it located?**

The SRY gene (also known as the testis determining factor), which is located on the short arm of the Y chromosome, is felt to be the gene that initiates differentiation of the indifferent gonad into a testis.

○   **At what stage of gestation does descent of the testis occur?**

Descent of testis into the scrotum occurs in late gestation, usually between 30 and 40 weeks. Descent may not be complete until after birth, especially in premature infants.

○   **What is the percentage of boys with cryptorchidism at birth in full-term male infants?**

Approximately 3%.

○   **What urological finding is associated with cystic fibrosis?**

Agenesis of the vas deferens is found in a high percentage of males with cystic fibrosis.

○   **What urachal anomalies can you name other than patent urachus?**

Anomalies that may be seen as urachal remnant variants include urachal cyst, urachal sinus, urachal diverticulum, and alternating urachal sinus.

◯ **Briefly outline a proposed embryologic origin for a communicating hydrocele of the cord, and define how this would differ from the origin of a communicating hydrocele.**

A communicating hydrocele represents a persistence of the patent processus vaginalis, a tonguelike extension of the peritoneum.

A communicating hydrocele of the cord requires a distal occlusion of the processus vaginalis, which must be accompanied by a relative narrowing of the processus proximal to the occluded processus. The area between the occlusion and the partial occlusion then traps peritoneal fluid to form a cystic dilation of the processus. Since the proximal portion of the processus remains open, these cystic structures may change in size.

◯ **What is the abdominal wall structure from which the cremasteric muscle and fascia develop?**

They develop from the internal oblique muscle.

◯ **Describe the embryologic mishap that would explain why most males with penopubic epispadias have urinary incontinence.**

Epispadias is at the most minimal end of the spectrum of the epispadias–exstrophy complex, with cloacal exstropy being the most severe example. This complex results when the cloacal membrane ruptures prior to its closure (before the mesoderm surrounding the membrane and the mesoderm of the genital swellings has grown to the midline and closed the anterior abdominal wall). In penile epispadias, the only defect is the dorsal urethral closure, while in penopubic epispadias with incontinence (the most common form), the bladder neck is not completely formed and incontinence results.

◯ **A 5-year-old male presented with a symptomatic left inguinal hernia. At exploration, a solid reddish nodule is found in the cord adjacent to the testis. What might this represent?**

This may be an accessory spleen. Accessory spleens are common and may be located in several areas. They may be carried into the scrotum as the developing left testis descends, and may present as an isolated scrotal nodule or multiple nodules, or as splenogonadal fusion, in which a very elongated spleen is attached like a long tongue extending from the spleen into the inguinal canal.

◯ **How does vaginal atresia differ from vaginal agenesis?**

Vaginal atresia involves only the distal vagina. The mullerian structures are not affected. The uterus, cervix, and proximal vagina are all normal and intact.

Vaginal agenesis is the absence of a proximal vagina in a normal 46 XX female with normal hormones. A hymenal fringe and a small distal vaginal pouch are usually present.

◯ **What is Mayer-Rokitansky-Kuster-Hauser (MRKH) syndrome?**

Another name for vaginal agenesis.

◯ **What urological problems are most commonly associated with vaginal agenesis?**

Unilateral renal agenesis or ectopia of one or both kidneys occurs in 74% of patients.

◯ **What is penile torsion and how is it treated?**

Penile torsion is the term used to describe the rotation of the penis around the longitudinal axis. It is usually a congenital condition, but it can occur after penile surgery. No treatment is necessary, but in rare cases a surgical correction can be done by degloving and skin realignment. A Dartos flap can be used in severe cases.

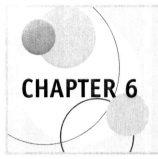

CHAPTER 6

Congenital Disorders of the Lower Urinary Tract

Tamer Aboushwareb, MD, and Anthony Atala, MD

○ **Describe the formation of trigone during development.**

The common excretory ducts (the portion of the nephric ducts distal to the origin of ureteric buds) dilate and become absorbed into the urogenital sinus. The right and left common excretory ducts fuse in the midline as a triangular area, forming the primitive trigone.

○ **How does the bladder appear in prune-belly syndrome?**

↑ collagen

The bladder usually appears massively enlarged with a pseudodiverticulum at the urachus. The urachus is patent at birth in 25% to 30% of children. Histologically, the bladder has an increased ratio of collagen to muscle fibers in the absence of obstruction.

○ **Why are indirect inguinal hernias frequent in exstrophy patients?**

Indirect hernia - exstrophy

This phenomenon is attributed to a persistent processus vaginalis, large internal and external inguinal rings, and lack of obliquity of the inguinal canal.

○ **What is the rate of occurrence of inguinal hernias in bladder exstrophy?**

In a review of 181 children with bladder exstrophy, Connolly and coauthors (1995) reported inguinal hernias in 81.8% of boys and 10.5% of girls.

○ **What is the primary anorectal defect in exstrophy?**

The perineum is short and broad and the anus is situated directly behind the urogenital diaphragm; it is displaced anteriorly and corresponds to the posterior limit of the triangular fascial defect.

○ **What is the average corporal length defect in exstrophy patients?**

It was found that the anterior corporal length of male patients with bladder exstrophy was almost 50% shorter than that of normal controls.

○ **How does the exstrophy patient's prostate compare to the normal age-matched control's prostate?**

The volume, weight, and maximum cross-sectional area of the prostate appears normal compared with published control values. However, in exstrophy patients, the prostate does not extend circumferentially around the urethra, and the urethra is anterior to the prostate in all patients.

○ **What is the classic picture of a female exstrophy patient?**

The vagina is shorter than normal, hardly greater than 6 cm in depth, but of normal caliber. The vaginal orifice is frequently stenotic and displaced anteriorly; the clitoris is bifid, and the labia, mons pubis, and clitoris are divergent. The uterus enters the vagina superiorly so that the cervix is in the anterior vaginal wall. The fallopian tubes and ovaries are normal.

○ **What is the incidence of reflux after surgical closure of the bladder in exstrophy patients?**

Reflux in the closed exstrophic bladder occurs in 100% of cases, and subsequent surgery is usually required at the time of bladder neck reconstruction. If excessive outlet resistance is gained at the time of either initial closure or combined epispadias and bladder exstrophy closure, and if recurrent infections are a problem even with suppressive antibiotics, ureteral reimplantation is required before bladder neck reconstruction.

○ **What are the most significant changes in the management of bladder exstrophy over the past two decades?**

Currently, bladder exstrophy is managed with (1) early bladder, posterior urethral, and abdominal wall closure, usually with osteotomy, (2) early epispadias repair, and (3) reconstruction of a continent bladder neck and reimplantation of the ureters when necessary. Most importantly, however, a definition of strict criteria for the selection of patients suitable for this approach has been created.

○ **What are the advantages incurred by osteotomy at the time of bladder closure?**

Pelvic osteotomy performed at the time of initial closure confers several advantages, including easy approximation of the symphysis with diminished tension on the abdominal wall closure and elimination of the need for fascial flaps. In addition, it allows placement of the urethra deep within the pelvic ring, enhancing bladder outlet resistance. Finally, it brings the large pelvic floor muscles near the midline, where they can support the bladder neck and aid in eventual urinary control.

○ **Why is the combined anterior osteotomy preferred to the classic posterior osteotomy?**

Besides the ease of approximation, combined osteotomy was developed for three reasons:

  1. Osteotomy is performed with the patient in the supine position, as is the urological repair, thereby avoiding the need to turn the patient.
  2. The anterior approach to this osteotomy allows placement of an external fixator device and intrafragmentary pins under direct vision.
  3. The cosmetic appearance of this osteotomy is superior to that resulting from the posterior iliac approach.

○ **When can you remove the external fixating device after primary closure?**

When good callus formation is seen on radiography, the fixating device and pins are removed with the patient under light sedation.

○ **In cases of small bladder strip at birth, which is preferable: rapid closure or closure after a reasonable waiting period?**

Ideally, waiting for the bladder template to grow for 4 to 6 months in the child with a small bladder is not as risky as submitting a small bladder template to closure in an inappropriate setting. This may result in dehiscence and allows the fate of the bladder to be sealed at that point.

○ **A young child presents with persistent UTI and apparent high-grade reflux after primary closure of the bladder. What is the proper management?**

Proper management is to begin long-term antibiotic therapy to control the infections. It may also be necessary to dilate the urethra or to begin intermittent catheterization.

○ **When is combined closure of exstrophy and epispadias repair considered?**

Combined closure of exstrophy and epispadias repair is considered in patients who have had closure surgery delayed beyond the newborn period or in patients in whom the initial newborn closure fails.

○ **What is the primary goal of bladder neck reconstruction procedures?**

The primary goal of this procedure is urinary continence, which is defined as a 3-hour dry interval. If this is not achieved within 2 years after bladder neck reconstruction, failure to achieve continence has resulted.

○ **What are the key determinants of management in bladder exstrophy?**

- Size and quality of bladder template.
- Extent of pubic diastasis and malleability of the pelvis.
- Need for osteotomy.
- Length and width of urethral plate.
- Penile size.
- Associated anomalies.

○ **What is the innervation pattern of the corporal bodies and bladder in cloacal exstrophy patients?**

Enervation to the duplicated corporal bodies arises from the sacral plexus, travels through the midline, perforates the interior portion of the pelvic floor, and courses medially to the hemibladders.

○ **What is the rate of occurrence of intestinal tract abnormalities in cloacal exstrophy?**

Omphalocele was reported to occur between 88% and 100% of cases, with most studies reporting omphalocele in more than 95% of cases.

○ **What is the most common mullerian defect in cloacal exstrophy?**

The most commonly reported müllerian anomaly is uterine duplication seen in 95% of patients.

○ **What procedures are performed in the one-stage repair of cloacal exstrophy?**

- Excision of omphalocele.
- Separation of cecal plate from bladder halves.
- Joining and closure of bladder halves followed by urethroplasty.
- Bilateral anterior innominate and vertical iliac osteotomy.
- Gonadectomy in males with un-reconstructible phallus.
- Terminal ileostomy/colostomy.
- Genital revision if needed.

○ **What is the two-stage repair of cloacal exstrophy?**

First stage (newborn period)
- Excision of omphalocele.
- Separation of cecal plate from bladder halves.
- Joining of bladder halves.
- Gonadectomy in male with un-reconstructible phallus.
- Terminal ileostomy/colostomy.

Second stage
- Closure of joined bladder halves and urethroplasty.
- Bilateral anterior innominate and vertical iliac osteotomy.
- Genital revision if needed.

○ **What is the incidence of vesicoureteral reflux in epispadias patients?**

The ureterovesical junction is inherently deficient in complete epispadias, and the incidence of reflux has been reported to be between 30% and 40%.

○ **What are the primary objectives of repair of male epispadias?**

The objectives of repair of penopubic epispadias include achievement of urinary continence with preservation of the upper urinary tract and the reconstruction of cosmetically acceptable genitalia.

○ **What is megacystis?**

The term *megacystis* is often used to describe any condition leading to a distended fetal bladder in utero, without referring to the cause of the dilation. Historically, congenital megacystis was thought to be caused by bladder neck obstruction, leading to massive bilateral vesicoureteral reflux (VUR) and a thin bladder wall.

○ **How sensitive is prenatal ultrasound in the diagnosis of posterior urethral valves?**

Ultrasonography is sensitive in detecting fetal hydronephrosis, but the specific diagnosis of posterior urethral valves is more difficult.

○ **What is the most important diagnostic study for posterior urethral valves?**

Voiding cystourethrography (VCUG) remains the most important study in diagnosis of posterior urethral valves because it defines the anatomy and gross function of the bladder, bladder neck, and urethra.

○ **What is the gold standard treatment in the management of posterior urethral valves?**

In general, primary ablation is the preferred surgical procedure to treat posterior urethral valves. Vesicostomy is reserved for very small or very ill infants, but vesicostomy remains an excellent alternative treatment in these difficult situations.

○ **What are the prognostic indicators of future renal function in posterior urethral valves patients?**

There are four basic predictors of renal function in patients with posterior urethral valves: ultrasound appearance, serum chemistries, age at diagnosis, and presence of reflux.

○ **How is nocturnal polyuria explained in patients with nocturnal enuresis?**

Nocturnal polyuria can be either absolute, which is usually associated with a derangement of the circadian rhythm of antidiuretic hormone secretion, or relative, mainly due to a reduced functional bladder capacity during sleep at night.

○ **What is the definition of hypospadias?**

Hypospadias, in boys, is defined as a group of three anomalies of the penis: (1) an abnormal ventral opening of the urethral meatus that may be located anywhere from the ventral aspect of the glans penis to the perineum, (2) an abnormal ventral curvature of the penis (chordee), and (3) an abnormal distribution of foreskin with a "hood" present dorsally and deficient foreskin ventrally. The second and third characteristics are not present in all cases.

○ **What are the current theories explaining congenital penile curvature?**

Currently, three major theories are proposed for the cause of penile curvature. These include (1) abnormal development of the urethral plate; (2) abnormal, fibrotic mesenchymal tissue at the urethral meatus; and (3) corporal disproportion or differential growth of normal dorsal corpora cavernosal tissue and abnormal corporal tissue ventrally.

○ **Higher maternal serum levels of man-made organochloro compounds (PCBs and similar chemicals) appears to correlate with what congenital urological abnormalities in newborn children?**

Undescended testes and hypospadias. The theory is that the chemical burden in the mother affects her endocrine function.

○ **In bilateral undescended testes, how often are the abnormal testis locations bilaterally identical and symmetrical?**

Approximately two thirds of the time.

○ **During what gestational week does the foreskin develop?**

At approximately the 20th week of gestation.

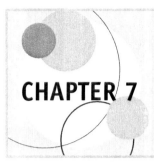

CHAPTER 7

Congenital Disorders of the Upper Tracts

Kevin M. Feber, MD, and Evan J. Kass, MD

○ **True or False: Potter syndrome is pathognomonic for bilateral renal agenesis.**

False. The findings that accompany Potter syndrome can be found in other conditions in which fetal oligohydramnios is present, including autosomal recessive polycystic kidney disease, posterior urethral valves, and prune-belly syndrome.

○ **What is the embryological basis and the characteristic findings of the Mayer Rokitansky–Kuster–Hauser syndrome and how does it usually present?**

During fetal development the mullerian ducts are adjacent to the wolffian ducts. Mullerian duct abnormalities may result in vaginal agenesis as well as malformation of the ipsilateral uterine horn or fallopian tube. The close proximity of the wolffian and mullerian duct structures may result in renal agenesis or ectopia. Initial clinical presentation is often primary amenorrhea with cyclical abdominal pain. Ovarian function is normal.

○ **Patients found to have a missing vas deferens during an infertility workup should be screened for what abnormality and how?**

Ipsilateral renal agenesis. A renal ultrasound is useful for this purpose.

○ **What is the long-term prognosis for a baby born with a solitary kidney?**

The patient is at increased risk for developing proteinuria, hypertension, and renal insufficiency over the course of his or her lifetime; however, the patient's life expectancy is normal.

○ **What is the most common additional urologic abnormality associated with a horseshoe kidney?**

Up to 33% of patients with a horseshoe kidney have evidence of significant ureteropelvic junction obstruction.

○ **The cephalad migration of a horseshoe kidney is limited by what structure?**

The inferior mesenteric artery.

○ **What is the normal direction of rotation of the human kidney as it ascends out of the pelvis?**

The kidney normally rotates 90 degrees ventromedially during ascent. Therefore, the renal pelvis, which was originally directed anteriorly, becomes directed medially.

○   **True or False: Most crossed ectopic kidneys are fused with their mate.**

True. Approximately 90% of crossed ectopic kidneys are fused with a normally placed mate.

○   **What is the most common cause of hydronephrosis in the fetal kidney?**

Ureteropelvic junction obstructions are the etiology of up to 80% of cases of fetal hydronephrosis.

○   **True or False: Most cases of prenatally diagnosed ureteropelvic junction obstruction require urgent surgical intervention following delivery.**

False. Debate continues surrounding the management of prenatally diagnosed ureteropelvic junction obstructions. Most often surgery is not necessary or can be performed on an elective basis after an appropriate evaluation and period of observation.

○   **In what percent of patients with ureteropelvic junction obstruction does the contralateral kidney demonstrate evidence of ureteropelvic junction obstruction?**

In patients found to have ureteropelvic junction obstruction, evidence for bilateral obstruction exists in 10% to 40% of cases.

○   **In what percentage of patients with ureteropelvic junction obstruction does vesicoureteral reflux coexist?**

Severe vesicoureteral reflux coexists in 10% of cases, whereas minor degrees of vesicoureteral reflux have been documented in as many as 40% of cases.

○   **Define and differentiate the terms dysplasia, aplastic dysplasia, and familial adysplasia.**

Dysplasia refers to the histologic findings of focal, diffuse, or segmentally arranged primitive structures that result from abnormal metanephric differentiation. Aplastic dysplasia is a small quantity of tissue that is nonfunctional and dysplastic by histologic criteria. Familial adysplasia is a term that identifies multiple persons in a single family with renal agenesis, renal dysplasia, multicystic dysplasia, or renal aplasia.

○   **What is the most common type of renal cystic disease?**

Multicystic dysplasia.

○   **A child is discovered to have a multicystic dysplastic kidney. This patient's contralateral kidney should be screened for what abnormalities?**

The contralateral collecting system should been screened for vesicoureteral reflux, which is present in 18% to 43% of cases, and for ureteropelvic junction obstruction, which has been demonstrated in 3% to 12% of cases.

○   **What is the average amount of renal parenchyma drained by the upper pole of a duplicated collecting system?**

About one-third of total renal parenchyma is drained by the upper pole of a duplicated collecting system.

○   **A ureteric bud arising on the mesonephric duct in an abnormally caudal location predisposes to what abnormality?**

The ureteral orifice will ultimately reside in a more cranial and lateral position within the bladder and be predisposed to vesicoureteral reflux.

○ **The upper pole ureter of a duplicated collecting system is predisposed to what abnormality?**

Obstruction with subsequent hydronephrosis.

○ **What is the Meyer–Weigert rule?**

The inferior and medial ureteral orifice in a duplicated collecting system drains the upper pole collecting system and tends to obstruct, whereas the superior and lateral ureteral orifice drains the lower pole collecting system and tends to reflux.

○ **True or False: Ectopic ureteral orifices in female patients are often associated with duplicated collecting systems.**

True. More than 80% of ectopic ureters in female patients are associated with duplicated collecting systems.

○ **Do male patients with ectopic ureteral orifices tend to have duplicated collecting systems?**

No. Ectopic ureteral orifices in boys drain single collecting systems in the majority of cases.

○ **A boy with a duplicated collecting system is found to have an ectopic ureter. Where will the terminal portion of the ectopic ureter most likely be found? the ectopic ureteral orifice will most likely be found within the vagina.**

Ectopic ureters in males terminate in the posterior urethra in approximately 50% of cases and the seminal vesicles in about 30% of cases.

○ **True or False: In a girl with continuous urinary incontinence found to have an ectopic ureter?**

False. The ectopic ureteral orifice will most often be found within the urethra or at the vestibule.

○ **What is Chawalla's membrane?**

Chawalla's membrane is a two-layered cell structure that transiently divides the ureteral bud from the urogenital sinus at approximately 37 days gestation. Incomplete dissolution of this membrane is believed to be the etiology of ureterocele formation.

○ **Ureteroceles tend to occur in patients of what race and sex?**

Ureteroceles are significantly more common in Caucasians and occur four times more frequently in females than in males.

○ **What is a pseudoureterocele?**

A radiographic finding in which a dilated ectopic ureter coursing behind the bladder impinges on the bladder wall giving the appearance of an ureterocele.

○ **What is the most common cause of urethral obstruction in a young girl?**

A prolapsing ureterocele.

○ **What is the length to diameter ratio in a normal nonrefluxing pediatric ureter?**

5:1

○ **What is the embryology of a circumcaval ureter or preureteral vena cava?**

The inferior vena cava develops from a plexus of fetal veins. Normally, the inferior vena cava forms from the right supracardinal vein as the right subcardinal atrophies. If the right subcardinal vein fails to atrophy and becomes the inferior vena cava, a segment of ureter becomes trapped behind the vena cava.

○ **What is the most common etiology of renal calculi in children?**

Hypercalciuria as a side effect of furosemide or glucocorticoid therapy.

○ **What is a pseudotumor of the kidney?**

A hypertrophied column of Bertin that may be sufficiently large to compress and deform the adjacent collecting system.

○ **What is the usual clinical course of classic congenital mesoblastic nephroma?**

Classic congenital mesoblastic nephroma is a benign tumor and treatment is limited to surgical excision.

○ **What is a nephrogenic rest?**

A nephrogenic rest is an abnormal focus of nephrogenic cells. Although these cells can be induced to form Wilm's tumor, the majority of nephrogenic rests involute and do not result in tumor formation.

○ **What hepatic abnormality is associated with autosomal recessive polycystic kidney disease?**

Congenital hepatic fibrosis.

○ **What are the ultrasound characteristics of autosomal recessive polycystic kidney disease?**

As a result of the enormous number of interfaces created by the tightly compacted, dilated collecting ducts, the kidneys appear large and homogeneously hyperechogenic.

○ **What neurological, gastrointestinal, and cardiac anomalies are associated with autosomal dominant polycystic kidney disease?**

Circle of Willis and Berry aneurysms, colonic diverticula, and mitral valve prolapse.

○ **Juvenile nephronophthisis and medullary cystic disease are transmitted by what modes of inheritance?**

Juvenile nephronophthisis is usually transmitted as an autosomal recessive trait, whereas medullary cystic disease is transmitted as an autosomal dominant trait.

○ **What are the characteristics of Alport's syndrome?**

Hereditary nephritis, high frequency hearing loss, ocular abnormalities, microhematuria, and proteinuria.

○ **What is sirenomelia and what renal defect is associated with it?**

It's a rare congenital syndrome in which the lower extremities are fused together. It occurs in approximately 1 in 60,000 to 100,000 births and is almost always fatal due to the associated renal agenesis. If kidney function is preserved, survival is possible but extremely rare. There is only one long-term survivor known.

○ **Is UPJ obstruction in children more common in boys or girls?**

Boys, by a ratio of about 5:2.

○ **In children with UPJ, which side is involved more often or is it a tie?**

It is more commonly found on the left than the right, with a ratio of 5:2. Bilateral disease happens in approximately 15% of cases.

○ **What is Fraley's syndrome?**

Fraley originally described this syndrome in 1966 as a condition where an aberrant crossing vessel causes clinical obstruction and hydronephrosis of the upper pole infundibulum resulting in significant renal pain or hematuria. This is usually identified on IVP or renal angiography, but may also be diagnosed with CT or MR angiography. Stones, pain, infection, and hematuria are commonly associated with the syndrome. It does not necessarily require surgical repair, only if symptomatic or clinically necessary.

○ **Describe the process of normal renal formation and the defect that may cause the agenesis of a kidney?**

An orderly branching ureteral bud is required for complete formation of the adult kidney. Between the fifth and seventh weeks of gestation, the ureteral bud arises from the mesonephric (wolffian) duct. A normal metanephric blastema needs to be present to induce the ureteral bud to branch into major and minor calyces. Agenesis of the kidney results when the ureteral bud fails to develop or the nephrogenic ridge is absent.

○ **In a patient with a normal left kidney and a right pelvic kidney, what is the location of both adrenal glands?**

The adrenal glands are both normally positioned.

○ **What are the six potential locations of an ectopic kidney?**

Pelvic, iliac, abdominal, thoracic, contralateral, or crossed.

○ **In a horseshoe kidney, are the calyces normal in number and orientation?**

The calyces are normal in number but have an atypical orientation. Since the kidney does not rotate, the calyces are oriented posteriorly and the pelvic axis stays in the obliquely lateral or vertical plane.

○ **Identify three specific causes of significant hydronephrosis caused by UPJ obstruction in patients with a horseshoe kidney?**

The obstruction results from one or more of the following:

1) the high insertion of the ureter into the renal pelvis.

2) its aberrant course over the isthmus.

3) the kidney's anomalous blood supply.

○ **What is a calyceal diverticulum?**

A transitional epithelium lined cystic cavity located within the renal parenchyma and connected to an adjacent minor calyx by a narrow channel or infundibulum.

○ **In a patient with a complete ureteral duplication with a refluxing lower pole moiety and a normal upper pole moiety who is undergoing ureteral reimplantation, should the ureters be reimplanted separately or together?**

The two ureters share a common blood supply that runs longitudinally between the two ureters. Both ureters should be reimplanted together in a common sheath reimplantation.

○ **In a female, what anomalies may result from incomplete or altered Müllerian development caused by mesonephric duct maldevelopment?**

Complete absence of the ipsilateral horn and the fallopian tube with a unicornuate uterus is the most common anomaly. A bicornate uterus with incomplete development of the horn on the affected side can also occur. When there is partial or complete fusion of the müllerian ducts in the midline, a didelphic or septated uterus with a solitary or duplex cervix may result.

○ **What test should be ordered if, during a physical examination, the vas deferens or body and tail of the epididymis are missing? What disorder would be suspected?**

An abdominal ultrasound to evaluate for unilateral renal agenesis.

○ **When does the kidney reach its adult location?**

The kidney reaches its adult location by the end of the eighth week of gestation.

○ **In crossed fused ectopia, how are the two renal units joined?**

The inferior aspect of the normal kidney is usually attached to the superior pole of the ectopic kidney. Ninety percent of crossed ectopic kidneys are fused.

○ **In fusion anomalies, how do the ureters insert into the bladder?**

The ureter from each kidney is usually orthotopic.

○ **The mullerian ducts stop developing at approximately what age of gestational development?**

The mullerian ducts cease development at around 5 weeks of gestational age.

○ **Medullary Sponge Kidney (MSK) has been associated with what urological problems?**

Recurrent UTIs, renal leak-type hypercalciuria, hypocitraturia, and nephrolithiasis.

○ **What renal pelvis pressure reading suggests obstruction when performing a Whitaker test?**

More than 22 cm of H_2O pressure suggests obstruction.

○ **What is the most common congenital urinary malformation?**

Renal agenesis.

○ **True or False: Symphysiotomy (division of the isthmus) is routinely recommended after pyeloplasty in patients with horseshoe kidney.**

False. Due to the abnormal vasculature, the kidneys tend to resume their previous position, so a symphysiotomy is no longer recommended. It also increases the risk of bleeding, fistula formation, and renal infarction.

○ **Compared to normal kidneys, horseshoe kidneys have a higher incidence of what urologic problems?**

Hydronephrosis, UPJ obstruction, stones, urinary tract infections, and tumors.

○ **What tumors are associated with horseshoe kidneys and which one of these is the most common?**

Renal cell, carcinoid, and Wilms tumors are all associated with horseshoe kidneys. Of these, renal cell is the most common.

○ **True or False: Temporary placement of a double J stent is a useful therapeutic clinical test for patients with flank pain and equivocal UPJ obstruction.**

True. Studies suggest that a 3-week trial with a double J stent can be useful in identifying those cases most suitable for surgical intervention.

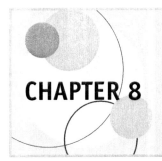

CHAPTER 8 Prune-Belly Syndrome

Mark R. Wakefield, MD, FACS, and Julie M. Riley, MD

○ **What are alternate, perhaps less stigmatizing, names for prune-belly syndrome?**

Prune-belly vividly describes the clinical appearance of most patients with the syndrome. However, many clinicians consider the negative connotations to be stigmatizing and socially undesirable. Thus, several alternatives have been proposed. Eagle–Barrett syndrome recognizes one of the original descriptions of a series of nine patients in 1950. Abdominal wall deficiency syndrome is a descriptive nomenclature. Triad syndrome emphasizes the three components of the classic syndrome. Nonetheless, prune-belly syndrome remains the common terminology, in part because of its intensely descriptive nature.

○ **What are three classic features that characterize prune-belly syndrome?**

Triad syndrome refers to the following three specific features of prune-belly syndrome:

1. Urinary tract dilation, specifically megaureter.
2. Abdominal wall deficiency.
3. Cryptorchidism.

The defective abdominal musculature gives the typical appearance of a wrinkled prune, with laxity of the anterior abdominal wall. The testes are both nonpalpable. The urinary tract dilation includes tortuous, dilated ureters, as well as varying degrees of an enlarged smooth-walled bladder and dilated prostatic urethra.

○ **What is the approximate incidence of prune-belly syndrome?**

The true incidence is not well known. The estimated incidence is similar to that of bladder extrophy. The reported range is 1 per 29,000 to 40,000 live births. With increasing prenatal diagnosis and termination, the incidence has been decreasing. The classic triad syndrome only occurs in males. However, variations that include two of the three features can occur in males and females. The incidence is uncertain for patients with incomplete prune-belly syndrome, but probably is one-fourth as common as the classic syndrome. Furthermore, approximately 15% of patients with incomplete prune-belly syndrome were females.

○   **What is the incidence of prune-belly syndrome in females?**

Of all prune-belly syndrome cases, 3% to 4% occur in females.

○   **What is the most common genetic karyotype in patients with prune-belly syndrome?**

Normal. However, several genetic defects are associated with prune-belly syndrome. These include Turner syndrome, Monosomy 16, Trisomy 13, and Trisomy 18.

○   **To what does pseudo-prune-belly syndrome refer?**

Incomplete prune-belly syndrome refers to patients with two of the three classic findings of the triad. For females, this would include the dilation of the urinary tract and lax abdominal wall musculature, but not the undescended testes. Pseudo-prune-belly syndrome refers to those males with ureteral dilation and undescended testes but normal abdominal wall.

○   **What percentage of patients will have atypical presentation of prune-belly syndrome?**

An incomplete form of prune-belly syndrome is present in as many as 25% of patients. Most will have the typical urinary tract finding of dilated ureters, but will have either normal abdominal wall musculature (pseudo-prune-belly syndrome) or descended testes. Females with incomplete prune-belly syndrome are even less common, affecting less than 5% of patients with the syndrome. In females the urinary tract dilation may be less severe.

○   **What are some proposed embryologic etiologies of prune-belly syndrome?**

There are several theories explaining the embryogenesis of prune-belly syndrome. Each theory has both supporting experimental and empiric evidence, but none been proven. These theories are not mutually exclusive.

Urinary tract obstruction may result from a transient urethral membrane at a critical phase of development. Abdominal wall laxity then results from outward compression from the dilated urinary tract. The migration of the testicles is blocked by the enlarged bladder. Primary prostatic maldevelopment with hypoplasia of the prostatic urethra is another possible cause of urinary tract obstruction. A final postulated cause is felt to be due to transient obstruction at the glanular and penile urethral junction. In any case, fetal urinary ascites may or may not occur.

Primary mesodermal maldevelopment may also explain prune-belly syndrome. Failure of myoblast precursors to differentiate and/or migrate appropriately may explain the abnormal development of the abdominal wall. The laxity of the abdominal wall may then be the primary event. The decreased intra-abdominal pressures then result in urinary tract dilation and undescended testicles. However, if the developmental defect occurs early enough (third week of gestation), then all of the abnormalities may be explained by a common event in the mesenchymal tissues.

Persistence of the yolk sac has been implicated in the abdominal wall abnormalities resulting in redundant tissues. The allantoic diverticulum becomes overdeveloped and becomes incorporated into the urinary tract as redundant tissues.

○   **Which is the prevailing theory?**

Mesodermal arrest. This is thought to occur between the sixth and the tenth gestational week although it could occur as early as 3 weeks gestation.

○   **Histopathology of the abdominal wall muscles is suggestive of what type of etiology: developmental arrest or muscular atrophy?**

Developmental arrest. The lack of aponeurotic layers support this etiology.

○ **What are the three categories of prune-belly syndrome?**

Category I has marked oligohydramnios secondary to dysplasia or severe bladder outlet obstruction. Prognosis is very poor in this group as most are either stillborn or die within the first few days of life. Little intervention is warranted in this group.

Category II shows moderate renal insufficiency and moderate to severe hydroureteronephrosis. This would include patients with urethral atresia and a patent urachus. The goal of treatment in this group is to stabilize renal function. The treatment in this category has the most controversies.

Category III consists of patients with mild or incomplete forms of prune-belly syndrome. There is no pulmonary insufficiency seen. Invasive treatment is necessary in those patients with recurrent infections.

○ **Fetal ascites may be transient in prune-belly cases. Why?**

It is reabsorbed, usually before birth.

○ **What is the role of prenatal diagnosis with fetal ultrasound in prune-belly syndrome?**

In general, prenatal diagnosis of prune-belly syndrome has not been reliable. There are high false-positive and false-negative rates of prenatal diagnosis. The typical intrauterine appearance of prune-belly syndrome is bilateral hydronephrosis with an enlarged noncycling bladder. Earlier fetal ascites and oligohydramnios may also be suggestive of prune-belly syndrome. However, the differential diagnosis of these findings includes posterior urethral valves, vesicoureteral reflux, bilateral ureteropelvic junction obstruction, neurogenic bladder, and megacystitis/megalourethra syndromes.

○ **Late presentations of prune-belly syndrome are typified by what characteristics?**

Although the typical appearance of the abdomen in neonates with prune-belly syndrome usually lead to prompt diagnosis, some children present at a later age. These children often have less severe forms of the syndrome. These children may present with difficulty sitting from a supine position as a result of weaker abdominal muscles. Walking may be delayed due to difficulty with standing and balance. Older children will have a characteristic potbelly with loss of wrinkling of the skin due to stretching of the abdominal viscera.

○ **What diagnostic evaluation in patients with prune-belly syndrome should be avoided?**

A voiding cystourethrogram should be avoided in the early prenatal period. Instrumentation of the urinary tract puts the patient at increased risk of infection and sepsis. The diagnosis should be suspected based on physical examination findings. The dilated bladder and ureters are often palpable due to the lax abdominal wall. Although used previously to confirm diagnosis, intravenous pyelogram does not image the urinary tract well due to poor concentrating ability of neonatal kidneys and dilution of contrast in the dilated urinary tract. Abdominal ultrasound can be useful in assessing the degree of urinary tract dilation. Serial assessment of serum electrolytes, renal function, and urine culture are important diagnostic tests. A renal scan is necessary when renal function stabilizes to evaluate renal function and drainage.

Some experts, however, recommend an early VCUG despite the risks because it is the best way to identify reflux and urethral stenosis. Bladder size can be determined as well as the presence of any urachal remnants.

○ **What is the most common nongenitourinary anomaly in patient with prune-belly syndrome?**

Thoracic cage malformations, including pectus excavatum and pectus carinatum, occur in more than 75% of patients with prune-belly syndrome. The chest wall malformations are likely due to the restrictive effects of oligohydramnios. In the most severe form, pulmonary hypoplasia can occur with associated pneumothorax and high neonatal mortality rate. Most patients, however, have only mild pulmonary dysfunction, often only evident on formal pulmonary function testing. Prune-belly syndrome patients will have a less forceful cough due to weaker abdominal musculature placing them at increased risk for postoperative respiratory distress, pneumonia, and bronchitis. Other common anomalies include cardiac (10%), gastrointestinal (30%), and orthopedic deformities (50%).

○ **What is the most common anomaly of the musculoskeletal system in patients with prune-belly syndrome?**

Skin dimples on the knee or elbow are the most common abnormality of the musculoskeletal system, excluding the typical abdominal wall defects. The skin dimples occur in 45% of patients. More severe anomalies include varus deformity of the feet (club foot), which occurs in 25% of patients, congential hip dislocation (5%), spinal dysmorphism (5%), and rarely severe lower extremity hypoplasia. Skin dimples are likely a result of compression from oligohydramnios. Other etiologies have been proposed: ischemia from compressed iliac vessels or a common defect in mesenchymal development at 3 weeks gestation.

Cardiac abnormalities occur in 10% of patients with prune-belly syndrome. The most common cardiac abnormalities in prune-belly syndrome are patent ductus arteriosus, ventricular septal defect, atrial septal defect, and tetralogy of Fallot.

Malrotation of the midgut occurs more frequently in patients with severe prune-belly syndrome. Other gastrointestinal anomalies, including gastroschisis and omphalocele, have been described in patients with prune-belly syndrome.

○ **In addition to the classic triad of findings, what are the common anomalies of the urinary system in prune-belly syndrome?**

The penile urethra is usually normal, although a megalourethra is associated with prune-belly syndrome. The prostatic urethra is hypoplastic in most patients with prune-belly syndrome. The bladder neck is wide open and tapers to the normal membranous urethra. The prostatic urethra appears dilated as a result of the prostatic hypoplasia. The prostatic utricle and ejaculatory ducts are dilated. The bladder is enlarged but usually does not have trabeculation. The patent urachus may persist, especially if there is urethral atresia. The ureters are involved with the proximal ureters typically being less dilated. The kidneys are afflicted by varying degrees of hydronephrosis and renal dysplasia.

○ **What is the likelihood of renal failure among patients with prune-belly syndrome?**

One-third of patients will progress to renal failure.

○ **What causes renal failure in patients with prune-belly syndrome?**

Renal failure in patients with prune-belly syndrome results from the reflux of infected urine and subsequent pyelonephritis. High-grade obstruction or high-pressure reflux may result in severe renal dysplasia at birth, as seen in some neonatal autopsy studies. However, most patients with prune-belly syndrome have low pressure vesicoureteral reflux. As long as the urine remains sterile, the risk of renal failure appears to be low, despite the high incidence of reflux and dilation of the upper tract.

○ **What is the role of renal transplantation in patients with prune-belly syndrome?**

Renal transplantation in patients with prune-belly syndrome is as successful as transplantation for other indications in children. Special attention must be directed toward management of the urinary tract prior to transplantation. Adequate bladder emptying with clean intermittent catheterization is often necessary and is preferable to urinary diversion.

○ **How common is vesicoureteral reflux in patients with prune-belly syndrome?**

Vesicoureteral reflux occurs in as many as 85% of the patients with prune-belly syndrome. The reflux tends to be low pressure. Most children with prune-belly syndrome do not outgrow this reflux. Nonetheless, surgery to correct the reflux is usually reserved for those patients with recurrent pyelonephritis, whose reflux is refractory to more conservative therapies such as vesicostomy. Ureteroneocystostomy is associated with a high risk of ureterovesical obstruction and recurrence of reflux in patients with prune-belly syndrome.

○ **What are the typical characteristics of the kidney in patients with prune-belly syndrome?**

Fifty percent of patients with prune-belly syndrome will have dysplastic kidneys. Dysplasia shows either Potter type II or IV. Type II is more indicative of mesenchymal defect whereas type IV is related to obstruction. The renal pelvis is often dilated. The degree of dilation is not proportional to the degree of dysplasia. Renal infection, not the degree of obstruction or reflux, poses the greatest risk.

○ **What are the typical characteristics of the ureters in patients with prune-belly syndrome?**

The ureters in patients with prune-belly syndrome are dilated in 80% of the cases. The proximal ureters tend to be spared with increased dilation and tortuosity in the distal segments. The ureters may have decreased smooth muscle and an altered collagen matrix, which leads to a loss of luminal coaptation and ineffective peristalsis. The proximal ureters are more suitable for reimplantation when indicated because of improved proximal peristalsis. The distal ureters have poor blood supply and show smooth muscle deficiency with fibrous degeneration.

○ **What are the typical characteristics of the bladder in patients with prune-belly syndrome?**

The bladder in patients with prune-belly syndrome is enlarged. The bladder is thick walled, but is typically smooth with minimal trabeculation or diverticula. There is an increased ratio of collagen to muscle fibers in the bladder. Dilation of the urachus may result in pseudodiverticulum at the dome of the bladder. The intertrigonal ridge is wide with laterally placed ureteral orifices. The bladder neck is open and funnels into the prostatic urethra.

○ **What are the urethral abnormalities associated with prune-belly syndrome?**

Dilation of the posterior urethra is seen in patients with prune-belly syndrome that is secondary to prostatic hypoplasia. This prostatic hypoplasia leads to ejaculatory failure and retrograde ejaculation is very common.

Urethral atresia is also associated with prune-belly syndrome. A patent urachus must be present in order for survival. Prune-belly syndrome is also associated with a megalourethra. There are two types of megalourethra. A fusiform deformity consists of a deficiency of both the corpus spongiosum and cavernosum. When the patient voids the entire phallus dilates. A scaphoid deformity is a deficiency of only the corpus spongiosum with preservation of the glans and corpus cavernosum. The ventral urethra is seen to dilate with voiding.

○ **Are posterior valves associated with prune-belly syndrome?**

Occasionally.

○   **What is the significance of a patent urachus in prune-belly syndrome?**

A patent urachus is present in 25% to 30% of patients with prune-belly syndrome. It is frequently found in the setting of urethral obstruction. Early deaths do occur when patients with urethral obstruction do not have a patent urachus so it may allow for survival in some patients.

○   **What does cystometrogram evaluation in patients with prune-belly syndrome typically demonstrate?**

Bladder function in patients with prune-belly syndrome is variable. Initial urodynamic evaluation with cystometrogram will usually demonstrate a high-capacity bladder with normal compliance, decreased sensation, and poor contractility. Bladder pressures during voiding are low. Emptying is often incomplete. Despite this, 50% of patients void spontaneously with normal voiding pressures and flow rate and low postvoid residual. Bladder herniations are common.

○   **What is the typical location of the undescended testicles in patients with prune-belly syndrome?**

The testicles are usually located at the pelvic brim. Early orchiopexy is usually possible. The Fowler–Stevens technique is often necessary for the testicles to reach the scrotum. Testicular autotransplantation with microvascular anastomosis has also been performed.

○   **What is the cause of infertility in patients with prune-belly syndrome?**

Infertility of patients with prune-belly syndrome is multifactorial. Failure of emission or retrograde ejaculation is common. Prostatic and seminal fluids may be insufficient. Spermatogenesis may be altered. Early orchiopexy, electroejaculation, and intracytoplasmic sperm injection may allow for fertility in some patients. Intra-abdominal testes tend to develop progressive tubular fibrosis. Human chorionic gonadotropin (HCG) therapy does not help in these cases.

○   **What are the growth characteristics of patients with prune-belly syndrome?**

In general, the growth of children with prune-belly syndrome depends upon their renal function. With impaired renal function, there is significant growth delay. Nonetheless, growth retardation occurs in more than one-third of patients with normal renal function.

○   **What is the initial management of prune-belly syndrome?**

The initial management of patients with prune-belly syndrome has evolved and now relies upon the recognition of the syndrome and generally involves noninvasive therapies. Stabilization of the associated cardiopulmonary complications is paramount, as they are often more serious in the neonatal period. Usually the child is able to spontaneously void but this may be facilitated by bladder massage. Prophylactic antibiotics are indicated as vesicoureteral reflux can be assumed to exist. Catheter drainage or other instrumentation should be considered cautiously, as the possibility of urinary tract infection is a significant risk. If the patient has persistent azotemia or acidosis, urinary tract diversion may be necessary. Stomal stenosis appears to be more common in children with prune-belly syndrome; therefore, a large caliber (28F) vesicostomy is advisable. Occasionally, percutaneous nephrostomies are needed in the setting of sepsis. Cutaneous ureterostomies may be necessary if the ureters are obstructed distally due to extreme tortuosity. Urethrotomy to improve urinary drainage is now limited to the few patients with anatomic urethral obstruction. Circumcision is advisable in order to reduce the risk of infection.

○ **What are the long-term treatment options for patients with prune-belly syndrome?**

The treatment of patients with prune-belly syndrome must be individualized. However, in general, most patients can be treated conservatively with delayed surgical reconstruction. Prophylactic antibiotics are indicated in the initial treatment of vesicoureteral reflux, which is present in more than 85% of patients. If recurrent pyelonephritis ensues, ureteral reimplant may be necessary. The proximal ureters are utilized as their function is less impaired than the distal ureter. If tapering of a redundant ureter is needed, imbrication may be advantageous in order to preserve ureteral blood supply. Reduction cystoplasty is usually limited to excision of urachal remnants. Orchidopexy should be performed early, often with a transabdominal approach. A staged procedure such as a Fowler–Stephens procedure may be needed in order for the testicles to reach the scrotum. Microvascular autotransplantation has also been employed. Abdominal wall reconstruction is primarily a cosmetic procedure but may improve pulmonary function.

○ **What are the common types of abdominal wall reconstruction?**

The three most utilized surgical procedures are the Randolph, Ehrlich, and Monfort techniques. The Randolph technique involves a transverse incision from the 12th rib to the pubic symphysis to the opposite 12th rib with a full-thickness removal of the skin, lower abdominal musculature, and peritoneum. Healthy fascia is approximated to the anterior iliac spines, pubic tubercle, and inferior fascia. The Ehrlich technique utilizes a vertical midline incision that allows for preservation of the umbilicus. The skin and subcutaneous tissues are elevated off the muscle and fascial layers and an overlapping, pants over vest, advancement of each side to the contralateral flank is performed, preserving the less affected lateral muscles and fascia. The Monfort technique uses a similar approach as the Erhlich technique but instead of a straight vertical incision, an elliptical incision is made to remove redundant skin. The underlying tissue and muscle is freed from the fascia and vertical incisions are made on the lateral fascia. These incisions are closed over the medial fascia. This procedure can also be performed laparoscopically.

○ **What is the prognosis for patients with prune-belly syndrome?**

The prognosis for patients with prune-belly syndrome has improved. Some infants are stillborn and as many as 25% of patients in some series died in the neonatal period due to urosepsis, renal failure, or most commonly concomitant cardiopulmonary disease. With improvement in neonatal intensive care, the neonatal mortality rate is less than 10%, death is most often due to renal failure as a result of severe renal dysplasia. Despite avoidance of urinary tract instrumentation and the use of suppressive antibiotics, urinary tract infections are common. More than 75% of patients will develop urinary tract infections; however, febrile infections and pyelonephritis is unusual, especially in those patients with good renal function. Renal failure occurs in 25% to 30% of patients with prune-belly syndrome. The presence of early renal insufficiency and urosepsis predict progression to renal failure. A nadir serum creatinine greater than 0.7 mg/dL predicts the development of renal failure. When needed, renal transplantation can be performed safely.

CHAPTER 9

Cryptorchidism: Diagnosis and Management

Jeffrey P. Wolters, MD, MPH, and Harry P. Koo, MD, FAAP, FACS

○ **What is the SRY gene? Where is it located and what is it thought to encode for?**

SRY stands for Sex determining Region on the Y chromosome. It is located on the short arm of the Y chromosome. It is thought to encode for the TDF (testis determining factor) protein.

○ **During sexual differentiation of the gonad into a testis, what are the first cells to differentiate in the testis and approximately when does that happen?**

The Sertoli cells differentiate at around 6 to 8 weeks.

○ **What is the primordial hormone of the fetal testis? When and where does it begin to get produced?**

Mullerian-inhibiting substance. It starts to get produced by the Sertoli cells around the eighth week of gestation.

○ **What cells in the testes are responsible for the production of testosterone in utero?**

Leydig cells.

○ **What two structures are the remnants of the regressed mullerian ducts?**

The appendix testis and the prostatic utricle.

○ **What two hormones are essential for testicular descent?**

Testosterone and DHT. Mullerian-inhibiting substance is *not* essential for descent as it was once thought to be.

○ **What is the name of the heterodimeric protein hormone that is secreted by Sertoli cells to cause normal feedback inhibition of FSH?**

Inhibin.

○ **What is the incidence of cryptorchidism in full-term neonates, 1 year olds, and adults, respectively?**

The incidence is 3%, 1%, and 1%, respectively, where it remains throughout adulthood.

○ **True or False: Spontaneous descent of an undescended testicle is rare after the first year of life.**

True.

○ **What is now believed to be the single greatest predisposing factor for cryptorchidism?**

Low birth weight, independent of length of gestation.

○ **Cryptorchidism is noted in what percentage of fathers and brothers respectively?**

Fathers: 1.5% to 4%; brothers approximately 6% to 7%.

○ **At 1 year of age, what percentage of cryptorchid testes have descended in premature infants and in full-term infants, respectively?**

It is 95% for premature infants and 75% for full-term infants. The majority of all descents will have occurred in the first 3 months of life.

○ **What percentage of cryptorchid children will have bilateral undescended testes?**

Ten percent.

○ **What percentage of cases of cryptorchidism are accompanied by epididymal anomalies?**

Ninety percent. It is thought that the cranial gubernaculum develops an abnormal embryologic attachment. Resultant anomalies can range from simple elongation to aberrant fusion, complete disjunction, or even total absence. Therefore, even in the setting of normal germ cell development, fusion anomalies can have a significant negative impact on fertility.

○ **True or False: Due to the embryologic association of the ureteric bud and the wolffian duct, an ultrasound of the upper urinary tracts is recommended in patients with true cryptorchidism.**

False. The incidence of upper tract abnormalities in cryptorchidism is no greater than the general population, so routine ultrasound evaluations of the upper tracts is not needed except in cases of suspected intersex.

○ **When does testicular descent typically begin and finish?**

Descent typically begins in the 23rd week of gestation when the processus vaginalis elongates into the scrotum. At 24 weeks, descent is complete in 10% of fetuses, at 27 weeks 50%, at 28 weeks 75%, and at 34 weeks 80%.

○ **What is the difference between a cryptorchid and an ectopic testis?**

A cryptorchid testis is located along the normal path of descent but has failed to reach a dependent position in the scrotum. Ectopic testes descend normally through the external inguinal ring but then migrate away from the normal pathway.

○ **What is the most common location for a cryptorchid testis.**

The inguinal canal.

○ **What are some possible locations for an ectopic testis and which of these is the most common?**

Ectopic tests can be found in the perineum, the femoral canal, suprapubic, and transverse scrotal locations; however, the most common location is the superficial inguinal pouch.

○ **The superficial inguinal pouch is also known as the Denis–Browne pouch. What two tissue layers does it lie between?**

The external oblique fascia and Scarpa's fascia.

○ **What options are available for medical therapy for cryptorchidism?**

HCG (human chorionic gonadotropin) and GnRH (gonadotropin releasing hormone).

○ **What is the overall efficacy of hormonal treatment?**

<20%.

○ **What is the mechanism of action and dosage of hCG?**

Stimulation of Leydig cells resulting in increased plasma testosterone levels, thus promoting testicular descent. Injections are given twice a week over a period of 2 to 4 weeks. A total dose of at least 10,000 IU and preferably less than 15,000 IU is usually needed.

○ **Above 15,000 IU of hCG, deleterious side effects become more common. What are some of these?**

Increased rugation and pigmentation of the scrotum, transient increase in penile size, and development of pubic hair. It also can cause changes in testicular histology.

○ **What is the mechanism of action and dosage for GnRH?**

GnRH stimulates the anterior pituitary to release LH that promotes testicular descent. GnRH is administered transnasally at a dose of 1.2 mg daily for 4 weeks.

○ **Can hCG and GnRH be used together?**

Yes.

○ **What percentage of cryptorchid testes are nonpalpable?**

Twenty percent.

○ **What percentage of "nonpalpable testes" are absent on surgical exploration?**

Approximately 30%.

○ **What type of problem is thought to cause an absent (vanishing) testis?**

It is though to be sequelae of a compromising intrauterine vascular event.

○ **What is the role of imaging versus physical examination by a urologist with respect to localizing a nonpalpable testis?**

A good physical examination by a urologist is more valuable and reliable than US, CT, and MRI. While CT and MRI may discern the gonads in older children, they both have a significant false negative rate that makes them poor choices to verify absence.

○ **What is the best approach to locating a nonpalpable testis?**

The first-line intervention is a thorough examination under anesthesia. This will often offer the surgeon a better opportunity to reaffirm or primarily establish testicular position. If the testis(es) remains nonpalpable, a diagnostic laparoscopy should be performed.

○ **What are the three possible findings that could be appreciated during a diagnostic laparoscopy for undescended testis?**

1) Absent (vanishing) testis (i.e., blind ending vessels above the internal ring).

2) Cord structures entering the internal ring.

3) Intra-abdominal testis.

○ **What are the four main risks associated with an undescended testis?**

1) Subfertility—20% to 30% of patients with unilateral cryptorchidism and 75% to 80% of patients with bilateral cryptorchidism. *(Note: these rates were established when surgical intervention occurred during school age and not between 6 and 12 months of age as per the current guidelines.)*

2) Neoplasia—testicular cancer (risk is approximately 10 times greater).

3) Hernia—a patent processus vaginalis is present in approximately 90% of all cryptorchid testes.

4) Testicular torsion—is more common in undescended testes.

○ **Is orchidopexy protective against subsequent testicular cancer?**

No. The relative risk of cancer in a patient with a history of treated or persistent cryptorchidism is 3.6.

○ **What is the most common tumor in an abdominal cryptorchid testis, before and after orchidopexy?**

Before orchidopexy: Seminoma
After orchidopexy: Nonseminomatous germ cell tumors

○ **What is the recommended age to start treatment for cryptorchidism and why?**

Between 6 and 12 months of age. Spontaneous descent usually occurs by 3 months of age.

○ **A 12-year-old boy is noted to have a solitary left testicle on routine physical for the youth basketball league. His mother states that he underwent a diagnostic laparoscopy as a toddler that revealed blind ending cord vessels on the left side. What are the preferred recommendations to this boy's mother with respect to playing a contact sport and future imaging?**

Contact sports are permissible but a cup should be worn. If the exploratory history of blind ending vessels is accurate, then no further imaging is necessary.

○ **Physical examination under anesthesia performed on a 9-month-old boy reveals a nonpalpable left testis. Diagnostic laparoscopy reveals the left testicular vessels and vas coursing distal to the internal inguinal ring. What is the next course of action and what is the most likely finding?**

The next step is to perform a left inguinal exploration. The most likely finding at that time would be presence of a testicular remnant.

○ **In the scenario of the preceding question, if a testicular remnant is discovered what should be done and why?**

The remnant should be excised due to its potential for future malignant degeneration.

○ **What percentage of atrophic remnants has viable testicular elements, and thus potential for malignant conversion?**

13%.

○ **True congenital absence of one testis is extremely rare. What clinical sign is needed to differentiate testicular agenesis versus vanishing testis syndrome?**

Ipsilateral mullerian structures.

○ **A 4-year-old boy undergoes a left inguinal exploration for a presumed palpable testis at a level just above the external ring. At the time of exploration, the vas deferens in noted to end blindly just past the level of the internal ring. What is the next step and why?**

Laparascopic or extended abdominal exploration. A blind ending vas is not definitive evidence of an absent testis. Abdominal exploration needs to be performed to identify either an abdominal testis, or testicular remnant, or definitive evidence of blind ending vessels.

○ **What are the four KEY steps in performing a standard orchiopexy?**

1) Isolation of testis and cord structures.

2) Repair of patent processus vaginalis by high ligation of the hernia sac.

3) Complete mobilization of the spermatic cord without vascular compromise ensuring tension free placement in the scrotum.

4) Creation of a subdartos pouch within the hemiscrotum to receive the testis.

○ **If when attempting a standard orchidopexy for a testis located in the inguinal canal, the gonad can only be mobilized to the upper scrotum, what maneuver could be employed to gain additional cord length and how is this performed?**

The Prentiss maneuver: Take down the floor of the internal ring. Divide the inferior epigastric vessels and transversalis fascia thereby allowing the testis and cord to make a direct path to the pubic tubercle. The floor of the inguinal canal is then closed over the cord, superimposing the internal and external inguinal rings.

○ **A newborn is being evaluated for proximal hypospadias and bilateral nonpalpable testes. What potentially life-threatening condition needs to be considered and urgently evaluated?**

Congenital adrenal hyperplasia (CAH) from 21-hydroxylase deficiency must be ruled out in newborns with bilateral cryptorchidism and ambiguous genitalia.

○ **What medical treatment has been shown to improve fertility index in prepubertal cryptorchid boys?**

Studies have shown that a 4-week course of GnRH nasal spray prior to orchidopexy has a significant beneficial effect on the fertility index, although it is unclear if this benefit persists into adulthood. Optimal results were found in boys where orchiopexy was done before the age of 18 months.

○ **How should a retractile testicle be followed?**

Children with retractile testis should be monitored annually until puberty or until the testes have clearly descended permanently.

○ **Cryptorchid patients have a decreased synthesis of what hormone in the first year of life?**

Mullerian-inhibiting substance.

○ **There are several histopathologic hallmarks among the testes of cryptorchid boys that can be appreciated between 1 and 2 years of age. These include Leydig cell hyperplasia, Sertoli cell degeneration, delayed appearance of gonocytes, failure of primary spermatocyte development, as well as reduced total germ cell counts. Which of these abnormalities is first appreciable and at what point?**

Leydig cell hypoplasia—from the first month of life.

○ **Of the options in the preceding question, which is the most frequent histologic finding in the cryptorchid testis of a 4-year-old boy?**

Decreased number of germ cells.

○ **Elevation of what hormone in previously cryptorchid men has been correlated to eventual decreased paternity rates?**

FSH.

○ **A 20-hour-old infant has a right scrotal mass that does not transilluminate. What is the most likely diagnosis?**

Extravaginal torsion of the spermatic cord.

○ **Carcinoma in situ (CIS) is present in approximately 1.7% to 3% of previously cryptorchid testes and postulated to have originated within the fetal gonocytes. What is the risk for subsequent development of testicular cancer in gonads that harbor CIS?**

At least 50%.

CHAPTER 10
Megaureter, Ectopic Ureter, and Ureterocele

Madhu Alagiri, MD

○ **True or False: The ureter during embryologic development undergoes solidification and later recanalization.**

True. In the first 7 to 8 weeks of gestation, the fetal ureter looses its lumen and recanalizes. The reason for this is unknown, but it may help to explain the presence of ureteral dilation especially if the recanalization process is prolonged.

○ **True or False: The mesonephric duct is necessary for the development of the ureter.**

True. The ureteral bud arises from the mesonephric duct to interact with the metanephric blastema to form the future collecting system and renal parenchyma.

○ **What happens if the mesonephric duct is absent or maldeveloped?**

Absence or maldevelopment of the mesonephric duct will lead to ipsilateral renal agenesis along with absence of genital duct structures such as the vas deferens and seminal vesicles.

○ **True or False: The presence of hydroureteronephrosis on antenatal ultrasound usually indicates obstruction and can be the precursor to an obstructing megaureter.**

False. Hydroureteronephrosis and hydronephrosis are common findings on antenatal ultrasound. The findings are usually benign and are referred to as physiologic hydronephrosis without obstruction. However, true obstruction or high-grade vesicoureteral reflux may be present and further studies such as serial ultrasounds, voiding cystourethrogram, and diuretic renal scans may be necessary.

○ **What is the most common site for the termination of an ectopic ureter in a male.**

The ectopic ureter can terminate in a variety of places but always proximal to the urethral sphincter. The most common site of termination is the prostatic urethra.

○ **True or False: When considering a heminephrectomy for an atrophic, upper-moiety renal segment associated with an ectopic ureter, small accessory arteries and veins to the lower moiety can be divided with impunity because of the extensive arterial and venous collateral circulation.**

False. While the venous drainage to the kidney is redundant, care should be taken to preserve all accessory arteries to the lower pole segment since arterial collateral circulation is not present. Division of these vessels will result in tissue ischemia.

○ **A newborn child presents with a history of a 3-cm upper pole cyst first noted on routine antenatal ultrasound. What is the likely diagnosis and best course of action?**

The large "cyst" is most likely the hydronephrotic dysplastic remnant of a duplex system. An obstructing ectopic ureter, which has since involuted, may have been responsible for the findings. Serial ultrasounds can help to determine if the cyst is involuting.

○ **Describe an alternative to reimplanting an ectopic ureter in a duplex system and indicate its advantages.**

An ectopic ureter is often dilated and may need to be tapered prior to reimplantation. Additionally, in a duplex system, the ipsilateral ureter would also have to be reimplanted in a common sheath. As an alternative, the ectopic ureter can be connected to the normal ureter or renal pelvis as in ureteroureterostomy or ureteropyelostomy. This approach would avoid the bladder and precludes reimplanting the normal ureter.

○ **Define the "drooping lily" sign seen on a voiding cystourethrogram and describe its clinical significance.**

A drooping lily sign refers to the finding of reflux into a lower moiety of a duplex system. The renal pelvis of the lower moiety is laterally displaced and the calyces are directed laterally and inferiorly giving rise to the appearance of a drooping lily on the radiograph.

○ **True or False: Grade V vesicoureteral reflux has minimal chance for spontaneous resolution except for the newborn male infant.**

True: Male infants with high-grade vesicoureteral reflux have a markedly increased chance of fully resolving. This subset should therefore be placed on observation protocols rather than considered for immediate surgical correction.

○ **True or False: A Cohen cross-trigonal reimplantation may prevent future retrograde endoscopic instrumentation of the affected ureter.**

True. The Cohen cross-trigonal approach is a commonly used and highly successful method for correcting vesicoureteral reflux. The procedure places the affected ureteral orifice on the contralateral trigone. This makes transurethral instrumentation of the transplanted ureter often difficult or impossible.

○ **True or False: Bilateral extravesical ureteral reimplantation has a significant incidence of postoperative urinary retention.**

True. The extravesical reimplantation is a very effective and minimally invasive method for the correction of urinary reflux. In cases of bilateral repair, there is a well-described incidence of temporary urinary retention requiring catheterization. The etiology is unknown but may be related to damage to the perivesical nerve plexus during dissection.

○ **True or False: A duplex system with upper and lower moiety reflux is identified on a screening voiding cystourethrogram. This would indicate that both the upper and lower moieties are completely duplicated and both are refluxing.**

False. Upper and lower moiety reflux is often seen on a voiding cystourethrogram with apparent full duplication. However, full duplication is rarely present. Instead, the bifurcation of the ureters occurs close to the bladder and is easily missed on the radiograph.

○ **Describe the megacystis–megaureter anomaly associated with high-grade vesicoureteral reflux.**

Megacystis–megaureter refers to a large bladder and dilated ureters caused by the yo-yo reflux of urine between the bladder and ureters. During voiding, the bladder contracts and sends much of the urine up into the refluxing ureters. When the bladder relaxes after voiding, the urine rushes back into the bladder. The bladder never truly empties and thus can be quite capacious.

○ **True or False: To prevent bacterial colonization of the introitus and vagina in a child with vesicoureteral reflux, nitrofurantoin should be used as antibiotic prophylaxis.**

False. While nitrofurantoin is an excellent choice for antibiotic prophylaxis with its low tissue and intestinal levels, it does not significantly affect introital or vaginal flora. Trimethoprim-sulfamethoxazole would be the preferred choice because it is present in vaginal secretions.

○ **A 5-year-old girl with a notable history for urine holding and fecal retention presents with a febrile urinary tract infection. Diagnostic studies indicate uncomplicated moderate-grade urinary reflux. In addition to antibiotic prophylaxis, what else should be considered in the initial management?**

This child has elimination dysfunction with both urine and fecal holding. Aggressive management of these issues with timed voiding and dietary changes can often mitigate future urinary infections and minimize or resolve vesicoureteral reflux.

○ **True or False: An ectopic ureter may be mistaken for an ureterocele on ultrasound evaluation.**

True. An ectopic ureter and ureterocele can both look like a cystic mass in the bladder on ultrasound. The ureterocele is usually thin walled and the ectopic ureter tends to have a thicker wall but this may not always be the case.

○ **True or False: Antenatal detection of ureteroceles is the most common mode of diagnosis.**

True. With the advent of prenatal ultrasound as a routine part of perinatal care, the infant is often diagnosed prior to birth. Prior to the use of ultrasound, infants and children would present later in life with infection and obstruction.

○ **True or False: Endoscopic incision of a ureterocele is a common first step in managing this disorder.**

True. Endoscopic incision can often correct the obstruction associated with ureteroceles, but may create a patulous opening allowing high-grade reflux to occur.

○ **Describe the upper tract approach for ureterocele repair and provide its main advantages.**

The upper tract approach involves a heminephrectomy and partial ureterectomy for a nonfunctional renal segment, or in the case of a functioning upper moiety, a ureteropyelostomy. The primary advantages to this approach are that it avoids bladder surgery, can be definitive, and will correct the primary source of morbidity, which is renal obstruction.

○ **Describe the lower tract approach for ureterocele repair and its primary advantages.**

The lower tract approach refers to correction of ureterocele by entering the bladder, removing the ureterocele, and then reimplanting the ureter. The advantages to this approach are that it can be less morbid by reducing the risk to the lower moiety renal segment. A refluxing ipsilateral ureter can be corrected at the same time. The primary disadvantage is that it may still leave a nonfunctioning renal segment that may require further surgery.

CHAPTER 11

Urological Emergencies in the Newborn

John H. Makari, MD, MHA, MA, Patrick H. McKenna, MD, and Fernando Ferrer, MD, FAAP, FACS

○ **How often does prenatal sonography detect a significant fetal anomaly?**

One percent of pregnancies.

○ **How many of these are genitourinary and how many are hydronephrosis?**

25% are genitourinary; of these, 50% are hydronephrosis.

○ **What is the significance of bilateral hydronephrosis?**

This may indicate vesicoureteral reflux, fetal ureteral folds, or megaureters. Posterior urethral valves must also be considered in a male fetus, especially if there is evidence of a dilated bladder.

○ **What is the cause and significance of oligohydramnios?**

Abnormal or deficient fetal kidneys will produce less urine, which leads to oligohydramnios. Therefore, a screening ultrasound evaluation of the fetal kidneys is reasonable if oligohydramnios is found. Oligohydramnios may also be caused by rupture of amniotic membranes, inadequate urine production, obstructive uropathy, or postterm gestation. In relationship to the urinary tract, it results from renal agenesis or dysplasia, obstruction, or hypoperfusion of the kidneys. Oligohydramnios may lead to pulmonary hypoplasia. The second trimester is the most critical for fetal lung maturation.

○ **Which are potentially more dangerous: obstructive or nonobstructive lesions of the kidneys?**

In association with hydronephrosis, obstructive lesions are more dangerous, especially if bilateral. However, bilateral renal dysgenesis (caused by diseases such as autosomal recessive polycystic kidney disease, multicystic dysplastic kidney) may be lethal.

○ **Renal pelvic diameter measurements can be helpful in determining the significance of hydronephrosis. What measurements would be considered significant?**

Specific measurements are somewhat controversial. An AP diameter greater than 7 mm in the second trimester and 10 mm in the third trimester are some guidelines. Smaller is better.

O   **A distended bladder that does not empty suggests which diagnosis?**

Posterior urethral valves, prune-belly syndrome, urethral atresia, or neuropathic bladder (e.g., spina bifida).

O   **Which of these is the most dangerous?**

Urethral atresia has the highest mortality rate among these.

O   **A 23-year-old pregnant female presents for evaluation of prenatally detected unilateral hydronephrosis. There is no oligohydramnios. What would be your consideration and recommendation to the patient?**

Prenatal fetal hydronephrosis is the most commonly diagnosed fetal urologic abnormality. While the overall incidence of hydronephrosis on prenatal sonography is between 1% and 1.5%, the incidence of clinically significant hydronephrosis is between 0.2% and 0.4%. With normal amniotic fluid levels, close follow-up throughout the pregnancy and in the neonatal/newborn period as well as through the first year of life are required. The majority of cases of prenatal low-grade hydronephrosis may stabilize and resolve within the first year of life.

O   **This woman delivered a 7 lb, 3 oz otherwise healthy male infant. Postnatal sonography confirms the presence of unilateral hydronephrosis. What further evaluation do you recommend?**

Careful physical examination with an emphasis on observing the infant's active voiding is an important first step. The infant should be started on antibiotic prophylaxis as the incidence of urinary tract infection is approximately 3% to 4% in the first 6 months of life. A voiding cystourethrogram (VCUG) and nuclear renogram (DTPA or MAG 3) should also be scheduled. Recent work suggests a conservative approach to nuclear renography in patients with mild hydronephrosis.

O   **A 32-week prenatal sonogram of a male fetus followed for hydronephrosis reveals increasing bilateral hydronephrosis, a dilated bladder, and new-onset marked oligohydramnios. What is your recommendation?**

Posterior urethral valves leading to bilateral hydronephrosis with oligohydramnios is the most likely etiology, and this situation potentially represents a rare urologic indication for induction of labor or fetal intervention. Fetal lung maturity should be evaluated with a lecithin/sphingomyelin amniotic fluid ratio prior to a final recommendation. If fetal surgical intervention is considered, fetal renal function should be estimated by the urinary sodium chloride, osmolality, and β_2 microglobulin obtained by fetal bladder aspiration. A high-grade obstruction of a single system also requires a similarly rapid response. The outcomes for fetal intervention with respect to improvement of renal function are mixed.

O   **Consultation is requested for an otherwise healthy term infant with a palpable right-sided abdominal mass. Prenatal sonography was not performed. How do you proceed with your physical examination?**

A general examination must begin with initial attention to subcutaneous nodules (neuroblastoma) or dehydration, particularly with hematuria (as seen in renal vein thrombosis). The patient should be placed in the lateral decubitus position for kidney palpation by supporting the flank with one hand and palpating the upper quadrant subcostally with the opposite hand. Care should be taken to avoid extensive abdominal manipulation after the initial examination to prevent the rare occurrence of rupture as seen in cases of Wilms' tumor/mesoblastic nephroma. Transillumination of the flank mass may distinguish cystic from solid lesions. Following a complete physical examination, including careful blood pressure measurements, abdominal sonography is indicated.

O   **What are causes of nonobstructive fetal hydronephrosis?**

Vesicoureteral reflux (incidence of 15%–20% in white and less than 1% in black patients with prenatal hydronephrosis) and fetal ureteral folds are common causes of mild or transient ureteral dilatation noted on prenatal sonography.

○ **A prenatal sonogram detects oligohydramnios and the presence of multiple small cysts (1–2 mm in diameter). Liver sonography demonstrates periportal fibrosis. What are the most likely diagnosis and prognosis?**

Hepatic fibrosis with a polycystic kidney is consistent with autosomal recessive polycystic kidney disease of the infantile form. Postnatal sonography typically reveals bilaterally large, echogenic kidneys with poor corticomedullary differentiation. (Contrast urography would reveal severely delayed function and a nephrogram with an alternating radially oriented sunray pattern.) Infantile presentation typically leads to death by 2 months of age.

○ **What is the most likely cause of an abdominal mass in a healthy-appearing male infant and how can it be differentiated from the second most common cause of neonatal abdominal masses?**

Hydronephrosis due to UPJ obstruction is the most common cause of neonatal abdominal mass. Multicystic dysplastic kidney (MCDK) is the second most common cause of the neonatal abdominal mass and can be distinguished from UPJ obstruction by the technetium^{99m} DMSA renal scan. The renal scan usually demonstrates some function in the hydronephrotic kidney and nonfunction of the MCDK.

○ **An infant is diagnosed with a multicystic dysplastic kidney on the right side based on the "cluster of grapes" appearance on sonography and lack of function by DMSA renal scan. What is of concern regarding the contralateral kidney?**

The contralateral kidney and collecting system must be carefully studied in cases of MCDK. Contralateral vesicoureteral reflux is the most commonly encountered abnormality with an incidence of 20% to 40%. Contralateral hydronephrosis due to ureteropelvic junction obstruction occurs in approximately 10% of infants with multicystic kidney disease.

○ **A 1-month-old female infant is admitted to the neonatal intensive care unit with failure to thrive and respiratory distress. Physical examination reveals a large right-sided abdominal mass. Sonography reveals an enlarged right kidney with multiple noncommunicating cystic structures. A renal scan reveals no perfusion to the affected side and normal function of the left kidney. What treatment would you recommend?**

This clinical scenario is consistent with the findings of multicystic kidney disease (MCKD). Symptoms including respiratory distress, failure to thrive, hypertension, or hemorrhage are indications for nephrectomy in certain cases of MCKD. However, a subset of these patients may be managed by aspiration of the dominant cyst(s) as the cystic fluid tends not to reaccumulate. Aspiration can typically be done by sonographic guidance and may provide immediate or even long-term management.

○ **A clinically stable, otherwise healthy term neonate is diagnosed with left MCDK by sonography. The right kidney is noted to be free of reflux with intact renal function. Is there a role for observation? Must a nephrectomy be performed?**

In the absence of hypertension, feeding, or developmental problems due to mechanical or obstructive complications, immediate surgical excision is unnecessary. Concern for onset of hypertension, malignant degeneration of the MCDK to Wilms' tumor, or less commonly, renal cell carcinoma remains an argument for prophylactic removal of these nonfunctioning moieties. The minimal morbidity of a procedure accomplished through a small incision and the freedom from regular follow-ups or sonography are additional factors favoring nephrectomy. Noninterventional follow-up and the ability to sonographically follow MCDKs, as well as the high incidence of near-complete involution favor observation in these cases. One must remember, however, that while the cystic fluid found within MCDKs may be resorbed, the cyst wall is a persistent remnant. MCDK should be followed sonographically until at least age 5; nephrectomy should be performed if there is an increasing solid component.

○   **A term infant is noted to have a fixed, unilateral mass extending to the midline. Also noted are multiple bluish skin nodules. What is the most likely diagnosis and treatment?**

This clinical picture most likely represents neuroblastoma, an embryonal tumor of neural crest origin. Neuroblastoma is the most common solid abdominal mass and the most common malignant tumor in infancy. For low-stage tumors (I–II), surgical excision remains the treatment of choice. For stage III and higher disease, chemotherapy and radiation therapy are employed as multimodal therapies. As an exception for higher stage disease, surgical excision is often the standard of care without irradiation or chemotherapy in cases of stage IV-S disease (hepatic metastases, skin nodules, and bone marrow involvement).

○   **A lower abdominal mass is palpated in a newborn female. Examination of the perineum reveals a mass in the introitus. The mass persists following placement of a urethral catheter. What is the most likely diagnosis?**

A lower abdominal mass in an otherwise healthy female patient is most likely due to hydrometrocolpos or distension of the vagina and uterus.

○   **What anatomical abnormalities most commonly lead to hydrometrocolpos?**

An imperforate hymen is the most common cause of hydrometrocolpos. A less common etiology is a high transverse vaginal septum, which can be associated with a persistent urogenital sinus. In cases of a high transverse vaginal septum, the external anatomy may appear deceptively normal but sonography of the abdominal mass will reveal a cystic midline structure posterior to the bladder without septation.

○   **Three days following Gomco clamp circumcision, a newborn infant develops brisk bleeding from the incision. What is the risk of hemorrhage and how should it be treated following circumcision?**

Hemorrhage occurs in approximately 1% of cases. The incidence is highest at 3 days after birth due to the physiologic depression of plasma levels of vitamin K–dependent clotting factor. If conservative measures such as compression with an epinephrine-soaked gauze sponge or thrombin application fails, hemostatic suture placement is required.

○   **Consultation is requested approximately 7 days following a neonatal circumcision. Examination of the penis reveals dehiscence of the incision line with complete exposure of the ventral penile shaft. Treatment options include?**

Healing by secondary intention is the preferred approach following such a dehiscence. In rare cases, extensive denudation of skin may require skin grafting to prevent secondary chordee or scarring. Other acute complications of neonatal circumcision include infection, laceration, glans amputation, urinary retention, and necrosis. Nonacute complications of neonatal circumcision include excessive residual skin, skin asymmetry, epithelialized skin bridges, epidermal inclusion cysts, skin tethering/chordee, concealed (buried) penis, phimosis, meatal stenosis, urethrocutaneous fistula, and lymphedema.

○   **Consultation is requested for a glans amputation during a neonatal circumcision. How should this be managed?**

As with all acute complications during circumcision, immediate attention and treatment is the best management. Generally, glans amputation is partial. The amputated portion should be wrapped sterilely and kept cool on ice. It should not be submerged in saline. Operative attachment with long-lasting absorbable sutures (e.g., PDS) should be performed. Generally, viability of the amputated portion is improved when repair occurs within hours of the injury, but has been documented in delays up to 18 hours.

○ **A 9-day-old infant undergoing a sepsis workup is noted to have a palpable right-sided abdominal mass with associated gross hematuria. What is the most likely diagnosis?**

The most likely diagnosis is renal vein thrombosis (RVT). Sixty to seventy percent of patients with renal vein thrombosis have findings of a palpable mass with associated gross hematuria and proteinuria.

○ **A 2-day-old infant born to a diabetic mother has polyuria (10 mL/kg/h). Is the child at risk for compromised renal function?**

Yes. Infants of diabetic mothers experiencing an osmotic diuresis as well as infants with profuse diarrhea, sepsis, acute hypoxia, and hypotension are at risk for RVT. Renal vein thrombosis often occurs due to low renal perfusion pressures and increased blood viscosity secondary to extracellular volume contraction with resultant sludging of blood in renal venules.

○ **A 4-day-old infant with a palpable abdominal mass, gross hematuria, and thrombocytopenia undergoes an abdominal Doppler sonogram that confirms the diagnosis of unilateral RVT without caval thrombus. Appropriate treatment includes?**

Vigorous hydration, electrolyte management, and treatment of underlying cause are critical for patient well being. Aggressive anticoagulation and thrombolytic therapy are employed in certain situations. Thrombolytic agents such as urokinase, streptokinase, and tissue plasminogen activator are utilized for bilateral RVT.

○ **Following successful treatment of RVT, what sequelae may develop?**

Fibrosis of the kidney, renovascular hypertension, nephrotic syndrome, and chronic pyelonephritis are all possible sequelae of RVT. Hypertension in association with an atrophic kidney is often renin-mediated and a nephrectomy is curative.

○ **A 35-week gestation newborn is anuric for 36 hours following birth. Physical examination is unremarkable. Should a workup for acute renal failure commence?**

No. 92% and 99.4% of term newborns void within 24 hours and 48 hours of birth, respectively. Acute renal failure is suspected only if anuria persists more than 48 hours.

○ **The same infant persists with urine output of 0.7 mL/kg/h and a serum creatinine of 1.1 mg/dL at 72 hours. There is no history of oligohydramnios. What is the most common cause of oliguria in the newborn and how is it treated?**

Prerenal renal failure secondary to inadequate perfusion is the most common cause of oliguria in the newborn. Hypotension from sepsis, maternal antepartum hemorrhage, or surgical bleeding may lead to renal hypoperfusion. Similarly, congestive heart failure due to cardiac anomalies or dehydration may also lead to renal ischemia. Neonatal intensive care admission with volume expansion will rapidly reverse prerenal renal failure. Oligohydramnios is usually present in infants with anuria or oliguria due to postrenal causes.

○ **A term infant in the neonatal intensive unit has multiple unsuccessful attempts at umbilical artery catheterization. Consultation is requested 24 hours later for apparent new-onset neonatal ascites. What is the likely diagnosis and recommended treatment?**

Urachal laceration due to attempted umbilical arterial catheterization is the most common cause of neonatal intraperitoneal bladder rupture. Evaluation should consist of a VCUG and possibly a diagnostic paracentesis. While management may be conservative for most cases of neonatal ascites, initial operative management is recommended in cases of intraperitoneal bladder rupture.

○ **A term male infant is admitted to the intensive care unit immediately postpartum with hypotension and tachycardia. Physical examination is remarkable for a penis of only 1.5 cm stretched penile length. The external genitalia are otherwise normal. Electrolyte studies reveal hyponatremia, hyperkalemia, and hypoglycemia. What is the most likely diagnosis and how must the infant be treated?**

This critically ill infant with obvious micropenis (penile length 2.5 standard deviations below the mean, or less than 2.0 cm in a newborn male) must be evaluated for panhypopituitarism. Following intravenous glucose and electrolyte replacement, serial serum glucose, sodium and potassium evaluations are necessary. Serial gonadotropin and testosterone measurements from birth through 3 months of age will eventually document a neonatal luteinizing hormone (LH) surge in normal infants.

○ **A 1300-g preterm infant is being treated for respiratory distress syndrome (RDS) in the neonatal intensive care unit (NICU). Abdominal x-rays reveal bilateral 0.7 mm renal stones. The etiology of this condition includes?**

Furosemide, commonly used in the treatment of RDS and other conditions common to premature infants in the NICU setting, is associated with nephrolithiasis. Furosemide causes a hypercalciuric state with a secondary increased resorption of calcium in the proximal tubule and subsequent renal stone formation. Excessive calcium and glucose intake in specialized formulas for premature infants is another recognized cause of neonatal nephrolithiasis.

○ **A premature infant in the NICU with a patent ductus arteriosus receives furosemide at 2 mg/kg/d for 4 weeks. An abdominal x-ray reveals bilateral nephrocalcinosis. What is the most appropriate treatment?**

Furosemide-induced renal parenchymal stone disease rarely requires surgical intervention. The administration of hydrochlorothiazide, reduced calcium intake, and cessation of furosemide therapy often results in resolution of nephrolithiasis. Nephrocalcinosis may be followed with serial sonography. A baseline calcium-to-creatinine ratio of less than 0.2 portends a higher rate of resolution. In cases of discrete, massive calculus formation, shock wave lithotripsy, or open surgical intervention may be warranted.

○ **Umbilical artery catheterization is performed on a premature infant in the neonatal intensive care unit (NICU). Twenty-four hours later the infant has gross hematuria and hypertension. The hypertension is refractory to aggressive medical management. What is the diagnosis and the most appropriate treatment?**

A recognized complication of umbilical artery catheterization is renal artery thrombosis, either alone or as part of an extensive aortoiliac thrombus. The clinical diagnosis can be confirmed by Doppler sonography and radionuclide imaging, if necessary. While aggressive medical therapy combined with thrombolysis has a role in the treatment of many cases of renal artery thrombosis, nephrectomy would be indicated in this life-threatening case.

○ **A 38-week gestational age male infant is delivered following prolonged labor with meconium aspiration. Aggressive resuscitation efforts are successful. On day 3 of life, an abdominal mass is palpated on the right side. What is the likely sonographic finding and what is your diagnosis?**

Sudden increases in intra-abdominal pressure during prolonged labor may result in adrenal hemorrhage with the observed physical findings. Adrenal hemorrhage typically involves the right adrenal gland and sonographic findings initially demonstrate a hyperechoic or solid mass over the superior pole of the kidney. With time, the lesion may become hypoechoic and decreases in size. This finding should not be confused with neuroblastoma, the most common adrenal malignancy of infancy, which typically has a solid appearance on sonography but may be cystic or have a mixed echogenic pattern.

○   **A term male infant is noted to have multiple genitourinary anomalies at birth consistent with the classic bladder exstrophy/epispadias complex. How must the exstrophic bladder be maintained prior to surgical intervention?**

The mucosa of the bladder must be protected while the candidacy for surgery is discussed. Noncontact care may consist of placing the child in an incubator without a diaper and with saline mist to keep the mucosa moist. Alternatively, the bladder mucosa may be protected by a plastic wrap to prevent the mucosa from sticking to clothing or to the diaper. The umbilicus should be ligated with silk suture, rather than a plastic umbilical clamp, when exstrophy is recognized antenatally or postnatally. Broad spectrum antibiotics may be started to sterilize the bladder wall prior to surgical intervention.

○   **A 39-week-old term infant has a firm right scrotal mass at birth. The mass is painless and does not transilluminate. The overlying skin is erythematous and indurated. What is the most likely cause and what other entities should be considered in the differential diagnosis?**

The most common cause of a scrotal mass at birth is testicular torsion. The differential diagnosis for the described presentation includes hydrocele, incarcerated inguinal hernia, scrotal hematoma, tumor, meconium, trauma, and more rarely ectopic spleen or adrenal tissue.

○   **How is neonatal testicular torsion anatomically different from testicular torsion in adolescents?**

Neonatal testicular torsion is extravaginal since the tunica vaginalis is not adherent to the surrounding dartos fascia of the scrotal wall until 4 to 8 weeks of age. Torsion in the neonate, therefore, involves the testis, spermatic cord, and overlying tunica vaginalis. Testicular torsion in the adolescent, meanwhile, is intravaginal as the tunica vaginalis is fixed to the dartos fascia.

○   **An infant with a firm scrotal mass at birth is diagnosed with testicular torsion. The infant is hemodynamically stable and the contralateral testis is normal. Is surgical exploration and detorsion with orchidopexy necessary?**

It is well known that successful testicular salvage in the event of neonatal testicular torsion is exceedingly rare. Exploration with an intent of salvage alone is not justified. The role of scrotal exploration with contralateral testicular fixation due to the potential for asynchronous torsion until the tunica vaginalis adheres to the scrotal wall remains controversial. Clearly, however, if bilateral torsion is suspected, then exploration despite the low incidence of salvage is necessitated.

○   **A male infant delivered at an estimated 34-weeks gestational age without prenatal care demonstrates failure to thrive and neonatal ascites. The infant is noted to have a diminished, dribbling urinary stream. What is the most likely diagnosis?**

The most common cause of bladder outlet obstruction in the male newborn is posterior urethral valves. An abdominal mass, failure to thrive, and neonatal ascites are among the most common presenting symptoms. Clearly the widespread use of prenatal sonography has directed early investigation in patients with posterior urethral valves.

○ **Prenatal sonography at 22 weeks reveals bilateral hydroureteronephrosis with a distended bladder consistent with posterior urethral valves. Attempts at placement of a vesicoamniotic shunt are unsuccessful. Labor is induced at 32 weeks. What is the initial management at birth?**

Recognition of prenatal hydronephrosis suggests the need for repeat sonography at birth to establish a baseline view of the renal collecting systems. When a suspicion of posterior urethral valve exists, bladder catheterization should be performed and the patient should be placed on prophylactic antibiotics. A voiding cystourethrogram should be performed when the patient is stable. When a posterior urethral valve is present, voiding cystourethrography often demonstrates a thick trabeculated bladder with a dilated posterior urethra.

○ **A 35-week gestational age male infant with an apparent posterior urethral valve (PUV) on voiding cystourethrogram (VCUG) has tense abdominal distension with a fluid wave and a urine output of 0.2 mL/kg/h despite aggressive fluid resuscitation. What is the most likely diagnosis?**

Neonatal urinary ascites occurs in 7% of male infants with PUV. The diagnosis is based on clinical and radiological evidence and can be confirmed by a diagnostic tap of the ascites. When bladder outlet obstruction is suspected, catheter drainage is initiated followed by drainage of ascites only if respiratory compromise is suspected.

○ **A 32-week gestational age infant is delivered after induction of labor for oligohydramnios and hydronephrosis. A cystic mass is noted on the ventral surface of the penoscrotal junction. What finding is expected on the voiding cystourethrogram (VCUG)?**

A cystic mass at the penoscrotal junction especially with dribbling urinary stream is likely the rare finding of anterior urethral valve. VCUG will likely show a large ventral diverticulum due to a crescentic cusp on the ventral aspect of the urethra. Vesicoureteral reflux may also be seen with this condition.

○ **A term male infant is brought to the emergency department with fever, irritability, and weight loss. The infant is uncircumcised. Until what age is the infant more at risk for urinary tract infection (UTI) than circumcised male infants?**

Regardless of phimosis, the presence of foreskin predisposes an infant to UTI until approximately 6 months of age versus age-matched circumcised males. Colonization of the newborn prepuce diminishes as a risk factor beyond 6 months of age.

○ **An uncircumcised male infant is referred for a clean-catch urine culture revealing 50,000/mL *Staphylococcus epidermidis*. Is a voiding cystourethrogram (VCUG) indicated?**

Further evaluation in this child should not commence until a repeat culture is obtained using urine specimen collected in another manner. While plastic bag collected urine cultures are useful if negative, a confirmation must be sought with a catheterized specimen or suprapubic aspirate. If, however, a single organism with a colony count greater than 100,000/mL in a symptomatic infant is obtained, then a UTI should be treated even in a plastic bag obtained urine specimen.

○ **On initial examination, a term infant has left-sided cryptorchidism and a midshaft hypospadias. What is the incidence of a disorder of sex development in this patient with these findings?**

Phenotypic males with cryptorchidism and hypospadias are estimated to have a 20% to 30% incidence of disorders of sex development. Similarly, male phenotype with bilateral impalpable testes and perineal hypospadias alone should initiate an investigation for disorders of sex development.

○ **What familial risk factors increase risk of disorders of sex development in infants?**

Most disorders of sex development result from autosomal recessive inheritance and inquiry as to siblings with abnormal genitalia, infant death, or abnormal events at puberty is necessary. Maternal ingestion of androgenic medication. (Danazol), progestational agents, or drug abuse should also be carefully and investigated.

○ **A term infant with severe hypospadias and unilateral cryptorchidism is suspected to have a disorder of sex development. What is the most common disorder of sex development with this presentation?**

The most common disorder of sex development in patients with severe hypospadias, a testis on one side, and a nonpalpable undescended testis is mixed gonadal dysgenesis. This patient likely has a testis on one side and streak gonad on the contralateral side.

○ **Physical examination of a 37-week-old infant shows a hypertrophied clitoris and partially fused, rugated labioscrotal folds. The karyotype is 46 XX. What is the diagnosis and the most likely cause?**

The infant likely has a 46 XX disorder of sex development (previously referred to as "female pseudohermaphrodite"). This group constitutes 60% to 70% of all disorders of sex development in the neonatal period. Congenital adrenal hyperplasia is the etiology in the majority of patients with a 46 XX disorder of sex development.

○ **An infant is suspected of having congenital adrenal hyperplasia (CAH). What life-threatening condition must be considered and how is it diagnosed?**

A potentially lethal metabolic consequence associated with a disorder of sex development (DSD) is the salt-wasting form of CAH, which does not typically manifest in electrolyte disturbances until 1 to 2 weeks postnatally. Therefore, the etiology of DSD must be determined prior to discharge. CAH results from 21-hydroxylase deficiency in 95% of cases. The more common form leads to overvirilization and aldosterone deficiency in three-fourths of patients, while virilization alone is present in approximately one-fourth of patients with 21-hydroxylase deficiency. Salt wasting may also be present in patients with the much rarer causes of CAH, 11β-hydroxylase deficiency (5% of patients with CAH, less often manifests salt wasting) and 3β-hydroxysteroid-dehydrogenase deficiency (less than 1% of patients with CAH, almost always manifests salt wasting).

○ **A 2-week-old infant is brought to the emergency department with profound hypotension and hyperkalemia. Genital examination demonstrates virilization. What treatment should be administered?**

The salt-wasting form of congenital adrenal hyperplasia should be suspected and must be aggressively treated initially with a bolus infusion of 20 mL/kg normal saline. Cortisol replacement is started with a hydrocortisone sodium succinate bolus at 50 mg/m^2 followed by an infusion of 50 to 100 mg/m^2 added to intravenous fluids. For this critically ill infant, deoxycorticosterone (DOCA) at 1 to 2 mg should be injected intramuscularly every 12 to 14 hours.

○ **A 1-week-old female infant is evaluated in the emergency department for failure to thrive. Physical examination reveals hypertension and virilization of the genitalia with hypertrophy of the clitoris. An arterial blood gas sample is consistent with metabolic acidosis and the potassium level is 6.5 mg/dL. What is the most likely diagnosis?**

Congenital adrenal hyperplasia (CAH) resulting from 11β-hydroxylase deficiency is most consistent with this presentation and constitutes 5% of cases of CAH. A deficiency at this enzymatic level results in accumulation of 17-hydroxyprogesterone and androgens as well as the potent mineralocorticoid deoxycorticosterone. Hyperkalemic acidosis, hypervolemia with hypertension are presenting features.

○ **A term female infant is oliguric at 48 hours of age. Physical examination reveals a palpable, distended bladder and an erythematous interlabial mass. Renal sonography reveals hydronephrosis of the left upper pole. What is the most likely diagnosis?**

The most common cause of urethral obstruction in the female infant is an obstructing ureterocele. In addition, 80% of ureteroceles are associated with the upper pole ureter of a minimally functioning duplicated system. The sonographic findings are consistent with an ureterocele arising from a duplicated collecting system.

○ **Antenatal sonography of a 25-week gestational age female fetus reveals right-sided hydronephrosis and an intravesical cystic dilatation consistent with an ureterocele. Follow-up postnatal sonography, however, demonstrates persistent hydronephrosis but no obvious ureterocele. What are likely technical errors during sonography that may confound the diagnosis?**

There are common errors in sonographic technique that may render the diagnosis of ureteroceles difficult. If the bladder is overdistended, then the ureterocele may become effaced and be invisible on sonography and even on voiding cystourethrogram. Additionally, if on cystourethrography, the injected contrast is too concentrated, the ureterocele may become obscured on radiologic imaging. If the bladder is completely empty at time of sonography, on the other hand, a large ureterocele may mimic the wall of the bladder and distinction between the bladder wall and ureterocele may be difficult.

○ **A neonate is noted to have deficiency of abdominal wall musculature, diffuse dilatation of the urinary tract, and hydronephrosis. The patient is without cardiopulmonary complications and clinically stable. Does this patient require acute urological intervention to address the upper tract dilatation?**

Rarely does a case of group 2 prune-belly syndrome described above require urgent urological intervention. Sonography and serial electrolytes are used to assess parenchymal reserve and extent of uropathy. A diuretic renal scan should be performed. Patients presenting with group 1 characteristics, on the other hand, including oligohydramnios, pulmonary hypoplasia, cardiac anomalies, urachal abnormalities, or pneumothorax require intervention for the cardiopulmonary abnormalities prior to other aspects of care.

○ **The neonate with prune belly syndrome described in the previous question may be expected to have up to an 85% rate of vesicoureteral reflux. Should a VCUG be immediately performed to determine the grade of reflux and subsequent treatment?**

Instrumentation of a neonate with prune belly syndrome is associated with a high risk of infection and should be performed only with antibiotic prophylaxis.

○ **An infant is found to have an imperforate anus on newborn examination. What urologic evaluation should be performed?**

Urologic anomalies are frequently found in patients with anorectal malformations. In patients with anorectal lesions occurring above the levator muscles ("high" lesions), urologic abnormalities are present 60% of the time; they are present 20% of the time in patients with lesions below the levator muscles ("low" lesions). The most common urologic findings are vesicoureteral reflux, neuropathic bladder, renal agenesis or dysplasia, and cryptorchidism. Evaluation should include renal–bladder sonography, voiding cystourethrography, and urodynamic evaluation in patients with high lesions or those with spinal abnormalities.

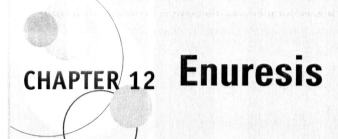

CHAPTER 12 Enuresis

Sang Won Han, MD, Hye Young Lee, MD, MS, and Koon Ho Rha, MD, FACS, PhD

○ **A normal 7-year-old boy suddenly develops daytime urinary frequency every 20 minutes without incontinence. His symptom is limited to daytime only, and no enuresis was reported. Medicosurgical history, physical examination, urinalysis, and brief ultrasound of the kidneys and bladder are normal. What is the most appropriate management option?**

The daytime urinary frequency syndrome is a benign condition, which occurs in otherwise normal children who have no associated daytime incontinence or nighttime symptoms. The etiology is generally unknown and a conservative approach is not unreasonable. Symptoms usually resolve in 2 to 4 months and are characteristically unaffected by anticholinergic drugs.

○ **An otherwise normal 6-year-old boy wets his bed two or three times a week at night. He has no urinary symptoms during the daytime. What is the most likely cause of his nocturnal enuresis?**

Nocturnal enuresis has historically been thought to be due to maturational delay. Additional support for the concept of maturational lag comes from observation of a generalized but not pathologic immaturity in many younger enuretics, who may show a tendency toward passivity, late walking, and other minor evidences of developmental delay. Anatomic abnormalities such as ureterocele may rarely be responsible for both diurnal and nocturnal wetting.

The more recent theories about nocturnal enuresis suggest there are three causes: overproduction of urine, smaller than expected bladder capacity for age, and difficulty in arousal from sleep.

○ **Urinary overproduction in enuretic children would be due to what?**

- Abnormal circadian secretion of vasopressin.
- Increased natriuretic factor secretion.
- Increased dietary sodium.
- Defect in renal aquaporin-2 receptors in the kidney.

○ **What percentage of nocturnal enuresis patients have a significantly smaller bladder than normal for their age?**

Approximately 20%.

○ **What percentage of nocturnal enuresis patients have a problem with arousal from sleep?**

Approximately one-third.

127

○ **How many patients with nocturnal enuresis will demonstrate overactive bladder?**

Approximately two-thirds.

○ **True or False: Treatment of nocturnal enuresis with overactive bladder with an anticholinergic is no better than placebo.**

True. But adding an anticholinergic to other remedies in difficult cases may be helpful. A buzzer alarm alone will cure approximately two-thirds.

○ **A 7-year-old boy has been taking imipramine for 3 months due to enuresis. What is the most potent pharmacologic effect of imipramine on the lower urinary tract?**

Three major actions of imipramine in the urinary tract are antimuscarinic action, direct inhibition of bladder smooth muscle, and analgesic effect. It also causes CNS sedation and blockade of norepinephrine reuptake. However, the most important bladder action is the direct relaxant effect.

○ **The only diagnosis that can be excluded in a 4-year-old boy with incontinence based on history alone is what?**

Primary enuresis. The diagnosis of enuresis can only be made after 5 years of age.

○ **A 6-year-old girl has been suffering from marked urinary frequency and urgency for 2 weeks. Physical examination is normal, and her urinalysis and culture are normal. The next step should be?**

Observation. In the case of a pediatric benign condition, evaluation should be minimal if no significant complication is eminent. In most cases, spontaneous improvement is the rule.

○ **The mother of a 5-year-old boy who still wets his bed at night was concerned about the chance of recovery by the age of 15. What is the percentage of recovery you can tell this mother?**

Ninety-nine percent.

○ **The parents of a 6-year-old girl who still wets her bed at night tell the pediatrician that her older brother was also an enuretic. What percentage of children at age 5 are enuretic?**

Approximately 15% of normal children will still wet at night at 5 years of age. Enuresis is defined as an involuntary discharge of urine. The term is often used alone, imprecisely, to describe wetting that occurs only at night during sleep. It is more accurate, however, to refer to nighttime wetting as nocturnal enuresis and to distinguish it from daytime wetting or diurnal enuresis. The age at which enuresis becomes inappropriate depends on the statistics of developing urinary control, the pattern of wetting, and the sex of the child. Nocturnal enuresis occurring after the age of 5 or by the time the child enters grade school is generally considered a cause for concern.

○ **What is the spontaneous resolution rate for nocturnal enuresis without treatment?**

The spontaneous resolution rate is approximately 15% per year.

○ **Parents of an infant boy are curious about enuresis, since both of the parents were enuretic themselves. What percentage of patients with nocturnal enuresis have a positive family history for the same condition?**

Between 50% and 75%.

○   **What is the first event in the development of bowel and bladder control?**

In terms of continence, children develop nocturnal bowel continence before daytime bowel or bladder continence. The enuretic seldom exhibits an abnormality in bowel function or bladder function during the day and control of bladder function at night is the last event to occur. The usual sequence of development is (1) nocturnal bowel continence, (2) daytime bowel continence, (3) daytime bladder continence, and (4) after several months, nocturnal control of bladder function.

○   **A pediatrician consulted urology for a urodynamic evaluation of a 6-year-old boy with primary nocturnal enuresis. What is the finding you are most likely to find?**

A significant proportion of children with severe nocturnal enuresis show a marked reduction in functional bladder capacity when compared with age-matched controls. This may be related to the high prevalence of underlying bladder dysfunction, particularly of detrusor overactivity at night, in enuretic children.

○   **An otherwise normal 6-year-old boy wets his bed two or three times a week at night. What may be some of the contributing factors in his condition?**

Enuresis is caused by nonorganic disturbances affecting normal development, such as social factors and stress, which can modify urinary control. An increased prevalence of enuresis has been found in children from deprived environments and retardation in skeletal maturation, which may reflect delayed maturation of regulatory central nervous system functions.

○   **True or False: Nocturnal enuresis is generally considered a sleep disorder.**

False. It has been proposed that enuresis is a sleep disorder but recent studies indicate that enuretic sleep patterns are not appreciably different form the sleep patterns of normal children, and that most enuretics do not wet as a consequence of sleeping too deeply.

○   **Enuretic children are known to have normal bladder capacity under anesthesia, but exhibit decreased functional capacity. What is the predicted average bladder capacity in an 8-year-old boy and what is the formula used to estimate pediatric bladder capacity?**

The most widely accepted formula for the predicted bladder capacity in children is:

Bladder capacity (mL) = [age (years) + 2] × 30

Thus, if a child is 8 years old: $(8 + 2) \times 30$ or 300 mL

○   **A 6-year-old boy with enuresis, frequency and urgency, uninhibited detrusor contractions, and decreased functional capacity had been taking various remedies for his enuresis. After a thorough evaluation of his condition, the physician recommended anticholinergics. For which of his conditions has anticholinergic therapy proven most effective?**

Anticholinergic medication in this setting will have greatest impact on uninhibited bladder contractions but will probably not help his nocturnal enuresis very much.

○ **A 6-year-old boy had been taking various remedies for his enuresis. He has evidence of bladder hyperactivity, frequency and urgency, detrusor instability, day and night incontinence, as well as pure nocturnal enuresis. For which of his conditions has anticholinergic therapy been proven most ineffective?**

Pure nocturnal enuresis. Anticholinergic drug therapy has only been effective for enuresis in just 5% to 40% of patients. However, since anticholinergics eliminate uninhibited bladder contractions and increase bladder capacity, this therapy may be effective selectively for enuretic patients with symptoms of bladder hyperactivity, such as urgency, frequency, and day and night incontinence, while it is most effective in patients with proven uninhibited bladder contractions.

○ **True or False: A 7-year-old daughter of diplomat who just returned from Sweden told her physician that she had been satisfied with desmopressin (DDAVP) in the treatment of her enuresis. DDAVP can be administered both as a nasal spray or in oral form for the treatment of enuresis in the United States.**

False. The nasal spray form has been banned for the treatment of enuresis in the United States since December 2007 after 2 children using the nasal spray form died from hyponatremia and 59 others developed seizures. The pill form is still allowed.

○ **Is limiting fluid intake before bedtime a reasonable first step in controlling enuresis.**

Simply limiting fluids to reduce urine output is not generally effective. However, the importance of antidiuretic hormone (ADH) levels is now elucidated. Measurements of urinary and serum ADH demonstrate an absence or reversal of the normal circadian rhythm in enuretics who have lower than normal excretion of nocturnal ADH> desmopressin (DDAVP), a synthetic analog of ADH, became available. It has an effect lasting 7 to 10 hours. DDAVP has been shown to be more effective than placebo in treating enuresis, with effective rates up to 60%, especially in older children. Patients on DDAVP are 4.5 times as likely to say dry overnight as controls. Limitations are the relatively high cost of the drug and the potential for recurrence upon discontinuation.

○ **An 8-year-old boy had been taking imipramine before camping for 2 years and is very satisfied. How does imipramine work in controlling enuresis and would you expect imipramine to have an antidepressant effect at antienuretic doses?**

Imipramine taken at antienuretic doses will have impact on REM and light NREM sleep. It will also have anticholinergic effects as well as change the sympathetic input to the bladder, but there will not be any significant antidepressant action. The medication is known to be a weak anticholinergic agent with direct antispasmodic activity, alpha sympathetic inhibitory action, and norepinephrine reuptake inhibition.

○ **How well does imipramine work in the treatment of enuresis and how frequently is it used?**

Imipramine, a tricyclic antidepressant, is the most widely used antienuretic agent worldwide, but it's currently recommended only as a secondary agent. Enuresis can be eliminated in more than 50% of children and will be improved in another 15% to 20%, however, up to 60% of patients will relapse upon discontinuation. Its peripheral effects increase bladder capacity by (1) weak anticholinergic activity (ineffective in abolishing uninhibited detrusor contractions); (2) direct antispasmodic activity (not apparent at clinically effective antienuretic doses); and (3) complex effect on sympathetic input to the bladder (prevents norepinephrine action on alpha receptors and enhances its effect on beta receptors by inhibiting norepinephrine reuptake). Imipramine's effects on the central nervous system include its antidepressant activity and its action on sleep. Imipramine significantly alters sleep patterns by decreasing the time spent in REM sleep and increasing the time spent in light NREM sleep. It is unlikely that the effect of imipramine against enuresis is related to antidepressant activity because such effect requires much higher dosages and its onset would be significantly delayed.

○ **What is the most effective treatment for enuresis currently available?**

Management of enuresis has been divided into pharmacologic therapy and behavior modification. Modification of behavior has been quite successful but only for the very motivated parents and child. Bladder training was developed to increase functional bladder capacity, but has not seen much success. Another method of alternative behavior modification is responsibility reinforcement, such as reward and motivation. This also requires active and willing participation of the child to succeed.

It has been reported that the most effective therapy of treating enuresis is conditioning therapy, as in the bell alarm (buzzer alarm) method. Superior results have been reported with this method compared to other forms of behavioral therapy, as well as pharmacologic therapy with DDAVP. Imipramine is used as a second-line therapy.

○ **A 20-year-old army recruit was referred to an Army hospital after his confession of enuresis. He had not been free of bed-wetting throughout his life. What advise can you give him regarding diet to help minimize his problem?**

This patient has primary enuresis. Enuresis is found in more than 1% of the adult population, often with overt abnormalities on urodynamic studies such as uninhibited bladder activity. The extent of the investigation is usually more thorough than those carried out in younger enuretics. Cessation of compounds that might increase nocturnal urine output, such as caffeine, should be strongly advised before recommending other forms of treatment.

○ **A 6-year-old girl is being evaluated for both nocturnal and diurnal enuresis. Workup with history and physical examination, neurologic examination, urinalysis, and urine culture are normal. What is the next appropriate step?**

Most children with enuresis do not have a definite lesion. A careful history, physical examination, and urinalysis with culture are needed for all children with bed-wetting and are usually sufficient. Radiographic studies such as IVP or VCUG are not normally recommended. In patients with diurnal enuresis, normal history and physical examination, no evidence of neuropathy and a negative urine examination, the urinary tract anatomy should be screened. This can be accomplished noninvasively and satisfactorily with an ultrasound examination of the kidneys, ureters, and bladder before and after voiding.

○ **A 7-year-old girl with urgency and diurnal incontinence wets her bed about three times a week. Workup with history and physical examination, neurologic examination, urinalysis, and urine culture are normal. Radiographic imaging studies including abdominal ultrasonogram and voiding cystourethrogram are negative. What is the primary treatment?**

Diurnal enuresis occurs in 5% of 7-year-old children. In most children, the underlying problem is infrequent voiding. Timed voiding programs alone will be successful in the majority of children but require several months to be effective. Anticholinergics such as oxybutynin can be tried along with timed voiding.

○ **A 6-year-old girl with diurnal enuresis also has severe constipation and fecal soiling. However, radiographic studies of her spine and neurologic examination are normal as well as urinalysis and no residual urine is noted. What is the most appropriate treatment?**

This girl presents typical findings of dysfunctional elimination syndrome. It has been observed that a large fecal impaction may induce significant detrusor instability and other bladder dysfunctions, which in turn will result in urgency, UTI, and reflux. A high incidence of enuresis in children with UTIs and constipation has been reported. The evidence available so far strongly suggests that there is an important relationship between constipation, detrusor instability, reflux, UTIs, and enuresis. With neurologic abnormalities and urinary tract infection ruled out, timed voiding along with treatment of constipation can improve not only fecal soiling but also diurnal enuresis. Anticholinergics in this condition are not recommended as they are likely to aggravate constipation and may cause urinary tract infections.

○ **A 4-year-old girl who is toilet-trained complains of urinary incontinence. She says her underwear becomes wet right after she finishes voiding. What is the most likely diagnosis?**

The most likely diagnosis is vesicovaginal reflux. This best describes postvoid dribbling, which is typically when urine gets trapped in the vagina during voiding and dribbles out soon after standing in otherwise normal toilet-trained girls with no other associated urinary symptoms. Vesicovaginal reflux itself is harmless and tends to resolve with age but it can create a damp environment prone to infection. Therefore, the child may be taught to empty her vagina by simply voiding with her thighs apart and leaning forward after voiding before getting up.

○ **What percentage of secondary nocturnal enuresis is due to psychological factors and what specific disorder is involved most often?**

Approximately 50%. Anxiety-provoking factors predominate.

○ **How significant is the benefit of treating the psychological factors to improving the outcome over just treating the nocturnal enuresis directly?**

There is no significant proven benefit in treating the underlying anxiety disorder compared to just treating the enuresis.

○ **What percentage of children with attention deficit hyperactivity disorder (ADHD) also have nocturnal enuresis and is it reasonable that they would occur together?**

Twenty percent of ADHD cases also have enuresis. Both problems are believed to involve the same brain stem area abnormality so it's likely they would occur together.

○ **What percentage of ADHD children with nocturnal enuresis will have urodynamic evidence of overactive bladder dysfunction?**

Approximately 50%.

○ **Overactive bladder associated with nocturnal enuresis responds best to which therapy?**

Buzzer alarm behavioral therapy works best, except in children who also have ADHD.

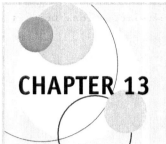

CHAPTER 13

Disorders of Sexual Development

Richard N. Yu, MD, PhD, James Mandell, MD, and David A. Diamond, MD

○ **What structure undergoes condensation and shortening to promote descent of the testis?**

The gubernaculum that anchors the testis to the genital region condenses to allow descent.

○ **What transcription factor is critical for gonadal differentiation toward the male lineage?**

SRY (sex determining region on the short arm of the Y chromosome), also known as the testis determining factor (TDF).

○ **What happens if the testis determining factor is missing or damaged?**

The gonad becomes an ovary.

○ **At what stage in fetal development does the gonad differentiate to become a testis or ovary?**

Between the sixth to eighth week of gestation, the indifferent gonad differentiates into testis or ovary.

○ **What cell type is responsible for producing mullerian-inhibiting substance (MIS)?**

The fetal Sertoli cells produce MIS.

○ **What soluble factor superfamily does mullerian-inhibiting substance belong to?**

Transforming growth factor beta (TGFβ).

○ **Which active steroid hormone is important for Wolffian duct induction and proliferation?**

The presence of testosterone results in the proliferation of the Wolffian duct system and the development of the efferent ductules, rete testis, epididymis, vas deferens, and seminal vesicles.

○ **What enzyme converts testosterone into dihydrotestosterone?**

The conversion is mediated by 5-alpha-reductase.

○ **Mullerian-inhibiting substance (MIS) prevents the development of which female reproductive structures?**

MIS prevents the development of the oviduct, uterus, cervix, and upper third of the vagina.

○ **What is the most common cause of disorders in sexual development (DSD) in children in North America and Europe?**

The most common cause is Klinefelter's syndrome.

○ **What physical findings are most suggestive of DSD?**

Nonpalpable gonads and severe hypospadias.

○ **What laboratory tests are most often used to confirm the presence of congenital adrenal hyperplasia?**

The most efficient tests include fluorescence in situ hybridization (FISH) or karyotype analysis and plasma 17-hydroxyprogesterone >500 mg/dL.

○ **What are the two most common enzyme defects resulting in congenital adrenal hyperplasia?**

21-hydroxylase deficiency (90% of cases) and 11-beta hydroxylase deficiency (5% of cases). Both enzyme defects result in elevated plasma levels of 17-hydroxyprogesterone. 11-beta hydroxylase deficiency specifically results in elevated plasma levels of 11-deoxycortisol and 11-deoxycorticosterone.

○ **What imaging studies are the most helpful in defining the anatomy associated with a DSD?**

Use of the abdomino-pelvic ultrasound (to look for the presence of a uterus) and a fluoroscopic genitogram to look for a vaginal connection to the urogenital sinus are extremely helpful.

○ **What is the typical appearance of a patient with complete androgen insensitivity syndrome (CAIS) and why?**

These patients appear as normal phenotypic females with normal development of secondary sexual characteristics. Development of the external male genitalia does not occur due to the lack of the androgen receptor dependent.

○ **What is the typical development of the internal genitalia in patients with CAIS?**

On examination, these patients have a short, blind-ending vagina with no internal mullerian duct structures. Since MIS is present during embryogenesis, the mullerian duct structures do not develop.

○ **What is the most common demonstrable defect seen in patients with CAIS?**

The most common finding is the absence of high-affinity binding of dihydrotestosterone.

○ **What are the common clinical presentations that most often lead to the diagnosis of CAIS?**

Primary amenorrhea (peripubertal) and female patients with bilateral inguinal hernias. Approximately 2% of females presenting with these findings will have CAIS. Females with clinically significant hernias may benefit from vaginoscopy at the time of surgery to confirm the presence of a cervix.

○ **What is the most common karyotype in patients with ovotesticular DSD (true hermaphroditism)?**

The most common karyotypic finding is 46 XX.

○ **What are the most common gonadal malignancies associated with a dysgenetic gonad and the presence of a Y chromosome?**

The most common malignancies are gonadoblastomas and dysgerminomas.

○ **What is the most common karyotypic finding in Klinefelter's syndrome?**

An additional X chromosome (47 XXY or 46 XX, XXY).

○ **What is the histopathologic finding in patients with pure gonadal dysgenesis?**

Bilateral streak gonads and underdeveloped mullerian structures are found.

○ **During development, when does the gonad develop into a testis?**

During the second month.

○ **What is anti-mullerian hormone (AMH)?**

Anti-mullerian hormone is the same as mullerian-inhibiting substance.

○ **True or False: An ovotesticular DSD often has a degree of Wolffian development near the testicular tissue even when joined to an ovary.**

True. The gonad contains both ovarian and testicular elements. The paracrine effect of the testicular element on the Wolffian duct results in the development of this tissue to varying degrees.

○ **The external genitalia of both sexes are identical through how many weeks of gestation?**

Seven weeks.

○ **What is the incidence of a DSD condition when two impalpable testes are found on examination?**

Fifty percent.

○ **Congenital adrenal hyperplasia is associated with what potentially lethal condition?**

Salt-wasting nephropathy occurs in 75%. If not recognized, the resulting hypotension can cause vascular collapse and death.

○ **A perfectly normal-appearing, phenotypic male presents with an inguinal hernia on one side and an impalpable testis on the other. Karyotype is 46XY. What DSD problem is most likely?**

Isolated deficiency of mullerian-inhibiting substance.

○ **What is the controversy regarding management of CAIS?**

Whether or not to leave the gonads in situ until the child completes pubertal development.

CHAPTER 14

Neurogenic Voiding Dysfunction

George P.H. Young, MD, FACS, and
Joseph E. Jamal, MD

○ **What are the pathways and influences involved in normal micturition?**

Voluntary control is exerted by the cerebral cortex by release of tonic inhibitory signals to the pontine micturition center (PMC). The PMC initiates voiding by stimulation of parasympathetics at S2-S4 causing detrusor contraction. The PMC also inhibits sympathetic fibers T11-L2 causing relaxtion of the bladder neck and proximal urethra. Finally, the PMC inhibits the somatic fibers of the pudendal nerve causing relaxation of the external sphincter.

○ **Neurogenic control of the bladder in infants is by what part of the central nervous system also known as the primitive voiding center?**

Sacral reflex center.

○ **Where does the pudendal nerve originate?**

Nucleus of Onuf. This nucleus is a collection of sacral somatic nerve cells that originate from the lateral border of the ventral horn of the sacral spinal cord (S2-S4).

○ **Explain the functions of the pudendal nerve.**

It controls the external urethral sphincter. The pudendal also innervates the penis as well as the ischiocavernosus and bulbocavernosus muscles. The pudendal and pelvic nerves also receive postganglionic axons from the caudal sympathetic chain ganglia.

○ **Over stimulation of the pudendal nerve produces what urological problem?**

Urinary retention.

○ **What can cause overstimulation of the pudendal nerve?**

Trauma to the suprasacral–infrapontine spinal cord.

○ **What cord segment is evaluated with the bulbocavernosus reflex?**

This test evaluates the integrity of the S2-S4 segments.

○ **Briefly summarize the parasympathetic innervation of the bladder?**

Parasympathetic efferents originate from the pelvic nerves S2-S4. The ganglions are located near the organ and the neurotransmitter is acetylcholine. The receptors are muscarinic (M2/M3) and stimulation results in bladder contraction.

○ **Where are the parasympathetic postganglionic neurons located?**

In the detrusor wall as well as the pelvic plexus.

○ **What is the most common type of muscarinic receptor in the bladder?**

The M2 type is the most common type as it accounts for approximately 80% of the bladder's muscarinic receptors. Its exact function in the bladder is unknown, but it is thought to be involved with the neuromodulation of bladder compliance. The M2 receptors are primarily cardiovascular where they help mediate heart rate and cardiac output.

○ **Which muscarinic receptor is most involved with cholinergic stimulation of the detrusor?**

M3, even though it only represents about 20% of the total muscarinic receptors in the bladder. M1 receptors are primarily located in the central nervous system and salivary glands. They deal with cognition and saliva production. This is why a selective M3 antimuscarinic agent should theoretically have fewer central nervous system and dry mouth side effects than nonselective agents. The M5 receptors are primarily located in the ciliary muscle of the eye.

○ **What is the pathway of the sympathetic innervation of the bladder?**

Sympathetic preganglionic nerves exit from the lumbar spinal cord to synapse in the sympathetic chain ganglia. The postganglionic sympathetics then travel through the inferior splanchnic nerves to the inferior mesenteric ganglia. They finally travel in the hypogastric nerve to the pelvic plexus and the urogenital organs.

○ **What is the role of sympathetic innervation of the bladder and outlet?**

Together they promote bladder storage via the hypogastric nerve (T10-L2). Alpha (bladder base and prostate) and beta (bladder body) receptors exist on the bladder and alpha receptors are on the prostatic capsule. Beta activation results in inhibition of muscle contraction. Alpha activation results in increased outlet resistance.

○ **What types of afferent fibers exist in the bladder?**

Myelinated (Aδ) and unmyelinated (C) axons.

○ **How do they differ?**

- Aδ bladder afferents are finely myelinated axons located in the detrusor smooth muscle and sense bladder fullness (tension).
- C bladder afferents have unmyelinated axons, are located in the detrusor mucosa, and most are mechanoinsensitive (hence the term "silent C fibers"). These fibers can be recruited after injury/inflammation to form new functional afferent pathways (becoming mechanosensitive) that can cause pain and urge incontinence.

○ **What is capsaicin?**

A vanilloid, capsaicin stimulates and desensitizes unmyelinated C fiber axons to produce pain and release neuropeptides. Resiniferatoxin (RTX) is an ultrapotent analog of capsaicin.

○ **How is capsaicin involved with spinal cord injuries?**

Although normal micturition is associated with myelinated Aδ afferent fibers, after spinal cord injury a capsaicin-sensitive unmyelinated C fiber–mediated spinal reflex may develop, resulting in detrusor overactivity.

○ **What is the distinction between the smooth and the striated urinary sphincters?**

The smooth sphincter refers to a physiological rather than an anatomic sphincter. It is located at the smooth musculature of the bladder neck and the proximal urethra. Control is involuntary. In contrast, the striated sphincter is anatomic and includes the skeletal muscle surrounding the membranous urethra in men and the middle segment of the urethra in females. This sphincter also includes the striated muscle surrounding the urethra in both men and women. The outer portion of this sphincter is under voluntary control.

○ **The rhabdosphincter contains what specific type of muscle fiber?**

Striated, slow-twitch (type I) muscle fibers.

○ **According to Wein, what are the three factors necessary for (A) normal bladder and urine storage to occur, and (B) normal bladder emptying to occur?**

The factors necessary for urine storage:

1. Accommodation of urine at low pressure with appropriate sensation.

2. A closed outlet at rest and one that remains so with increases of intra-abdominal pressure.

3. No involuntary bladder contractions.

Requirements for normal emptying:

1. A contraction of adequate magnitude and duration.

2. Lowering of outlet resistance when this contraction occurs.

3. No anatomic outlet obstruction.

○ **What is the order of processes in micturition?**

Afferent activity from the bladder activates the PMC, which first acts to inhibit the spinal guarding reflex. The pudendal nerve mediates relaxation of the striated external sphincter. This is followed by relaxation of the bladder neck/proximal urethra by sympathetic fibers from T11-L2. Almost simultaneously the detrusor contracts and detrusor pressure rises via the S2-S4 parasympathetic efferents.

○ **The first recordable event of the micturition reflex is?**

Cessation of sphincter EMG activity.

○ **Define "detrusor hyperreflexia."**

Detrusor hyperreflexia is defined as detrusor overactivity (DO) due to a disturbance of the neural control mechanisms. Without evidence of a relevant neurological disorder, the term "detrusor hyperreflexia" cannot be used, and instead the term "detrusor instability" is used.

○ **What are the three hypotheses to explain detrusor overactivity (DO)?**

1. Neurogenic—DO may arise from generalized, nerve-mediated excitation of the detrusor muscle from various sources. Cerebral damage can reduce suprapontine inhibition. Spinal cord lesions can damage axonal pathways allowing primitive spinal bladder reflexes to occur. New reflexes secondary to C fiber bladder afferent neurons can disrupt normal sacral activity. Over time, sensitization of peripheral afferents in the bladder can trigger detrusor overactivity.

2. Myogenic—DO contractions result from a combination of an increased likelihood of spontaneous contraction and enhanced propagation of activity between muscle cells. Patchy denervation commonly occurs in DO, which can affect smooth muscle cell spontaneous contractions, and ultimately propagation over a wider area of detrusor.

3. Peripheral autonomous activity—This hypothesis suggests that increased bladder sensation results from increased localized detrusor contraction and that detrusor overactivity is due to enhanced coordination of modular activity through the myovesical plexus.

○ **What is overactive bladder (OAB)?**

OAB is a symptomatic diagnosis that is usually secondary to detrusor overactivity. DO is a diagnosis that requires urodynamic testing. The quantification of OAB symptoms should be by frequency–volume chart and validated questionnaires.

○ **From cranial to caudal, explain how neurological lesions typically effect voiding dysfunction.**

- CNS lesions result in detrusor hyperreflexia. Normally, the CNS inhibits reflex contraction of the detrusor. Loss of this tonic detrusor inhibition, (due to stroke, Parkinson disease (PD), MS, brain tumors) results in detrusor overactivity (DO) with normal coordination of detrusor and sphincter, and normal sphincter tone and sensation. (Please note MS can have ANY manifestation depending on the location of the lesion.)
- Pontine micturition center (PMC)—lesions above the PMC are described above, with coordinated DO. Below the PMC, the detrusor and external urethral sphincter become uncoordinated, resulting in detrusor–sphincter dyssynergia (DSD).
- Spinal cord lesions above S2 are upper motor neuron (UMN) lesions and result in DSD. All spinal cord injuries can result in spinal shock. Spinal cord injuries above T6 may result in autonomic dysreflexia.
- Neurological lesions below S2 can be due to spina bifida, MS, surgeries (APR), myelodysplasia, disc herniation, and results in acontractile detrusor, and therefore retention.

○ **The sacral spinal cord begins at what level and ends at which spinal cord level?**

It is important to distinguish between spinal column segment (bone level) and the corresponding cord level. The sacral spinal cord begins at the column level of T12-L1. It terminates as the cauda equina at spinal column level L2.

○ **After the cerebral shock phase wears off, what type of bladder condition is found most often?**

Detrusor hyperreflexia with coordinated urethral sphincter activity. This occurs because the pontine micturition center (PMC) is released from cerebral inhibitory control. Clinically, this causes frequency, urgency, and urge incontinence.

○ **How is the above situation treated?**

Foley catheter or intermittent catheterization during cerebral shock phase. Anticholinergic medications afterward.

○ **Spinal shock typically lasts how long?**

Six to twelve weeks.

○ **What is the voiding pattern observed in a complete cord injury above the sacral reflex?**

Most commonly, these lesions result in urge incontinence from detrusor hyperreflexia, absent sensation below the level of the lesion, smooth sphincter synergy, and striated sphincter dyssynergia. Lesions above the sympathetic outflow tract T7 or T8 (spinal column level of T6) may also result in smooth sphincter dyssynergia.

○ **A diver suffers from a complete spinal cord injury at the level of T8. What pattern of voiding would be expected immediately following the accident?**

The immediate result is a period of spinal shock. There is generally bladder areflexia and acontractility. Some EMG activity may be present at the external sphincter but there is no voluntary control. Urinary retention is the most common finding initially, and is typically managed with a Foley catheter. The areflexic period generally lasts 6 to 12 weeks but may persist up to 1 to 2 years.

○ **While performing cystoscopy on a patient with a high cervical cord injury, he develops hypertension, flushing, sweating, and bradycardia. What is the problem and what should be done?**

This is a classic description of autonomic hyperreflexia. It arises from massive autonomic discharge in patients with cord injuries above the sympathetic outflow tract (T6). Prevention is based on use of spinal anesthesia and the use of oral Nifedipine (10 mg) 30 minutes prior to the procedure. Initial management of symptoms is withdrawal of the stimulus, alpha blockade, and bladder decompression with foley catheter.

○ **Who first described autonomic dysreflexia (aka hyperreflexia) and when?**

Anthony Bowlby in 1890.

○ **Can autonomic dysreflexia occur during the spinal shock period?**

Usually not. It generally occurs only when reflexes begin to return.

○ **What is the rate of autonomic dysreflexia in individuals with a T6 or higher injury?**

Usually about 50% to 90%.

○ **Autonomic dysreflexia not caused by bladder distension is most likely from what cause?**

Fecal impaction.

○ **What immediate pharmacological therapy should be started in autonomic dysreflexia?**

Immediate release nifedipine and nitroglycerine paste. The nifedipine should be the bite-and-swallow rather than sublingual form.

○ **Is terazosin useful in the prevention of autonomic dysreflexia?**

Yes, but other agents are preferred.

○ **What diseases result in peripheral neuropathy resulting in urinary retention?**

Diabetes, AIDS, polio, Guillain–Barre syndrome, tabes dorsalis, and pernicious anemia.

○   **After a stroke, what percentage develop acute urinary retention?**

Twenty-five percent.

○   **Describe the effects on voiding following a cerebrovascular accident.**

The effects on micturition are divided into acute and long term. The initial period of shock may be associated with urinary retention secondary to detrusor areflexia. The most common long-term sequela is detrusor hyperreflexia. Sensation and compliance are generally intact.

○   **What effect does Alzheimer disease (AD) have on voiding?**

Alzheimer dementia involves the loss of gray and white matter in the frontal lobes. Incontinence may ensue and may be secondary to detrusor hyperreflexia with voluntary sphincter activity or may be due to loss of awareness to void.

○   **Does outlet obstruction exist in patients with Parkinson disease (PD)?**

Voiding dysfunction exists in 35% to 70% of patients with PD. The most common symptoms are urgency, frequency, nocturia, and urge incontinence. The most common finding on urodynamics is detrusor hyperreflexia with smooth sphincter synergy. In contradistinction to patients post-CVA, those patients with PD generally do not have outlet obstruction and subsequently respond poorly to prostatectomy. This may be due to poorly sustained bladder contractions and poor sphincter relaxation.

○   **In what way is PD different from a stroke urodynamically?**

Both demonstrate detrusor hyperreflexia but PD patients usually have a weakened sphincter as well.

○   **How does multiple sclerosis (MS) affect voiding?**

MS is a demyelinating disease that most commonly involves the posterior and lateral columns of the cervical spinal cord. Fifty to ninety percent of these patients have voiding dysfunction at some point. The most common finding is detrusor hyperreflexia. Thirty to sixty-five percent of these patients have striated sphincter dyssynergia.

○   **In MS, how often is detrusor areflexia found?**

Twenty to fifty percent.

○   **What is diabetic cystopathy?**

This is a term that describes the effects of diabetes on the urinary bladder. The most recent evidence points to both a sensory and motor dysfunction. Urodynamically, these bladders demonstrate impaired sensation, increased capacity, decreased contractility, and impaired flow patterns. Pressure/flow studies can differentiate poor bladder emptying from outlet obstruction. Timed voiding plays a pivotal role in therapy.

○   **Diabetic cystopathy typically occurs how long after the onset of diabetes?**

Ten years.

○ **What is Shy–Drager syndrome?**

This disorder results from cell loss and gliosis in the cerebellum, substantia nigra, intermediolateral columns of the spinal cord, and Onuf's nucleus. Clinically, patients demonstrate orthostatic hypotension, anhidrosis, and certain degrees of parkinsonian symptoms plus autonomic dysfunction. Diagnostically, these individuals are identified by the uncommon findings of an open bladder neck (in contrast to PD patients) and striated sphincter denervation on EMG.

○ **Patients with Shy–Drager syndrome should avoid what type of urological surgery?**

TURP, because the rate of total incontinence is high.

○ **TURP should generally be avoided in what disease states?**

In addition to Shy–Drager syndrome, TURP should be avoided if possible in PD patients due to high rates of incontinence.

○ **What is Fowler syndrome?**

Urinary retention in a young woman without anatomic cause or obvious neurological dysfunction, occurring intermittently with normal voiding in between. It is characterized by retaining urine for over a day but without urgency despite a bladder capacity of 1 L. MRI of the brain and the entire spinal cord is normal. Diagnosis is based on EMG abnormalities of the striated urethral sphincter.

○ **Name and define the four types of incontinence.**

1. Stress urinary incontinence manifests as leakage secondary to increased intra-abdominal pressure due to weak pelvic support.

2. Urge incontinence is leakage with the urge to void, usually associated with advanced age, neurological diseases (multiple sclerosis, stroke, upper motor neuron diseases, brain tumors), idiopathic.

3. Overflow incontinence patients leak when they have a full bladder, with constant leaking or dribbling. These are commonly associated with grade III or IV prolapse, previous surgeries (APR), lower motor neuron diseases (detrusor areflexia).

4. Global incontinence is a constant leakage requiring extensive workup.

○ **In patients with neurogenic voiding dysfunction, what urodynamic finding has the highest correlation with the development of upper tract damage?**

Detrusor–sphincter dyssynergia correlates highest with the upper tract damage.

○ **In patients with bladder outlet obstruction, what is the opening pressure on pressure–flow studies?**

These patients have opening pressures greater than 80 cm H_2O.

○ **A Valsalva leak point pressure less than what is diagnostic of intrinsic sphincter deficiency?**

A pressure less than 60 cm H_2O is evidence for intrinsic sphincter deficiency.

○ **What are the general factors that contribute to urinary incontinence in women?**

Predisposing factors such as anatomy and collagen status. Inciting factors such as childbirth and previous surgery. Promoting factors such as infection and obesity. Decompensating factors such as aging.

○ **How do Kegel exercises reduce incontinence?**

These exercises not only produce a direct physical obstruction to urinary leakage, but they also can help abolish uninhibited detrusor contractions. This is accomplished by stimulation of afferent sacral nerves at low frequencies (below the pain threshold of C fibers). This causes inhibition of efferent pelvic nerve firing thereby reducing detrusor activity.

○ **Kegel exercises stimulate the activity of which pelvic nerve?**

Pudendal nerve.

○ **What is the failure rate of pelvic floor biofeedback?**

Biofeedback works by bringing to conscious control that which was previously unconscious. The most important factor in the success of therapy is a well-motivated patient. In fact, attrition rates remain as high as one-third even in well-established centers.

○ **Why is pharmacotherapy using acetylcholine-like drugs not clinically useful in facilitating bladder emptying?**

These drugs are rapidly hydrolyzed by cholinesterases thereby limiting their efficacy.

○ **What are the urodynamic parameters used to diagnose bladder neck obstruction in women?**

While validated nomograms do not exist, the following findings are highly suggestive of obstruction: sustained detrusor contraction of normal or high pressure, poor flow of urine, and lack of bladder neck funneling on fluoroscopy. All of these findings must be accompanied by a synergic external urethral sphincter for bladder neck obstruction to exist.

○ **What are some of the causes of urinary retention in females?**

Etiologies of retention in women include: MS, spina bifida occulta, viral sacromyeloradiculitis, lumbar disc protrusion, cauda equina syndrome, bladder neck obstruction, pseudomyotonia, and reflex sympathetic dystrophy.

○ **What factors may contribute to urinary incontinence following radical prostatectomy?**

Any one combination of the following or may contribute to incontinence:
- Residual outlet obstruction.
- Detrusor instability.
- Sphincter incompetence.
- Preexisting neurologic disease.

○ **Two days following a lumbar laminectomy, a 61-year-old male is in urinary retention. What is the treatment?**

Disc disease is commonly associated with voiding dysfunction. The most common finding is that of detrusor areflexia. Generally, patients present with symptoms of poor emptying. Interestingly, laminectomy may not improve the bladder dysfunction. Treatment in this male would consist of catheter placement and urodynamic studies.

○ **When evaluating incontinence in geriatric patients, what does the mnemonic DIAPPERS refer to?**

Delirium, **I**nfection, **A**trophic vaginitis, **P**sychological problems, **P**harmaceuticals, **E**xcess urine output, **R**estricted mobility, **S**tool impaction.

○ **What is the most common type of urinary incontinence in the elderly?**

Urge incontinence is the most common cause of urinary incontinence in the elderly. Many conditions that are prevalent in this population predispose them to this type of incontinence including CVA, PD, spinal cord injury, MS, and BPH.

○ **Is urinary incontinence a normal consequence of aging?**

While age-related changes are present in the elderly and predispose them to incontinence, this should not be considered a normal part of aging and a thorough evaluation is indicated.

○ **What broad categories of medications may be associated with urinary incontinence?**

ACE inhibitors, alcohol, α-adrenergic agonists and antagonists, calcium channel blockers, diuretics, narcotics, sedatives and hypnotics, and vincristine.

○ **What are the indications for urodynamics testing in the incontinent patient?**

Any patient who reports a history of a failed incontinence procedure or previous radical pelvic surgery, patients with mixed symptoms (including both stress and urge), history of a neurologic disorder, and most importantly any patient in whom stress incontinence is not demonstrated on physical examination.

○ **What are common therapies designed to treat bladder storage deficits of bladder etiology, in order of invasiveness?**

Behavioral therapy/biofeedback, pharmacological therapy (anticholinergics, TCAs, calcium antagonists, potassium channel openers, prostaglandin inhibitors, β-adrenergic agonists, α-adrenergic antagonists, DMSO, capsaicin, resiniferatoxin, botulinum toxin), bladder overdistension, electrical stimulation/neuromodulation, interruption of innervation (selective sacral rhizotomy), augmentation cystoplasty.

○ **What are common therapies designed to treat bladder storage deficits due to bladder outlet related issues in order of invasiveness?**

Behavioral therapy/biofeedback, electrical stimulation, pharmacological therapies (α-adrenergic agonists, TCAs, β-adrenergic agonists/antagonists), vaginal supportive devices (pessaries), periurethral bulking agents (collagen, synthetics), vesicourethral suspension, sling procedures (both with prolapse repair if needed), artificial urinary sphincter, bladder outlet reconstruction, myoplasty.

○ **What are common therapies designed to aid in bladder emptying due to bladder contractility problems in order of invasiveness?**

Valsalva/credé, bladder training, pharmacological therapies (parasympathomimetics, prostaglandins, α-adrenergic antagonists, opioid antagonists), electrical stimulation (neuromodulation), reduction cystoplasty, bladder myoplasty.

○   **What are common therapies designed to aid in bladder emptying due to bladder outlet problems in order of invasiveness?**

- At the site of obstruction: pharmacological therapies (α-adrenergic antagonists, 5a-reductase inhibitors, LHRH agonists/antagonists, antiandrogens), prostatectomy, bladder neck incision/resection, urethral stricture repair, urethroplasty.
- At the smooth sphincter: pharmacological therapies (α-adrenergic antagonists, β-adrenergic agonists), transurethral resection/incision, Y-V plasty.
- At the striated sphincter: behavioral therapy/biofeedback, pharmacological therapy (benzodiazepines, baclofen, dantrolene, α-adrenergic antagonists, botulinum toxin injection), urethral overdilation, surgical sphincterotomy, pudendal nerve interruption.

○   **How does neuromodulation work on both storage and emptying functions?**

Two theories:

1. Inhibition of afferent fibers from the bladder that affect sensation and micturition reflex arcs in the spinal cord.
2. Direct stimulation of efferent fibers via the pudendal nerve to the external sphincter cause sphincter closure and reflexive detrusor relaxation.

○   **Where is the lead for a sacral nerve stimulator placed, and how does it work?**

Sacral nerve stimulators (e.g., InterStim) are used for refractory urge incontinence, overactive bladder, and idiopathic urinary retention for patients who have failed conservative therapy. The lead is placed in the S3 foramen, where both the pelvic plexus and pudendal nerve run.

○   **How is the correct placement of a sacral stimulator lead determined clinically and what is the appropriate response that is observed?**

The lead is tested by a clinical nerve stimulation test. The appropriate motor response is dorsiflexion of the great toe and bellows contraction of the levator muscles in the perineal area (anal wink).

○   **What are the clinical indications for a sacral nerve stimulator (SNS)?**

SNS can be used for both storage dysfunction (e.g., urgency–frequency and urge incontinence) and emptying dysfunction (nonobstructive urinary retention). There are no defined preclinical factors, such as urodynamic findings, that can predict which patients will respond to sacral neuromodulation.

○   **How often do the nerves from the S2-S4 sacral foramina differ?**

The detrusor is innervated primarily by S3 and to a lesser extent by S2 and S4. Rectal stimulation is by means of all three roots equally. Erectile stimulation is mainly by S2 with a small contribution from S3 but none from S4.

○   **What are the contraindications to sacral neuromodulators?**

Contraindications include significant bone abnormalities in the spine or sacrum that may prohibit access to the foramen, inadequate mental capacity of patients who could not manage the device, physical limitations that prevent voiding (functional incontinence), future need of MRI, and noncompliance. SNS are not contraindicated and can be used in specially selected patients with multiple sclerosis, spinal cord injury, and chronic cystitis, and even in certain pediatric cases.

○ **What is the most common complication associated with sacral nerve stimulators?**

The InterStim device is relatively new; however, pain at the neurostimulator site was the most common complaint (15% of patients) after 1 year of follow-up. Lead migration occurs in roughly 12% of SNS procedures performed previous to the newer InterStim device with its tined leads. Surgical revision was required in 33.3% of InterStim cases to resolve an adverse event. Explantation for lack of efficacy occurred in 10.5%. Infection of the battery site warrants explantation of the entire system.

○ **How does botulinum toxin (Botox) work?**

Botox blocks the release of acetylcholine and other transmitters from presynaptic nerve endings. Injection into the detrusor impairs contractility, and results in temporary muscle atrophy at the injection sites. The desired chemical denervation is a reversible process, and axons are regenerated in about 3 to 6 months. Additionally, Botox has also been shown to suppress afferent nerve activity by inhibiting the release of substance P and CGRP from sensory terminals.

○ **When can Botox be used?**

There are a number of potential uses for Botox. Careful workup is necessary to determine when it will be most efficacious. With detrusor overactivity, Botox can result in improvements in symptoms of frequency, urge incontinence, and the sense of urgency. Botox can also improve bladder capacity, volume at first reflex detrusor contraction, bladder compliance, and decreases in detrusor pressures during bladder filling and voiding. Recently, Botox has been used to treat pelvic floor spasticity as well as patients with nonneurogenic overactive bladder and even interstitial cystitis. Its efficacy has also recently been shown in benign prostatic hyperplasia, where injections into the prostate can induce prostatic atrophy by inducing apoptosis, inhibiting proliferation, and downregulating α_{1A}-adrenergic receptors.

○ **What are some of the differences between sacral nerve stimulators and Botox injections?**

The FDA has approved neuromodulation for use in urge-incontinence, urge-frequency syndrome, and idiopathic urinary retention. Botox injections have not been FDA approved for any use in the urinary tract. Some patients may prefer a trial of Botox injections. Its advantages include a lower initial cost, simpler procedure, and no need for permanent implant or possible revisions. Its main disadvantage is that it only lasts 3 to 9 months, requiring repeat administration. Currently, long-term response to neuromodulation is better established than Botox, as there is no direct comparison study.

○ **What is Hinman syndrome?**

Initially known as nonneurogenic neurogenic bladder or subclinical neurogenic bladder. It describes a form of bladder–sphincteric dysfunction in children that was characterized by a combination of bladder decompensation with incontinence, poor emptying, and recurrent urinary infections. Most children also have significant bowel dysfunction, including encopresis, constipation, and fecal impaction.

○ **What is Ochoa (urofacial) syndrome?**

Children with this syndrome exhibit all the classic features of dysfunctional voiding, including urinary incontinence, recurrent UTIs, constipation, reflux, and upper tract damage, but they also have a peculiar painful or apparently crying facial expression during smiling. It has autosomal recessive inheritance and has been located on chromosome 10. Urodynamic studies characteristically showed a sustained contraction of the external sphincter during voiding. The resulting severe bladder–sphincter dysfunction is often associated with a dismal outcome.

O   **What is dysfunction elimination syndrome in children?**

It is a term used to recognize that many children with dysfunctional voiding and recurrent UTIs often have associated bowel dysfunction, including constipation, fecal impaction, and encopresis. Any gross distention of the rectum by impacted feces can result in mechanical compression of the bladder and bladder neck, leading to urinary obstruction. In addition, it has been observed that large fecal impaction may induce significant detrusor instability and other bladder dysfunctions, which in turn will result in the urge syndrome, UTI, and reflux.

O   **What percentage of clinical problems seen in pediatric urology are the result of neurologic lesions that affect lower urinary tract function?**

25%.

O   **What is the most common cause of neurogenic bladder dysfunction in children?**

Abnormal development of the spinal canal and internecine spinal cord. Myelomeningocele accounts for more than 90% of all open spinal dysraphic states, with a spectrum of neurologic lesions depending on which neural elements have everted with the meningocele sac.

O   **Where is the most common location of a meningocele?**

The bony vertebral level provides little information regarding the exact neurologic level or lesion produced. The most common site of meningocele is the lumbosacral spine (47%), followed by lumbar (26%), then sacral (20%).

O   **What are the most common abnormalities of the lower urinary tract found to coexist with VUR in children?**

Detrusor overactivity and uncoordinated detrusor–sphincter function during micturition. These abnormalities may occur secondary to urinary infection or can be acquired during the period when voluntary control of micturition is being established. Remember, reflux from incompetence of the ureterovesical junction may be worsened by detrusor instability, and patients with this dysfunction often have bilateral high-grade reflux and injured upper renal tracts.

O   **What medications are used to treat children with overactive bladder?**

- Antimuscarinic agents, such as oxybutynin, are the gold standard and act by reducing the frequency and intensity of involuntary contractions, resulting in an increase in the functional bladder capacity. The nonselective pattern of activity and penetration of the blood–brain barrier are known to induce systemic and central side effects.
- α-adrenergic blockers are used in patients with evidence of bladder neck dysfunction for relaxation of the bladder neck.
- Tricyclic antidepressants, such as imipramine, have been found to be effective for increasing urine storage by both decreasing the detrusor contractility and increasing outlet resistance. They should be used judiciously in children because of the high incidence of side effects.

CHAPTER 15 **Urodynamics**

Gamal M. Ghoniem, MD, FACS

○ **True or False: A high postvoid residual urine volume correlates with both the symptoms and urodynamic findings associated with bladder outlet obstruction.**

False. A high postvoid residual volume does not necessarily mean bladder outlet obstruction. This condition can be present in association with any physical bladder outlet obstruction or it can be present in association with a poorly contracting bladder. Conversely, this condition may not be present in patients with severe bladder outlet obstruction if they have enough detrusor function to overcome the outlet obstruction. Elevated postvoid residual volumes when present do not necessarily lead to infection.

○ **A 40-year-old female had a uroflow with Q_{max} of 50 mL/s, a mean of 25 mL/s, and a configuration that looks like a bread loaf standing on end. The most likely single diagnosis is?**

Sphincteric incontinence with low outlet resistance.

○ **What are the two events most likely to produce a similar electromyographic pattern?**

Striated sphincter dyssynergia and Valsalva voiding both produce similar EMG patterns of increased activity. Patients with these conditions void in the absence of coordination between the detrusor muscle and the sphincteric unit.

○ **During the act of volitional voiding what would you expect a normal EMG pattern to look like?**

During the act of normal volitional voiding the EMG should be silent.

○ **At initiation of normal voiding, which event happens first?**

The initial measurable event upon voiding is decreased EMG activity. This precedes an increase in detrusor pressure and a decrease in maximum urethral pressure.

○ **What is the relationship between pressure and flow during normal micturition in men and women?**

Normal urinary flow in young healthy males should be 15 to 25 mL/s and the associated detrusor pressure should be less than 40 cm H_2O. Women typically void with similar or slightly higher peak flow rates but the associated detrusor pressures are lower and usually approximately 20 cm H_2O. Interestingly, identical results on repeated measurements are difficult to obtain with repeated pressure flow studies in the same healthy individual.

○ **What does an intermittent flow pattern in an individual with normal deep tendon and bulbocavernosus reflexes and normal perineal sensation most likely indicate?**

Intermittent flow in an otherwise normal individual is most suggestive of abdominal straining. The neurologically intact patient cannot have neurogenic detrusor overactivity or detrusor sphincter dyssynergia.

○ **A patient with incontinence shows evidence of low compliance by urodynamics. The Valsalva leak point pressure is 20 to 30 cm H_2O. What would you tell the patient her risk of upper tract deterioration is?**

Valsalva leak point pressures less than 40 cm H_2O will actually protect the upper tracts from pressure-induced hydronephrosis and subsequent deterioration in renal function. The lower the leak pressure, the less likely upper tract deterioration will happen, when bladder compliance is low.

○ **In phase 2 (the tonus limb) of the cystometrogram, bladder compliance is most dependent upon which factor?**

Viscoelastic properties of the detrusor. Other neural factors like cerebral inhibition of reflex bladder activity and intact thoracolumbar spinal cord are more active in the final phase.

○ **What is the most important parameter in uroflowmetry with volumes between 150 and 350 mL: maximum flow rate or average flow rate?**

Maximum flow rate is most indicative of normal detrusor function.

○ **A patient, with no evidence of neurologic disease, has evidence of involuntary detrusor contractions during the filling phase of a CMG. What is your diagnosis? Idiopathic detrusor overactivity or poor compliance?**

Idiopathic detrusor overactivity. In the presence of neurological disease, identical findings on a CMG would lead to the diagnosis of neurogenic detrusor overactivity.

○ **What is the Valsalva leak point pressure?**

The Valsalva leak point pressure is the pressure at which passive urethral resistance is overcome by increasing abdominal pressure and urine leaks through an otherwise closed sphincter. Normal is 60 cm water or more. This is not a measure of detrusor function and the result can be affected by the presence of a large cystocele.

○ **How is detrusor pressure (P_{det}) calculated ?**

P_{ves}–P_{abd} (vesical pressure–abdominal pressure). The detrusor pressure is important in recognizing pressure increases due to abdominal and not true vesical pressure, e.g., straining.

○ **What does high bladder compliance relate to?**

Bladder accommodation. High compliance does not relate to high leak pressure.

○ **What does the static infusion urethral pressure profile most accurately predict?**

Intrinsic sphincter deficiency. It does not predict striated sphincter dyssynergia or urethral obstruction.

○ **What is the most common urodynamic findings seen in patients with CVA?**

Neurogenic detrusor overactivity, normal compliance, smooth sphincter synergia, and striated sphincter synergia.

○ **True or False: In patients with cerebral infarction, the upper tracts are at minimal risk of deterioration.**

True. Immediately following the injury, these patients often manifest detrusor areflexia. As they convalesce, patients with cerebral lesions (CVA, subdural hematoma, closed head injuries, brain tumors, etc.) most commonly develop neurogenic detrusor overactivity. They can have uninhibited motor neurogenic bladders with neurogenic detrusor overactivity. The bladder activity in these patients is characterized as complete coordinated incontinence. These patients void at normal pressures, but in an uninhibited manner with coordination between the detrusor muscle and sphincter mechanism. In these cases, there is no detrusor sphincter dyssynergia, and high-pressure voiding is not a common finding.

○ **When do you most likely see pseudodyssynergia?**

In a patient with a cerebrovascular accident. In these patients, the sensation is intact.

○ **A 72-year-old male develops urgency, frequency, and urge incontinence following a CVA. Prior to his CVA, he complained of a decreasing stream and hesitancy. His postvoid residual is 130 mL. What is the most likely cause of his high residual?**

Benign prostatic hyperplasia with bladder outlet obstruction would be the most likely explanation for his elevated postvoid residual volume. CVA causes neurogenic detrusor overactivity.

○ **Are suprapontine lesions (stroke, dementia, etc.) usually associated with detrusor sphincter dyssynergia?**

No. They are usually associated with neurogenic detrusor overactivity or detrusor areflexia, phasic idiopathic detrusor overactivity, or detrusor overactivity

○ **A 21-year-old male patient with cerebral palsy and severe mental retardation has day and night incontinence. What is the most practical and informative urodynamic evaluation?**

A postvoid residual plus renal ultrasound. In this situation, with an uncooperative patient, videourodynamic studies, pressure-flow studies, or even simple cystometry are not likely to impact your management.

○ **What are the urodynamic findings in a complete spinal cord transection at cord level T10 after spinal shock has disappeared?**

Neurogenic detrusor overactivity, striated sphincter dyssynergia, and smooth sphincter synergia.

○ **What are the urodynamic findings in patients with voiding dysfunction secondary to Shy–Drager syndrome?**

An open bladder neck at rest, decreased detrusor compliance, striated sphincter denervation.

○ **Are uninhibited detrusor contractions diagnosed by filling CMG always due to bladder outlet obstruction?**

No. They can be caused by neurologic diseases that affect upper motor neuron function.

○ **What are the urodynamic findings generally associated with autonomic hyperreflexia?**

Neurogenic detrusor overactivity, striated sphincter dyssynergia, and smooth sphincter dyssynergia. Lesions above T6 are usually associated with smooth sphincter dyssynergia.

○ **Which condition is detrusor striated sphincter dyssynergia most frequently associated with?**

Suprasacral spinal cord injury. It is absent in Parkinson disease, stroke, myelomeningocele, and radical pelvic surgery.

○ **What is the most common urodynamic abnormality in patients with voiding dysfunction secondary to multiple sclerosis?**

Neurogenic detrusor overactivity. The second most common dysfunction is striated sphincter dyssynergia.

○ **At approximately which vertebral column level does the sacral spinal cord begin and end?**

T12-L2.

○ **Two weeks after an abdominoperineal resection, a 70-year-old male with minimal voiding symptoms prior to his surgery has a postvoid residual of 400 mL. What are the most likely urodynamic abnormalities and what is the preferred management strategy?**

Detrusor areflexia and low compliance will result from pelvic nerve injury, and the best management would be CIC with or without anticholinergics.

○ **What is the most common cause for upper urinary tract deterioration in the SCI patient?**

Striated sphincter dyssynergia. This results in elevated detrusor pressures, high residual urine, hydronephrosis with secondary urinary infections, and renal failure.

○ **What is the best treatment for a T10 paraplegic with type I striated sphincter dyssynergia, grade 1 reflux, a postvoid residual of 250 mL, no hydronephrosis, normal compliance, and unsustained detrusor contractions?**

Intermittent catheterization. The description fits a safe reservoir; only CIC is indicated.

○ **A C5-6 SCI female patient has low bladder compliance, an incompetent bladder neck, urethral erosion, and grade 1 hydronephrosis. What would be the best treatment?**

A bladder neck closure or obstructive sling with ileovesicostomy.

○ **A C5-C6 male SCI patient has no change in postvoid residual urine following external sphincterotomy. What is the most likely reason?**

Impaired bladder contractility. Less common conditions like inadequate sphincterotomy, smooth muscle dyssynergia, and urethral stricture can cause large residuals.

○ **During cystoscopy, a C7 quadriplegic patient complains of sweating and headache. His blood pressure has rapidly risen to 210/120. What is the best initial management?**

Empty the bladder. In this emergency situation, the offending cause, i.e., distention, should be treated immediately, and usually this is enough to control the autonomic hyperreflexia. Other measures, like oral nifedipine or even phentolamine intravenously, are not effective enough in controlling this serious situation. Unattended, serious complications like stroke can occur.

○ **A C5 quadriplegic on external condom catheter drainage has recurrent episodes of autonomic dysreflexia. Urodynamic evaluation shows high-pressure detrusor contractions and prolonged external sphincter dyssynergia. What is the best option for management?**

A bladder augmentation with subsequent clean intermittent catheterization will minimize the future morbidity in this individual.

○ **What is the main indication for pressure–flow studies?**

To help distinguish detrusor hypocontractility from urethral obstruction low-flow conditions, with or without large residual urine, which can result from any of these conditions.

○ **What percent of men with symptoms of prostatism are found to have urodynamically proven outlet obstruction?**

30%.

○ **What study yields a definitive diagnosis of bladder outlet obstruction?**

Detrusor pressure/flow study is the gold standard for the diagnosis of bladder outlet obstruction.

○ **What is the clinical presentation of tethered cord syndrome?**

Patients typically present in infancy with detrusor areflexia and urinary retention.

○ **What are the characteristics of diabetic cystopathy?**

An increased bladder capacity, impaired detrusor contractility, and decreased bladder sensation with diminished urinary stream.

○ **What are the factors that lead to a favorable outcome following prostatectomy in patients with Parkinson disease?**

Normal intravesical voiding pressures with decreased flow rate, voluntary urethral sphincter contractions which can interrupt the urinary stream, adequate voluntary detrusor contractions, and perceived urgency. However, decreased detrusor contractility is not favorable. Alternative minimally invasive measures using thermotherapy, radiofrequency, or laser may be considered.

○ **What are the strong indications for a urodynamic evaluation?**

MS, spina bifida, sacral agenesis, high imperforate anus, and monitoring of a patient with spinal cord injury are all indications for a urodynamic evaluation.

○ **What is the estimated bladder capacity of a healthy 2-year-old male?**

120 mL. A simple formula to use is age in years $+ 2 =$ capacity in ounces.

○ **What is the initial management of the newborn with myelodysplasia?**

The initial management should include: serum electrolytes, BUN, serum creatinine, measurement of residual urine, renal sonogram, and VCUG. The urodynamic studies the day prior to spinal closure are not indicated.

○ **When should urodynamic studies be performed for myelomeningocele patients?**

Urodynamics are helpful in the newborn period as a baseline study. This is important in order to assess the relative risk of the upper tracts based upon the bladder dynamics and to monitor any changes during the course of the disease.

○ **Why has vesicostomy been demonstrated to be effective in initial management in infants born with posterior urethral valves?**

A vesicostomy is a simple and safe procedure in infancy, bringing the dome of the bladder to the skin. This results in upper tract decompression in 90% of the cases. Reflux is not a problem because voiding pressures are eliminated. The risks of urethral injury are avoided, since valve ablation may be delayed. In addition, vesicostomy dosen't cause a permanent reduction in bladder capacity.

○ **A 3-year-old boy received a vesicostomy at 4 months of age secondary to posterior urethral valves. He now presents with progressive hydronephrosis and a serum creatinine of 2.5 mg/dL. A CMG revealed low bladder compliance. What is the next best step in management?**

A high urinary diversion would be appropriate. Other management strategies, such as augmentation cystoplasty and vesicostomy closure or CIC, are usually not effective.

○ **To further characterize the cause of a 350-cc residual urine in a 60-year-old, non–insulin-dependent diabetic, what is the most informative study?**

A simultaneous detrusor pressure/flow study.

○ **A 50-year-old female with urgency and frequency following a suspension procedure voids with a detrusor pressure of 50 cm H$_2$O at a peak flow of 12 mL/s. The most likely diagnosis is:**

Urethral obstruction. Storage (irritative) bladder symptoms with high voiding pressures are indicative of outlet obstruction after a suspension procedure.

○ **A 53-year-old female underwent needle suspension 1 year ago. She complains of continuous urinary incontinence in upright positions. Seventeen years ago, she underwent abdominal hysterectomy and retropubic suspension. Videofluorourodynamics show an open bladder neck with minimal hypermobility, no involuntary contractions, and good bladder capacity, with low Valsalva leak pressure. What is the best operative option?**

A pubovaginal sling procedure. The patient has intrinsic sphincter deficiency (ISD) and would not benefit from repeat suspension.

○ **A 55-year-old man has had a detubularized right colon orthotopic continent diversion. He has done well for 1 year, but now complains of increasing incontinence. Pouch urodynamics revealed several pressure spikes. What is the mechanism most likely responsible for his incontinence?**

A return of coordinated bowel contractions.

○ **Why is nocturnal enuresis common with orthotopic diversions?**

Because of loss of the spinal reflex arc recruiting external sphincter contraction.

○ **How can you best describe cecal contractions?**

Intermittent high-pressure contractions. They are usually massive contractions and not peristaltic.

○ **What is the new classification of detrusor activity?**

According to the International Continence Society updated terminology, "detrusor overactivity" is now classified as "idiopathic detrusor overactivity" (replacing detrusor instability term), or "neurogenic detrusor overactivity" (replacing detrusor hyperreflexia term).

○ **How can you differentiate between striated external sphincter and smooth muscle internal sphincter dyssynergia in spinal cord injury (SCI) patients?**

Using fluoro-urodynamics. In the case of internal sphincter dyssynergia, the bladder neck will be closed and detrusor pressure will be high with possible trabeculations, diverticula, and reflux. Similar findings can be found in external sphincter dyssynergia with the exception of an open bladder neck and dilated posterior urethra.

○ **Identify the name and site of the spinal cord micturition center.**

Onuf's nucleus in the sacral spinal cord (S2 anterior horn).

○ **What are the most likely urodynamic and videourodynamic findings in a 42-year-old woman with urinary incontinence, high residual urine volume, hydronephrosis, and urinary tract infection 18 months after a low anterior resection for rectal cancer?**

Detrusor hypoactivity, decreased compliance, open bladder neck, and fixed external sphincter tone. These changes are secondary to peripheral detrusor denervation involving both sympathetic and parasympathetic nerve fibers as a result of her surgery.

○ **A neurologically normal 40-year-old woman with no previous anti-incontinence surgery presented with lower urinary tract symptoms (LUTs) and urge incontinence. Her urodynamic study showed P_{det} of 55 cm H_2O and corresponding Q_{max} of 8 mL/s. She has 150 mL residual urine. What is her diagnosis and best management?**

The patient has functional bladder outlet obstruction (BOO). Alpha blocker medication.

○ **What is the reason for not obtaining a leak pressure measurement in a postprostatectomy incontinence (PPI) patient who demonstrated stress incontinence on physical examination?**

Such patients often have scarred urethras that won't leak with the relatively large urethral catheter used. The leakage can only be demonstrated conclusively when the catheter is removed.

○ **What percentage of overactive bladder (OAB) patients in clinical practice remain on antimuscarinic therapy beyond 1 year?**

Less than 30%. The reasons are side effects, cost, and lack of efficacy.

○ **At what point does nocturia significantly affect quality of life (QOL) scores?**

It begins to have an effect at two times per night. At three or more episodes, it's considered a major bother.

○ **What percentage of urology residents have never actually personally performed a full urodynamics examination?**

Approximately 70%.

CHAPTER 16 Urethral Strictures

Jeremy B. Myers, MD, and Tom F. Lue, MD

○ **What portions of the urethra make up the anterior versus the posterior urethra?**

The designation of the anterior and posterior urethra refer to a developmental division between the distal and proximal urethra. The anterior urethra is composed of the fossa navicularis, the pendulous (penile urethra), and the bulbar urethra. The pendulous urethra is bounded distally by the fossa navicularis and proximally by the penile scrotal junction. The bulbar urethra begins at the junction of the pendulous urethra and is proximally defined by the urogenital diaphragm. The posterior urethra is composed of the short membranous urethra, starting at the urogenital diaphragm and ending at the prostate, and the prostatic urethra, which travels through the prostate to the bladder neck.

○ **What is the arterial blood supply to the anterior urethra?**

There are two arteries that supply blood to the anterior urethra. The bulbar artery arises from the internal pudendal artery and enters the urethra at the proximal bulb. The second artery is the dorsal penile artery, which also arises from the internal pudendal artery. This artery courses along the dorsal aspect of the corporal bodies giving off penetrating arteries to the anterior urethra along its course.

○ **How is the distal urethra perfused when the urethra is transected during trauma or an anastomotic urethroplasty?**

If the bulbar artery is transected, the blood supply to the distal urethra is maintained by penetrating arteries from the dorsal penile artery as well as retrograde flow via the connection between the distal bulbar artery and the dorsal penile artery located in the glans.

○ **What is the blood supply for a pedicled penile skin flap?**

The dorsolateral and ventrolateral artery arise from the external pudendal artery, which in turn arises from the femoral artery.

○ **What is the blood supply to the scrotal skin?**

Superiorly, it is also supplied by branches of the external pudendal artery arising from the femoral artery. Inferiorly, a posterior scrotal artery arises from the perineal artery, which in turn arises from the internal pudendal artery, and ultimately the hypogastric artery.

○   **Increased urinary pressure behind a tight urethral stricture can have what effect on the urethra?**

Spongiofibrosis, which is the scarring process in the corpus spongiosum underlying the visually evident stricture, may develop for a considerable distance both proximally and distally due to cracking of the epithelium and underlying scar tissue as high-pressure urine is forced by the strictured area.

○   **Where is a dorsal onlay graft or flap placed versus a ventral onlay graft or flap?**

Dorsal refers to the dorsum of the urethra, similar to the dorsum of the penis. So a dorsal onlay graft or flap would rest against the ventral aspect of the corpora cavernosa; these corporal bodies serving as its roof and vascular bed of the graft. A ventral onlay graft or flap lies on the ventral aspect of the urethra. If a free graft is used, the corpora spongiosum is closed above it to provide a vascular bed to nourish the graft.

○   **What process occurs after a graft placement which allows for survival of the graft?**

There is a two-step process, lasting approximately 96 hours, called imbibition and inosculation. In the first step, imbibition, which lasts about 48 hours, the graft absorbs its nutrients passively from the graft bed or "imbibes" these nutrients. The second step is called inosculation and is the process of connection of vessels from the graft bed to the graft and ingrowth of capillaries.

○   **True or False: Congenital urethral strictures are common etiologies of stricture disease.**

False. Congenital urethral strictures are rare and are probably overestimated. Histopathologically they differ from acquired strictures in that their walls consist of smooth muscle rather than scar tissue. They form as a result of inadequate fusion of the anterior and posterior urethra.

○   **True or False: Urethral stricture development secondary to gonorrhea tends to result in discreet lesions within the bulbar urethra.**

False. While infectious strictures tend to develop within the bulbar urethra, they also tend to involve considerable length of the urethra and underlying spongiosum.

○   **Urethral stricture following cardiothoracic surgery with bypass may occur in up to 22% of cases. Which portion of the urethra is most at risk for stricture development?**

Pendulous urethra. Etiology may be related to local tissue ischemia/hypoxia during the bypass portion of the operation.

○   **Prior to repair of a completely obliterative urethral stricture, optimal radiographic evaluation includes which studies?**

In addition to a retrograde urethrogram, a voiding cystourethrogram is essential to identify the proximal extent of the stricture.

○   **True or False: Substitution urethroplasty tends to fail earlier than anastomotic repair.**

False. Anastomotic repair tends to fail within the first year, while substitution urethroplasty has been shown to fail at a rate of 5% per annum with a 60% successful outcome rate after 10 years.

○   **In substitution urethroplasty, what factors lead to increased restenosis rates?**

Tubularized flaps have a higher restenosis rate than patch flaps. In addition, the use of scrotal skin has a higher failure rate when compared to penile shaft or preputial skin.

○ **When treating a urethral stricture with progressive weekly dilations, what is the largest caliber dilator that should be used?**

Current recommendations are: do not exceed a 24F dilator.

○ **When treating a urethral stricture with visual urethrotomy, the 12-o'clock position incision was made too deep. What specific complication can occur?**

Peyronie's-like reaction resulting in chordee and erectile dysfunction.

○ **Is there any difference between internal urethrotomy and simple dilation outcomes in the treatment of urethral strictures?**

There is no proven efficacy difference between the two methods of treatment.

○ **What is the reported success rate of urethral dilation or internal urethrotomy and does it decrease with successive similar treatments?**

The success rate for initial dilation or urethrotomy is approximately 40% to 60%. This declines with secondary procedures to approximately 20% to 30% and has 0% long-term success for three or more procedures.

○ **What factors predict stricture recurrence postdilation or internal urethrotomy?**

Long strictures >2 cm are unlikely to have a durable positive response. Prior dilation or internal urethrotomy lowers success rates substantially, as well as the presence of balanitis xerotica obliterans.

○ **What is the optimal time for a urethral catheter after internal urethrotomy?**

Three to five days. Longer periods of catheterization have not been shown to help. Self-catheterization for dilation does seem to improve outcomes.

○ **Why is anastomotic urethroplasty generally inappropriate for treating pendulous urethral strictures?**

The resulting urethral shortening is sufficient to cause ventral chordee.

○ **What is the disadvantage of using scrotal skin for urethral reconstruction?**

A high incidence of dermatitis, which can lead to restenosis. Also, the genital skin is hair bearing, which can lead to stone formation and encrustation within the neourethra.

○ **Which type of bulbar urethral stricture lends itself best to anastomotic urethroplasty?**

Short strictures usually <2 cm in length and due to trauma.

○ **What are the signs of a traumatic urethral injury from pelvic fracture during the acute evaluation in the emergency department?**

Blood at the meatus, inability to void, failure to pass a catheter, and a high ballottable prostate all are signs of urethral injury or disruption.

○ **When should repair of pelvic urethral distraction injury be undertaken?**

Three months is generally considered to be a sufficient period of time to allow for resolution of tissue edema, periurethral hematoma, and "stabilization" of the injury. Immediate repair is associated with recurrent stricture and a higher rate of erectile dysfunction.

○ **What maneuvers can gain length for an anastomotic repair of a long posterior urethral defect?**

Maneuvers that can aid in bringing together the urethra for long posterior urethral defects are extensive mobilization of the bulbar urethra, separation of the proximal corporal bodies, partial pubectomy, and possibly rerouting the urethra around one of the corporal bodies.

○ **Retrograde urethrography may exacerbate a urethral stricture by what mechanism?**

Excessive pressure may cause extravasation of contrast material and lead to worsened periurethral fibrosis.

○ **What are the two specific contraindications to using an indwelling urethral stent?**

Patients who have undergone prior substitution urethral reconstruction, particularly with skin, and patients with deep spongiofibrosis.

○ **When performing substitution urethroplasty over fibrosed spongiosum, which is considered superior: graft or flap substitution?**

Flap substitution. In cases where the underlying blood supply is in question, a flap, which carries its own blood supply, has a more predictable outcome.

○ **Meatal strictures associated with balanitis xerotica obliterans are best managed with what approach?**

A formal meatal reconstruction is usually necessary as dilation in this condition rarely results in a long-term response.

○ **Which has a higher success rate and why: skin island onlay flap or a tabularized flap?**

The skin island flap is better. Tubularized flaps tend to form anastomotic strictures.

○ **How should a stricture of the membranous urethra be managed in a patient who has had a previous TURP?**

Unfortunately, membranous urethral strictures are not uncommon after TURP. DVIU or urethral reconstruction carries a high risk of incontinence since there is no bladder neck sphincteric mechanism. If incontinence develops, an artificial sphincter may be the only way to restore continence. Therefore, management is usually serial self-intermittent catheterization as a form of continuing urethral dilation therapy.

○ **What is the incidence and treatment of bladder neck contractures after radical prostatectomy?**

The incidence is 5% to 15% and the initial treatment of choice is dilation or internal urethrotomy. For recurrent strictures of the bladder neck, men may need further endoscopic procedures such as placement of a urethral stent or formal repair and reanastomosis.

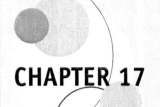

CHAPTER 17 Prostatic Hyperplasia

W. Bruce Shingleton, MD

○ **The development of the transition zone of the prostate begins at what week of embryologic development?**

This occurs at week 16 of development of the fetus.

○ **What effect do finasteride and dutasteride have on serum testosterone levels?**

There is no change in serum testosterone levels. Dutasteride may lower serum dihydrotesterone.

○ **What percent of patients with BPH will have symptom improvement or stabilization without treatment?**

Up to 50% of patients with BPH will have symptom stabilization or improvement regardless of whether treatment is started.

○ **What percent of the ejaculate arises from the prostate gland?**

Prostatic secretions constitute 15% of the total ejaculate volume.

○ **What is the average weight of the prostate in an adult male aging 40 years?**

At this age, the mean weight of the prostate is approximately 20 g.

○ **The prostate is in contact with how many and what fascial layers?**

The three fascial layers which abut the prostate include Denonvilliers posteriorly, the endopelvic fascia cranially, and the lateral pelvic fascia.

○ **What artery provides the major source of blood for the prostate?**

The prostatovesicular artery arising from the inferior vesical artery is the main source of arterial blood to the prostate.

○ **The plexus of Santorini drains into what major veins?**

This venous complex drains into the hypogastric veins.

○ **The urethra divides the prostate into what areas?**

The urethra demarcates the prostate into the fibromuscular (ventral) and glandular (dorsal) areas.

○ **The transition zone constitutes what percentage of the prostate?**

The transition zone comprises 4% to 5% of the glandular prostate.

○ **What is the largest zone of the prostate?**

Typically, the peripheral zone is the largest zone accounting for approximately 75% of the prostate gland.

○ **The fibromuscular stroma is composed of mainly what type of tissue?**

Smooth muscle fibers are the main component of the fibromuscular stroma.

○ **What cell types are present in the acinar epithelium?**

There are two cell types: glandular cells and basal cells.

○ **BPH is the most common cause of what urologic symptom?**

Gross painless hematuria. BPH is commonly associated with gross painless hematuria in men older than 60 years. When present, one must perform a complete evaluation to rule out neoplasm as an etiology.

○ **Dutasteride and finasteride have what effect on prostatic tissue levels of 5 alpha-DHT?**

Both decrease 5 alpha-DHT prostatic tissue levels.

○ **Dutasteride and finasteride produce what side effects in regard to sexual function?**

The side effects include decreased libido, decreased ejaculatory volume, and erectile dysfunction.

○ **The majority of alpha-1 adrenoceptors are located where in the GU tract?**

The alpha-1 receptors are located mainly in the bladder neck and prostate.

○ **Postobstructive diuresis is thought to be due to what factor?**

The obstruction results in altered function of the collecting duct cells manifested as a loss of renal concentrating ability with resultant diuresis. The ability to acidify the urine is also often impaired with an obstructive process. The ensuing postobstructive diuresis will resolve once the collecting ducts have regained their ability to conserve a fluid load and the renal medullary interstitium has regained its osmotic gradient.

○ **What is the reported incidence of urethral stricture after TURP?**

Urethral strictures have a reported incidence of 2.7% to 20% following TURP.

○ **During a transurethral resection of the prostate (TURP) a large venous sinus is opened. What are the next steps to be performed?**

Lower the height of the irrigation fluid to decrease further fluid absorption. Diligent efforts to endoscopically gain control of the bleeding should be undertaken, but can be difficult. Therefore, it may be necessary to quickly finish the resection and place a Foley catheter with appropriate traction, which will usually tamponade the bleeding. Serum electrolyte studies are appropriate to monitor for TUR syndrome (dilutional hyponatremia), and intravenous Lasix should be administered to help minimize the dilutional hyponatremia that can be associated with the unroofing of a large venous sinus.

○ **True or False: Transurethral incision of the prostate (TUIP) is useful regardless of the size of the prostate?**

False. Success with this technique is typically limited to a prostate 30 g or less in size.

○ **What alternative minimally invasive treatment modalities are available for use in anticoagulated patients?**

Laser prostatectomy and transurethral electrovaporization (TUVP) have been successfully used in anticoagulated patients for the treatment of BPH.

○ **Define the temperature range for hyperthermia and thermotherapy of the prostate?**

Temperatures >44.5°C constitute thermotherapy and temperatures <44°C are termed hyperthermia.

○ **The outer zone of the prostate is of what embryologic origin?**

The endoderm gives rise to the outer (peripheral) zone of the prostate.

○ **What percent of men develop symptoms secondary to BPH?**

Fifty percent of men with BPH will have symptoms as they age.

○ **How many isoenzymes exist for 5-alpha-reductase?**

There are two isoenzymes: type I and type II, with type II being the major isoenzyme in the prostate.

○ **What two growth factors are important in the development of BPH?**

Transforming growth factor alpha and epidermal growth factors have been identified as the major growth factors in the development of BPH.

○ **Does androgen ablation have any effect on the cell population of the prostate?**

Epithelial cells are mainly affected by a decrease in androgens and show varying degrees of atrophy as compared to stromal cells.

○ **What alpha-receptor subtype is most numerous in the prostate?**

Alpha 1A is the most prevalent alpha-receptor subtype in the prostate.

○ **What is the relationship between symptoms score and degree of obstruction as determined by pressure flow study?**

Various studies have shown no correlation between symptom score and pressure study regarding degree of obstruction.

○ **What is one disadvantage of Nd:YAG or "Green light" laser prostatectomy versus TURP?**

There is no tissue specimen available for histologic examination in patients treated by laser.

○ **Does treating BPH with hyperthermia cause a temporary rise in serum PSA?**

In a review of clinical trials of hyperthermia treatment, posttreatment PSA was not significantly elevated following hyperthermia treatment for BPH.

○ **True or False: Electrovaporization of the prostate (TVP) requires a longer operative time than TURP?**

True. During TVP, only a small segment of the prostate is treated at a given interval versus a larger surface area covered by each pass of the loop of the resectoscope resulting in longer operative time for TURP.

○ **What is the danger of using distilled water during transurethral surgery?**

Intravascular hemolysis will occur with the use of distilled water.

○ **What is the danger of increasing the height of irrigation fluid during transurethral surgery?**

Fluid absorption during TURP has been estimated at 20 cc/min of resection time. The height of the irrigant will cause increased fluid absorption across open venous sinuses.

○ **Prostatic secretions include:**

A high level of zinc is present in prostatic secretions.

○ **What is the anatomic female equivalent to the prostate gland?**

The Skene glands in the female urethra are the homologue to the male prostate.

○ **What typical female malignant neoplasm can arise in the prostate?**

Endometrial carcinoma can occur at the prostatic utricle.

○ **What is the site of origin for endometrial carcinoma of the prostate?**

The utricle is the site of endometrial carcinoma in men.

○ **The treatment of TUR syndrome includes:**

Symptomatic dilutional hyponatremia must be managed aggressively. The total body sodium deficit is calculated using the following formula: $(0.6 \times$ weight in kilograms$) \times ($desired serum Na^+ – the measured serum $Na^+) =$ total body Na^+ deficit. This value divided by 513 mOsm/L gives the liters of 3% saline that must be administered to correct the total body sodium deficit. One-half the total body deficit should be corrected in the first 2 hours and the remainder over the next 6 hours. Failure to correct the Na^+ deficit can have lethal results.

○ **What drugs penetrate into the prostatic fluid?**

Trimethoprim-sulfamethoxazole and fluoroquinolones are the only drugs that achieve therapeutic levels in the prostatic parenchyma.

○ **Where are Cowper's glands located?**

They are located within the urogenital diaphragm.

○ **The blood supply to the prostate arises from how many groups of arteries?**

Two: a urethral and capsular group.

○ **Lymphatic drainage of the prostatic urethra is to what lymph nodes?**

The obturator and external iliac lymph nodes are the main lymphatic drainage group.

○ **True or False: Saline is safe and effective to use for irrigation during transurethral surgery?**

False. Saline irrigation results in dissipation of electric current and renders the resectoscope useless, unless a bipolar unit is used.

○ **Bacterial prostatitis is caused by what gram-positive organism?**

The gram-positive organism is *Enterococcus*.

○ **Where are prostatic calculi located within the prostate?**

The calculi are located between the prostatic adenoma and the surgical capsule.

○ **Do they have any clinical significance?**

No.

○ **What are they made of?**

Usually calcium phosphate.

○ **When were the technical improvements to create the modern resectoscope first completed?**

In 1932 by Dr. Joseph McCarthy.

○ **Who first described the prostate anatomically and who named it prostate?**

Vesalius described it in 1538. Caspar Bartholin named it "prostate" in 1611.

○ **What advances to the resectoscope were designed by Dr. Theodore M. Davis?**

Thicker cutting loop, insulated outer sheath, and the dual foot pedal.

○ **Who provided the first correct and detailed description of the prostatic blood supply and when?**

Ruben Flocks in 1937.

○ **Who is credited with the first description of modern TURP technique?**

Reed M. Nesbit who published his technique in 1943 in his book *Transurethral Prostatectomy*.

○   **What is the difference between the Stern-McCarthy and Iglesias resectoscopes?**

The Stern-McCarthy uses a rack and pinion action while the Iglesias uses a spring.

○   **What is the 5-year risk for a reoperation after TURP?**

Approximately 5%. This increases to 13% at 10 years.

○   **The average TURP removes how much tissue?**

It removes 22 g.

○   **What is the average age?**

Sixty-nine years.

○   **Does prostate doubling time increase or decrease with age?**

Decreases.

○   **What portion of the male population develops a prostate of 100 g or more?**

Four percent.

○   **On an average, how much does the prostate grow each year?**

0.6 cc/y with a mean decrease in urinary peak flow rate of .2 mL/s/y.

○   **How many patients with BPH present with some degree of renal failure?**

Ten percent.

○   **What is the only absolute indication for an open prostatectomy?**

Need for an additional open bladder procedure.

○   **What is the usual maximum operating time limit for TURP to minimize complications?**

Ninety minutes is the maximum time but less than 60 minutes is best.

○   **What is the maximum size prostate that can be treated by TURP?**

There is no arbitrary size limit. It depends on the skill of the surgeon and the 90-minute time limit.

○   **Contraindications to TURP are:**

Active anticoagulation, recent MI, dysfunctional external sphincter, recent radiation therapy to the prostate, and active urinary tract infection. Shy–Drager syndrome and Parkinson's are relative contraindications.

○   **Where is the external sphincter muscle closest to the bladder neck?**

At 12-o'clock position.

○ **What is the danger if the verumontanum is accidentally resected?**

While ejaculatory duct obstruction is possible, the main danger is loss of the distal urethral landmark.

○ **What is the maximum recommended height of the irrigating fluid above the bladder during TURP?**

It is 60 cm. Fluid absorption substantially increases beyond this height.

○ **What technique can be used to perform a TURP when contractures, penile prosthesis, or deformity prevent access through the penis?**

A perineal urethrostomy.

○ **Where is the prostate tissue thinnest?**

At 12-o'clock position.

○ **Symptoms of dilutional hyponatremia generally do not occur until the serum sodium reaches what level?**

Until serum sodium reaches 125 mEq or less.

○ **What percentage of patients develop some degree of dilutional hyponatremia?**

Approximately 2%.

○ **What is the main advantage of Bipolar TURP?**

It can be used with normal saline irrigation.

○ **What are the most common mistakes made in TURP surgery?**

- Failure to do a perineal urethrostomy when indicated.
- Elevation of irrigating fluid to over 60 cm in height above the bladder.
- Not quitting early if it appears clear that finishing the resection would take much longer than 90 minutes. These partial resections usually do quite well if at least one side of the prostate has been completed.

○ **What should be done if the seminal vesicles are opened or perforated during a TURP?**

Nothing. They will usually heal without incident.

○ **What should be done at the end of the TURP just before placing the catheter?**

Carefully inspect for bleeding vessels. Lowering the irrigation flow and pressure will allow additional bleeding sites to become visible. Make sure all prostate chips have been evacuated. Carefully check any bladder diverticula for chips. Finally, inspect the ureteral orifices and external sphincter muscle to make sure there was no inadvertent injury.

○ **True or False: The most difficult procedure for a urologist to learn to do well is the TURP.**

True.

○   **What should be done if bleeding is encountered during a TURP and the bleeding source cannot be found?**

Check the opposite side of the prostate capsule. Many bleeding vessels will "Ricochet" off the opposite sidewall. Next, do a careful, methodical inspection of the lining of the prostate and bladder neck. Fill the bladder. This will tilt the inferior bladder neck and distal trigone forward and expose additional potential bleeding points.

○   **Many TURP techniques begin the resection at 12-o'clock position. Is this a good practice?**

Probably not. The intention is to allow the lateral lobes to fall down into the prostatic urethra making the resection easier. However, the prostate thickness is thin here, which allows early perforation. Also, there is no direct visualization of the key distal landmark, the verumontanum and so there is a greater risk of an inadvertent injury to the external sphincter muscle which is most proximal at this position. Starting at the median lobe or lateral lobes would be safer.

○   **Where in the prostatic cell is testosterone converted to 5-alpha-dihydrotestosterone?**

This conversion occurs in the cytoplasm.

○   **Is BPH an inherited, genetic disorder?**

Although not usually thought of as being a genetic disorder, BPH clearly shows inheritable characteristics. Patients with a positive family history tend to develop symptoms at an earlier age and they tend to have larger prostate glands (82 vs. 55 g).

○   **True or False: Proscar (finasteride) reduces the risk of acute urinary retention more than Avodart (dutasteride)?**

False. The risk reduction is reportedly the same for both (57%).

○   **What are the significant differences between finasteride (Proscar) and dutasteride (Avodart)?**

Dutasteride is both a type 1 and type 2 inhibitor of 5 alpha reductase. Finasteride affects only type 2. Dutasteride has a 5-week half-life, while finasteride is just 8 hours. The average reported shrinkage of the prostate with dutasteride is 27% but only 18% with finasteride.

○   **Of the two, is dutasteride or finasteride more effective clinically?**

They are essentially equivalent. Dutasteride might be effective in slightly smaller prostates than finasteride.

○   **Nocturnal urinary overproduction is an etiological factor in what percentage of men with nocturia?**

Up to 70%.

○   **Is there a role for angiography in managing hematuria after TURP?**

Yes, if the hematuria is not well controlled by other means and is severe enough to warrant a more aggressive approach. Superselective unilateral arterial embolization has been reported to be highly successful in selected cases of severe hemorrhage after TURP that could not be controlled otherwise.

○   **A 72-year-old male presents with urinary retention and a TURP is performed. During the surgery, despite your exemplary technique, excessive bleeding is encountered. The entire prostatic fossa is oozing heavily and the patient is bleeding from various places including IV sites, lips, mouth, and nose indicating some type of coagulopathy. The platelet count is normal and stable, but the fibrin split products are extremely high. What is going on and what's the treatment?**

The patient has primary fibrinolysis, probably from prostate cancer. Fibrinolysins from the cancer are released during the TURP and resulted in the coagulation disorder. The lack of any thrombocytopenia suggests the diagnosis. Treatment is with intravenous Amicar.

○ **True or False: Evaluation of a patient for BPH requires a prostate examination and PSA.**

True. It is necessary to determine if there is evidence of prostate cancer in the patient.

○ **What is the most common cause of lower urinary tract symptoms?**

Benign prostatic hyperplasia.

○ **True or False: Postvoid residual urine volume should be monitored regularly if a patient elects medical therapy for treatment.**

True. The patient may develop significant elevated volumes without clinical symptoms.

○ **True or False: The newer minimally invasive treatments for BPH are a substantial improvement over TURP.**

False. Current studies indicate the therapies are at best equivalent to TURP but not better. TURP is more flexible in that it can be done on patients with any size or shape prostate, depending only on the skill and experience of the resectionist.

○ **What is the role of intraprostatic stents in the management of BPH?**

At the present time, it is a temporary treatment for urinary retention.

○ **True or False: Radiofrequency ablation of the prostate (TUNA) can deliver an improvement in symptoms up to at least 1 year.**

True, but long-term results from studies are lacking.

○ **True or False: Transurethral microwave therapy should not be used in patients with prostate size over 100 g.**

True, although clinical studies have been done showing a benefit in those patients.

○ **What specific receptor does tamsulosin work on?**

Alpha 1a.

○ **What are the main side effects of alpha blockers?**

Dizziness and asthenia.

○ **What is the mechanism of action for BPH phytotherapeutic agents such as saw palmetto?**

It is unknown at this time.

○ **Is medical or surgical therapy indicated for the initial treatment of uncomplicated BPH?**

Medical therapy is the recommended first option.

○ **True or False: Lower urinary tract symptoms (LUTS) is not specific for BPH.**

True. As men age, different diseases can cause voiding symptoms but BPH remains the most common.

○ **True or False: A patient with BPH who develops an elevated serum creatinine should have a renal US.**

True. Renal insufficiency is rare in patients with BPH, but can occur and requires radiographic evaluation. Bilateral symmetrical hydronephrosis in patients with azotemia is strongly suggestive of urinary retention.

○ **What percentage of men older than age 50 will someday develop symptomatic BPH?**

At least 50%.

○ **What percentage of men with BPH will ultimately undergo surgery for it?**

Twenty-nine percent.

○ **What is the minimal average percentage amount of tissue removal by TURP needed to alleviate BPH symptoms?**

Approximately 30%.

○ **When should routine PSA testing be stopped?**

If the PSA is less than 3 by age 75, most experts agree that routine testing can be discontinued.

○ **True or False: Holmium laser ablation and photoselective laser vaporization of the prostate have similar efficacy.**

True.

○ **What are the expected reductions in PSA and prostate volumes in holmium laser ablation and photoselective laser vaporization of the prostate?**

Each is expected to demonstrate a 35% to 40% reduction in both PSA and prostate volumes.

CHAPTER 18 Female Incontinence and Vesicovaginal Fistula

Ja-Hong Kim, MD, and Shlomo Raz, MD

○ **Define urinary incontinence.**

Urinary incontinence is the complaint of any involuntary leakage of urine and is considered to be a *storage* symptom. This is often socially embarrassing and impacts negatively on a patient's quality of life. It is important to identify the fluid lost as urine and not fluid from another source, that is, peritoneal or uterine. Also, one must be sure that the urine is coming per urethra and not from a urinary fistula or ectopic ureter. Furthermore, urinary leakage may need to be distinguished from sweating or vaginal discharge.

○ **What are other storage symptoms as defined by the International Continence Society?**

- Increased daytime frequency is the complaint by the patient who considers that he/she voids too often by day.
- Nocturia is the complaint that the individual has to wake at night one or more times to void.
- Urgency is the complaint of a sudden compelling desire to pass urine, which is difficult to defer.
- It is important to further characterize these symptoms with 24-hour bladder diary recording micturition episodes, voided volumes, and fluid intake.

○ **Describe the symptoms associated with the various types of urinary incontinence.**

- Urge urinary incontinence is the complaint of involuntary leakage accompanied by or immediately preceded by urgency.
- Stress urinary incontinence is the complaint of involuntary leakage on effort or exertion, or on sneezing or coughing.
- Mixed urinary incontinence is the complaint of involuntary leakage associated with urgency and also with exertion, effort, sneezing, or coughing.
- Continuous urinary incontinence is the complaint of continuous involuntary loss of urine.
- Nocturnal enuresis is the complaint of involuntary loss of urine that occurs during sleep.
- Postvoid dribble is term used to describe involuntary loss of urine after voiding, usually after rising from the toilet.
- Overflow incontinence is any involuntary loss of urine associated with overdistension of the bladder.

○ **Can stress incontinence induce urge incontinence?**

Yes. Urgency may result from compensatory responses initiated in the incontinent patient. For example, once the initial symptom of stress incontinence is noticed, the patient may urinate frequently to keep the bladder empty, thus reducing the chance of stress-related incontinent episodes. As the bladder accommodates to these lower volumes, decreased bladder capacity and/or compliance may ensue. Subsequently, when the bladder distends beyond its reduced functional capacity, the patient experiences sensory urgency, frequency, and urinary incontinence. Alternatively, urgency may be a product of urine passage into the proximal urethra with stress leakage. Correction of the stress incontinence may eliminate the urgency.

○ **List the components of normal urinary continence in response to increases in abdominal stress.**

Normal continence in the female is a product of several forces working together. These forces include the proper *anatomic location* of the sphincteric unit, the critical functional and anatomic *urethral length*, the *mucosal coaptation* of the urethral surface, and the increased urethral pressure generated by *reflex pelvic contractions* at the time of stress. Failure of one of the components of this delicate balance will not invariably produce stress incontinence because of the compensatory effect of the other forces.

○ **Describe the urethral "washer effect."**

The female urethra consists of a 4-cm tube of inner epithelium and outer muscularis. The infolded epithelium is enclosed by a rich vascular sponge, which in turn is surrounded by a fibromuscular and smooth muscle coat. This submucosa, consisting of loosely woven connective tissue scattered throughout with smooth muscle bundles and an elaborate vascular plexus, provides a compressive "washer effect" vital to the mechanism of continence. The effectiveness of this washer is thought to be estrogen dependent.

○ **List the structures that provide normal pelvic support.**

- The fascia of the pelvic floor may be collectively referred to as the *levator fascia*. Although the fascia works in an integrated fashion to provide pelvic support, certain areas of the fascia have been separately described because of their importance in supporting individual female pelvic structures.
- The *pubourethral ligaments* connect the midportion of the urethra with the inner surface of the inferior pubis. Laterally, this midportion of the urethra is supported by segments of the levator fascia just below their attachments to the pubis. Collectively, these may be referred to as the *midurethral complex*.
- The *urethropelvic ligaments* (periurethral fascia) connect the proximal urethra and bladder neck laterally to the tendinous arch of the obturator muscle.
- The *vesicopelvic ligaments* (pubocervical fascia) connect the bladder base laterally to the tendinous arch of the obturator muscle.
- The *cardinal-sacrouterine ligaments* connect the uterine cervix and isthmus to the sacral vertebrae.
- The *broad ligaments* connect the uterine body to the pelvic sidewall.

○ **Describe outlet abnormalities associated with urinary incontinence.**

Urethral hypermobility: The pelvic floor fails to support the vesical neck and proximal urethra. This results in either the vesical neck and proximal urethra being situated *below* the inferior margin of the symphysis pubis at rest or they descend from a position situated *above* the inferior margin of the symphysis pubis during stress.

Intrinsic sphincter deficiency: The internal urethral sphincter fails to maintain continence even at low detrusor pressures (0–60 cm H_2O) with resultant leakage of urine per urethra.

○   **Define detrusor overactivity.**

Detrusor overactivity is a urodynamic observation characterized by involuntary detrusor contractions during the filling phase, which may be spontaneous or provoked. It can be further classified as either *neurogenic detrusor overactivity* when there is a relevant neurological condition (previously termed "detrusor hyperreflexia") or *idiopathic detrusor overactivity* when there is no defined cause (previously termed "detrusor instability").

○   **Is urge incontinence the same as detrusor overactivity?**

Yes. Urge incontinence implies involuntary bladder contractions. These may not be identifiable on urodynamics given that patients can suppress involuntary contractions.

○   **What is bladder compliance?**

Bladder compliance describes the relationship between bladder volume and detrusor pressure and is dependent upon the viscoelastic properties of the detrusor. Compliance is calculated by dividing the change in volume by the change in detrusor pressure during two specific points at the time of filling cystometry: (1) at the start of the bladder filling and (2) at cystometric capacity or immediately before the start of any detrusor contraction that causes significant leakage. The result is expressed in mL/cm H_2O.

○   **Distinguish between abdominal, Valsalva, and detrusor leak point pressures (LPP).**

Abdominal/Valsalva LPP: Intravesical pressure at which urine leakage occurs due to increased abdominal pressure in the absence of a detrusor contraction. In the normal patient, urine loss should never occur during abdominal straining even at high pressures.

Detrusor LPP: Lowest detrusor pressure at which urine leakage occurs in the absence of either a detrusor contraction or increased abdominal pressure. In the normal patient, urine exits the urethra at relatively low bladder pressures during voiding. A detrusor LPP greater than 40 cm H_2O has been used to identify patients with neurologic abnormality who may be at risk for upper tract damage. Detrusor LPP can be measured during involuntary detrusor contraction in patients with detrusor overactivity.

○   **What is the role of the history?**

Because urinary symptoms may be similar despite disparate etiologies, the history is often nondiagnostic when considering female urinary incontinence. There is a 30% error in diagnosing stress urinary incontinence if only the history is used. Evaluation of the incontinent female must include a history, physical examination, and adjuvant testing. However, because more than one symptom is often present, it is essential to determine the relative severity of each complaint. It is important to focus on the *chief presenting symptom* in deciding the next diagnostic or therapeutic step.

○ **Describe the key components of initial evaluation of female urinary incontinence.**

- Q-tip test: Assesses mobility of the urethra. With stress, the tail of the applicator will transcribe an arc of 0 to 30 degrees in most women. Movement of greater than 35 degrees suggests urethral hypermobility.
- Stress testing: Assesses urethral leak with stress. With the bladder full, the patient is asked to cough or strain. The patient with stress incontinence will immediately lose urine as a brief, small squirt associated with the stress. The position is variable. Eighty percent of patients will leak in the lithotomy position, an additional 10% of patients will leak at an incline of 45 degrees, while the final 10% of patients will only leak in the standing position.
- Speculum examination: Assesses concomitant pelvic floor defects. Urethral hypermobility may be measured with a Q-tip, but a speculum exam is necessary to evaluate the anterior vaginal wall, the vaginal apex, an enterocele, a rectocele, the anal sphincter, and the perineal body.
- Bladder diary: Measures the voided volumes, daytime frequency, incontinence episodes, pad usage, and other information such as fluid intake, degree of urgency, and leakage during a full 24-hour period.
- Pad testing: Assesses the quantity of urine lost during incontinence episodes; methods range from a short provocative test to a 24-hour pad test. Increase of >15 g in pad weight gain is considered abnormal.
- Postvoid residual: Assesses volume of urine left in bladder after voiding by either an ultrasound bladder scanner or straight catheterization.

○ **What are the indications for urodynamic testing?**

- When there is component of both stress and urge urinary incontinence.
- When results of simpler diagnostic tests have been inconclusive.
- When empirical treatments have proved unsuccessful.
- When the patient complains of incontinence but it cannot be demonstrated clinically.
- In symptomatic patients who have previously undergone corrective surgery.
- In patients with a history of prior radical pelvic surgery.
- In patients with known or suspected neurologic disorders.

○ **What are the indications for cystoscopy?**

In all patients with urgency as a complaint, bladder pathology such as bladder stone, bladder cancer, and carcinoma in situ must be ruled out. All patients with hematuria should undergo cytologic examination, cystoscopy, and upper tract evaluation. Patients with pure stress urinary incontinence may undergo preoperative cystoscopy to evaluate for incidental coexisting disease.

○ **Describe several radiographic evaluations useful in assessing female urinary incontinence.**

- Cystogram with voiding films (VCUG): Often obtained videourodynamics, these tests are useful in comparing resting and straining films. Lateral films are helpful in identifying urethral position at rest and hypermobility with straining. These standing lateral films are also useful in assessing the degree of cystocele if present. Urinary leak may be observed on the lateral straining films.
- Ultrasound: Useful in identifying urethral mobility and prolapse, ultrasound can be performed transabdominally, transrectally, or transvaginally. The quality of the examination is highly dependent upon the skills of the ultrasonographer.
- MRI: Usually reserved for cases of more severe prolapse, the dynamic MRI of the pelvis is very helpful in identifying cystocele, uterine prolapse, and rectocele. It is also useful in revealing any concomitant pelvic pathology when hysterectomy is being considered as part of pelvic repair. Use of the HASTE sequence MRI is particularly helpful in identifying urologic pathology.

○ **What is the role of Kegel exercises and estrogens in female urinary incontinence?**

- Kegel exercises: If performed properly and diligently, Kegel exercises can strengthen the levator musculature, which can lead to an increase in urethral pressure, better urethral reflex response to stresses, reduction of cystocele, and improved cough-urethra pressure transmission in stress urinary incontinence. These exercises are also useful for urge incontinence. By increasing pudendal activity to the sphincter muscles, this may in turn stimulate a reflexive inhibitory input to the detrusor, thereby suppressing involuntary bladder contractions.
- Estrogens: Lack of estrogen causes the urethral mucosa and underlying blood vessels to atrophy, leading to a decreased compressive washer effect. In women who are estrogen deficient, estrogen causes hypertrophy and thickening of the urethral mucosa and engorgement of the blood vessels beneath.

○ **Identify several behavioral modifications for a woman with urge incontinence.**

- Timed voiding: Instruct the patient to void on a timed schedule. The specific interval should be based on voiding before the development of urgency. Increase the interval after several weeks without urgency.
- Prompted voiding: Instruct the patient not to delay voiding. Additionally, the patient must concentrate on completely relaxing and emptying the bladder during the void.
- Fluid restriction: Limit the fluid intake for patients to 4–6 glasses per day. Avoid caffeine-containing beverages and fluid consumption after dinner.
- Avoidance of bladder irritants: Eliminate bladder irritants such as alcohol and caffeine, which can exacerbate lower urinary tract symptoms and have a diuretic effect.

○ **List the various pharmacologic treatments for a woman with urge incontinence.**

- Anticholinergics: Antagonize the muscarinic receptors of the bladder resulting in increased total bladder capacity, decreased amplitude of bladder contraction, and increased bladder volume before first bladder contraction.
- Antispasmodics: Primarily cause relaxation of detrusor smooth muscle in addition to anticholinergic effects and local anesthetic effects.
- Tricyclic antidepressants: Unique in the ability to increase urethral outlet resistance due to adrenergic stimulation on the smooth muscle of the bladder neck and proximal urethra in addition to anticholinergic effects and a sedative action that may be related to antihistaminic properties (e.g., imipramine hydrochloride, amitriptyline hydrochloride).
- Calcium channel blockers: Uncommon as first-line agents, calcium channel blockers inhibit the inflow of calcium after membrane depolarization and have the potential of relaxing the smooth muscle of the bladder (e.g., nifedipine).

○ **What are the treatment options in patients with refractory urge incontinence?**

- Botox injection: Inhibits acetylcholine release from cholinergic nerve terminals to suppress unstable contractions.
- Bladder augmentation: Allows for increased total bladder capacity and physical interruption of the overactive detrusor muscle. It is used as a last resort after exhausting all possible pharmacologic interventions for urge incontinence.
- Sacral neuromodulation: Uses electrical stimulation of the sacral nerve root, which results in afferent inhibition of sensory processing in the spinal cord. Studies suggest it has a conditioning effect on neural excitability and can restore neural equilibrium between facilatatory and inhibitory influences although the exact mechanism of action in each of these conditions may be different.

○ **Surgical implanted sacral neuromodulation devices or sacral nerve stimulation is targeted at which sacral nerve?**

Optimally, the S3 sacral nerve root. Only one side is typically treated. Approximately 75% of otherwise intractable cases of urge incontinence report significant improvement with this therapy. Approximately 50% are completely dry.

○ **Is sacral nerve stimulation useful in urinary retention? Can it be used in men?**

Yes to both.

○ **Tricyclic antidepressants like imipramine are reasonably effective in what proportion of patients with incontinence?**

Improvement is reported in approximately 60%.

○ **How does capsaicin work?**

Intravesical capsaicin desensitizes unmyelinated afferent nerves. It is most useful in patients who demonstrate bladder hypersensitivity on an ice water test. Improvement of 40% to 100% has been reported.

○ **How effective is intravesical oxybutynin?**

It is much more effective than oral forms. Plasma and tissue levels are higher but side effects are low as hepatic metabolism is avoided.

○ **What is the role for needle suspension for stress urinary incontinence?**

Needle suspension prevents urethral descent with stress. It has been effective in the treatment of urethral hypermobility but does not affect incontinence due to intrinsic sphincter deficiency.

○ **What is the role for urethral bulking agents for stress urinary incontinence?**

Various materials have been injected in the urethra either through the periurethral or transurethral methods as a bulking agent to treat urinary incontinence. The ideal injectable agent should be biocompatible, nonantigenic, noncarcinogenic, and nonmigratory. It is effective in the treatment of intrinsic sphincter deficiency, but does not affect incontinence due to urethral hypermobility.

○ **What is the role for suburethral sling for stress urinary incontinence?**

Suburethral (pubovaginal) sling procedures effectively prevent urethral descent with stress and improve the urethral washer effect. Therefore, slings are equally effective for urethral hypermobility and intrinsic sphincter deficiency. However, there are increased postoperative risks of retention with detrusor instability.

○ **An elderly woman presents with urinary urgency and frequency. Ultrasound evaluation determines her postvoid residual to be 350 mL. What is the diagnosis?**

This patient has detrusor overactivity with impaired contractility, which generally presents commonly in the elderly patient. Treatment is difficult since pharmacologic treatment of the detrusor overactivity often exacerbates the retention. This optimally requires clean intermittent catheterization that is often difficult in the elderly population. It is important to rule out large cystocele or other co-existing anatomic abnormalities which can "kink" the urethra and cause increased bladder outlet resistance.

○ **A 46-year-old woman, gravida 4, para 4, presents with urgency, frequency, and urinary incontinence. Physical examination is normal, Marshall test is negative, and urodynamic evaluation reveals a normally compliant bladder without involuntary bladder contractions. What is the diagnosis?**

This patient has classic urge incontinence. It is important to focus on the chief presenting symptom in evaluating a patient with urinary incontinence. Despite the obstetrical history and the lack of involuntary bladder contractions, the diagnosis remains urge incontinence.

○ **A woman presents with complaints of urgency and precipitous voiding shortly following a cough or sneeze. What is the diagnosis?**

This patient has stress-induced urge incontinence. Stress incontinence is the involuntary loss of urine during coughing, sneezing, or increases in intra-abdominal pressure. The described patient loses urine after the intra-abdominal pressure has returned to normal and continues to empty her bladder precipitously. This suggests an involuntary bladder contraction occurring due to the stress stimulus.

○ **A woman presents with urodynamically demonstrated stress incontinence with urinary urgency. What is the treatment of choice?**

Treatment of the stress incontinence. Urgency may result from compensatory responses initiated by the incontinent patient. Alternatively, urgency may be a product of urine passage into the proximal urethra with stress leakage. In 65% of patients with mixed stress and urge incontinence, correction of the stress incontinence will resolve the urgency. However, if the urgency component is successfully treated medically, many patients are satisfied without the surgery.

○ **A woman presents with urinary incontinence immediately following only repair of a large cystocele. What is the diagnosis?**

Stress urinary incontinence. The full bladder contributes to normal continence by creating a valvular effect through limited posterior rotation of the bladder base against a well-supported urethra during stress. Cystoceles exacerbate this valvular effect and may mask underlying urethral dysfunction. Correction of a large cystocele in this setting leads to incontinence due to either urethral hypermobility or intrinsic sphincter deficiency.

○ **Immediately following a needle bladder neck suspension, a woman complains of persistent stress urinary incontinence. What is the diagnosis?**

Intrinsic sphincter deficiency. Needle suspension corrects urethral hypermobility but is ineffective against intrinsic sphincter deficiency. Bulking urethral injections correct intrinsic sphincter deficiency but are ineffective against urethral hypermobility. Suburethral sling procedures correct both deficiencies.

○ **When performing a sling procedure, where should the central body of the mesh be located?**

At the mid to distal urethra, not the proximal urethra.

○ **Does vaginal surgery for stress incontinence have a significant impact on postoperative sexual function in women?**

When measured with a validated tool and compared with preoperative assessments, it does not appear that vaginal surgery for stress incontinence has any significant negative impact on sexual function in women.

○ **What is transient urinary incontinence?**

It's acute incontinence caused by a nonurological problem such as a change in medication.

○ **True or False: The only true cause of urinary stress incontinence is intrinsic sphincteric deficiency (ISD), which may or may not be associated with vesicourethral hypermobility?**

True. Sphincteric dysfunction may be caused by neurological factors, muscular degeneration, or trauma. Congenital problems may also be present.

○ **What is the classic presentation of a vesicovaginal fistula?**

Continuous urinary leakage after pelvic surgery.

○ **What are the predisposing factors for vesicovaginal fistula?**

Prior pelvic surgery or malignancy, radiation therapy, endometriosis, prior cervical conization or vaginal fulguration procedures, use of pessaries, steroid use, lack of estrogen effect, congenital deformities of any of the pelvic structures, and history of voiding problems or neurogenic bladder.

○ **What other symptoms may present in the immediate postoperative period if a vesicovaginal fistula is present?**

Excessive abdominal pain, extravasation with distension, hematuria, UTI, and excessive drainage from the wound or vagina are common complaints.

○ **True or False: A painless, watery discharge of varying amounts from the vagina developing 7 to 14 days after pelvic surgery suggests a vesicovaginal fistula.**

True. This is another way in which vesicovaginal fistulae may present.

○ **True or False: Excision of the fistulous tract and interposition of a well vascularized tissue flap are important considerations in vesicovaginal fistula repair.**

False. It is not necessary to excise the fistulous tract as most cases heal well without it. If excision of the fistula would cause too much collateral damage to the surrounding tissue or blood supply, it is OK to leave it. Interposition of a tissue flap is necessary only in cases of previous surgery, radiation therapy, or obstetrical injury.

○ **True or False: The preferred surgical repair for vesicovaginal fistula is transabdominal.**

False. The transvaginal route is preferred for most fistula repairs. Only the most complex repairs will need a different approach.

○ **What is the optimal timing of formal vesicovaginal repair?**

That depends on the risk factors and etiology of the fistula. In uncomplicated cases caused by iatrogenic injury, a period of 2 to 3 weeks may be sufficient; 3 to 6 months is recommended for injuries caused by obstetrical trauma; and 12 months is needed in cases of radiation therapy.

CHAPTER 19

Upper Urinary Tract Obstruction

Udaya Kumar, MD
and David M. Albala, MD

○ **In evaluating upper tract obstruction, which is the radiopharmaceutical of choice?**

^{99m}Tc-mercaptoacetyltriglycine (MAG3). It is more efficiently excreted by the kidney than DTPA, delivers a lower dose of radiation to the kidney than OIH, and provides better visualization of the anatomy of obstruction than other agents.

○ **What is the basis of the Whitaker test?**

It provides urodynamic evidence of mechanical obstruction of the upper tract at a given flow rate. As it is an invasive test, it is only used in cases with extreme dilatation of the upper tract or when renal function is too poor for adequate diuretic response.

○ **What are the phases in pressure changes in the ureter after unilateral occlusion of the ureter?**

Following unilateral occlusion, there is a rise in both ureteric pressure and renal blood flow for 1 to 1.5 hours. Then in phase 2, there is a continued rise in ureteric pressure while renal blood flow declines (5 hours). In the final phase, both renal blood flow and ureteric pressure fall.

○ **What are the causes of postobstructive diuresis?**

Postobstructive diuresis occurs after relief of bilateral ureteric obstruction or obstruction of a solitary kidney. It may be classified as physiologic, when caused by retained urea, sodium, and water, or pathologic when caused by impaired concentrating ability or sodium absorption.

○ **What is the embryological basis of the retrocaval ureter?**

The persistence of the posterior cardinal vein as the major portion of the inferior vena cava causes medial migration of and compression of the right ureter.

○ **What are the types of retrocaval ureter?**

There are two types. Type l, or the "low loop type," is the most common and the dilated proximal portion assumes a reverse J shape. Type II or the "high loop" is rarer. In this case, the ureter passes behind the vena cava at the level of or just above the UPJ.

○ **How common is hydronephrosis in pregnancy?**

Unilateral or bilateral hydronephrosis occurs by the third trimester of pregnancy in 90% to 95% of asymptomatic patients. In more than 80% of patients, right-sided hydronephrosis predominates.

○ **True or False: In the treatment of ureteric obstruction due to endometriosis, hormonal therapy is the treatment of choice.**

False. Surgery is more likely to be successful. The choice of surgery depends on the extent of ureteric involvement and the patient's desire to have more children. Ureterolysis with unilateral or bilateral oophorectomy and hysterectomy may be required. In severe cases, nephrectomy may be needed.

○ **How common is ureteral injury following hysterectomy?**

In routine hysterectomy, the incidence varies from 0.5% to 3% and is bilateral in one of every six cases. After radical hysterectomy, the incidence varies from 10% to 15%.

○ **How is ureteral involvement in Crohn's disease treated?**

Rarely is ureterolysis required for ureteral involvement in Crohn's disease. Medical or surgical therapy for Crohn's disease is usually effective in resolving ureteral involvement. It may also be indicated in some cases of severe retroperitoneal fibrosis with encasement of the ureter.

○ **What are the causes of retroperitoneal fibrosis (RPF)?**

Two-thirds of cases are idiopathic. Other causes include prolonged use of methysergide and other ergot derivatives. RPF can occur secondary to other disease processes of the retroperitoneum like hemorrhage, urinary extravasation, trauma, perianeurysmal inflammation, radiation therapy, surgery, inflammatory, bowel disease, collagen disease, and fat necrosis.

○ **What are the symptoms of retroperitoneal fibrosis?**

In approximately 90% of cases, there is a characteristic pain with a girdle-type distribution. The pain is dull and noncolicky. Later it becomes severe and unrelenting. The pain may be relieved by aspirin and not by narcotics. Rarely, there may be features of compression of the great vessels. Uremia is a late feature.

○ **What are the features of retroperitoneal fibrosis on intravenous urography?**

There is medial deviation of the ureters on IVU. Although this finding is present in up to 20% of normal studies, in RPF the displacement extends higher than the normal variant. There is usually associated obstruction and hydronephrosis. CT or MRI is most useful in establishing a diagnosis.

○ **How is retroperitoneal fibrosis treated?**

Any suspected medication like methysergide is withheld. If the patient is uremic, renal drainage should be established with ureteral stenting or nephrostomy tube placement. Steroid therapy may be useful in some but bilateral ureterolysis is required in most cases.

○ **What is pelvic lipomatosis?**

Pelvic lipomatosis is a proliferative disease of unknown etiology involving the mature fatty tissues of the pelvic retroperitoneum. It occurs exclusively in men in the third to sixth decade of life and is more common in African American men. This benign condition may lead to compression of the pelvic viscera including the ureters.

○ **What conditions may be associated with pelvic lipomatosis?**

It may be associated with cystitis cystica, cystitis glandularis, adenocarcinoma of the bladder, chronic UTI, hypertension, superficial thrombophlebitis, VU reflux, RPF, nontropical chyluria, and Proteus syndrome.

○ **How is pelvic lipomatosis diagnosed?**

Plain KUB x-ray may show the radiolucent area in the bony pelvis. On IVP, the bladder base is noted to be elevated and the bladder itself takes on a pear shape. CT is useful to confirm the diagnosis.

○ **How common is bilaterality in UPJ obstruction?**

Bilateral UPJ obstruction is seen in 10% to 40% of cases.

○ **True or False: UPJ obstruction occurs more commonly in males and on the left side.**

True. The ratio of male to female is more prominent in infancy (2:1). Left-sided lesions are more common. In infancy, about two-thirds of UPJ obstructions are on the left.

○ **How common is the finding of an aberrant lower polar vessel in UPJ obstruction?**

The incidence varies from 15% to 52%. Although some cases are no doubt caused by aberrant vessels, especially in adults, in most cases it is felt to be a concomitant finding rather than the cause.

○ **Vesicoureteric reflux and UPJ obstruction are found together in what proportion of cases?**

In approximately 10% (minor degree of reflux has been quoted in up to 40%). Severe cases of VU reflux can cause marked tortuosity of the ureter and secondarily give rise to UPJ obstruction.

○ **What are the congenital anomalies associated with UPJ obstruction?**

UPJ obstruction in the contralateral kidney (10%–40%), renal dysplasia and multicystic disease of the contralateral kidney, unilateral renal agenesis, duplicated collecting system, VU reflux, and the VATER complex.

○ **What is the investigation of choice for UPJ obstruction?**

A diuretic renogram is one of the best noninvasive methods to determine if a dilated upper tract is obstructed or not. The conventional renographic criteria for obstruction that warrant surgical repair are a flat or rising washout curve after furosemide administration, a half-time greater than 20 minutes and differential function less than 40%. Dynamic contrast MR urography is the newest imaging modality for UPJ obstruction. It provides anatomic and functional detail without the radiation exposure. A transit time (time between enhancement of renal cortex and appearance of contrast in the ureter) longer than 590 seconds is felt to indicate obstruction on MR urography.

○ **What test is useful to determine whether a hydronephrotic kidney is salvageable or not?**

A quantitative renal scan using technetium-99-DMSA is useful in determining whether a patient will benefit from pyeloplasty or not. If a kidney contributes less than 10% of the overall renal function, it should probably be removed.

○ **How is resistive index (on ultrasound examination) defined?**

(Peak systolic velocity − lowest diastolic velocity)/peak systolic velocity.

○ **What is the basis for the use of resistive index (RI) in the diagnosis of obstructive uropathy?**

A decrease in renal blood flow and an increase in renovascular resistance are hallmarks of obstructive uropathy. There is more reduction in diastolic than systolic blood flow, causing a rise in RI.

○ **What conditions other than obstructive uropathy can cause RI to be elevated?**

Values above the normally accepted 0.70 may be found in children, especially infants, in medical renal diseases, dehydration, hypotension, and in patients with a low heart rate.

○ **What are the determinants of the curve obtained during diuretic renography?**

The curve depends on the tracer used, the patient's hydration status, the dose and timing of the administration of the diuretic, and the overall renal function. The shape, size, and distensibility of the renal pelvis, its outlet resistance, gravity, and bladder filling also influence the curve.

○ **What are the patterns of curves described on the diuretic renogram?**

Type I (normal), type II (obstructed), type IIIa (dilated unobstructed), and type IIIb (equivocal).

○ **Can urinary biochemical markers be used in the diagnosis of upper tract obstruction?**

Epidermal growth factor, the renin–angiotensin system, monocyte chemoattractants, and transforming growth factors (TGF-β_1) have been implicated in patients with UPJ obstruction. Transforming growth factors (TGF-β_1) is elevated in patients with UPJ obstruction. There was 80% sensitivity for obstruction reported in pediatric patients undergoing pyeloplasty. The utility of these markers is yet to be determined.

○ **What are the ultrasound findings of UPJ obstruction in the neonate?**

The pelvis is seen as a large medial sonolucent structure, surrounded by smaller, rounded sonolucent structures representing the dilated calyces. Sometimes, the infundibular communications between the dilated calyces and the renal pelvis may be seen.

○ **True or False: It is difficult to distinguish antenatally between severe hydronephrosis and multicystic dysplastic kidneys (MDK).**

True. The ultrasound findings of MDK are lack of reniform shape of the kidney, multiple cysts of varying size, and no evidence of a collecting system. In severe hydronephrosis, the distinction may be difficult.

○ **What are the indications for intervention in UPJ obstruction?**

The presence of symptoms from obstruction, impairment of renal function, the development of infection or stones. Patients with solitary kidneys and bilateral UPJ obstruction should have intervention. The timing of repair in infants is controversial, as it is difficult to determine which kidneys are at risk.

○ **A dismembered pyeloplasty is not suitable for which UPJ obstruction cases?**

When the UPJ obstruction is associated with lengthy or multiple proximal ureteral strictures or when the renal pelvis is small, intrarenal, and relatively inaccessible.

○ **When is preoperative drainage of a kidney with UPJ obstruction indicated?**

When there is infection associated with obstruction, uremia due to obstruction in a solitary kidney or bilateral disease, and rarely in the patient with severe unrelenting pain.

○ **How is UPJ obstruction treated in the adult?**

Until recently, open surgery (i.e., pyeloplasty) was the only option. Minimally invasive alternatives now available include endopyelotomy (antegrade or retrograde), cautery wire balloon incision (Acucise device), and laparoscopic pyeloplasty.

○ **When an endopyelotomy is performed, where is the incision made?**

If a direct endoscopic incision is performed, a direct lateral cut is the safest. This appears to have the least likelihood of encountering a crossing vessel. In one study, a posterior-crossing vessel was found in 6.2% of cases, whereas no vessels were found crossing the UPJ laterally.

○ **What factors predict a poor outcome after endopyelotomy?**

Poor renal function, massive hydronephrosis, and the presence of a crossing vessel result in a reduced success rates.

○ **What are the possible complications of endopyelotomy?**

Hemorrhage is the most commonly encountered problem. Rarely ureteral avulsion, ureteral necrosis, arteriovenous fistula formation, hematoma, urinoma, and urinary infection have been reported.

○ **When hydronephrosis is noted in a horseshoe kidney, what is the likely cause?**

The obstruction is usually due to a UPJ obstruction and not due to pressure on the ureter from the isthmus.

○ **What are the basic techniques used in open pyeloplasty?**

There are two fundamental techniques; a pelvic flap is used in Culp and de Weerd, Scardino and Prince and Foley Y-V plasty operations. An Anderson–Hynes pyeloplasty is the dismembered type.

○ **Which part of the nephron is most resistant to damage from hydronephrosis?**

The glomerulus. Glomerular changes are not evident until 28 days of obstruction. In contrast, distal tubular and proximal tubular atrophy are seen at 7 and 14 days, respectively.

○ **How does urine exit the kidney in complete obstruction?**

In acute obstruction with high pressures, like ureteral calculi, urine exits through a rupture in the fornices. In low-pressure obstruction, urine exits via lymphatic channels and in chronic hydronephrosis, it is mostly into the renal venous channels.

○ **What is the incidence of UPJ obstruction?**

Urinary dilatation is detected in utero in 1 in 100 pregnancies; of these, significant uropathy is seen in 1 in 500. UPJ obstruction is responsible for 40% of these, placing the incidence of UPJ obstruction at 1 in 1250 births.

○ **What is the crescent sign on the excretory urogram in a patient with UPJ obstruction?**

The calyceal crescents represent transversely oriented collecting ducts and signify recoverable renal function.

○   **What are the causes of UPJ obstruction?**

Intrinsic:

- Congenital–adynamic muscular segment.
- Ureteral mucosal folds.
- High insertion of ureter into renal pelvis.

Extrinsic:

- Aberrant lower pole vessel.
- Retroperitoneal fibrosis.
- Retroperitoneal tumors.

Secondary:

- Renal calculi.
- Fibroepithelial polyps.
- Tumors.
- Failed pyeloplasty.

○   **Which is the most common cause of UPJ obstruction?**

Intrinsic causes are the most common, with an adynamic muscular segment (congenital) occurring frequently.

○   **Where is the most common site for ureteral strictures to occur?**

Ureteral strictures occur most commonly at the ureteropelvic junction. The second most common area of stenosis is at the ureterovesical junction.

○   **What is the appropriate treatment for failed endopyelotomy for UPJ obstruction?**

An open or laparoscopic pyeloplasty (including robotic assisted) are appropriate options depending on experience and expertise available.

○   **What is the appropriate treatment for a failed laparoscopic or open pyeloplasty?**

Endopyelotomy is a reasonable option after failure of pyeloplasty. However, long strictures, severe hydronephrosis, and poor renal function predict a poor outcome.

○   **What is the basis of endopyelotomy?**

Endopyelotomy uses the concept of a full-thickness incision of a narrow segment of ureter allowed to heal over a stent. The concept was first described in open surgery by Albarran in 1903 and popularized by Davis as intubated ureterostomy in 1943. Wickham and Kellett described endoscopic pyelolysis using the percutaneous approach.

○   **What approaches are available in performing endopyelotomy?**

Endopyelotomy can be performed antegrade using the percutaneous approach. Alternatively, it can be performed retrograde either using ureteroscopy (with laser or electrocautery) or using the Acucise balloon electrocautery. Unlike ureteroscopy or percutaneous approaches that are done under direct vision, Acucise endopyelotomy is performed using fluoroscopic guidance. The risk of a hemorrhagic complication is greater with the latter approach.

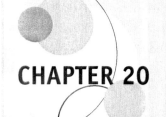

CHAPTER 20

Intestinal Segments in Urology

Sultan Saud Alkhateeb, MD, and Laurence Klotz, MD

○ **True or False: Ileal conduit is the standard form of urinary diversion.**

True. The ileal conduit was described in 1950 by Bricker and has remained a standard urinary diversion against which others are judged (Bricker, 1950). However, currently centers of excellence recommend that an orthotopic bladder be offered to most patients as the primary form of urinary reconstruction. Patients with advanced age or comorbidity should generally have an ileal conduit (Hautmann et al., 2007). Patients with prostatic urethral involvement should be considered for a conduit or a continent abdominal diversion.

○ **List the contraindications to an ileal conduit.**

Short bowel syndrome, inflammatory small bowel disease, and previous extensive radiation to the ileum.

○ **What is/are the absolute contraindication(s) to continent urinary diversion?**

Absolute contraindications to continent urinary diversion are compromised renal function with serum creatinine levels above 1.50 to 2.00 mg/dL, severe hepatic dysfunction, and patients in whom urethrectomy is indicated (usually because of urethral involvement by TCC) (Studer et al., 1998).

○ **A patient is considered for a continent diversion. His serum creatinine exceeds 2.0 mg/dL. How should he be evaluated to determine whether he is a candidate?**

Criteria for candidacy for a continent diversion include the ability to achieve a urine pH of 5.8 or less following an ammonium chloride loading test, a urine osmolality ≥ 600 mOsm/kg in response to water deprivation, a glomerular filtration rate >35 mL/min, and no more than minimal proteinuria. These tests are helpful in patients desiring continent diversion with borderline renal functions (i.e., serum creatinine between 1.50 and 2.00 mg/dL).

○ **Should extensive pelvic disease, a palpable mass, or positive lymph nodes preclude the use of neobladder because of the high propensity for pelvic recurrence or distant relapse?**

No. Convincing evidence suggests that a patient with an orthotopic diversion tolerate adjuvant chemotherapy less well. Local recurrence may be more problematic with a neobladder, but conversion to an ileal conduit if this occurs is a reasonable option. Patients can anticipate normal neobladder function until the time of death (Hautmann and Simon, 1999).

○ **True or False: Continent urinary diversions are better than incontinent diversions in terms of quality of life (QOL).**

False. Published evidence does not support an advantage of one type of reconstruction over the others with regard to QOL (Hautmann et al., 2007). Although the QOL studies have not demonstrated an advantage of orthotopic bladder replacement, many urologists believe that the QOL is improved. Patients usually prefer this option when offered.

○ **In terms of metabolic consequences, what bowel segment is preferably used for bladder reconstruction and why?**

Ileum is preferred to colon for bladder reconstruction. Chloride absorption and bicarbonate excretion are more pronounced in the colon, which leads to a higher risk of hyperchloremic metabolic acidosis, particularly in the presence of renal impairment (Davidsson et al., 1994).

○ **What is the advantage of stomach over other intestinal segments for urinary diversion?**

Stomach is less permeable to urinary solutes, it acidifies the urine, it has a net excretion of chloride and protons rather than a net absorption of them, and it produces less mucus.

○ **True or False: The jejunum is a good option as an intestinal segment for urinary intestinal diversion.**

False. The jejunum is usually not employed for reconstruction of the urinary system, because its use often results in severe electrolyte imbalance.

○ **What are the preferred methods of urinary diversion in patients with history of pelvic irradiation? Why?**

In patients with pelvic irradiation, it is preferable to avoid using the ileum because it is the bowel segment that is most affected by pelvic radiation. The preferred method of diversion is either a colon conduit or a continent cutaneous pouch using the colon (e.g., Indiana or Maintz pouch) (Leissner et al., 2000; Ravi et al., 1994).

○ **Which part of colon is the most appropriate segment as a colon conduit in patients undergoing a total pelvic exenteration?**

Sigmoid colon. No bowel anastomosis needs to be made.

○ **What is the contraindication to the use of sigmoid colon in addition to disease of the segment and extensive pelvic irradiation?**

If the internal iliac arteries have been ligated and the rectum has been left in situ, use of the sigmoid colon is contraindicated. It may result in sloughing of the rectum or its mucosa.

○ **What are the contraindications to the use of colonic segments?**

Inflammatory large bowel disease and severe chronic diarrhea.

○ **What are the main advantages of an ileocecal pouch (Indiana pouch)?**

The main advantage is, clearly, continence. In addition, the terminal ileum remains in the fecal stream (with the exception of the distal 15 cm), and it is avoided, especially following pelvic radiation.

○ **Where are the three vulnerable points involving the vascular supply to the colon located?**

Sudeck's critical point is located between the junction of the sigmoid and superior hemorrhoidal arteries with the midpoints between the middle colic and right colic arteries. Between the middle colic and left colic arteries are tenuous anastomotic areas. If the colon were transected in these regions, the anastomosis might be at risk because of compromised blood supply.

○ **What are the most common aerobic organisms in the bowel?**

Escherichia coli and *Streptococcus faecalis.*

○ **What are the most common anaerobic organisms in the bowel?**

Bacteroides species and *Clostridium* species.

○ **True or False: A mechanical bowel preparation reduces the concentration of bacteria as well as the total number.**

False. The mechanical preparation reduces the amount of feces, whereas the antibiotic preparation reduces the bacterial concentration.

○ **What are the common adverse effects of antibiotic bowel preparation?**

Diarrhea. Pseudomembranous enterocolitis, monilial overgrowth resulting in stomatitis, malabsorption of protein, carbohydrate, and fat are the other disadvantages.

○ **True or False: The main reason for detubularization of the bowel segment used in urinary diversion is altering the shape of the reservoir from spherical to ellipsoid.**

False. Detubularized bowel segments provide greater capacity at lower pressure and require a shorter length of intestine than do intact segments; shape is of secondary importance (Colding-Jorgensen et al., 1993).

○ **Is there any advantage of nonrefluxing ureterointestinal anastomosis over refluxing anastomosis?**

No, there are no differences between nonrefluxing and refluxing ureterointestinal anastomosis with regard to symptomatic UTI, number of ureterointestinal anastomotic strictures, and incidence of glomerular filtration rate (GFR) deterioration (Kristjansson, 1995a, 1995b).

○ **True or False: The pressure within the renal pelvis in refluxing conduit diversions is elevated above normal.**

False. Peristaltic ureteral contractions dampen pressure transmission from the intestine to the renal pelvis, as a result it is not elevated above normal.

○ **Which of the small bowel antirefluxing procedures has the lowest incidence of stricture as an ureterointestinal anastomosis?**

LeDuc procedure (mucosal trench). It has also the highest success rate in preventing reflux.

○ **Is ureteral stenosis in a patient with a ureterointestinal anastomosis more common on one side than the other? Why?**

Ureterointestinal anastomotic strictures occur more commonly with the left ureter. Blood supply to the ureter may be compromised where the ureter crosses over the aorta beneath the inferior mesenteric artery. Additionally, aggressive stripping of adventitia and angulation of the ureter at the inferior mesenteric artery can result in ischemia and subsequent stricture formation.

○ **What technical steps are used to avoid ischemia to the distal ureter in order to decrease the chance of ureteroenteric strictures? And what would be the options of management in case they develop?**

Mobilization of the ureter should be limited and the distal pelvic portion discarded. If placement of the left ureter under the free edge of the left colonic mesentery causes angulation against the inferior mesenteric artery, the ureter may be brought through a higher avascular window within the colonic mesentery.

   The options of management for ureteroenteric strictures include retrograde or antegrade endoscopic or percutaneous dilatation, or dilation and incision. Stents are left routinely. Success rates are 20% to 50% versus 44% to 63% for incision-based techniques. Open surgical repair is a more invasive procedure, but it has a success rate >90% (Hautmann et al., 2007).

○ **How long are patients at risk for ureterointestinal strictures?**

Late strictures (>10 years) are not uncommon. Patients are at risk for ureterointestinal strictures for the life of the anastomosis.

○ **What is the optimal site for a stoma in a jejunal conduit?**

Left upper quadrant. The portion of jejunum to be utilized should be as distal as possible.

○ **Which type of abdominal stoma is preferable when a collection device is worn?**

Protruding stoma. It has a lower incidence of stomal stenosis and fewer peristomal skin problems.

○ **What is the potential complication of the abdominal stoma placed lateral to the rectus sheath?**

Parastomal hernia. Ideally, the stoma should be placed through the belly of the rectus muscle.

○ **Which stomas are associated with an increased likelihood of parastomal hernias?**

The incidence of parastomal hernias for end stomas is 1% to 4%, compared to 4% to 20% for loop stomas.

○ **What are the options if an ileal conduit won't reach the skin?**
  • Turnbull stoma (i.e., loop ileostomy).
  • Excise mesentery from the terminal part of the loop.
  • Mobilize the base of mesentery.
  • Redo the loop.

○ **Which part of colon is the most appropriate segment for a conduit in patients requiring an intestinal pyelostomy?**

Transverse colon. It is an excellent segment when an intestinal pyelostomy needs to be performed.

○ **Which part of colon is the most appropriate segment to use as a colon conduit in patients who have received extensive pelvic irradiation.**

Transverse colon. This segment of bowel typically lies outside the treated field in patients undergoing pelvic irradiation. The isolated segment will be well supplied by the middle colic artery.

○ **True or False: Routine postoperative use of nasogastric decompression is necessary in all patients following intestinal urinary diversion.**

False. The routine use of nasogastric decompression is unnecessary. Several studies showed that patients who did not receive a routine nasogastric tube fared better in terms of complications such as fever, atelectasis, and pneumonia, and advanced more quickly to a regular diet (Inman et al., 2003).

○ **True or False: In the early postoperative period, irrigation of the continent urinary reservoir is essential.**

True. In the early postoperative period, indwelling catheters must be carefully irrigated to prevent initial mucous buildup within the diversion. After removal of the indwelling catheter, patients with good spontaneous voiding and complete emptying usually pass the mucus spontaneously in the urine. In contrast, patients with incomplete emptying and those performing CIC may need to irrigate to remove retained mucous (Varol and Studer, 2004).

○ **What is the etiologic agent of pseudomembranous enterocolitis?**

Clostridium difficile. C. difficile elaborates cytotoxin A and cytotoxin B that cause diarrhea and enterocolitis.

○ **What are the common causes of the bowel obstruction following construction of intestinal anastomoses?**

Adhesions and recurrent cancer.

○ **True or False: The incidence of postoperative bowel obstruction in patients who have segments isolated from the colon is less than that occurring with ileum.**

True. Postoperative bowel obstruction occurs in approximately 10% of patients who have bowel segments isolated from the ileum for urinary tract reconstruction compared to 4% of patients who have bowel segments isolated from colon.

○ **What are the complications of intestinal anastomoses?**

Stenosis, obstruction, pseudo-obstructions (Ogilvie syndrome) (acute colonic pseudo-obstruction characterized by massive colonic dilatation in the absence of mechanical cause), intestinal leak, hemorrhage, fistulas, wound infections, pelvic abscesses, sepsis. One percent of these complications require operations.

○ **Which factors contribute to a potential anastomotic breakdown?**

Poor blood supply, local sepsis, drains placed in direct contact with an anastomosis, and performance of an anastomosis on previously irradiated bowel. Poor blood supply and local sepsis cause ischemia, whereas drains placed on the anastomosis increase the likelihood of an anastomotic leak.

○ **What are the most commonly isolated bacterial species from intestinal urinary reservoirs? Should they ever be treated?**

They are *E. coli, Pseudomonas, Klebsiella, Proteus,* and *Enterococcus* species (Mansson et al., 1986). They should not be treated as long as they are asymptomatic (Akerlund et al., 1994).

○   **Which patients with asymptomatic bacteriuria and an intestinal diversion should be treated?**

Only patients with predominant cultures of *Proteus* or *Pseudomonas* should be treated. Other bacteria should not be treated unless symptomatic.

○   **What are the consequences of persistent infection in intestinal segments?**

Strictures and renal deterioration. Persistent infection of the intestine exposed to urine may result in strictures, bacterial seeding of the upper tracts, and renal deterioration.

○   **What is the most common cause of stone formation in conduits and pouches?**

Foreign body such as staples or nonabsorbable sutures. Persistent infection, lowered pH, stasis, and hypercalciuria are the other factors.

○   **What are the rates of spontaneous pouch rupture? And how would you manage it?**

Spontaneous pouch ruptures occurs in approximately 1.5% to 4.3% cases. It should be considered in all patients with continent urinary diversion who present with acute abdominal pain. The pouch should be catheterized to check for urinary retention or hematuria and a CT scan is the preferred radiological investigation (Mansson et al., 2003; Nippgen et al., 2001).

   The overall clinical features of the patient dictate the choice between conservative treatment with drainage and antibiotics versus surgical exploration (Baseman et al., 1997; Choong et al., 1998).

○   **What are the most common complications of an ileal conduit and how frequent are they?**

Stomal and peristomal complications include skin lesions, stenosis, and retraction of the stoma. These were reported to occur in up to 31% of cases. Parastomal hernia is seen in 10% to 15% of cases (Iborra et al., 2001). Upper urinary tract deterioration is seen in 34% of cases. This is caused by chronic bacteriuria, reflux, and obstruction (Singh et al., 1997).

○   **True or False: Continent urinary diversions have a higher overall complication and reoperation rates in contrast to ileal conduits.**

False. There is no difference between continent urinary diversions and ileal conduits in terms of overall complication and reoperation rates (Parekh et al., 2000; Gburek et al., 1998).

○   **What should the upper level of sustained bladder pressure be in a patient with a continent neobladder?**

40 cm H_2O. Sustained pressures over 40 cm H_2O put the upper tract at risk.

○   **What is the most common complaint of a patient with an orthotopic diversion?**

Nocturnal enuresis. The loss of native bladder and its reflexes and the production of an increased urine volume are responsible for this complaint.

○ **What are the patterns of day time incontinence following orthotopic urinary diversion? How would you manage patients with a persistent, severe form of daytime incontinence?**

Daytime continence is achieved earlier postoperatively compared with nighttime continence and 85% to 90% of patients with orthotopic bladder will be continent during the day at 1 year from surgery, those rates may decrease 4 to 5 years postoperatively, in part because of decreased tone of the urethral sphincter with advanced age (Madersbacher et al., 2002).

Persistent severe incontinence after orthotopic urinary diversion may be treated by periurethral collagen injection, definitive placement of a urethral sling, or an artificial urinary sphincter (Tchetgen et al., 2000).

○ **What are the patterns of nighttime incontinence following orthotopic urinary diversion? And how would you manage persistent forms of nighttime incontinence?**

Nighttime continence requires a 6- to 12-month postoperative interval to reach maximum levels as the capacity and the compliance of the diversion increase. The reported prevalence of persistent nighttime leakage is between 27% and 50% at 1 year from surgery. The treatment of persistent enuresis consist of limiting fluid intake after the evening meal, voiding before going to sleep, and timed voiding once or twice during the night. Use of imipramine hydrochloride 25 mg at bedtime is reported to decrease nighttime leakage in up to 25% of patients (El Bahnasawy et al., 2000).

○ **Which is the most common electrolyte abnormality in patients who have an ileal conduit?**

Hyperchloremic metabolic acidosis. It is seen as a late complication in 13% of patients.

○ **What is the mechanism of hyperchloremic acidosis in patients with ileal diversions?**

Ionized transport of ammonium is responsible for hyperchloremic acidosis in patients with ileal diversions. When ammonium substitutes for sodium in the Na/H antiport, NH_4 is coupled with the exchange of bicarbonate for chloride. So, NH_4 is absorbed across the lumen into the blood in exchange for H_2CO_3. In addition, potassium channels in bowel lumen may contribute to ammonium entry to the blood.

○ **What are the symptoms of the electrolyte abnormality that occurs with ileal and colonic diversions.**

Easy fatigability, anorexia, weight loss, polydipsia, and lethargy. Exacerbation of diarrhea is often seen in patients with a ureterosigmoidostomy.

○ **True or False: Normal serum pH and bicarbonate exclude metabolic acidosis in patients with intestinal urinary diversion.**

False. Normal serum pH and bicarbonate do not exclude severely compensated metabolic acidosis, blood gas analysis and body weight measurement are required. If possible, these patients should not be given hydrogen antagonists and/or proton pump inhibitors, because these contribute to systemic acidosis by preventing hydrogen excretion with subsequent bicarbonate preservation on the cellular side (Mills and Studer, 1999).

○ **What is the optimal management of hyperchloremic metabolic acidosis in a patient with intestinal urinary diversion?**

The key to successful management is proper diagnosis by exclusion of urinary infection and sepsis, as well as awareness of the salt-losing syndrome. Proper treatment includes catheter reinsertion to insure good drainage and to minimize further chemical reabsorption, rehydration with intravenous normal saline, and correction of acidosis with sodium bicarbonate at a dose of 1.3 g tid. Patients with incomplete emptying and those with reduced renal function are most vulnerable to these metabolic problems (Racioppi et al., 1999).

○ **What is the consequence of the treatment of metabolic acidosis by NaHCO₃ alone?**

Severe hypokalemia. The treatment must involve both correction of the acidosis with bicarbonate and replacement of potassium. Potassium citrate may be helpful.

○ **What is the treatment of persistent hyperchloremic metabolic acidosis in patients with ileal conduits if an excessive sodium load is undesirable?**

It has been shown in animal models that both chlorpromazine and nicotinic acid result in inhibition of cyclic AMP, which impedes chloride ion transport, so HCO_3 levels increase (Koch and McDougal, 1985). These agents used alone do not correct the acidosis in humans, but they limit its development and thus reduce the need for alkalinizing agents. Chlorpromazine may be given in a dose of 25 mg tid and should be used with care in adults because there are many untoward side effects, including tardive dyskinesia. Nicotinic acid may be given in a dose of 400 mg tid or qid and should not be used in patients with peptic ulcer disease or significant hepatic insufficiency (Dahl and McDougal, 2007).

○ **Which kind of urinary diversion has the highest possibility of hypokalemia?**

Ureterosigmoidostomies. Ileal segments reabsorb some of the potassium when exposed to high concentrations of potassium in the urine whereas colon does not.

○ **What are the causes of hypokalemia in patients with intestinal urinary diversion and what would be the treatment?**

The potassium depletion is probably owing to renal potassium wasting as a consequence of renal damage, osmotic diuresis, and gut loss through intestinal secretion. Treatment with potassium citrate is often effective especially for patients with colonic reservoir (Koch et al., 1990).

○ **What kinds of electrolyte abnormalities are seen in patients with a jejunal conduit?**

Hyponatremic, hypochloremic, and hyperkalemic metabolic acidosis. Sodium chloride replacement and thiazides are the treatment of choice.

○ **What is the likely diagnosis of a patient with a jejunal conduit who has lethargy, nausea, vomiting, dehydration, muscular weakness, and an elevated temperature?**

Metabolic disturbance. Hyponatremia, hypochloremia, hyperkalemia, azotemia, and acidosis are seen in patients with jejunal conduits.

○ **How effective is IV hyperalimentation for the treatment of the metabolic disturbances in a patient with a jejunal conduit?**

Administering hyperalimentation solutions may exacerbate the syndrome.

○ **Which electrolyte abnormalities are seen when the stomach is used for urinary diversion?**

Hypochloremic, hypokalemic metabolic alkalosis. This is a more significant problem if the patient has concomitant azotemia.

○ **True or False: Hypergastrinemia may occur following gastric pouch orthotopic bladder formation.**

True. Hydrochloric acid produced by the parietal cells in the body of the stomach has a negative feedback on antral gastrin secretion. When the body of the stomach is removed this negative feedback mechanism may be impaired.

○ **What are the most likely causes of altered sensorium in a patient with a urinary diversion.**

Magnesium deficiency, drug intoxication, hyperammonemia, or diabetic hyperglycemia (this is not a consequence of the intestinal diversion).

○ **What are the causes of magnesium deficiency in patients with intestinal urinary diversion.**

Magnesium deficiency is usually due to nutritional depletion, but it may result from renal wasting, altered calcium metabolism, acidosis, and sulfate metabolism (McDougal and Koch, 1989).

○ **In which type of urinary diversion is altered sensorium most commonly found?**

Ureterosigmoidostomy. It has been reported for those with ileal conduits as well.

○ **True or False: Acute changes in ammonia load results in significant changes in serum ammonia levels when hepatic function is normal.**

False. The hepatic reserve for ammonia clearance is great, and it is unlikely that acute changes in ammonia loads results in significant changes in serum ammonia levels when hepatic function is normal. Patients who have ammoniogenic coma with clinically normal.

Liver functions generally have a significant infection with a urease-producing bacterium. Often, the infection is associated with obstruction of the urinary tract. Direct access of bacteria and endotoxin to the liver via the portal circulation results in altered hepatic metabolism without significant alteration in hepatic enzyme concentrations (McDougal, 1992).

○ **What is the treatment of ammoniagenic coma?**

Draining the urinary intestinal diversion to prevent urine exposure to the intestine for extended periods of time, administration of neomycin to reduce the ammonia load from the enteric tract, and limitation of protein consumption should be done to limit the patient's nitrogen load. In severe cases, arginine glutamate 50 g in 1000 mL of 5% dextrose in water intravenously to complex the ammonia in the gut and to prevent its absorption. Additionally, lactulose may be given orally or per rectum.

○ **True or False: Serum concentrations of urea and creatinine are less accurate measures of renal function after enteric diversion.**

True. Urea and creatinine are reabsorbed by both the ileum and the colon.

○ **What is the most accurate means of determining renal function in patients with a urinary diversion?**

Measurement of renal function with serial serum determination of 51Cr-EDTA after bolus injection is the most accurate method of determining renal function. This agent crosses the intestinal mucosa in negligible quantities.

○ **Which classes of drugs can be problematic in patients with urinary intestinal diversion regarding drug toxicity?**

Drugs that are absorbed by the gastrointestinal tract and excreted unchanged by the kidney. This includes phenytoin, certain antibiotics, and methotrexate.

○ **What is the mechanism of hypocalcemia in intestinal urinary diversion?**

Hypocalcemia is a consequence of depleted body calcium stores and excessive renal wasting. Chronic acidosis is buffered by carbonate in the bone, with subsequent release of calcium into the circulation. The kidneys clear the released calcium, resulting in a gradual decrease in body calcium stores. Renal tubular absorption of calcium is also inhibited directly by sulfate and enhanced by acidosis. Treatment consists of calcium therapy (McDougal and Koch, 1989).

○ **What is the cause of bone demineralization in intestinal urinary diversion? Could it be prevented?**

The cause is complex, but long-term changes in acid–base balance are likely the major contributory factor. Other causes are vitamin D resistance and excessive calcium loss by the kidney. It has been shown in animals with urinary diversion that oral supplementation with bicarbonate can prevent demineralization even in the absence of significant systemic acidosis (Inman et al., 2003). Some institutions now recommend oral sodium bicarbonate at a dose of 1.3 g tid when base deficit is >2.5 mmol/L (Stein et al., 1997).

○ **A patient with urinary diversion has hip pain, lethargy, and proximal myopathy. What is the diagnosis?**

Osteomalacia.

○ **What are the abnormalities in serum chemistry in a patient who develops osteomalacia?**

The calcium is either low or normal, the alkaline phosphatase is elevated, and the phosphate is low or normal.

○ **In a patient with osteomalacia, you've corrected the acidosis and provided dietary calcium. What is the next step?**

1-α-hydroxycholecalciferol should be administered. This is a vitamin D metabolite that is more potent than vitamin D_2.

○ **Loss of which bowel segment may cause vitamin B_{12} and bile salt malabsorption?**

Terminal ileum.

○ **What is the effect of vitamin B_{12} deficiency?**

Vitamin B_{12} deficiency results in macrocytic anemia and neurological degeneration.

○ **What length of time is required for the depletion of vitamin B_{12} stores in the complete absence of absorption in a patient who has an extensive terminal ileum resection?**

Three to four years. Partial malabsorption may take up to 30 years to become clinically manifest.

○ **What are typical neurological manifestations of vitamin B_{12} deficiency?**

Peripheral neuropathy, optic atrophy, subacute combined degeneration of the spinal cord, and dementia.

○ **Loss of which segment of bowel is associated with folic acid malabsorption?**

Jejunum. In addition, malabsorption of fat and calcium may be seen.

○ **True or False: In patients with ileal neobladder, vitamin B$_{12}$ and folic acid levels should be measured on a regular basis starting 2 years after surgery.**

True. According to a recent recommendation by a WHO consensus conference on bladder cancer, vitamin B$_{12}$ and folic acid levels should be routinely measured starting from year 2 after surgery (Hautmann et al., 2007).

○ **What is the lipid profile effect of a patient in whom 60- to 100-cm ileum are removed from the fecal stream?**

Serum cholesterol decreases, while triglycerides increase.

○ **What are the major consequences of lipid malabsorption seen in patients with ileal resection?**

A deficiency of the fat-soluble vitamins (A, D, E, K) and an increase in incidence of gallstones and renal stones.

○ **In which part of the intestinal segments used for urinary diversion does the least net water movement occur?**

Stomach. It is followed by the colon, ileum, and jejunum, respectively.

○ **What is the most common histologic type of cancer seen in association with urinary intestinal diversion?**

Adenocarcinoma, especially following ureterosigmoidostomy. These patients should be followed by stool occult blood and/or colonoscopy after 5 years postdiversion.

○ **A 27-year-old male with spina bifida undergoes an ileal conduit undiversion. How should the defunctionalized intestinal conduit segment be managed?**

Excision of the segment is appropriate. If left in situ, it has malignant potential.

○ **A patient is diagnosed with a recurrent invasive lesion in the urethra following radical cystectomy and neobladder construction. What is your treatment?**

Urethrectomy. Convert to a continent diversion, if possible, or remove the reservoir and convert to a conduit.

○ **Which kind of neobladder is the most amenable for conversion of a patient to a conduit?**

Studer neobladder. It has a 15- to 20-cm isoperistaltic proximal ileal limb.

○ **What is the preferred method of delivery in a pregnant women with intestinal urinary diversion?**

Elective cesarean section before the onset of labor is the preferred method of delivery in patients with urinary diversion, especially with an orthotopic bladder substitution. Vaginal delivery may result in damage to the pelvic floor muscles and subsequently affect continence mechanisms.

Cesarean section should be preformed through a high incision. The mesentery of the reservoir is usually pushed away from the gravid uterus. An experienced reconstructive urologist should be involved and have time to review thoroughly the patient's reconstructed anatomy before the case (Hensle et al., 2004).

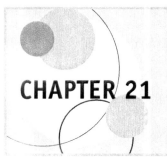

CHAPTER 21

Urinary Diversion and Undiversion

Christopher L. Coogan, MD, and Frederick L. Taylor, MD

○ **What is the electrolyte abnormality most commonly seen when stomach is used in the urinary tract?**

Hypochloremic metabolic alkalosis. This is secondary to the HCl secretion by the stomach segment, involving the H^+/K^+ ATPase secretory mechanism of the gastric mucosa.

○ **What is the electrolyte abnormality most commonly seen when jejunum is used in the urinary tract?**

Hyponatremic, hypochloremic, hyperkalemic metabolic acidosis. This has been termed the "jejunal conduit syndrome." This syndrome can be quite debilitating, resulting in nausea, anorexia, lethargy, fever, and even death. The more proximal the segment used, the more likely the syndrome is to develop, secondary to the increased surface area available, due to increased villi and microvilli. The jejunum should be used only when there are no other acceptable segments available for use.

○ **What is the electrolyte abnormality most commonly seen when ileum or colon is used in the urinary tract?**

Hyperchloremic metabolic acidosis. This is caused by the substitution of ammonium for sodium in the Na/H transport. Therefore, ammonium chloride is absorbed into the bloodstream in exchange for carbonic acid (CO_2 and H_2O).

○ **What is the cause of the altered sensorium occasionally associated with intestinal conduits?**

Magnesium deficiency, drug intoxication, or abnormalities of ammonia metabolism. This should be treated with drainage of the urinary intestinal diversion (Foley or rectal tube), administration of neomycin (to reduce the enteric ammonia load), minimizing protein intake, and treating the underlying condition.

○ **True or False: Continent urinary diversions are generally associated with fewer metabolic abnormalities.**

False. Given the longer dwell time of urine in contact with the intestinal segment used, both neobladders and continent urinary diversions are associated with a higher risk of electrolyte and metabolic abnormalities.

○ **True or False: Mechanical bowel preparation results in a reduction in bacteria per gram of enteric contents.**

False. Mechanical bowel preparation will reduce the total number of bacteria in the gut, but not their concentration.

○   **What is the most common stomal complication following urinary diversion?**

Stomal stenosis. The incidence is reported to be 20% to 25% for ileal conduits and 10% to 20% for colon conduits. Other complications include bleeding, bowel necrosis, dermatitis, parastomal hernias, and stomal prolapse.

○   **Which segment of bowel is most suitable for nonrefluxing ureterointestinal anastomoses?**

Colon. Numerous anastomoses (Leadbetter and Clarke, Goodwin, Strickler, and Pagano) employ the seromuscular strength of the tenia to create a backing for the submucosal tunnel needed for the antireflux procedure.

○   **What type of ureteroileal anastomosis carries the highest risk of ureteral stricture?**

Antirefluxing ureteroileal anastomosis. In general, antirefluxing anastomoses carry a higher risk of stricture that persists for the life of the conduit.

○   **Which method of repair (open or endourologic) of ureteral anastomotic strictures has the higher success rate and by how much?**

Although open and endourological methods of repair have been successful, open repair carries a higher success rate (approximately 75% vs. 60% for endourological methods).

○   **What is the most common site of ureteral stricture after ileal conduit formation not at the ureteroileal anastomosis?**

The left ureter as it crosses over the aorta. As the left ureter crosses over the aorta and underneath the inferior mesenteric artery it is both extrinsically compressed and angulated, which may result in stricture formation. In addition, aggressive stripping of the periureteral adventitia may result in vascular compromise at this level, also predisposing to stricture.

○   **Briefly describe the Bricker ureterointestinal anastomosis.**

The Bricker anastomosis is a refluxing end-to-side anastomosis. It involves spatulating the distal end of the ureter, and stitching the full thickness of the bowel to the full thickness of the ureter. This anastomosis boasts both technical ease as well as a low complication rate (see figure).

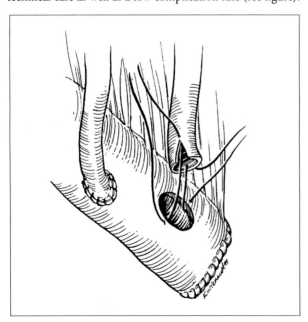

○   **Briefly describe the Wallace ureterointestinal anastomosis.**

The Wallace anastomosis is a refluxing end-to-end anastomosis. Different techniques are described, but the concept is that the ureteral ends are spatulated and sewn together into a common opening. This "common ureter" is then anastomosed to the end of the intestinal segment used. It has a lower stricture rate due to the wide anastomosis, but is not recommended for patients with extensive carcinoma in situ or a high likelihood of recurrence in the ureter. Recurrence in the distal aspect of one ureter could block the egress of both ureters, causing bilateral obstruction (see figure).

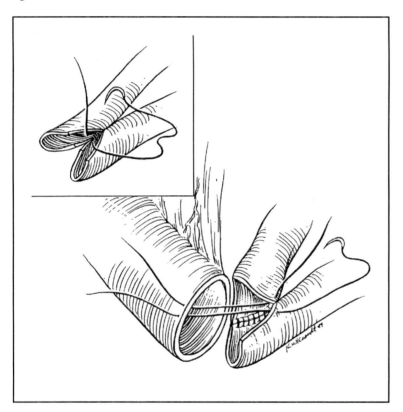

○   **What is the generally accepted cut-off value of serum creatinine at which continent diversions and orthotopic neobladders are no longer considered?**

2.0 mg/dL. Due to the extended dwell time of urine in contact with the intestinal segments used, continent diversions and orthotopic neobladders should be considered only for those patients with good renal function.

○   **What renal parameters must be met to consider continent diversion in a patient with a serum creatinine greater than 2.0 mg/dL?**

Urine pH 5.8 or less after ammonium chloride load, urine osmolality of 600 mOsm/kg or greater with water deprivation, GFR greater than or equal to 35 mL/min, and minimal protein in the urine.

○   **What percentage of patients with normal preoperative creatinine and GFR who undergo conduit diversion develop renal deterioration?**

Approximately 18% to 20% of patients with ileal conduit diversion will have progressive renal deterioration, which may lead to death from renal failure in approximately 6% of patients.

○   **What long-term effects can urinary intestinal diversion have on the bony skeleton?**

Osteomalacia. Osteomalacia (or renal rickets) has been reported most commonly with ureterosigmoidostomy, but also with colon and ileal conduits, and ileal ureters. It is thought to be secondary to acidosis, vitamin D resistance, and excessive calcium loss by the kidney.

○   **What type of reservoir requires nocturnal emptying?**

Ureterosigmoidostomy. Although all continent reservoirs may require nocturnal emptying to prevent overdistention, the increased risk of metabolic acidosis from ionized transport of ammonium via the Na^+/H^+ antiport in ureterosigmoidostomy necessitates nocturnal emptying.

○   **True or False: Approximately 75% of urine specimens from ileal conduits are infected.**

True. Intestine, in contrast to urothelium, generally lives symbiotically with bacterial flora. Most patients have no sequelae from their chronic bacteruria, and are not treated unless they develop symptoms.

○   **What bacterial infections from conduits or continent diversions should be treated?**

Cultures dominantly positive for *Proteus*, *Pseudomonas*, or *Klebsiella* species should be treated. Infections caused by *Proteus* and *Pseudomonas* have been linked to upper tract deterioration, and all three organisms are urea-splitting, making patients infected with these organisms more likely to form stones.

○   **What is the urinary diversion procedure that puts the patient at the highest risk for development of carcinoma of the intestinal segment?**

Ureterosigmoidostomy. Following ureterosigmoidostomy, as many as 40% of patients will develop tumors at the ureterosigmoid anastomosis given sufficient time. Approximately half of the tumors are adenocarcinoma and the rest are benign polyps. The mean latency period between ureterosigmoidostomy and the diagnosis of tumor is 26 years.

○   **If performing undiversion following ureterosigmoidostomy, what must be done to minimize the risk of tumorigenesis?**

The distal ureteral stumps must be removed from contact with the colonic epithelium. Adenocarcinoma has been reported to occur when the ureterointestinal anastomoses were left in situ, even when the diversion is defunctionalized.

○   **Briefly describe the Mitrofanoff procedure.**

The Mitrofanoff procedure is the creation of a continent, catheterizable urinary diversion. It is usually performed with the appendix, which is anastomosed to the conduit (or bladder) in a tunneled fashion (similar to a ureteroneocystostomy). The other end of the appendix is brought out to the anterior abdominal wall, and is utilized for clean intermittent catheterization.

○   **In patients who have received extensive pelvic radiation, which intestinal segment is preferred for creation of a conduit?**

The transverse colon. Given its position within the abdominal cavity, it is the most likely to have remained unaffected by previous pelvic radiation.

○   **What is the blood supply of the appendix?**

The appendiceal artery, a branch usually off of the ileocolic artery, which arises from the superior mesenteric artery.

○   **What is the source of continence for orthotopic neobladders?**

In both the male and female, the preserved striated external sphincter is the source of continence. Daytime continence rates of greater than 95% can be expected if this mechanism is surgically spared.

○   **What are the two phenomena thought to be responsible for nocturnal enuresis following orthotopic neobladder procedures?**

First, the spinal reflex arc that recruits external sphincter contraction is gone, as the native bladder (and therefore the afferent nerves) has been removed. The other hypothesis is that there is a significant reabsorption and recirculation of urinary constituents and metabolites that stimulate increased urinary volume, resulting in nocturnal enuresis.

○   **Briefly describe the ureterointestinal anastomosis described by Studer and colleagues.**

The Studer ileal neobladder incorporates a novel approach to prevent reflux. The proximal limb of small bowel is left intact for a length of 20 to 25 cm, and the neobladder is constructed from the distal 35 to 40 cm of ileum. The ureters are then anastomosed to the intact proximal limb in a standard (Bricker) ureterointestinal refluxing anastomosis. This proximal limb of ileum retains its peristaltic integrity, effectively dampening back-pressure on the upper urinary tract (see figure).

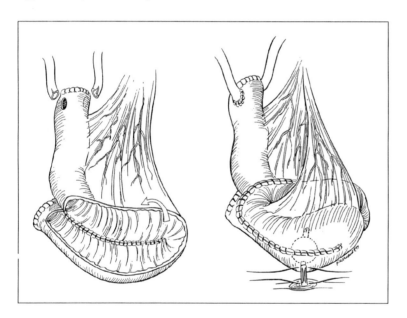

○   **What tumor location in women is a contraindication to orthotopic neobladder formation after radical cystectomy?**

Bladder neck involvement. Patients with bladder neck involvement often have involvement of the anterior vaginal wall, and orthotopic neobladder formation could compromise the margins of resection.

○   **What tumor location in men is a contraindication to orthotopic neobladder formation after radical cystectomy?**

The prostatic urethral stroma. It is recommended that all men being considered for an orthotopic neobladder undergo formal transurethral resection of the prostatic urethra, and are candidates only if the prostatic stroma is free of disease. Currently, some advocate frozen sections of the urethral margin to assess suitability for a neobladder.

○ **What are the four basic methods of achieving continence in a urinary diversion?**

The Mitrofanoff principle, the ileocecal valve, the nipple valve, and the hydraulic valve.

○ **What is the continence mechanism in an Indiana pouch?**

The buttressed ileocecal valve. Neourethral pressure profiles show that the continence zone is confined only to the area of the ileocecal valve, rendering imbricating sutures necessary only for this area.

○ **True or False: The appendix is removed during formation of the Indiana pouch.**

True. The buttressed ileocecal valve is the continence mechanism of the Indiana pouch. The appendix is removed, as it may serve as a nidus for infection and abscess formation.

○ **Describe the Benchekroun hydraulic ileal valve.**

Twelve to fourteen centimeter of ileum is selected and reverse intussusception is performed such that serosa covers the entire segment and mucosa apposes mucosa. The ends are then sutured in position, allowing space between sutures to allow the mucosal surface to fill with urine as pouch pressures increase. The blunt serosal end is secured to the abdominal wall, and catheterization is done so that the catheter passes through a serosally lined channel into the conduit. When pressures rise in the conduit, urine flows into the mucosal space of the valve, coapting the serosal surface, ensuring continence (see figure).

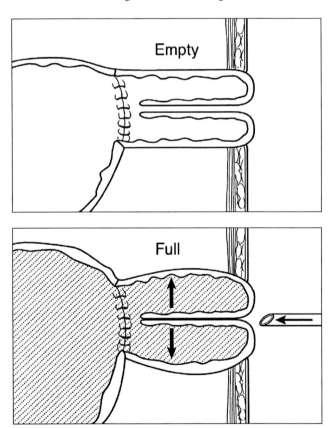

○ **What is the most common complication of the Benchekroun hydraulic ileal valve?**

Stomal stenosis. Stomal stenosis requiring surgical revision has been reported in up to 73% of patients undergoing this procedure. Devagination of the valve is another complication, with a reported incidence of up to 36%.

○ **What is the "pipe stem" deformity of the ileal conduit, what is the cause and how should it be treated?**

The "pipe stem" deformity of an ileal conduit is the radiographic appearance on loopogram of strictured areas along the course of the loop. This results in a thin, noncompliant loop with decreased peristalsis and propulsion of urine with subsequent deterioration of the upper urinary tracts. The cause is vascular insufficiency. Treatment usually requires replacement of the entire loop.

○ **What is the incidence of stones in patients with ileal conduits?**

Approximately 20%. The etiology of stone formation is multifactorial. Staples and nonabsorbable sutures may act as a nidus for stone formation. There is an increased incidence of bacteruria following intestinal diversion, which may also cause stone formation.

○ **True or False: Patients with continent diversions are at increased risk of reservoir stones.**

True. This is secondary to the increased urinary excretion of calcium, magnesium, and phosphate in continent diversions as compared to ileal conduits. Also, patients with long segments of ileum used for reconstruction (continent diversions and orthotopic neobladders) may have secondary hyperoxaluria.

○ **What is "pouchitis"?**

Pouchitis is a condition described in continent urinary diversions that is manifested by pain in the region of the pouch and increased pouch contractility. This may result in temporary failure of the continence mechanism. Antibiotic treatment usually results in resolution of these symptoms.

○ **What is the continence mechanism of the Kock pouch?**

The surgical principle used in achieving continence by the Kock pouch is the intussuscepted nipple valve. This surgical procedure is felt to be the most technically difficult to perform of all of the continence mechanisms.

○ **What are the most common complications of the Kock pouch?**

Nipple failure resulting in loss of continence is the most common complication following Kock pouch formation. This can be expected in 10% to 15% of cases even in the hands of the most experienced surgeons.

○ **What is the continence mechanism of the Penn pouch?**

The Mitrofanoff principle. The Penn pouch was the first conduit to utilize the Mitrofanoff principle, using the appendix tunneled into the tenia of the ascending colon.

○ **What is a potential drawback to the use of the appendix as a continence mechanism?**

The appendix has a small luminal diameter, allowing catheterization only with a 12F or 14F coudé catheter. Since intestinal reservoirs produce large amounts of mucus, this often makes irrigation and emptying difficult. Also, the appendix may be surgically absent or of insufficient length for use.

○   **What are the contraindications to ureterosigmoidostomy?**

Hydronephrosis, pelvic radiation, neurogenic bladder, renal, or hepatic dysfunction. Dilated upper tracts are more subject to reflux and obstruction, which can be deleterious to renal function. Previous pelvic radiation will likely involve both the sigmoid and the pelvic ureters. Patients with neurogenic bladder usually have associated functional bowel abnormalities as well. Renal insufficiency is a contraindication to any continent diversion. Patients with hepatic dysfunction should not undergo ureterosigmoidostomy because of the risk of ammonia intoxication.

○   **What is essential in the preoperative evaluation of patients selected for rectal bladder urinary diversion or ureterosigmoidostomy?**

Anal sphincter integrity testing. Patients should be required to retain an enema solution of liquid and solid material in an upright and ambulatory position without soilage for a specified amount of time. Some investigators recommend a 500 mL mixture of thin oatmeal that the patient is asked to retain for 1 hour.

○   **Which patients should undergo routine urinary cytology after continent urinary diversion?**

All patients undergoing continent diversion. Malignancy has been reported in all bowel segments exposed to urine. Thus, urinary cytology should be monitored in all patients undergoing continent diversion regardless of whether or not diversion was performed for a malignant condition.

○   **Which patients should undergo routine colonoscopy after continent urinary diversion?**

All patients whose urine and fecal streams are mixed. In addition to routine cytology in all patients whose urine stream is diverted via an intestinal segment, patients whose urine and fecal streams are mixed should undergo routine colonoscopy to evaluate for intestinal malignancies.

○   **True or False: Renal insufficiency is a contraindication to urinary undiversion.**

False. Many candidates for undiversion will likely have renal insufficiency, either secondary to their underlying pathology or the diversion itself. If transplantation becomes necessary in these patients, it is better done into a functioning lower urinary tract than a urinary diversion.

○   **With what intestinal segment is the "hematuria–dysuria" syndrome associated?**

Stomach. Following gastrocystoplasty, the urine is markedly acidic, which can lead to bladder pain, dysuria, hematuria, and skin erosion in approximately 30% of patients.

○   **What is the gastrointestinal consequence of the loss of the ileocecal valve?**

In the short-term, this results in frequent bowel movements and diarrhea. Most patients recover bowel regularity following intestinal adaptation or pharmacologic therapy, but some patients have steatorrhea or diarrhea refractory to medical management following loss of the ileocecal valve.

○   **True or False: Refluxing ureterointestinal anastomoses have a higher incidence of renal deterioration than nonrefluxing anastomoses following conduit formation in patients with normal ureters.**

False. In patients with normal peristaltic contractions of the ureter, there does not seem to be detrimental pressure transmission to the renal pelvis in patients with refluxing anastomoses. Additionally, the presence of nonrefluxing anastomoses does not prevent bacterial colonization of the renal pelvis.

○ **What are the contraindications to ileal conduit formation?**

The contraindications to ileal conduits are short bowel syndrome, inflammatory disease of the small intestine, and previous radiation to the pelvis.

○ **What type of continent diversion has the smallest immediate postoperative capacity?**

Ileal pouches. Ileal pouches (e.g., Kock or T-pouches) have immediate postoperative volumes of approximately 150 mL. In contrast, right colon pouches routinely have an immediate postoperative capacity of approximately 300 mL. This information is essential for patients to catheterize themselves with appropriate frequency during the initial postoperative period.

○ **What is the most common composition of stones formed in urinary diversions?**

The stones are usually of mixed composition and may be made up of struvite, calcium oxalate, calcium phosphate, and uric acid. Foreign materials may act as a nidus for stone formation within the diversion.

○ **What type of continent reservoir is most likely to form stones?**

The Kock pouch. Another unique complication of the Kock pouch is the higher incidence of stones, secondary to the use of staples on the intussuscepted nipple valve.

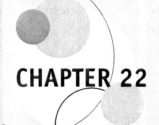

CHAPTER 22 # Male Infertility

Howard H. Kim, MD, and
Marc Goldstein, MD, DSc (hon), FACS

NUMBERS TO REMEMBER

○ **What are the WHO reference values for count, concentration, motility, and morphology on semen analysis?**

A total count of 40 million spermatozoa per ejaculate or more, concentration of 20 million per mL or more, progressive motility of greater than or equal to 50%, and 30% or more normal forms by WHO criteria define baseline criteria for normal fertility.

○ **What percentage of couples are infertile and how often is a male factor present?**

Fifteen percent of couples are infertile, and in fifty percent of cases, a male factor is present.

○ **What percentage of infertile men have varicoceles?**

Thirty to forty-five percent.

○ **What percentage of infertile men have no known cause for their infertility even after a thorough workup?**

25% to 30%.

○ **What percentage of infertile men have azoospermia and what percentage of these men have obstructive azoospermia?**

10% to 15% of infertile men and <1% of all men have azoospermia. Obstruction accounts for 40% of all cases of azoospermia.

○ **What percentage of infertile men have chromosomal abnormalities?**

Six percent.

○ **What percentage of men with nonobstructive azoospermia have Y chromosome microdeletions?**

Three to thirteen percent.

○   **What percentage of men with unilateral and bilateral cryptorchidism have oligozoospermia on semen analysis?**

Thirty percent of men with unilateral and fifty percent of men with bilateral cryptorchidism have oligozoospermia on semen analysis.

○   **A couple has one 4-year-old child and is now having difficulty conceiving again. The male partner has oligoasthenozoospermia and normal hormonal testing. What abnormality can be expected on physical examination?**

A varicocele is found in up to 80% of men with secondary infertility. A varicocele has been shown to cause progressive worsening of semen parameters.

○   **What percentage of patients undergoing varicocelectomy for infertility can expect to have improvement in semen parameters and which parameters are most often improved?**

Approximately 70% of patients have improvement in semen parameters after varicocelectomy. Sperm motility is most often improved followed by count and then morphology.

○   **What is the live birth rate for in vitro fertilization (IVF) with intracytoplasmic sperm injection (ICSI) for male factor infertility?**

Approximately 30% to 40% per cycle.

○   **What is the most important predictor of IVF/ICSI outcomes?**

Age of the female partner.

○   **What percentage of men develop significant antisperm antibodies after vasectomy?**

Sixty percent.

○   **What percentage of men who have undergone vasectomy eventually seek reversal?**

Six to ten percent.

ANATOMY AND PHYSIOLOGY

○   **The pituitary hormones FSH and LH act on which cells in the testis and what are the specific mediators of feedback inhibition from these cells to the pituitary gland?**

FSH acts on the Sertoli cell and inhibin is the mediator of its feedback inhibition; LH acts on the Leydig cell and testosterone is the chemical mediator of feedback inhibition.

○   **Which cells in the testis form the blood–testis barrier and exclude sperm from recognition by the immune system?**

Tight junctional complexes between adjacent Sertoli cells create the blood–testis barrier making the seminiferous tubule an immunologically privileged site.

○   **Autonomic innervation of the testis is provided by which nerve or nerves?**

The superior spermatic nerve and the inferior spermatic nerve.

○ **A germ cell undergoes how many meiotic divisions before producing a mature sperm?**

Germ cells undergo multiple mitotic divisions to produce many primary spermatocytes, which then undergo two meiotic divisions to first produce secondary spermatocytes and then spermatids.

○ **Aside from sperm transportation, what is the most important function of the epididymis?**

Sperm maturation occurs along the length of the epididymis resulting in mature sperm capable of fertilizing oocytes.

○ **Prostate specific antigen (PSA) plays what role in male fertility?**

The protein secreted by prostate epithelium is a protease enzyme involved in semen liquefaction.

○ **Which substance produced in the seminal vesicle is the major energy source for sperm metabolism?**

Fructose.

○ **What is the role of the acrosome and where is it located?**

The acrosome forms a cap on the sperm head and contains the enzymes necessary for drilling into the zona pellucida of the oocyte.

○ **Do the testis, epididymis, and vas deferens share the same embryological origin?**

No. The testis develops from coelomic epithelium of the genital ridge and underlying mesenchyme. Primordial germ cells migrate to this area. The epididymis and vas deferens, however, develop from the Wolffian (mesonephric) duct.

○ **What is the normal adult testicular size?**

Testes measure 15 to 25 cm^3 in volume and 4.5 to 5 cm in longitudinal length in young healthy men.

○ **When evaluating the ejaculatory ducts by TRUS, what is their normal size parameters?**

They are usually 2- to 8-mm wide and 2- to 3-cm long.

○ **In performing a subinguinal varicocelectomy, the internal spermatic artery is inadvertently ligated and divided. By what blood supply might the testis still survive?**

The deferential artery and the cremasteric artery also supply blood flow to the testis.

○ **A patient develops retrograde ejaculation after RPLND for testis cancer. Which nerves were likely injured and which class of medications may be used to treat the problem?**

Thoracolumbar sympathetic nerves control closure of the bladder neck during seminal emission via norepinephrine. α-adrenergic agonist drugs have been used to stimulate closure of the bladder neck.

○ **Prolactin release is restricted by what natural chemical?**

Dopamine from the hypothalamus.

○ **What is the effect of thyrotropin-releasing hormone and vasoactive intestinal peptide on prolactin secretion?**

They stimulate prolactin release.

○ **What is the total length of the seminiferous tubules of a normal testis?**
The length is 250 m.

○ **Sperm maturation from spermatogonium to mature sperm takes how long?**
Seventy-five to ninety days.

○ **At what age do men lose 50% of their Sertoli and Leydig cells?**
Age 50 for Sertoli cells, age 60 for Leydig cells.

○ **What are the glands of Littre?**
Another name for the periurethral glands.

○ **What is the average length of the vas deferens?**
The average length is 30 to 35 cm.

○ **What is the origin of the deferential artery?**
The internal iliac (hypogastric) artery or its branches, the superior or inferior vesicle artery.

○ **Blood entering the testis is 2°C to 4°C lower than rectal (body) temperature as a result of what mechanism?**
Countercurrent heat exchange system of the testicular vasculature.

DIAGNOSIS

○ **What physical finding is most predictive of active sperm production in the testis?**
Testicular size and consistency.

○ **What is the most common finding on physical examination of infertility in men?**
Varicocele.

○ **A patient presents with azoospermia, low ejaculatory volume, and a semen pH of 6.5. Postejaculation urine is negative for sperm. The vasa deferentia are palpable. What is the next test that should be performed and what is the most likely diagnosis?**
Transrectal ultrasound of the prostate should be performed to rule out ejaculatory duct obstruction.

○ **When is a testis biopsy indicated in men with azoospermia?**
Normal serum FSH level, normal testes and palpable vasa on physical examination.

○ **Men with nonobstructive azoospermia can have DNA microdeletions in which genes on which chromosome?**
The AZF (AZoospermia Factor) genes on the Y chromosome.

◯ **Which AZF deletion has the best prognosis for successful testicular sperm extraction in men with nonobstructive azoospermia?**

AZFc. Men with complete AZFa or AZFb deletions have never had sperm successfully retrieved from their testes.

◯ **Men with congenital absence of the vas deferens (CAVD) can have mutations in which gene?**

The cystic fibrosis transmembrane conductance regulator (CFTR) gene on the long arm of chromosome 7.

◯ **A patient is found to have unilateral congenital absence of the vas deferens. The presence of which organ needs to be confirmed?**

The ipsilateral kidney may be absent due to lack of development of the mesonephric duct.

◯ **A patient with primary infertility is found to have a normal sperm count, but zero motility. Viability staining shows that the sperms are alive. Semen culture and antisperm antibody testing are negative. Which syndrome or disease should be suspected?**

Immotile cilia syndrome. If the patient also has chronic sinusitis, bronchiectasis, and situs inversus, he has Kartagener's syndrome.

◯ **A patient seen for infertility complains of a new onset right varicocele. What pathological entity should be suspected?**

An imaging study should be obtained to rule out a right-sided retroperitoneal mass.

◯ **A patient with Klinefelter's syndrome has a small number of sperm in his ejaculate. What would his karyotype most likely reveal?**

46, XY/47, XXY mosaic.

◯ **A patient with azoospermia has extremely small testicular size (6 cm³ volume) and an FSH of 26. The most likely diagnosis is?**

Primary testicular failure or hypergonadotropic hypogonadism. Also called nonobstructive azoospermia.

◯ **A patient with a history of unilateral testicular torsion presents with primary infertility. A semen analysis reveals normal volume and count, but significantly low motility as well as sperm agglutination. There is no evidence of infection. What condition should be suspected and by what test is it confirmed?**

In a patient with torsion, cryptorchidism, infection, obstruction or trauma, and the above-noted semen parameters, antisperm antibodies should be suspected. The direct immunobead assay is used to test for antisperm antibodies.

◯ **A patient presents with primary infertility. On examination, he has normal male secondary sex characteristics and slightly decreased testicular size. Semen analysis reveals normal volume and pH, but azoospermia. FSH is slightly elevated; LH and testosterone are normal. What are the most likely histologic findings on testis biopsy?**

Germ cell aplasia or Sertoli cell-only syndrome in which the seminiferous tubules are lined by Sertoli cells but no germ cells or maturation arrest in which germ cells are present but do not progress to mature spermatozoa.

○   **A patient with azoospermia is found to have very low levels of FSH, LH, and testosterone. He also reports anosmia. What is the diagnosis?**

This patient with hypogonadotropic hypogonadism has Kallmann's syndrome.

○   **A patient with primary infertility reports having had the mumps at age 6. Is this a clinically significant factor in his infertility?**

No. Prepubertal mumps does not appear to affect the testis while postpubertal mumps orchitis can result in significant testicular damage and atrophy.

○   **A bodybuilder who abuses anabolic steroids presents with azoospermia. What is the mechanism for this failure of sperm production and is it reversible?**

Exogenous androgenic steroids suppress gonadotropin secretion and interfere with spermatogenesis. This form of hypogonadism is usually reversible after discontinuation of steroid use, but in some cases it is permanent.

○   **A tall, thin patient presents for infertility evaluation. He is found to have gynecomastia. What will his testicular examination reveal? What will his semen analysis show and what is the underlying cause for his condition?**

This patient with Klinefelter's syndrome will have small, firm testes and azoospermia on semen analysis. His karyotype of 47, XXY results from nondisjunction of the meiotic chromosomes of the gametes of either parent.

○   **What commonly inhaled controlled substance is associated with infertility and by what mechanism?**

Marijuana can lead to a decrease in sperm concentration, motility, and abnormal morphology as well as decreased serum testosterone levels and gynecomastia. The drug alters the hypothalamic-pituitary–gonadal axis.

○   **How long does the process of spermatogenesis take? How long does it take for sperm to appear in the ejaculation?**

It takes 74 days for a mature sperm to develop from a primitive germ cell or spermatogonia. Including ductal transit time, the time from spermatogenesis to ejaculation is approximately 3 months.

○   **A 13-year-old boy is found to a have a grade II left-sided varicocele on a school sports physical examination. His testes are of equal, normal size and consistency. GnRH stimulation test reveals a normal LH and FSH response. Would you recommend elective varicocelectomy at this time?**

Fifteen percent of all males have a varicocele and only a small percentage of these men will have difficulties with fertility. With no evidence of decreased testicular volume and no exaggerated FSH release in response to GnRH, elective surgery would not be indicated at this time.

○   **A patient with primary infertility is found to have increased numbers of WBCs in the semen. What is this called and what are the possible causes? What needs to be tested for? Can seminal WBCs have an adverse affect on sperm function?**

Pyospermia (or leukocytospermia) may be due to either a genital tract infection or an inflammatory immunologic response. Cultures to rule out urinary and genital tract infection should be performed. The etiology may never be determined and pyospermia can resolve without specific treatment. Increased ejaculation is sometimes suggested. Seminal WBCs can produce reactive oxygen species (ROS) that adversely affect sperm function.

○ **How does testicular radiation exposure lead to infertility? How long after radiation therapy can it take for spermatogenesis to return and how long should a patient wait before trying to conceive after gonadal exposure to radiation?**

Ionizing radiation is lethal to sperm by increasing free radical formation. It also alters sperm head morphology and damages sperm chromatin structure. It can take up to 5 years for spermatogenesis to return. Direct effects on DNA can result in numerical and structural chromosomal abnormalities; therefore, conception should be avoided for 2 years.

○ **Describe the underlying cause of male infertility in Prader–Willi syndrome and Laurence–Moon–Biedl syndrome.**

Both have hypogonadotropic hypogonadism.

○ **What causes a fertile eunuch and how is the condition treated?**

Isolated LH deficiency. FSH is usually normal. Examination findings are large testes, lower ejaculate volumes, and eunuchoid body habitus. Treatment is hCG therapy.

○ **When is transrectal ultrasound used in the evaluation of male infertility?**

In men with azoospermia or severe oligozoospermia, palpable vasa deferentia, and low semen volume to rule out ejaculatory duct obstruction. It is also used to check the seminal vesicles.

○ **A 15-year-old boy is referred to you with a grade III left varicocele, an 18-cm³ volume right testis and a 12-cm³ volume left testis. What do you recommend?**

Left varicocelectomy. Grade III varicoceles are found in 20% of cases (3% of postpubertal boys) and pose the greatest risk for future infertility. Catch-up growth occurs in 80% of boys after varicocele repair.

○ **Which test should be performed on the female partner of a man with congenital absence of the vas deferens (CAVD)?**

Screening for cystic fibrosis transmembrane conductance regulator gene (CFTR) mutations.

○ **Men with obstructive azoospermia usually have what blood abnormally?**

Circulating antisperm antibodies.

○ **A low serum testosterone level is most often associated with what subjective/clinical disorder?**

Decreased libido.

○ **What are the prognostic indicators for a successful pregnancy after a vasectomy reversal?**

Partner age and fertility status, presence of sperm granuloma, and short obstruction interval.

SEMEN ANALYSIS AND LABORATORY ASSAYS

○ **Using Kruger strict criteria, what is the clinically significant threshold of normal forms that predicts good fertilization without ICSI?**

Four percent.

○ **Define oligozoospermia.**

Less than 20 million sperms per mL.

○ **What morphologic semen characteristics comprise the "stress pattern" often seen in patients with a varicocele?**

Increased numbers of sperm with tapered heads, immature germ cells, and amorphous sperm cells.

○ **The laboratory reports an increased number of round cells on semen analysis. What do these cells represent?**

Round cells are either prematurely released immature germ cells or white blood cells representing inflammation or infection. Immunohistochemical staining and the Endtz test can distinguish between the two.

○ **A patient is found to have a normal sperm count and zero motility. Which two laboratory tests can help distinguish between immotile and dead sperm?**

The hypoosmotic swelling test and viability staining can be used. Living sperm experience bulging of the plasma membrane and curling of the tails from fluid absorption under hypoosmotic conditions. Both tests reflect the integrity of the plasma membrane in living versus dead sperm.

○ **What semen parameters suggest the eventual need for ICSI?**

Less than 5% motility, less than 4% normal morphology, and less than 2 million sperms per mL. Patients with sperm extracted directly from the epididymis or testis proceed directly to ICSI.

○ **True or False: A semen fructose level less than 120 mg/dL suggests ejaculatory duct obstruction?**

True.

○ **How much binding in an immunobead test would be considered a positive test for antisperm antibodies?**

More than 15% to 20%.

○ **What is CASA?**

Computer **A**ided **S**emen **A**nalysis. It is quite labor intensive and expensive. Also, it is less useful with very low or very high counts. It's most useful as a research tool.

TREATMENT

○ **A patient is undergoing a vasectomy reversal. Fluid expressed from the proximal end of the vas is thick and pasty and no sperm are seen on microscopy. What is the next step the surgeon should undertake?**

Perform a vasoepididymostomy instead of a vasovasostomy.

○ **An azoospermic patient who had a hernia repair as a child resulting in obstruction of the inguinal vas deferens and a normal ipsilateral testis has an atrophic opposite testis with a normal vas deferens. What surgical procedure may restore sperm to the ejaculate?**

A crossover vasovasostomy.

○ **An azoospermic patient who previously underwent surgery for a pituitary tumor is found to have undetectable levels of FSH and LH. What form of therapy may restore spermatogenesis?**

Treatment with intramuscular hCG and recombinant FSH can replace absent LH and FSH and initiate spermatogenesis.

○ **A patient with azoospermia is found on transrectal ultrasound of the prostate to have a midline cystic structure causing dilation of the ejaculatory ducts and seminal vesicles. What is the origin of this structure and what procedure may restore sperm in the ejaculate?**

The cyst is likely a Mullerian duct remnant. Transurethral resection of the ejaculatory ducts (TURED) may unroof the obstructing cyst and allow sperm to be present in the semen.

○ **A patient with neuropathy secondary to diabetes mellitus develops anejaculation. If he fails α sympathomimetic oral therapy, the next option to obtain sperm is?**

Electroejaculation. If unsuccessful, then consider either microsurgical vasal or epididymal sperm aspiration to obtain sperm for use with IVF.

○ **A patient with azoospermia and bilateral varicoceles underwent a testicular biopsy that revealed late maturation arrest. What treatment option may result in the appearance of sperm in the ejaculate?**

Bilateral varicocelectomy has been reported to reverse late maturation arrest in some cases, resulting in completion of spermatogenesis and appearance of adequate sperm in the ejaculate to allow for IVF/ICSI.

○ **A couple presents with primary infertility. The male partner has normal semen parameters. The female partner's evaluation is also negative. A postcoital test on two occasions, however, reveals no sperm in the cervical mucus. What assisted reproductive procedure may increase this couple's chance of conceiving?**

Intrauterine insemination (IUI) is a useful form of treatment for bypassing cervical female factor infertility.

○ **A patient with primary infertility and oligoasthenoteratozoospermia has low normal levels of FSH, LH, and testosterone. What form of empirical medical therapy may help improve his semen parameters?**

Clomiphene citrate (Clomid) has been used in these cases. While most patients experience an increase in FSH, LH, and testosterone, only a small subset of patients will achieve an improvement in semen parameters.

○ **A paraplegic with a cervical spinal cord injury has anejaculation. What is the preferred treatment option for sperm acquisition?**

Vibratory stimulation applied to the frenulum of the penis can result in antegrade ejaculation via the ejaculation reflex arc. If this fails, electroejaculation or microsurgical vasal or epididymal sperm aspiration can be used to obtain sperm.

○ **A patient who has undergone a vasectomy wishes to have a reversal. On examination, he has bilateral sperm granulomas and the sites of the vasectomy are high in the straight segments of the scrotal vasa deferentia. Are these findings more indicative of the need for vasovasostomy or vasoepididymostomy at the time of surgical exploration?**

Vasovasostomy. Sperm granuloma and longer vasal length proximal to the site of obstruction are associated with a lower incidence of secondary epididymal obstruction.

○   **A patient with primary infertility is found to have severe oligozoospermia with only 100 motile sperm in his ejaculate on repeat evaluations. Evaluation reveals no correctable or treatable conditions and empirical medical therapy fails to improve his count. What option is available for this patient to conceive his own biological child?**

Small numbers of sperm can be used to fertilize ova in an IVF cycle employing intracytoplasmic sperm injection (ICSI); individual sperm are directly injected into an individual ovum.

○   **A patient receives four courses of cisplatin-based chemotherapy for testicular cancer. Immediately after treatment he is azoospermic. What are the chances that spermatogenesis will return and how long can it take?**

His chances for recovery of spermatogenesis are 50% after 2 years and 80% after 5 years. It may take up to 1 year after treatment for sperm production to begin and several years to reach steady-state levels.

○   **When doing a testis biopsy, is one or both sides done?**

While one side may be sufficient for diagnosis, there is a 40% incidence of diagnostic discrepancies between the two sides, so bilateral biopsies are often recommended. Cryopreservation of some tissue may allow for IVF or ICSI to be performed later.

○   **What is the significance of palpable dilated veins with palpable reflux on valsalva one month after varicocele repair?**

Probably nothing. Ligated veins may remain enlarged due to thrombosis, which can take weeks to resolve.

○   **When would you first expect to see improvement in the semen parameters after varicocele ligation?**

By 3 months.

○   **Should a vasectomy and a varicocelectomy be done together?**

No, because of the possibility of testis atrophy. However, at least one study demonstrated good results for simultaneous vasectomy and varicocelectomy using microsurgical technique to preserve the deferential veins and prevent testicular atrophy.

○   **When the postcoital test indicates no sperm, very few sperm, and/or the semen analysis is only moderately abnormal. If IUI fails more than three times, consideration should be given to IVF/ICSI?**

When the postcoital test indicates no sperm, very few sperm, or in those with unexplained infertility. If IUI fails more than three times, consideration should be given to IVF/ICSI.

○   **How do clomiphene and tamoxifen work in male infertility and which patients are likely to benefit most?**

They are mild antiestrogens. They work best in men with low-normal testosterone levels and normal estradiol levels.

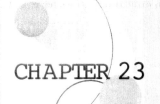

CHAPTER 23

Male Sexual Function and Dysfunction

Alan W. Shindel, MD, and Tom F. Lue, MD

○ **What is the anatomic arrangement of the penis?**

The dorsal penis contains two erectile bodies, the corpora cavernosa, which contain a central cavernosal artery that is principally responsible for penile engorgement during erection. There is a single erectile body (the corpus spongiosum) on the ventral portion of the penis that contains the urethra. Each corporal body is enclosed in a sheath of tough connective tissue called the tunica albuginea.

○ **What is Buck's fascia?**

Buck's fascia is the layer of connective tissue that covers both corpora cavernosa and the corpus spongiosum in separate fascial compartments. The dorsal artery, deep dorsal vein, and dorsal nerves of the penis lie beneath Buck's fascia.

○ **From which artery is the deep penile blood supply derived?**

The cavernous arteries responsible for penile erection receive blood from the internal pudendal artery, which in turn is a branch of the hypogastric artery.

○ **What is the anatomic relationship of the cavernous nerves to the prostate?**

The cavernous nerves, which are branches of the pelvic plexus, travel posterolateral to the apex of the prostate at the 5-o'clock and 7-o'clock positions.

○ **What is the mechanism of penile erection?**

During sexual stimulation, the neurotransmitter nitric oxide (NO) is released from the cavernous nerves to smooth muscle in the cavernous arteries and the corpora cavernosa. NO activates guanylate cyclase, which cleaves cellular GTP into cGMP. Through a complex cascade of events, cGMP leads to decreased intracellular concentration of calcium ions, which prompts relaxation.

With relaxation, the cavernous arteries and erectile tissues dilate, leading to increased penile blood flow and engorgement of the corpora. Swelling of the corporal sinuses compresses the emissary veins (which drain the corpora) against the tunica albuginea. Compression of these veins prohibits blood from escaping the corpora, producing a firm penile erection. With increasing sexual excitement, there is concomitant contraction of the bulbospongiosus and bulbocavernosus muscles. This leads to a pressure increase in the distal corpora cavernosa that may be as high as many hundreds of millimeters of mercury. There is also increased blood flow to the corpus spongiosum, causing engorgement of the ventral shaft and glans of the penis (rigid erection phase).

○   **What is the mechanism of penile detumescence?**

After sexual excitement has passed, nitric oxide (NO) release from the cavernous nerves declines. Concomitantly, the enzyme phosphodiesterase type 5 (PDE5) cleaves cGMP into 5′ GMP, which is not metabolically active. With the decline in cGMP concentration, intracellular calcium levels in the vascular smooth muscle rise and contraction occurs, leading to reversal of arterial dilation and blood drainage from the corpora.

○   **What is the physical sequence of events of ejaculation and which portion of the nervous system controls it?**

Ejaculation is divided into two phases, emission and ejection.

Emission is the phase during which the bladder neck closes and seminal fluid (from the prostate and seminal vesicles) is mixed with sperm from the epididymis in the posterior urethra and is under sympathetic nervous system control.

Ejection is expulsion of semen from the penis by rhythmic contractions of the bulbospongiosus muscle; ejection is mediated by the somatic nervous system.

○   **Which areas in the brain control erection and ejaculation?**

The medial preoptic area and the paraventricular nucleus of the hypothalamus have been identified as important supraspinal centers for erection and ejaculation.

○   **What is erectile dysfunction (ED)?**

ED is defined as the persistent inability to attain or maintain a penile erection sufficient for satisfactory sexual intercourse.

○   **According to data from the Massachusetts Male Aging Study, ED affects how many men older than 50 years?**

More than 50%. The prevalence of ED increases with age. Less than 10% of men in their twenties and thirties complain of the condition.

○   **What are the most common risk factors for ED?**

ED may be divided into organic, psychogenic, or mixed. Vascular risk factors are the greatest risk factors for ED (hypertension, hypercholesterolemia, diabetes, tobacco use, coronary artery disease). Nerve injury from pelvic surgery and or neuropathic conditions may contribute to ED. Deficiency of testosterone may lead to tissue atrophy in the penis as well as diminished libido.

Psychogenic ED often stems from depression, anxiety, relationship stress, or other nonorganic factors. Psychogenic factors frequently occur in men with organic ED and may complicate medical treatment; in many cases addressing nonorganic factors may be required even in cases of organic ED.

○   **What classes of antihypertensive medication are most often associated with ED?**

β-Blockers and thiazides. According to preliminary studies, ACE inhibitors and angiotensin receptor blockers may have a neutral or even positive effect on erectile function in hypertensive men.

○   **Are there subtypes of organic ED?**

Yes. Arterial insufficiency is defined as inadequate arterial response to sexual stimulation, leading to inadequate blood flow into the penis. Venous leak is a failure of the occlusive mechanism in which the emissary veins are compressed between the corporal body and the tunica. Mixed vascular ED is the coexistence of both venous leak and arterial insufficiency.

○ **Why is diabetes a particularly severe risk factor for ED?**

Neuropathy and vascular small vessel disease are common in men with diabetes. Diabetes is also associated with decreased levels of circulating testosterone and damage to endothelial and smooth muscle cells.

○ **Spinal cord injury patients can have either reflex erections from tactile stimulation or psychogenic erections. What cord level of injury separates the two groups?**

Patients with injuries above T10-12 may have reflexogenic erections (mediated by penile stimulation) and rarely have psychogenic erections, while patients with a level of injury below T12 may experience psychogenic erections but may not get reflex erections.

○ **What other sexual problems and conditions may occur in men and be commonly confused with and/or associated with ED?**

- Premature ejaculation: Persistent and recurrent ejaculation before or shortly after penile penetration associated with a lack of feeling of control over the process and leading to significant patient and/or partner distress.
- Hypoactive sexual desire disorder: Decreased interest or receptivity to sexual activity.
- Retarded/delayed ejaculation: Persistent and recurrent difficulty ejaculating and/or attaining orgasm despite ostensibly sufficient sexual stimulation.

○ **Which commonly used drugs have been associated with impairment in ejaculation and orgasm?**

Alcohol, tricyclic antidepressants (amitriptyline and imipramine), and selective serotonin reuptake inhibitors (SSRI) are the mostly commonly used drugs associated with impairment in ejaculation and orgasm.

○ **What is an appropriate initial evaluation for a man with ED?**

An assessment should be made for vascular risk factors as well as psychologic comorbidities. A basic electrolyte panel, hemoglobin A1c, resting blood pressure, and serum lipid profile are adequate for initial evaluation.

○ **What are the Princeton criteria?**

The Princeton criteria is an algorithm for stratifying ED patients with respect to their cardiac risk factors. Men with severe cardiac disease should undergo cardiac optimization prior to initiation of therapy for ED. Men with no or mild cardiac disease may safely start ED therapy without further investigation. Men in the intermediate category may need further evaluation by a cardiologist prior to starting ED therapy.

○ **What is dynamic infusion cavernosometry (DIC)?**

DIC is a procedure to diagnose venous leak as a cause of ED. A needle is placed into the corpora to inject a vasodilating agent. After 10 minutes and/or a penile erection has developed, sterile saline is infused. The rate of inflow necessary to maintain a set degree of axial rigidity in the penis is a measure of the integrity of the veno-occlusive mechanism of the penis; a high flow rate implies greater leak and suggests venous leak ED.

○ **Normal veno-occlusive function is suggested by what maintenance flow rate on dynamic infusion cavernosometry testing?**

A maintenance flow rate of 6 mL/min or less represents normal veno-occlusive function if maximal smooth muscle relaxation has been achieved.

○ **What is the role of cavernosography in the evaluation of erectile dysfunction?**

In a patient in whom venous leak is clinically suspected, contrast injection into the corpora demonstrates the sites of abnormal leaking veins. This test is seldom indicated in the modern era but still is useful for preop planning if venous surgery for the treatment of ED is contemplated.

○ **What is nocturnal penile tumescence (NPT)? When do nocturnal erections occur and how is the rigidity of these erections measured?**

NPT is the normal cycle of nighttime erections that occur during REM sleep in healthy males of all ages. Testing for NPT can be performed using a pressure monitor that fits around the penis. NPT testing is typically utilized to determine whether ED is psychogenic or organic; if normal nocturnal erections occur it is likely that there is a strong psychologic component to ED.

○ **What role does penile color Doppler ultrasound play in the diagnosis of ED?**

Color Doppler ultrasound after administration of a vasodilating agent permits accurate assessment of peak systolic velocity (PSV) and end diastolic velocity (EDV) in the cavernosal arteries. A PSV less than 30 to 35 cm/s is indicative of arterial disease while a persistent EDV greater than 5 cm/s predicts patients who may have venous leak. This is the preferred test for vasculogenic ED in the modern era.

○ **A 35-year-old male with ED due to a pelvic fracture and a 65-year-old male with ED secondary to long-standing hypercholesterolemia and hypertension undergo pelvic angiography. What are the expected findings?**

The younger man would likely have a focal stenosis or occlusion of the penile or cavernosal artery. The older man would likely have diffuse stenotic plaques.

○ **A patient is seen for a complaint of decreased libido. Physical examination is normal. What is an appropriate initial endocrine evaluation?**

A morning free and total testosterone level is a good initial screening test. If abnormal, it should be repeated along with prolactin, LH, and FSH levels.

○ **What formulations of testosterone supplementation are available in the United States?**

Testosterone can be administered by either depot IM injection, transdermal patch, transdermal gel, a transbuccal system, or slow release subcutaneous pellets. Oral testosterone pills are seldom utilized in the United States.

○ **What evaluation is required before starting a man on supplemental testosterone?**

It is essential to obtain basic electrolytes, liver function tests, a complete blood count, and a serum PSA. A digital rectal examination should be performed to rule out occult prostate cancer. Men with prostate or breast cancer, lower urinary tract symptoms referable to an enlarged prostate, severe heart failure, severe sleep apnea, and/or polycythemia should be cautioned that testosterone may exacerbate these problems and may not be a safe therapeutic option.

○ **How does hyperprolactinemia cause hypogonadism? How is it treated?**

Hyperprolactinemia leads to suppression of the normal pulsatile secretion of GnRH by the hypothalamus. This in turn leads to decreased LH and FSH secretion by the pituitary gland, which removes the stimulus for testicular production of testosterone. Dopamine agonists such as bromocriptine are used to treat hyperprolactinemia. If a prolactin-producing tumor is present, surgical resection may cure the disorder.

○ **What is the mechanism of action of phosphodiesterase type 5 (PDE5) inhibitors (sildenafil, vardenafil, tadalafil)?**

These drugs inhibit the breakdown of cGMP by PDE5, thereby prolonging smooth muscle relaxation in the cavernosal arteries and corporal bodies.

○ **What are the most common side effects of PDE5 inhibitors? What are contraindications to the use of PDE5 inhibitors?**

The most common side effects are headache, dyspepsia, facial flushing, back pain, and visual disturbances; side-effect profiles differ between drugs. PDE5 inhibitors should not be used in patients taking nitrates as this may cause severe hypotension. PDE5 inhibitors should also not be taken within 4 hours of α-blocker medications as this may also lead to significant hypotension.

○ **What are some ways to optimize the efficacy of PDE5 inhibitors?**

Patients should be instructed that the medication augments but does not cause penile erection. Sexual stimulation is required for these drugs to work. Sildenafil and vardenafil should not be taken after a high-fat meal, as this will slow absorption of the drug. All PDE5 inhibitors may be taken on demand for the treatment of ED. Tadalafil may be taken daily at a low dose for the chronic management of ED.

○ **Which drugs are most commonly used alone or in combination for intracavernosal pharmacologic injection therapy for ED?**

Prostaglandin El, phentolamine (an α-blocker), and papaverine (a nonselective phosphodiesterase inhibitor). Prostaglandin is the only one of these that is FDA approved, although it may be used in combination with the other two after compounding by a pharmacist. These medications are highly effective irrespective of sexual stimulation.

○ **What are the risks/side effects of intracavernosal injection therapy for ED?**

Fear of needles and penile pain limit the acceptability of this therapy for many patients, although many others find it highly satisfactory. Bleeding, pain, and infection are minor side effects that can be obviated with instruction of good injection technique. Priapism and corporal fibrosis are more serious complications, which may also occur.

○ **What is MUSE? How is it administered?**

MUSE is prostaglandin E1 in a pellet form for intraurethral placement. The patient is instructed to urinate, after which an applicator is placed into the distal urethra and the pellet is dislodged. The pellet dissolves and is absorbed into the corpus spongiosum. Venous channels then transfer the drug to the corpus cavernosum.

○ **What are the reported side effects of vacuum erection device use?**

Pain is the most common side effect followed by penile bruising and numbness. The penis may become cold, the ejaculate may be trapped in the urethra by the constriction band, and the base of the penis proximal to the band may pivot during intercourse. The constrictive band should not be left in place for more than 30 minutes.

○ **What are the advantages of vacuum erection devices?**

Vacuum erection devices are the least expensive, long-term treatment for ED. There is no risk of medication interactions. They can work in any type of ED. Since there is no medication involved and the process is strictly mechanical, they are highly reliable.

○ **Which patients are candidates for penile venous ligation surgery?**

Young patients with a history of primary (lifelong) ED, venous leak without arterial insufficiency, and a discrete area of venous leak demonstrated by cavernosography are potential candidates for venous ligation surgery. The procedure is unlikely to be effective in cases of diffuse venous leakage.

○ **Which artery is most commonly used as the source of new arterial blood to bypass obstruction in a penile artery during revascularization surgery?**

The inferior epigastric artery is the most commonly used source of new arterial inflow.

○ **A patient experiences undesired inflation of his three-piece inflatable penile prosthesis. What is the most likely cause?**

Autoinflation occurs when pressure around the reservoir is high enough to force fluid back through the pump into the cylinders at a time when inflation is not desired. This may occur due to inadequate dilation of the reservoir space during prosthesis placement or by scarring and formation of a compressive scar around the reservoir during healing. Most modern three-piece penile prosthetics are equipped with a lockout valve to eliminate or at least reduce this complication.

○ **What is the penile prosthesis SST deformity and how is it corrected?**

Downward bowing of the glans after penile prosthesis implantation is called the SST deformity (named after the airplane's nose). It is the result of either distal corporal underdilation or cylinder undersizing at the time of implantation or postoperative anatomic changes that leave the glans unsupported. Surgical correction includes redilating the corpora and resizing the device. Occasionally, glans fixation is required to add stability.

○ **Which patients are at highest risk of penile prosthesis infection?**

Patients with poorly controlled diabetes and immunocompromised patients. Patients with spinal cord injury are also at higher risk for infection as they may not have sensation to detect occult injury to the penis and/or prosthesis. Increased risk of infection is also associated with repeat implant operations and surgical revisions.

○ **After placement of a three-piece inflatable penile prosthesis a patient has bloody urine. There was no evidence of urethral injury during surgery. What has likely occurred and how is this complication best avoided?**

The patient has most likely sustained a bladder injury during reservoir placement. This type of injury is prevented by draining the bladder completely with a catheter prior to the retropubic dissection.

○ **During distal dilation of the corpora for placement of an inflatable penile prosthesis, a tear is made in the urethra with the dilator at the level of the urethral meatus. What is the best form of management?**

A cylinder should not be placed in the injured corpora. No direct attempt should be made to close the urethral tear. After it has healed over a catheter, a cylinder can be placed on that side 4 to 6 weeks later.

○ **A patient with a three-piece inflatable penile prosthesis is explored for suspected periprosthetic infection. At surgery, gross pus is found around the cylinders. What is the best form of management?**

The standard of care is to remove all components of the device and irrigate the wound thoroughly. The wound can be closed primarily with drains left in place. Prosthesis reimplantation can be attempted in 4 to 6 months, although there is likely to be significant corporal fibrosis after this much time. Successful salvage procedures have been developed that permit immediate replacement of a prosthesis in the case of low-grade infection or simple prosthetic erosion.

○ **What medical therapies are available for the treatment of premature ejaculation (PE)?**

There are no FDA-approved treatments for PE. Serotonin has an antiorgasmic effect in the central nervous system; for this reason selective serotonin reuptake inhibitors (SSRI) have been used to treat premature ejaculation. SSRI have been proven to increase ejaculatory latency in placebo-controlled trials. Topical application of an anesthetic ointment to the penis has also been demonstrated to be more effective than placebo in the treatment of PE.

○ **What medical therapies are available for the treatment of sexual desire disorders?**

Testosterone supplementation in hypogonadal men is the most common means of treating decreased libido. For men who are eugonadal or cannot take testosterone supplements, relationship counseling and/or treatment of psychiatric comorbidities (if present) may be beneficial.

○ **A man hears a "pop" as his penis buckles during intercourse. This is followed by pain, penile bruising, and swelling. What has occurred and how is it treated?**

The patient may have sustained a penile fracture due to rupture of the tunica albuginea of the corpus cavernosum followed by blood extravasation and subcutaneous hematoma formation (the eggplant sign). The preferred management is penile exploration and repair of the tunical tear.

○ **A patient with clinical evidence of a penile fracture and a ventral hematoma also has urethral bleeding. What concurrent injury should be suspected? How is it diagnosed and treated?**

This patient may have sustained an injury to the urethra as well as a cavernosal tear. He should have a retrograde urethrogram and/or flexible cystoscopy to diagnose the site and extent of the urethral injury. Surgical exploration should follow and the cavernosal, spongiosal, and urethral injuries repaired.

○ **A patient with sickle cell anemia presents to the emergency department with a 4-hour history of prolonged painful erection. What is the underlying mechanism and preferred management?**

The traditional belief has been that sludging of sickled red blood cells in the corpora leads to prolonged erection in men with sickle cell associated priapism. New evidence suggests that there may be an underlying defect of endothelial function and/or PDE5 activity in sickle cell disease. Treatment at the underlying sickle cell crisis should be initiated but management of priapism should not be delayed; corporal aspiration and/or injection of an α-adrenergic agent should be employed to bring about detumescence.

○ **A patient with idiopathic low-flow priapism fails to respond to repeated corporal aspiration, irrigation, and injection of an α-adrenergic agonist. What is the next appropriate form of treatment?**

Patients who fail conservative therapy need surgical intervention by penile vascular shunting. In cases of prolonged penile erection (greater than 24 hours), significant tissue damage has likely occurred and some degree of ED from prolonged ischemia is to be expected. In these situations, the shunt is undertaken for relief of pain from compartment syndrome more than for erectile function preservation. There are a variety of shunt procedures, discussion of which is beyond the scope of this chapter.

○ **What is stuttering priapism and how is it treated?**

Stuttering priapism is the condition of idiopathic recurrent priapism. It generally responds to intracavernosal vasoconstrictors and the patient may be instructed on self-administration of this therapy. When this is insufficient or the problem fails to resolve, a 6-month treatment with LHRH agonists to decrease serum testosterone has been effective. In many cases, these men maintain normal erectile function despite being on androgen suppression therapy.

○ **A patient reports penile engorgement after blunt perineal trauma. What is the likely mechanism? How is this best managed?**

This patient likely has high-flow priapism caused by a cavernosal artery to cavernosal tissue fistula. This can be diagnosed by penile color Doppler ultrasound or pelvic angiography. High-flow priapism is typically not painful and does not contribute to penile ischemia. Therefore, conservative management with observation ±compression can be attempted. Cavernosal arterial embolization or ligation of the fistula after 6 months have passed may also relieve the condition but ED is a potential complication of these treatments.

○ **What conservative nonsurgical options exist for the treatment of Peyronie's disease?**

There are numerous oral medical therapies for Peyronie's disease. Examples include vitamin E, arginine, carnitine, colchicine, trental, tamoxifen, and potassium para-aminobenzoate. Preliminary studies suggest that a penile extender (Fastsize) might be helpful. Unfortunately, none of these have emerged as consistently and universally effective. Arginine and trental appear to be the most promising at the moment. Intralesional injection of verapamil, interferon, and/or collagenase is advocated by some investigators.

CHAPTER 24

Peyronie's Disease and Penile Fractures

Stephen W. Leslie, MD, FACS

PEYRONIE'S DISEASE

○ **What is Peyronie's disease?**

Peyronie's disease is a fibrotic disorder of the penis in which a tough fibrous plaque forms in the tunica albuginea. These plaques may become calcified. PD is often but not always associated with penile pain and progressive deformity, either curvature or narrowing, during the "acute" phase. The "chronic" phase involves resolution of pain with stabilization of the deformity.

○ **What is the incidence of Peyronie's disease?**

Approximately 9% of the adult male population.

○ **Describe the pathophysiology of Peyronie's disease.**

While the pathophysiology of the disorder is not entirely clear, it is thought to be due to abnormal wound healing in men with some minimal level of penile trauma or injury, most often from sexual activity.

○ **Is Peyronie's disease genetic?**

There appears to be a genetic component as it tends to occur more frequently in relatives with the condition.

○ **Peyronie's disease is related to what other conditions associated with abnormal wound healing?**

It is associated with several other conditions related to abnormal wound healing such as Dupuytren's contractures and tympanosclerosis.

○ **What percentage of men with Peyronie's also have depression?**

Approximately 50%.

○ **How often is ED associated with Peyronie's disease?**

Approximately 30% of the time.

○ **What is the natural history of Peyronie's? How many patients will improve spontaneously, remain stable, or worsen over time?**

Approximately 12% to 13% will improve spontaneously, 40% to 50% will tend to remain stable, and the remainder will tend to get worse.

○ **What is the specific critical cytokine involved in Peyronie's disease, where is it normally found, and how does it work?**

Transforming growth factor β 1 (TGF β 1). It is an activator of collagen synthesis released by neutrophils and macrophages during wound healing.

○ **What is the differential diagnosis of Peyronie's? (Name at least five)**

- Penile fracture.
- Sarcoma (very rare).
- Fracture of the penile septum—with or without hematoma formation.
- Congenital curvature.
- Dorsal vein thrombosis.
- Cavernosal fibrosis.
- Leukemic infiltrate.

○ **Name three oral agents that were used for Peyronie's but are no longer recommended by most experts.**

Vitamin E, potaba, tamoxifen, and colchicine are no longer recommended. Vitamin E and tamoxifen do not appear to be effective, while potaba and colchicine have significant side effects with little or no benefit consistently reported.

○ **Name at least five other promising medical treatments for Peyronie's other than intralesional injections and surgery.**

Promising therapies currently include

- Arginine.
- Carnitine.
- Trental.
- Medical-grade penile extenders like Fastsize (www.fastsize.com).
- PDE5 inhibitors (Viagra, Levitra, and Cialis).
- Iontophoresis (with verapamil and dexamethasone).

○ **Name three intralesional agents that appear to be potentially useful for Peyronie's disease.**

1. Verapamil.
2. Interferon.
3. Clostridial collagenase.

○ **Which intralesional agent appears to be the most effective and what is the dosing regimen?**

Verapamil has shown the most benefit. Typically, verapamil is injected in 10-mg doses twice a week for 12 weeks. If no benefit is seen after 6 weeks, the dose is increased to 20 mg.

○ **What is the role of oral verapamil in the treatment of Peyronie's disease?**

Currently, oral verapamil plays no role in the treatment of Peyronie's disease. The reason is that the local concentration of verapamil necessary to inhibit fibroblast activity is many times greater than any safe level potentially possible with oral therapy.

○ **What is the optimal role of intralesional or oral steroids in this disorder?**

Steroids are not effective in this disease.

○ **What is the benefit of shock wave lithotripsy and radiation therapy in Peyronie's?**

Shock wave lithotripsy has not been effective. Low-dose radiation therapy has shown some benefit in relieving pain when used early in the disease, but it has no effect on the outcome.

○ **How effective is verapamil 15% topical gel for Peyronie's?**

There are conflicting reports, but the majority suggest it has little activity due to poor tissue penetration. Most experts do not recommend it currently.

○ **Which type of treatment, other than surgery, appears to be the most effective in treating Peyronie's?**

Intralesional verapamil injections have shown the best results of all nonsurgical therapies. However, the optimal combination of nonsurgical therapies is not yet clear.

○ **What is the rationale for using verapamil to treat Peyronie's?**

Verapamil appears to increase collagenase activity, decrease fibroblast proliferation in Peyronie's plaques, and affect cytokine expression. It is also thought that it can interfere with collagen and fibronectin transport, which are calcium-dependent processes.

○ **Peyronie's most commonly involves what aspect of the penis (dorsal, ventral, or lateral) and why?**

The dorsal midline is involved most often, probably from delamination during sexual activity. This causes an upward curvature.

○ **What surgical treatment options exist for a patient with symptomatic Peyronie's disease?**

Patients with a stable, nonpainful plaque and difficulty with penetration due to penile angulation are surgical candidates. Surgical options include penile plication, plaque incision or excision with grafting, and/or implant of a penile prosthesis. The more severe the curvature, the more aggressive the surgical procedure is likely to be.

○ **Describe the Yachia procedure.**

The Yachia procedure is a modification of the Nesbit plication for Peyronie's disease. Instead of excising a wedge of tissue from the tunica, the Yachia procedure uses longitudinal incisions in the tunica, which are then closed horizontally in a Heineke–Mikulicz fashion. (Simple plication procedures without incisions or wedge resections have demonstrated good results in patients with relatively mild curvatures. When doing these plications, a minimal amount of tissue in the actual plication seems to provide better patient satisfaction.)

O **When is the placement of a penile prosthesis most appropriate in Peyronie's patients?**

When there is significant preexisting ED and relatively severe curvature. In many cases, placement of a penile prosthesis alone is sufficient to provide adequate straightening. Manual modeling, where the penis is manually bent in the opposite direction of the curvature during surgery, sometimes provides durable improved straightening. If this is insufficient, then incisions and/or plaque excision with possible grafting will be needed.

O **Besides ED, what two additional disorders are associated with Peyronie's disease?**

Dupuytren's contractures and tympanosclerosis.

O **What is Van Buren's disease?**

Another name for Peyronie's disease. W.H. Van Buren published an early account in English of Peyronie's Disease in the *New York Medical Journal* in 1874.

O **What is the Space of Smith?**

The Space of Smith is the area between the erectile tissue and the tunica albuginea. It is usually obliterated in Peyronie's disease.

O **What is different about the scar tissue in Peyronie's disease compared to scar tissue elsewhere in the body?**

The scar tissue in Peyronie's retains fibrin within the mature scar. This does not occur elsewhere in the body. Peyronie's scar tissue tends to have less elastin and collagenase than most bodily scars and the collagen deposition is more disorganized.

O **Who first described Peyronie's disease and when? (Hint: It wasn't Peyronie!)**

Peyronie's disease was first described by Gabriel Fallopius in 1561 and first written about by Guilio Cesare Aranzi in 1587.

O **Who was Peyronie and when did he write about Peyronie's disease?**

Francois Gigot de la Peyronie, the personal physician of King Louis XV of France, did not write about "his" disease until 1743. When he did, he wrote an authoritative treatise on it and his name has been associated with the disorder ever since.

PENILE FRACTURES

O **What is the average thickness of the tunica albuginea of the penis when flaccid and during an erection?**

It averages 5 mm in thickness when flaccid, 2 mm when erect.

O **What is the "rolling sign" and when does it occur?**

The "rolling sign" occurs when the clot within the torn tunica overlying a penile fracture is palpable as an immobile, firm, tender swelling over which the penile shaft skin can be gently rolled.

O **What structure needs to be intact for the "rolling sign" to occur?**

Buck's fascia needs to be intact.

○   **In penile fractures, is Buck's fascia usually torn or usually left intact?**

Buck's fascia is usually intact.

○   **What is the "eggplant sign" and what problem does it indicate?**

This is the typical appearance of the penis immediately after a penile fracture with extensive hematoma formation and extravasation of blood.

○   **How does the clinical appearance of a penile fracture differ if Buck's fascia is torn compared to if it is intact?**

When Buck's fascia is intact, the hematoma from the fracture occurs deep to Buck's fascia and is relatively contained. When Buck's fascia is ruptured, blood will leak into the scrotum, perineum, and lower abdominal wall.

○   **What is the most common site for a penile fracture?**

The most common site of the tear is proximal, near the base of the penis.

○   **Describe the appearance of the actual defect in the tunica.**

The tears are almost always solitary, transverse, and unilateral.

○   **What is the expected incidence of urethral ruptures associated with penile fractures?**

Between 14% and 33%.

○   **What type and direction of force is most likely to cause a urethral rupture in association with a penile fracture?**

When the urethra is stretched during tumescence, it become vulnerable to rupturing from an angular force with dorsal bending.

○   **What predisposing factors lead to a greater risk of an associated urethral rupture?**

Periurethral fibrosis and urethral strictures.

○   **What is the most common cause of penile fractures?**

Bending during intercourse with forcible thrusting that misses the introitus and encounters bone. In the Middle East, the most common cause is forceful manipulation (65%).

○   **True or False: A penile fracture cannot generally occur in the flaccid penis.**

False. In approximately 3% of patients, the penile rupture occurs in the flaccid state, usually from direct blunt penile trauma.

○   **True or False: After a penile fracture, the angulation or deviation of the penis is generally toward the side of the tear in the tunica.**

False. The angulation is usually toward the side opposite the tear.

○ **When should a urethral injury be suspected in a penile fracture?**

When there is blood at or from the urethra, difficulty in voiding, inability to pass a catheter, and in the presence of factors predisposing to urethral injury as mentioned earlier. In actuality, every case of penile fracture should be suspect for a urethral rupture.

○ **What other clinical entity can present in an identical fashion to a penile fracture?**

Rupture of the deep dorsal vein of the penis.

○ **True or False: It is important to rule out a ruptured dorsal vein of the penis since its management is different than a penile fracture.**

False. Treatment is essentially the same, as both entities need surgical exploration.

○ **True or False: Cavernosography can be used to confirm the diagnosis of penile fracture and localize the tear in difficult cases.**

True, although this is rarely necessary as the clinical presentation is usually sufficient.

○ **What are the potential complications of cavernosography in penile fractures?**

Contrast-reaction fibrosis from extravasated contrast, infection, and priapism.

○ **What imaging studies, if any, are recommended in suspected penile fractures?**

Sonography is the recommended study if any imaging at all is needed. A retrograde urethrogram is indicated in cases of suspected urethral injury.

○ **How should penile fractures be treated?**

Immediate surgical exploration, evacuation of hematomas, and primary repair with buried, absorbable sutures through a circumferential subcoronal incision with degloving is the current recommended treatment. Complications of this approach include subcoronal skin necrosis, infections, abscess formation, transient distal edema, and penile curvature. A small, longitudinal skin incision has been suggested as an alternative surgical approach that would reduce some of the complications but this limits the ability to fully inspect the entire tunica and urethra.

○ **How should a concomitant urethral injury be handled and what complications are possible?**

A diverting cystostomy may be sufficient treatment for a partially torn urethra although a direct repair gives equally good results. A complete transaction requires an end-to-end anastomosis and cystostomy. Urethral strictures and corporourethral fistulas are possible complications when a urethral injury is involved with a penile fracture.

○ **What is the expected outcome of conservative (nonsurgical) treatment of penile fractures?**

Significant complications are likely including development of a firm, fibrous plaque similar to Peyronie's disease (which can occur in 30%–53% of patients treated conservatively), organized hematoma formation, cavernous fibrositis, penile angulation, ED, and delayed chordee.

CHAPTER 25

Adult Urinary Tract Infections

David M. Albala, MD, FACS and Udaya Kumar, MD

○ **How common are urinary tract infections in young women?**

UTIs occur in approximately 1% of schoolgirls (age 5–14). This proportion rises to 4% by young adulthood.

○ **Should patients with asymptomatic bacteriuria be treated?**

Pregnant women, children younger than of 4 years, patients with severe diabetes, and patients with *Proteus* infections should be treated regardless of symptoms.

○ **Which bacteria are urea splitting?**

Majority are *Proteus* and *Providentia* species. *Pseudomonas, Klebsiella, Staph. epidermidis,* and mycoplasma are also capable of producing urease. *E.coli* is not a urea-splitting organism.

○ **What is emphysematous pyelonephritis?**

It is a rare complication of pyelonephritis that can occur in diabetic patients. Nonresolving pyelonephritis despite therapy and the triad of fever, vomiting, and flank pain should be investigated. Presence of intraparenchymal gas on plain KUB or CT is diagnostic.

○ **What is significant bacteriuria?**

The number of bacteria that exceeds the number usually caused by contamination. 10^2 CFU/mL or more of a known pathogen in a patient with dysuria would be significant. Previously $\geq 10^5$ had been the cutoff limit. However, 20% to 40% of women with symptomatic UTIs had colony counts between 10^4 and 10^5.

○ **What are bacterial pili?**

Bacteria have surface structures called adhesins to mucosal surfaces. The most important adhesins are long filamentous appendages called pili fimbriae.

○ **What is phase variation?**

Changes in environmental growth conditions of bacteria can cause them to rapidly shift between piliated and nonpiliated phases.

○ **What patient genetic factors affect susceptibility to UTIs?**

Variation in bacterial adherence to vaginal, urethral, and buccal cell surfaces is genetically determined. Women with nonsecretor blood group phenotypes are more prone to UTIs.

○ **How common are *E. coli* infections?**

In the community setting, *E. coli* account for 85% of the UTIs. In the hospital setting, this proportion reduces to 50%.

○ **What tests are used to localize UTIs to the upper or lower tract?**

Fairley bladder washout and Stamey ureteral catheterization tests.

○ **How accurate are clinical signs in localizing UTIs to the upper or lower tract?**

Less than 50%. Fever and loin pain with significant bacteriuria, traditionally taught to be diagnostic of pyelonephritis, may occur with cystitis alone. Conversely, in patients with only bladder symptoms, the upper urinary tract is often involved.

○ **What is the recommended duration of therapy for uncomplicated UTIs?**

In a patient with a structurally normal urinary tract, a single dose or a 3-day course of antimicrobial treatment is adequate. Success rates are lower with single-dose therapy compared to multiday regimens. In men, all UTIs should be presumed complicated and treated for 7 days or more and an underlying cause sought.

○ **Is antibiotic prophylaxis necessary for TURP?**

No. If the preop urine shows no growth ($<10^2$ CFU/mL), prophylaxis is not necessary. In patients with significant growth, urethral catheters, risk of endocarditis, or whose bacterial status is unknown, prophylaxis is warranted. The risk of bacteremia is 50% if antimicrobials are not given when a UTI is present.

○ **What antibiotics are suitable as prophylaxis for transrectal biopsy of the prostate?**

Metronidazole with ampicillin or trimethoprim-sulfamethoxazole is often used. A fluoroquinolone is a suitable alternative.

○ **When are imaging studies needed in UTI?**

Infections in males, febrile infections, failure to respond to appropriate therapy, bacterial persistence, and suspected urinary obstruction warrant imaging studies.

○ **What are the common causes of unresolved bacteriuria during therapy?**
- Bacterial resistance to drug (resistance may develop during the course of therapy).
- Mixed bacterial growth with varying drug susceptibilities.
- Rapid reinfection with a new organism.
- Renal insufficiency.

- Papillary necrosis.
- Staghorn calculus.
- Self-inflicted infections or deception in taking medications.
- Urinary obstruction.

○ **What is bacterial persistence?**

Despite clearance of bacteriuria with appropriate antimicrobial treatment, the same organism can reappear in the urinary tract from a site within the urinary tract that was excluded from the high concentrations of the antimicrobial agent, e.g., a struvite stone.

○ **Which antibiotics are suitable for long-term, low-dose prophylaxis?**

Nitrofurantoin, TMP-SMX, TMP, cephalexin. A low dose of the antibiotic is given, typically at bedtime for 6 to 12 months.

○ **Are there alternatives to long-term, low-dose prophylaxis?**

Intermittent 3-day, self-start therapy or postintercourse therapy may be used instead.

○ **What does urinary microscopy show in patients with acute pyelonephritis?**

Numerous white cells and bacteria WBCs exhibit Brownian motion of cytoplasm (glitter cells); granular and leukocyte casts; bacteria may be seen in casts.

○ **True or False: Nitrofurantoin and TMP-SMX are generally ineffective against *Pseudomonas* species.**

True. TMP alone or with SMX is effective against most uropathogens except enterococci and *Pseudomonas* sp. Nitrofurantoin is ineffective against *Proteus* and *Pseudomonas* sp.

○ **Why does an infection with *Proteus* cause more concern than *E. coli*?**

Patients who have a protracted infection with *Proteus* risk formation of struvite calculi due to the alkalinization caused by the urea-splitting bacteria. This leads to precipitation of Ca, Mg, NH_4, and PO_4 salts. *E. coli* does not produce urease.

○ **True or False: Prophylactic antibiotics should be given to catheterized patients to reduce risk of UTI.**

False. This does not reduce risk of infections. In fact, they give rise to infections with organisms resistant to several antibiotics.

○ **What are the radiologic features of xanthogranulomatous pyelonephritis?**

It is usually unilateral. IVU shows renal calculi in 38% to 70% of cases, a nonfunctioning kidney in 27% to 80%, a renal mass in 62%, and a calyceal deformity in 46%. On CT scan, a large renal mass with the renal pelvis tightly surrounding a central calcification is seen.

○ **What are the diagnostic features of malacoplakia histologically?**

Large histiocytes called von Hausemann cells and small basophilic calculospherules called Michaelis-Guttmann bodies, which may be intra- or extracytoplasmic.

○ **Why should a hydatid cyst not be aspirated?**

The contents of a hydatid cyst are highly antigenic and may cause anaphylaxis if it ruptures and spills during aspiration.

○ **What is the initiator of gram-negative septic shock?**

Endotoxin, a lipopolysaccharide component of bacterial cell wall, activates the macrophages and humoral pathways in septic shock. Most of the toxicity of endotoxin is contributed by lipid A, which is bound to the core oligosaccharide.

○ **Why do postmenopausal women have UTIs more frequently?**

Lack of estrogen causes changes in vaginal pH and microflora including loss of lactobacilli and colonization with *E. coli*. In addition, some women may have residual urine after voiding.

○ **When is screening for bacteriuria worthwhile?**

The first trimester of pregnancy. There appears to be little advantage in screening healthy women.

○ **True or False: In women with bacteriuria, acute pyelonephritis occurs more commonly in pregnant women than in nonpregnant women.**

True. Nonpregnant women with screening bacteriuria (SCBU) rarely develop pyelonephritis in contrast to 28% of pregnant women with SCBU.

○ **Which antimicrobials are suitable for use in pregnancy?**

Penicillins (including ampicillin and synthetic penicillins) and cephalosporins are safe throughout pregnancy. Short-acting sulfonamides and nitrofurantoin may be used in the first two trimesters. The former can cause neonatal hyperbilrubinemia and the latter hemolytic anemia in newborn if used near term.

○ **What is the incidence of bacteriuria in the elderly?**

Greater than 20% of women and >10% of men older than 65 years have bacteriuria. Most are asymptomatic.

○ **What is the difference between bacterial persistence and unresolved bacteriuria?**

Unresolved bacteriuria implies that the urinary tract is not sterilized during therapy. Bacterial persistence means recurrence of infection with the same organism after initial clearance.

○ **What is the significance of squamous cells in urine?**

Numerous squamous cells in the urine would indicate preputial, vaginal, or urethral contamination.

○ **Why is plasmid-mediated (R factor) resistance important?**

It is more common than selection of resistant clones. The resistance is transferable and produces multiple resistant strains making therapy difficult.

○ **What problems do diabetic patients encounter with regard to urinary infections?**

Diabetic women appear to be more prone to UTIs. Diabetic patients often have glomerulopathy, with difficulty concentrating antimicrobials. They are also more prone to complications like papillary necrosis and emphysematous pyelonephritis.

○ **What is the classic presentation of septic shock syndrome?**

Fever and chills followed by hypotension, but this occurs only in 30% of cases.

○ **What is the earliest metabolic abnormality in septic shock syndrome?**

Metabolic alkalosis as a consequence of hyperventilation. This occurs even before chills or fever.

○ **What are the x-ray findings of malacoplakia?**

On IVU, enlarged kidneys with multiple filling defects (best appreciated on U/S or CT). On CT, the foci are less dense than parenchyma. Unifocal lesions are indistinguishable from other inflammatory lesions and neoplasia.

○ **What is the added advantage in using low-dose TMP-SMX prophylaxis in renal transplant patients?**

In the immunosuppressed patient, TMP-SMX not only prevents UTIs but also provides protection against *Pneumocystis carinii* pneumonia, listeriosis, and nocardiosis.

○ **How do you treat candiduria in the renal transplant patient?**

As untreated candiduria can lead to the formation of obstructing candidal fungal balls, they should be treated promptly with fluconazole or with low-dose amphotericin plus rucytosine if it fails.

○ **True to False: Steroids increase the risk of UTI.**

True. The incidence of UTI increases approximately threefold in patients on prolonged steroid therapy.

○ **Why are fluoroquinolones contraindicated in children and pregnant women?**

They have the potential to damage developing cartilage.

○ **Why are trimethoprim and fluoroquinolones particularly suited for UTI prophylaxis?**

Both drugs are actively secreted in the vagina and bowel, thereby inhibiting growth of uropathogens at these sites.

○ **What is the most reliable form of urine collection?**

Suprapubic aspiration is the least prone to contamination.

○ **What is the most common form of recurrent UTI in women?**

Reinfection (new infection from bacteria outside the urinary tract) is the most common cause.

○ **What is the basis for leukocyte esterase test?**

Leukocyte esterase is produced by neutrophils and catalyzes the hydrolysis of an indoxyl carbonic acid ester to indoxyl. The latter oxidizes a diazonium salt on the dipstick to produce a color change.

○ **How sensitive and specific is the nitrite dipstick test for bacteriuria?**

Specificity is more than 90% but sensitivity varies from 35% to 85%. The test is less reliable in detecting bacterial concentration $<10^5$. The most common cause of a false-positive test is contamination.

○ **Why is nitrofurantoin not suitable for the treatment of pyelonephritis?**

Nitrofurantoin is rapidly excreted in urine but does not achieve therapeutic levels in most body tissues including the kidney.

○ **What constitutes significant bacteriuria in a catheterized patient?**

A count of $>10^2$ CFU/mL implies significant bacteriuria since these counts usually persist or increase in a catheterized patient within 48 hours.

○ **What measures are useful in reducing catheter-associated UTIs?**

Use of closed catheter drainage reduces catheter-related UTIs from 90% at 4 days to 30% to 40%. Periodic instillation of a chemical, e.g., hydrogen peroxide into the collecting bag may delay the onset of infection.

○ **What is the most common organism associated with Fournier's gangrene?**

Either staphylococcal or streptococcal infections may be solely responsible, although it is increasingly recognized that mixed infections, including gram-negative and anaerobic organisms, are the rule rather than the exception.

○ **How is Fournier's gangrene treated and what is the mortality rate?**

Prompt treatment is critical as the mortality is 20% or more otherwise. Even with prompt therapy, the mortality rate is 5% to 6%. Intravenous hydration and multiple antibiotics with adequate surgical debridement are mainstays of treatment. Hyperbaric oxygen has been useful in some cases.

○ **How often is an orchiectomy necessary in Fournier's gangrene?**

Orchiectomy is almost never needed. The testicles have a separate blood supply and can often be preserved by placement in a thigh pouch even if the scrotum is removed.

○ **Which antibiotics are suitable for the treatment of chronic prostatitis?**

Nonlipid-soluble drugs are unable to reach prostatic acini. Lipid-soluble drugs, weakly basic antibiotics that are concentrated in the prostate are most suitable. Fluoroquinolones are the drugs of first choice. Trimethoprim-sulfamethoxazole, clindamycin, erythromycin, and doxycycline are also appropriate choices.

○ **Which bacteria are usually resistant to the carbepenems?**

Carbepenems (ertepenem, imipenem, and meropenem) are active against gram-positive pathogens, gram-negative pathogens, and anaerobic bacteria and maintain efficacy against most β-lactamase-producing bacteria. They are not effective against *P. aeroginosa*, methicillin-resistant *Staphococcus aureus,* and enterococci including vancomycin-resistant enterococci. Doripenem, the new carbepenem, and meropenem have activity against some strains of *Pseudomonas.*

○   **What issues complicate UTIs in patients with chronic renal insufficiency?**

Uremia impairs the immune system making it difficult to clear infections. The delivery of antibiotics to the urinary tract, including the kidneys, is compromised because of the reduced blood flow to the kidneys, low urine volume, and reduced renal drug-concentrating ability. Patients on dialysis are also more prone to acquiring secondary UTIs from elsewhere in the body.

○   **True or False: Circumcision is protective for HIV infection.**

True. It provides approximately 60% protection.

CHAPTER 26

Interstitial Cystitis and Other Inflammatory Conditions of the Lower Urinary Tract

J. Nathaniel Hamilton, MD, Timothy Yoost, MD, and Eric S. Rovner, MD

○ **How common is interstitial cystitis (IC) in the United States?**

Prevalence: 36.6 per 100,000 patients. Incidence: 2.6 per 100,000 women per year.

○ **What is the term preferred by the International Continence Society for interstitial cystitis?**

Painful bladder syndrome.

○ **Are there racial/ethnic differences in the prevalence of IC?**

Yes, 94% of patients are Caucasian. There appears to be a slightly higher incidence in Jewish women.

○ **Is the incidence of childhood bladder problems increased in patients with IC?**

Yes. The incidence is ten times higher in patients with IC than controls.

○ **What is the natural history of IC?**

Median presentation is at age 40. Spontaneous remission occurs in up to 50% of patients at a mean of 8 months. Patients may have complete and spontaneous relief from the symptoms, have a waxing and waning course, may be completely asymptomatic with intermittent "flares," or have a chronically progressive course of increasing symptoms over several years.

○ **What is the etiology of IC?**

Unknown. The most commonly cited hypotheses include (1) a pathogenic role of mast cells in the detrusor and/or mucosal layers of the bladder as a primary or secondary process, (2) a deficiency in the glycosaminoglycan layer (GAG) on the luminal surface of the bladder resulting in increased permeability of the surface layer and thus exposure of the underlying submucosal tissues to toxic substances in the urine, (3) an infection with a poorly characterized agent such as a slow growing virus or extremely fastidious bacterium which is unable to be cultured, (4) the production of a "toxic" substance in the urine, (5) neurogenic hypersensitivity or neurogenic inflammation mediated locally within the bladder or at the level of the spinal cord, (6) a manifestation of pelvic floor muscle dysfunction or dysfunctional voiding, and (7) autoimmune disorder.

○   **What percentage of patients with IC are female?**

Ninety percent.

○   **What other diseases have been associated with IC?**

Allergies (41%), irritable bowel (30%), inflammatory bowel disease (7%), Sjögren's syndrome, vulvar vestibulitis syndrome, systemic lupus erythematosus, fibromyalgia, and sensitive skin.

○   **What are the characteristic voiding symptoms of patients with IC?**

Irritative voiding symptoms including urinary urgency, urinary frequency (>8 per day by NIDDK criteria) with nocturia, and pain with negative urine cultures. Obstructive symptoms including a sensation of incomplete bladder emptying and double voiding may be present. Absence of nocturnal symptoms suggests an alternative diagnosis.

○   **What are the two subgroups of IC?**

IC is often divided into two distinct subgroups based on intraoperative findings at cystoscopy and bladder overdistension. These categories are the ulcerative (i.e., classic) and nonulcerative (i.e., Messing-Stamey) types.

○   **Which of the following excludes a diagnosis of IC: endometriosis, pyuria, hematuria, bladder overactivty on urodynamics, or ureteral calculus?**

None. All of these conditions may coexist in patients with IC Each of these may be related to a cause of lower urinary tract symptoms and should be properly investigated and treated prior to making a diagnosis of IC

○   **What percentage of patients with IC experience dyspareunia?**

Approximately 50% to 75%.

○   **What imaging studies are specific for IC?**

No known radiographic, ultrasonographic, or other imaging findings are specific for IC Unless indicated to help exclude alternative diagnoses, radiographic studies have only a limited role in the evaluation of IC Cross-sectional imaging including MRI, CT scan, and pelvic sonography, may be performed when clinically indicated to evaluate for a suggestive pelvic mass that is causing compression of the bladder or for an adjacent inflammatory process (e.g., diverticulitis). Cystography and voiding cystourethrography may be used to evaluate the bladder for other causes of irritative lower urinary tract symptoms, including intravesical masses, stones, bladder diverticula, urethral diverticula, urethral stricture, meatal stenosis, or findings suggestive of a neurogenic or nonneurogenic voiding dysfunction.

○   **Which urodynamic findings are common in IC?**

There is no urodynamic pattern that is pathognomonic for IC On filling cystometry, most patients have a hypersensitive bladder with small volume at first sensation to void and at capacity. Filling may be limited by an intense urge to void or pain. Bladder compliance, flow, and postvoid residual are normal.

○   **What percentage of IC patients demonstrate detrusor overactivity on urodynamic testing? What is the significance of this finding?**

Involuntary bladder contractions may be found in 14% of IC patients. This is not different from the general population. Other than excluding the patient from clinical trials adhering to the NIDDK criteria, there is no other significance.

○ **What are the common findings at cystoscopy in patients with IC?**

Prior to hydrodistention—normal appearing bladder and urethral lumen, and rarely a Hunner's ulcer (found in <10% of patients).

Following hydrodistention under anesthesia—glomerulations (petechial hemorrhages), submucosal hemorrhages, mucosal cracking, and bloody effluent upon drainage (terminal pinking).

○ **What are the findings during cystoscopy in a patient with "classic" IC as compared to the nonulcerative form of the disease?**

Classic IC (10% of IC patients)—reduced capacity under anesthesia (<400 mL during hydrodistention), ulcers, scars.

Nonulcerative disease (90% patients)—capacity >400 mL, no ulcers, scars, or mucosal cracking.

○ **What is the diagnostic utility of a bladder biopsy in IC?**

Although a higher proportion of IC patients will have detrusor mastocytosis as compared to normals, there are no histologic findings on bladder biopsy which are pathognomonic of IC In general, bladder biopsy is performed in patients being investigated for IC in order to eliminate carcinoma in-situ or occult malignancy as a cause for their lower urinary tract symptoms.

○ **What is the significance of the NIDDK criteria for a diagnosis of IC?**

These criteria were developed at an NIH sponsored consensus conference to ensure a relatively homogenous and uniform population of patients for accrual and inclusion into IC research studies. Fulfillment of these criteria is not necessary for the diagnosis of IC in clinical practice.

○ **What is the potassium chloride test?**

This is an in-office test used by some physicians in patients suspected of having a diagnosis of IC After the intravesical instillation of 45 mL KCl (400 mEq/L), 70% of patients with a diagnosis of IC will experience pain versus only 4% of normals. This is felt to be due to a defect in the GAG layer of the bladder in patients with IC Other conditions such as UTI may give a false-positive result.

○ **What is the role of hydrodistention in patients with IC?**

Hydrodistention is utilized both diagnostically and therapeutically in patients being evaluated for IC Following hydrodistention, it is generally felt that many patients with IC will manifest glomerulations, submucosal hemorrhages, mucosal cracking, and blood-tinged effluent upon drainage ("terminal pinking"). Furthermore, a significant number of patients have relief of their symptoms following hydrodistention.

○ **Apart from IC, which conditions may manifest glomerulations following hydrodistention?**

Neoplasia, infectious cystitis, radiation cystitis, chemical cystitis, and a defunctionalized bladder (patients on dialysis or after urinary diversion).

○ **Are there any proven beneficial dietary restrictions for IC?**

No. Many patients report improvement after altering their diet (changes in caffeine, alcohol, carbonated beverages, and juices), but in the only prospective randomized trials performed, there was no benefit to diet modification and no association with a certain diet.

○ **Name at least five oral agents that have been utilized clinically in the treatment of IC?**

Tricyclic antidepressants, sodium pentosanpolyphosphate (Elmiron), hydroxyzine (antihistamines), L-arginine, nalmephene, anticholinergic agents (oxybutinin, hyoscyamine, etc.), corticosteroids, antispasmodics, immunosuppressives, anti-inflammatories, and calcium channel blockers.

○ **What is the theoretical mechanism of action of amitriptyline in the treatment of IC?**

The tricyclic antidepressants such as amitripyline have a number of pharmacologic properties which may be of some theoretical benefit in patients with IC including anticholinergic effects, β-adrenergic effects (smooth muscle relaxation), strong H_1-antihistaminic activity, and central nervous system sedative effects.

○ **How is bladder hydrodistention performed?**

The bladder is filled to capacity at 80 cm H_2O under anesthesia for 8 minutes. The maximum pressure can be regulated by simply raising the height of the filling solution to 80 cm above the symphysis pubis of the patient.

○ **How effective is bladder hydrodistention in the management of IC?**

Symptomatic improvement can be expected in up to 30% to 60% of patients.

○ **What is the mechanism by which hydrodistention relieves the symptoms of IC?**

Unknown. Hypotheses include neuropraxis by mechanical trauma or epithelial damage from mechanical trauma.

○ **What is dimethylsulfoxide (DMSO) and how is it utilized to treat IC?**

DMSO is a product derived from the wood pulp industry. It has a number of pharmacologic properties, which may have some theoretical benefit in patients with IC including anti-inflammatory, analgesic, muscle relaxant properties, and mast cell histamine release. It is used as an intravesical lavage instilled on a weekly basis. It is sometimes administered in combination with steroids, alkalinizing agents, and heparin.

○ **How effective is intravesical DMSO in IC?**

Induces remission in up to 34% to 60% of patients. Progressive resistance may be seen after repeated treatments.

○ **What is neuromodulation therapy for IC?**

Sacral nerve stimulation, an approved therapy for urgency/frequency as well as urinary retention, has been explored in the treatment of IC and related urgency/frequency.

○ **What is the mechanism by which neuromodulation relieves IC symptoms?**

The primary mechanism underlying the effects of neuromodulation on voiding dysfunction including IC is unknown. It is hypothesized that electrical nerve stimulation in IC relieves pain by stimulating myelinated afferents to activate segmental inhibitory circuits. As a secondary effect, urinary frequency and urgency may also be reduced. Randomized, prospective, controlled trials demonstrating long-term efficacy of neuromodulation in IC are lacking.

○ **What is urethral syndrome?**

The urethral syndrome is a very nonspecific constellation of symptoms including urinary frequency, urgency, dysuria, and suprapubic discomfort without any objective findings of a urologic abnormality to account for the symptoms. The concept of the urethral syndrome, chronic or acute, is now essentially historic, as this terminology is no longer used.

○ **What is the percentage of patients who develop radiation cystitis after external beam therapy?**

Early radiation cystitis usually occurs at 3 to 6 weeks after therapy in approximately 20% of patients. Late hemorrhagic cystitis will occur in 3% to 12% of patients. The risk of radiation cystitis varies with the dose and mode of delivery of the radiation. Radiation changes including fibrosis and compliance changes may occur years following the radiation treatments.

○ **What is the risk of transitional cell carcinoma of the bladder after pelvic radiation?**

Two- to fourfold increased risk. When found, the tumors tend to be high-grade and locally extensive.

○ **What are the approximate maximum radiation doses tolerated by the bladder?**

Approximately 65 to 70 Gy. Above 80 Gy, mucosal and/or full-thickness changes occur.

○ **What three factors of radiation delivery affect the occurrence of radiation cystitis?**

1. Volume and area of bladder treated (the trigone is especially sensitive).
2. Rate of delivery. Dose >2 Gy/Fraction increases risk.
3. Total dose.

○ **Which histopathologic changes lead to hematuria after pelvic radiation?**

Progressive obliterative endarteritis resulting in mucosal ischemia, telangiectasias, submucosal hemorrhage, and ulceration. Chronically, interstitial fibrosis ensues.

○ **How effective is hyperbaric oxygen therapy for control of radiation cystitis?**

Resolution of hematuria occurs in >90% of patients. Promotes neovascularization and generalized vasoconstriction.

○ **How many hyperbaric treatments are usually necessary for control of symptoms related to radiation cystitis?**

Thirty treatments at 2 atm for 2 hours per treatment.

○ **What percentage of patients receiving cyclophosphamide will develop hemorrhagic cystitis in the absence of prophylactic measures?**

Up to 40% will develop hemorrhagic cystitis in low-dose chemotherapy protocols. This increased further in patients receiving high doses of cyclophosphamide in preparation for bone marrow transplantation.

○ **When is the usual onset of hemorrhagic cystitis in patients treated with cyclophosphamide?**

The hematuria usually develops acutely during therapy or shortly thereafter.

○ **Which metabolite of cyclophosphamide is thought to be responsible for hemorrhagic cystitis?**

Acrolein.

○ **Which agent(s) reduce the development of cyclophosphamide-induced hemorrhagic cystitis?**

Mesna—specifically binds acrolein. 20 mg/kg IM given at 0, 4, 8, and 12 hours after cyclophosphamide dosing.

N-acetylcysteine (Mucomyst)—oral, parenteral, or intravesical. Systemically reduces antineoplastic effect of cyclophosphamide.

Overhydration during administration of cyclophosphamide.

○ **What is the risk of bladder cancer after cyclophosphamide therapy?**

Ninefold increased risk with a short latency period (6–12 years). Most are muscle invasive at the time of diagnosis.

○ **What other drugs or derivatives are associated with hemorrhagic cystitis?**

Penicillins, danazol, busulfan, anilines, toluidine, and ether.

○ **What is the mechanism of action of epsilon aminocaproic acid (EACA) in treating hemorrhagic cystitis?**

Inhibits clot lysis by blocking plasminogen activation and fibrinolysis thereby promoting clot formation over bleeding surfaces.

○ **What is Alum and what is its mechanism of action in treating hemorrhagic cystitis? How is it administered?**

Potassium or ammonium aluminum sulfate (Alum) forms a salt–protein precipitate over the bleeding surface of the bladder. It is administered as a 1% intravesical lavage at 5 mL/min.

○ **What are the first steps for treatment if a patient on Alum bladder irrigation becomes confused or has an arrhythmia?**

Stop infusion and check serum aluminum as well as potassium or ammonia level depending on the solution used.

○ **What are the drawbacks of intravesical formalin for intractable hemorrhagic cystitis?**

Intravesical administration is quite painful requiring regional or general anesthesia. Reflux of formalin into the upper urinary tract may result in ureteral fibrosis, obstruction, and papillary necrosis.

○ **What x-ray study should be performed prior to the initiation of intravesical formalin for hemorrhagic cystitis?**

A cystogram should be performed to exclude vesicoureteral reflux, as reflux of the formalin into the upper tracts can have potentially devastating consequences.

○ **What is the mechanism of action of DDAVP (desmopressin) for intractable hemorrhagic cystitis?**

Increases factor VIII and von Willebrand factor levels.

○ **Which parasites have been associated with hemorrhagic cystitis?**

Echinococcus and schistosomiasis.

○ **Which viruses have been associated with hemorrhagic cystitis?**

Adenovirus types 11, 21, 35; papovarirus; influenza A; cytomegalovirus in immunodeficient states.

○ **What virus is associated with hemorrhagic cystitis following a bone marrow transplant?**

BK virus. A human polyomavirus that is present in approximately 60% of healthy adults and is usually acquired in childhood by the respiratory route.

○ **What percentage of bone marrow transplant recipients excrete BK virus in their urine?**

Up to 47%, and the infection usually represents reactivation of latent virus.

○ **What is the first-line treatment for BK cystitis?**

Supportive measures and hyperhydration. Catheter placement should be avoided if possible because of the immunocompromised state of the patient.

○ **What is the antiviral medication given to patients with refractory BK cystitis?**

Cidofovir (3–5 mg/kg in four to six doses).

○ **A 68-year-old female is referred with *de novo* urinary retention. Physical examination reveals a vesicular eruption over the mons pubis and right buttocks. What is the most likely diagnosis?**

Herpes zoster may result in detrusor underactivity secondary to sacral root involvement. Characteristically, it involves a vesicular rash along sacral dermatomes. Intravesical vesicles may be seen. Resolves spontaneously over 1 to 2 months.

○ **What is eosinophilic cystitis and how does it present?**

This is a pathologic diagnosis made on bladder biopsy in the setting of an eosinophilic infiltrate of the bladder lamina propria and detrusor. Nonspecific presentation: urgency, frequency, hematuria. A history of allergies and peripheral eosinophilia may be present. Occasionally, a mass may be palpable, mimicking sarcoma in children.

○ **What are the endoscopic findings in eosinophilic cystitis?**

Yellow raised plaques, necrotic ulcerated lesions, edema, and erythema.

○ **Which radiologic findings are associated with eosinophilic cystitis?**

Vesicoureteral reflux is seen in one-third of patients. Bladder wall thickening may be seen on bladder sonography or other cross-sectional imaging.

○ **How is eosinophilic cystitis treated?**

Treatment is generally nonspecific with steroids and antihistamines. It often has a self-limiting course.

○ **What bladder pathology is associated with schistosomiasis?**

Bladder cancer in the setting of *S. hematobium* has an early onset (40–50 years) and a high frequency of squamous cell carcinomas (60%–90%), with 5% to 15% adenocarcinomas.

○ **How do patients with malacoplakia present?**

Chronic urinary tract infections; 40% have associated systemic diseases such as immunodeficiency, malignancies, or autoimmune disease.

○ **What are the characteristic pathologic findings of genitourinary malacoplakia?**

Microscopically, infiltrates of bacteria-laden histiocytes (Michaelis-Gutmann bodies), lymphocytes, and plasma cells. Grossly, the lesions consist of raised yellow-brown plaques with hyperemic borders.

○ **What systemic diseases are associated with malacoplakia?**

Immunodeficiency states (especially organ transplantation patients on immunosuppressants), carcinoma, and autoimmune diseases.

○ **What is the role of bethanechol in the management of genitourinary malacoplakia and what is the proposed mechanism by which it exerts it effect?**

Along with intracellularly acting antibiotics such as trimethoprim-sulfamethoxazole and the fluoroquinolones, bethanechol is the most commonly utilized therapy for malacoplakia. It is generally felt that the Michealis-Gutmann bodies in malacoplakia represent incompletely digested bacterial material within the lysosomes of the histiocytes. Bethanechol increases the intracellular levels of cGMP promoting microtubule formation, which assists in lysosomal phagocytosis and digestion.

○ **Is there a gender difference in the incidence of emphysematous cystitis?**

Two-thirds of patients are female.

○ **Which factors predispose patients to develop emphysematous cystitis?**

Diabetes mellitus (50%), neurogenic bladder, chronic cystitis, bladder outlet obstruction, and immunodeficiencies.

○ **What are the most common pathogens in emphysematous cystitis?**

In decreasing frequency, *E. coli, Enterobacter, Klebsiella, Clostridia,* and *Candida.*

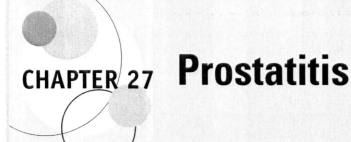

CHAPTER 27 Prostatitis

Durwood E. Neal, Jr., MD, and
Daniel S. Hoyt, MD

○ **How prevalent is prostatitis in the general population?**

Two to ten percent of men are currently experiencing prostatitis. It represents anywhere from 3% to 12% of urology office visits for men, and is the most common presenting diagnosis for men younger than 50 years. Prostatitis affects men of all ages, with the highest incidence between the ages of 20 and 49 years, but there is a second increase in incidence after the age of 65 years.

○ **What is the histologic definition of prostatitis?**

An increased number of inflammatory cells within the prostatic parenchyma.

○ **What is the most common histologic pattern of inflammation seen in prostatitis specimens?**

Lymphocytic infiltrate of prostatic stroma located immediately adjacent to the acini.

○ **Describe the four categories of the NIH prostatitis classification.**

1. Category I describes acute bacterial prostatitis seen in patients with acute febrile illness, a new onset of significant lower urinary tract symptoms, and possibly other systemic symptoms (chills, malaise, etc.).

2. Category II represents chronic bacterial prostatitis. Patients may have constant, long-term symptoms or have recurrent episodes of acute episodes of prostatitis with asymptomatic periods. The most important finding in category II prostatitis is recurrent documented UTIs.

3. Category III denotes chronic nonbacterial prostatitis, more recently termed chronic pelvic pain syndrome (CPPS). It is divided into IIIA (inflammatory CPPS) and IIIB (noninflammatory CPPS). IIIB has historically been referred to as prostatdynia.

4. Category IV refers to asymptomatic inflammatory prostatitis. It is a histologic diagnosis only, typically made after evaluation of semen, prostate chips, or prostate biopsy specimens.

○ **What is the most common category of prostatitis?**

Type III (chronic prostatitis/chronic pelvic pain syndrome), which accounts for 90% to 95% of cases of prostatitis.

○ **What family of bacteria is the most common cause of category I and category II prostatitis?**

The enterobacteriaceae family of rod-shaped, gram-negative organisms is the most common bacteria implicated in both acute and chronic prostatitis. It is usually a normal part of gastrointestinal flora. *E. coli* is the most common specific pathogen in bacterial prostatitis. Other genera are *Proteus, Serratia, Klebsiella,* and *Enterobacter.*

○ **What other pathogens have been implicated in bacterial prostatitis?**

Pseudomonas (gram-negative) and enterococci (gram-positive) have been found to be the causes of bacterial prostatitis. Various other organisms that are commonly found in the urethra of unaffected males have been theorized as possible causative pathogens, including *Staphylococcus* species, *Corynebacterium, Mycoplasma,* and *Ureaplasma.* Other postulated organisms include *Chlamydia, Candida* species, and nonculturable microorganisms.

○ **What role do prostatic calculi play in bacterial prostatitis?**

Although prostatic calculi do not lead to symptomatic bacterial prostatitis in every patient, it has been demonstrated that they can lead to persistent bacterial prostatitis that is recalcitrant to antibiotics. This is most likely related to bacterial aggregation and biofilm production along the surface and in the interstices of the stone.

○ **Intraprostatic ductal reflux has been implicated as an important mechanism in the development of which categories of prostatitis? Which anatomic portion of the prostate is most susceptible to ductal reflux and why?**

All categories of prostatitis are either initiated by or at least affected by ductal reflux of urine into the prostate. Reflux of bacteria into the prostate can lead to infectious prostatitis, and it has been postulated that even sterile urine leads to prostatic inflammation secondary to immunologic response, or the presence of chemical irritants in the urine itself. The ducts to the peripheral zone are more horizontally oriented and seem to reflux more easily than other regions of the prostate.

○ **What happens to the levels of fructose, citrate, and acid phosphatase in prostatic secretions during acute bacterial prostatitis?**

The levels of these entities are reduced during infection of the prostate. Protein synthesis is dramatically reduced, and the cells are unable to acquire citrate during episodes of bacterial prostatitis.

○ **What happens to the levels of zinc and calcium in prostatic secretions during acute bacterial prostatitis?**

These divalent cations are normally sequestered in the prostate cells by an active transport mechanism. These processes are reduced during active infection, and secretory levels drop.

○ **How is the pH of prostatic secretions affected during acute bacterial prostatitis?**

The secretions become more basic during an acute infection. Some studies have proposed that this increase in pH reduces the diffusion and/or efficacy of antibiotics in the prostate tissue.

○ **What happens to prostatic blood flow during acute bacterial prostatitis?**

Prostatic blood flow increases in acute infections of the prostate, much like any other organ. There is most likely vascular redistribution to the periphery as a result of edema in the central portion of the gland.

○ **What is the most widely used index for research and clinical evaluation of prostatitis?**

The NIH Chronic Prostatitis Symptom Index is a valid and reproducible instrument to evaluate the symptoms and quality of life in individuals with prostatitis. The NIH-CPSI has become the primary instrument used for the quantification of CP/CPPS and has already been used in multiple placebo-controlled clinical trials.

○ **In what clinical scenario should a DRE never be performed while evaluating prostatitis?**

None. Most experts agree that a DRE can be done during the evaluation of any category of prostatitis, even category I (acute bacterial prostatitis). However, category I patients should have a single, gentle DRE, since a vigorous examination or prostatic massage can exacerbate the illness.

○ **Describe the Meares-Stamey test for evaluation of men with prostatitis.**

This test involves the collection of urine and prostatic fluid specimens before, during, and after prostatic massage. The first collected sample is the initial 10 mL of voided urine (voided bladder 1 or VB1) that represents urethral flora, followed by a midstream urine sample collected after 200 mL has been voided (VB2) that represents bladder flora. At this point, prostatic massage is performed and the expressed prostatic secretions are collected (EPS), followed by the final voided urine sample (VB3). These samples are then sent for culture and microscopic analysis.

○ **In what clinical scenario is the Meares-Stamey test contraindicated in the evaluation of a patient with suspected prostatitis?**

Patients with suspected category I prostatitis should not undergo the Meares-Stamey test, since the required prostatic massage could lead to bacteremia and acute worsening of symptoms.

○ **How can the Meares-Stamey test differentiate between category IIIA and IIIB prostatitis?**

Category IIIA is diagnosed when no pathogenic bacteria are cultured, but greater than five WBCs per HPF are seen on EPS or VB3 or both. Category IIIB is diagnosed when no pathogenic bacteria are cultured, and there are no significant levels of WBCs in the EPS and VB3.

○ **Describe the preprostatic massage and postprostatic massage test (two-glass test) and how it compares to the Meares-Stamey test.**

The patient gives a midstream urine sample prior to undergoing prostatic massage, then a urine sample (the initial 10 mL) following massage. It has been found to be 96% to 98% as accurate as the Meares-Stamey test.

○ **In a patient with acute bacterial prostatitis being treated with appropriate intravenous broad-spectrum antibiotics, what diagnosis should be entertained if he continues to be febrile and highly symptomatic (chills, malaise) after 48 hours of therapy?**

Prostatic abscess should always be considered in patients with category I prostatitis who fail to respond to appropriate antimicrobial therapy. Urinary retention might also explain a failure of appropriate antibiotic therapy.

○ **What medical conditions place a patient at increased risk of developing a prostatic abscess?**

Immunocompromised patients (notably HIV-infected) are at a much greater risk of developing prostatic abscesses compared to the general population. Other important risk factors include urethral strictures, alcoholism, and chronic steroid use. Severely immunocompromised hosts are at an increased risk for prostatic abscesses caused by fungi.

○ **What are the best imaging modalities and what is the optimal treatment in a patient with a suspected prostatic abscess?**

CT scan is an acceptable imaging study to identify a prostatic abscess, but the gold standard is transrectal ultrasound. Transurethral unroofing of the abscess is considered the optimal treatment. Transperineal percutaneous drainage and transrectal drainage are other options.

○ **What is the appropriate antimicrobial management of a patient with category I prostatitis who presents with fevers, chills, and an elevated white blood cell count?**

Initial management with broad-spectrum parenteral antibiotics is considered the standard of care in acutely ill patients with category I prostatitis. Typically, a penicillin or penicillin derivative is coupled with an aminoglycoside. Once the patient has shown a good response to parenteral therapy, they can be switched to oral antibiotics, usually a fluoroquinolone, for 4 weeks.

○ **What other symptoms/complications should be addressed in patients with category I prostatitis?**

Many patients diagnosed with acute bacterial prostatitis experience varying degrees of urinary retention. α-Blockers might be needed for elevated postvoid residuals and acute LUTS, while suprapubic drainage might be required in those patients with more significant urinary retention during acute infection of the prostate. Avoidance of a urethral catheter is considered ideal when possible.

○ **What antibiotic class is usually recommended for category II prostatitis and why?**

Fluoroquinolones have been recommended as first-line therapy for chronic bacterial prostatitis. They show the best penetration into the prostate and seminal fluid (because of high lipid solubility), with the highest concentration by levofloxacin. The usual course is 4 to 6 weeks. Macrolides, sulfa/trimethoprim, and doxycycline are usually considered second-line therapies.

○ **What role, if any, does antibiotic therapy play in category III prostatitis?**

Patients with CP/CPPS with relatively new onset of symptoms (median of 4 weeks) might benefit from a course of antibiotics, but patients with longstanding symptoms almost never see benefit from prolonged courses of antibiotics.

○ **How long should patients with CP/CPPS be on α-blockers before they can expect to see a reduction in symptoms?**

A number of studies have shown that it takes a minimum of 6 weeks of α-blockade therapy before symptom amelioration begins to occur. Many men might need up to 3 months or more before they begin to see a significant improvement is symptoms.

○ **What anti-inflammatory agents have been found to reduce symptoms in men with CP/CPPS?**

NSAIDs and corticosteroids have been shown to have a modest effect on symptoms related to chronic prostatitis. Pentosan polysulfate has also shown promise. Newer cyclooxygenase-2 inhibitors have also been studied and appear to be promising treatment options.

○ **What other pharmacologic agents have been shown to be potential treatment options for men with CP/CPPS?**

Quercetin, a bioflavinoid OTC supplement, has been shown to offer significant symptom relief in a few small trials. Tricyclic antidepressents have also been studied and showed modest improvement in symptoms.

○ **What role does surgical treatment play in CP/CPPS?**

Most experts recommend against TURP for the management of CP/CPPS unless a specific indication is found. TUMT has been studied with promising but inconsistent results.

○ **What other nonpharmacologic therapy options have been suggested for CP/CPPS?**

Prostatic massage, once the mainstay of prostatitis treatment, is still a controversial treatment option. There is no clear consensus regarding its use in prostatitis, while others recommend frequent ejaculation as a treatment option. Biofeedback, pelvic floor physical therapy, and myofascial release have each been supported by small clinical trials.

○ **Which antibiotic used in prostatitis has the most significant effect on male fertility?**

Doxycycline has been found to reduce both sperm production and semen quality secondary to toxic metabolites.

○ **How many tubuloalveolar glands are typically found in the prostate?**

Approximately 20.

○ **What are spermine and spermidine?**

These are natural host defenses found in prostatic fluid, as well as prostatic antibacterial factor, a zinc-containing protein. They are more effective against gram-positive organisms.

○ **Category I prostatitis is a recognized complication of what rectal surgical procedure?**

Sclerotherapy for rectal prolapse.

○ **Prostatic inflammation is found most commonly in which zone of the prostate?**

In both human and nonhuman primates, the peripheral zone is most commonly involved with the inflammatory process. This is most likely the result of the horizontal orientation of the ducts.

○ **What happens to PSA during acute prostatitis?**

PSA is elevated in the serum, sometimes markedly, during episodes of category I prostatitis, as well during acute exacerbations of category II prostatitis. It can also be elevated during other categories of prostatitis, but the degree of elevation is not clear.

○ **Patients originally misdiagnosed as prostatitis may actually have what other disorder?**

Interstitial cystitis.

CHAPTER 28

Genitourinary Tuberculosis

Peter Langenstroer, MD, MS

○ **What is tuberculosis?**

Tuberculosis is a bacterial infection caused by *Mycobacterium tuberculosis*. It spreads from person to person by a pulmonary route followed by hematogenous seeding to the genitourinary tract.

○ **When was the first case of tuberculosis described?**

Tuberculosis is a disease that has been prevalent for many centuries. Dating back to 7000 BC, human skeletal remains have revealed pathologic findings consistent with TB infections.

○ **What are other historical names used for tuberculosis?**

Scrofula, consumption, phthisis, Kings-Evil.

○ **What is the incidence of TB worldwide?**

The worldwide incidence of TB is 10 million cases per year with 3 million deaths per year.

○ **What is the estimated number of people a TB infected person could subsequently infect?**

30.

○ **What are the two main mechanisms for eradication of TB?**

Case identification and treatment, and Bacillus Calmette-Guerin (BCG) vaccination.

○ **What are the problems associated with BCG vaccination?**

The duration of response is only 15 years. It has little effect on the incidence of infection and is ineffective in patients with prior TB infections. BCG also carries many potential side effects.

○ **What are the unique microbiologic characteristics of *Mycobacterium tuberculosis*?**

M. tuberculosis is an aerobic nonmotile bacterium with a high propensity to develop drug resistance. Its doubling time is slow at 24 hours. It can survive following phagocytosis in the lysosome of the macrophage.

253

○ **Describe the inflammatory response and typical histologic findings associated with genitourinary TB.**

The response is mainly via cell-mediated immunity. Lymphocytes and Langhans' giant cells make up the typical histologic findings of the TB granuloma.

○ **Do nontuberculosis mycobacteria cause pathogenic changes in the GU tract?**

This is very rare. Only a handful of cases have been reported. The mycobacteria involved include *M. kansasii, M. avium-intracellulare, M. xenopi,* and *M. fortuitum*.

○ **What test can be used to differentiate *M. tuberculosis* from nontuberculosis mycobacteria?**

p-nitro-α-acetylamino-β hydroxypropriophenone, the NAP test.

○ **What populations are at highest risk for developing TB?**

People living in underdeveloped countries, alcoholics, HIV patients, IV drug abusers, the homeless, and the elderly.

○ **What is the most common age group and gender to develop GU TB?**

GU TB is most commonly seen in the 20- to 40-year-old age group with a 2:1 male-to-female predominance.

○ **What is the classic triad of TB infections?**

Fatigue, weight loss, and anorexia.

○ **What percent of extrapulmonary TB is related to the GU tract?**

Worldwide, 14% of all cases of extrapulmonary TB are related to the GU tract, and approximately 6% in the United States.

○ **How does TB spread to the GU tract?**

GU TB is the result of metastatic spread of the mycobacterium via the blood stream. It usually results from a primary pulmonary focus. Only 25% of patients have a known history of TB.

○ **What is the mechanism that leads to TB of the lower urinary tract?**

Urinary excretion of the mycobacterium from the kidney causes seeding and infection of the lower urinary tract. Epididymal and prostatic TB are spread hematogenously.

○ **What are some of the clinical findings associated with GU TB?**

Sterile pyuria is the hallmark of GU TB. Other less specific signs are painless urinary frequency, nocturia, hematuria, hematospermia, suprapubic pain, and flank pain.

○ **How often is microscopic hematuria found in cases of GU TB?**

Microscopic hematuria is present in approximately 50% of cases.

○ **How should one culture the urine of a patient suspected of having GU TB?**

Five consecutive early morning urine specimens should be obtained and cultured on two separate media. Lowenstein–Jensen medium will isolate *Mycobacterium tuberculosis*, BCG, and nontuberculosis mycobacterium. Radiometric media such as BACTEC 460 is much faster and takes only 2 to 3 days for results.

○ **What is the quickest way to diagnose TB?**

PCR testing is highly sensitive, specific, and quick. Results are available in 6 hours.

○ **A 41-year-old woman native of India is referred to her urologist with irritative voiding and sterile pyuria. What is the differential diagnosis?**

Carcinoma in situ, genitourinary TB, and interstitial cystitis.

○ **What genitourinary organs are spared from TB infections?**

None. All organs of the genitourinary tract are targets for TB infections. However, TB of the penis, prostate, and urethra are rare.

○ **What are the primary medications currently used to treat GU TB?**

Rifampin, isoniazid, pyrazinamide, streptomycin, and ethambutol.

○ **What is the 2003 CDC recommendation for the medical treatment of uncomplicated GU TB?**

Isoniazid, rifampin, pyrazinamide, and/or ethambutol for 2 months and then isoniazid and rifampin for 4 additional months. At this time, a 6-month treatment regimen is the standard of care. Some authors recommend a three-drug regimen for 6 months.

○ **A 45-year-old woman has just completed her course of medical therapy for renal TB. She is asymptomatic and feels well. How should she be followed?**

She should be seen at 3, 6, and 12 months following completed treatment. At each visit she should have three consecutive morning urine specimens sent for TB cultures. Radiographic examination of her upper urinary tract would also be indicated. She should also return if symptoms recur.

○ **How long should one treat a patient with medical therapy for GU TB prior to embarking on a surgical intervention?**

Six weeks.

○ **What is a nonspecific test that can be used to monitor the effectiveness of treatment for TB?**

Erythrocyte sedimentation rate (ESR), if elevated prior to therapy, can be used to monitor the effectiveness of a specific treatment.

○ **Of the five most commonly used antituberculosis medications, (rifampin, isoniazid, pyrazinamide, ethambutol, and streptomycin), which drugs are bactericidal?**

Rifampin, isoniazid, pyrazinamide, and streptomycin.

○ **Following institution of isoniazid, rifampin, and pyrazinamide for GU TB, the patient notices the development of a pruritic macular rash. This is followed by generalized myalgias and conjunctivitis. Which drug is most commonly associated with this hypersensitivity reaction?**

Rifampin and streptomycin are most commonly associated with hypersensitivity reactions.

○ **Which anti-TB drugs are to be avoided in the presence of renal failure?**

Ethambutol and streptomycin are primarily renally excreted and should be avoided in this situation.

○ **A 62-year-old man receiving isoniazid, rifampin, pyrazinamide, and ethambutol for GU TB has developed visual changes since the initiation of medical therapy. What is the most likely cause of his new symptoms?**

Ethambutol can lead to optic neuritis. It is recommended that all patients receiving the drug undergo monthly visual examinations.

○ **Three weeks following initiation of medical treatment for GU TB, the patient is noted to have a rise in the liver enzyme panel. Jaundice is not present. How should this be managed?**

Most patients will have a transient elevation in the liver enzyme panel for the first few weeks of therapy. If jaundice develops, the medications should be withdrawn until the jaundice resolves. Medical therapy can then be reinstituted.

○ **Which of the antituberculosis drugs is ototoxic?**

Streptomycin.

○ **A 34-year-old woman on oral contraceptive medications becomes pregnant following the initiation of an antituberculosis regimen. What is the likely cause for the failure of her contraceptive?**

Rifampin can affect the metabolism of estrogen in oral contraceptive preparations. This can lead to an increased failure rate of these contraceptives. Women of childbearing age should use an alternative means of contraception while taking antituberculosis drugs.

○ **A 40-year-old man with the new diagnosis of GU TB has severe cystitis secondary to bladder involvement. Anticholinergic medications did not improve his symptoms. What can be added to the usual drug regimen in order to improve his symptoms?**

Prednisone can reduce the symptoms of acute TB cystitis. Prednisone may also be of benefit if a distal ureteral stricture is present; however, this issue remains controversial. Rifampin will significantly decrease the bioavailability of prednisone.

○ **A 32-year-old man is being evaluated for left flank pain and sterile pyuria. What is the appropriate workup?**

This individual should have a repeat urinalysis, urine cytology, urine culture for TB, cystoscopy, and an intravenous pyelogram or CT scan. Intravenous pyelograms are preferred. If a CT scan is done, it should be with intravenous contrast.

○   **On a plain film of the abdomen, the patient is noted to have a large left upper pole calcification. The intravenous pyelogram (IVP) reveals that he has minimal function of this kidney and blunting of his calices. His urine cultures reveal TB. What would be the indications for nephrectomy in this individual?**

A nonfunctioning kidney, associated renal cell carcinoma, uncontrolled hypertension, persistent severe flank pain, and patient noncompliance with the appropriate medical treatments are all indications for nephrectomy in the described setting.

○   **What is the likelihood of finding hypertension in a patient with renal TB compared to the general population without TB?**

Patients with renal TB are approximately twice as likely to have hypertension as the general population.

○   **If the kidney is entirely destroyed with caseous decay, how should it be managed?**

These kidneys are best managed by nephrectomy.

○   **When is the appropriate time to perform the nephrectomy?**

It is 4 to 6 weeks after the initiation of medical therapy.

○   **A 27-year-old woman with hypertension is found to have an atrophic right kidney from chronic renal TB. What is the likelihood that she will have an improvement in her hypertension with a nephrectomy?**

Approximately 65% of patients with significant unilateral renal involvement will have improvement in their hypertension.

○   **What are the common IVP (intravenous pyelogram)/CT findings of renal TB?**

The three most common findings are hydrocalycosis, hydronephrosis, and hydroureter. Additional findings include calcification, parenchymal loss, distorted calices, calyceal loss, and poorly functioning or nonfunctioning kidneys.

○   **A 21-year-old man with renal TB has a small renal calcification resulting from the infectious process. He has been adequately treated for his TB. How should his stone be managed?**

Calcification is associated with the normal tissue response from the destructive process and subsequent mineralization of the fibrous scar tissue. Small calculi can be observed. Larger calculi should be excised in a parenchyma sparing fashion.

○   **What are the common radiographic findings of TB in the ureter?**

Ureteral strictures, beading of the ureter, hydroureterosis from distal stenosis, ureterovesical obstruction, and vesicoureteral reflux.

○   **What is the most common portion of the ureter to be affected by TB?**

The ureterovesical junction.

○   **How does TB lead to vesicoureteral reflux?**

Scarring in the bladder at the level of the ureteral orifice can cause contraction of the surrounding tissue leading to a contracted rigid golf hole type ureteral orifice. This same process can also lead to stenosis of the ureteral orifice.

○   **A 50-year-old man was diagnosed with a distal ureteral stricture secondary to GU TB. He is placed on the standard medical regimen for GU TB. After 3 weeks of medical therapy he has no improvement in his ureteral obstruction. What is the next appropriate step in management?**

The addition of prednisone to his regimen would be indicated and should improve his ureteral stenosis.

○   **Following 3 more weeks of medical management, his obstruction persists. What are the remaining options for the treatment of his distal ureteral stricture?**

Accusize balloon dilation/incision, psoas hitch reimplantation, Boari flap reimplantation, and transureteroureterostomy.

○   **Describe the usual features of TB cystitis.**

The bladder lesions arise at the ureteral orifices. The lesions are velvety, red, inflamed, and edematous with granulations as a later finding. More advanced disease can affect the entire bladder.

○   **When is a bladder biopsy indicated in GU TB?**

Never. If the urine cultures are negative, the bladder biopsies will also be negative. If there is concern for a urothelial malignancy, then a bladder biopsy is indicated. Isolated tubercles away from the ureteral orifices should be biopsied for malignancy.

○   **A 55-year-old man was treated for severe GU cystitis with isoniazid, rifampin, pyrazinamide, and prednisone for 6 months. Following treatment, he remains disease free. However, he has severe persistent urgency, frequency, and nocturia. His bladder capacity is 120 mL. What would be the next appropriate therapy?**

Augmentation cystoplasty.

○   **A 20-year-old man presents with a superficial ulcer of his glans penis. Biopsy of the lesion rules out a malignancy but reveals TB. How could he have contracted this disease?**

Hematogenous spread from a primary pulmonary source or direct inoculation from the female genital tract.

○   **How does TB orchitis develop?**

TB orchitis is almost always a direct extension of TB of the epididymis. TB is spread to the epididymis via the blood stream.

○   **A 22-year-old HIV-positive man presents with scrotal swelling and a tender right testicle and epididymis. Upon palpation, he has beading of his associated vas deferens. He has a poorly defined fullness to the globus major of the epididymis that is directly associated with the testis. What would be the next step in the management of this patient?**

A scrotal ultrasound should be obtained to further delineate the fullness.

○   **The ultrasound reveals a solid mass involving the testis and epididymis as well as a small associated loculated hydrocele. What is the next step in the management?**

The patient should have tumor markers drawn and undergo a radical orchiectomy. This lesion may represent a testicular malignancy.

○ **A 40-year-old man with prior pulmonary TB has epididymal fullness that on ultrasound is consistent with TB. The testis is uninvolved. What technique could be used to evaluate for active TB in his scrotum?**

Fine needle aspiration can frequently yield active TB within the epididymis.

○ **What complication can arise from epididymal TB?**

Obstructive azospermia.

○ **A young couple wish to have children. Female factor infertility has been ruled out. The potential father was treated for pulmonary TB. His workup has revealed findings consistent with epididymo-orchitis related to his past history of TB. He is found to be profoundly azospermic. How should they proceed?**

Natural conception in unlikely is this setting. Most patients will require epididymal or testicular sperm aspiration followed by in vitro fertilization.

○ **Antituberculosis antibiotics should be used for how long in HIV-positive patients?**

Nine months is usually recommended.

○ **Patients with HIV account for what percent of the total TB population?**

Fifty percent. TB testing is recommended in all HIV patients.

CHAPTER 29

Medical Aspects of Urolithiasis

Elizabeth Phillips, MD, and Manoj Monga, MD

○ **How common is nephrolithiasis?**

The overall prevalence of stone disease is approximately 8%.

○ **How many Americans experience a bout of renal colic caused by nephrolithiasis annually?**

Approximately 1,200,000.

○ **How does region affect the incidence of nephrolithiasis?**

More common in the southeast United States and less common in the northwest.

○ **Is the worldwide incidence of kidney stones increasing, decreasing, or about the same and why?**

The rate of kidney stone disease is increasing worldwide. This is thought to be the result of more cultures adopting a Western diet as well as global warming contributing to increased dehydration.

○ **Is nephrolithiasis more common in men or women and by what ratio?**

The male:female ratio is 3:1. Roughly 4% of women and 12% of men will develop at least one stone at some point in their lifetimes.

○ **What type of calculus is equally common in men and women?**

Cystine and uric acid stones.

○ **What type of calculus is more common in women then men?**

Struvite stones are twice as likely to occur in women because of the higher incidence of urinary tract infections in females.

○ **What is the most common age at presentation with nephrolithiasis?**

A peak incidence for nephrolithiasis occurs from 25 to 40 years old.

○ **What is the current estimated yearly cost of kidney stone disease in the United States?**

More than 2 billion dollars a year and rising.

○ **What effect, if any, does obesity have on kidney stone formation?**

Obesity is a strong predictor of stone recurrence especially in first-time stone formers. Obesity causes changes in urine chemistry reflecting increased calcium, uric acid, sodium, and decreased citrate in the urine. Urine of obese patients has also been found to have a lower pH. Obesity is associated with a higher risk for both uric acid and calcium oxalate stones.

○ **How does obesity affect nephrolithiasis?**

Through purine gluttony, dietary excesses, diabetes, and insulin resistance.

○ **How might insulin resistance contributes to stone forming?**

Insulin resistance at the cellular level results in hyperinsulinemia, which in turn causes defects in renal production of ammonia, lowering the pH of the urine.

○ **What medications can be used to facilitate ureteral stone passage in urolithiasis?**

α_1-adrenergic antagonists facilitate stone passage. Tamsulosin and other α-blockers, used often in BPH, facilitate passage of stones less than 10 mm. The rate of stone passage increases approximately 30% with the use of α-blockers, and the need for narcotics and surgical intervention decreases. Steroids may be used to reduce ureteral edema for easier stone passage. In addition, calcium channel blockers such as nifedipine have been shown to cause ureteral dilatation and relaxation resulting in increased spontaneous stone passage rates.

○ **What percentage of patients require intervention for passage of a stone?**

It is 20% overall; 50% of patients with stones ≥5 mm. A proximal ureteral stone will have a lower chance of spontaneous stone passage (50%) than a distal ureteral stone (85%). In general, a stone 4 mm or less in size has a 90% chance of eventual passage.

○ **What is the average time to spontaneous stone passage?**

The time to spontaneous passage correlates with stone size. The average time to stone passage is 1 week for <2 mm, 2 weeks for 2 to 4 mm, and 3 weeks for >4 mm.

○ **How long should we wait for an asymptomatic stone to pass or move before considering doing a surgical procedure?**

Roughly 30 days. After that time, the risk of possible long-term complications, like strictures, increases. If the stone is symptomatic, intervention should obviously be done sooner.

○ **What are the indications for hospitalization in the acute setting of renal colic?**

Severe pain requiring continuing parenteral pain medication, fever and infection, intractable vomiting, renal insufficiency, and a solitary kidney. Urinary tract infection with an obstructed system or increased serum creatinine are the two indications for emergent decompression of the collecting system with ureteral stenting or placement of a percutaneous nephrostomy tube.

○ **What medication decreases the need for narcotics to control renal colic?**

Ketorolac (Toradol) IV has been demonstrated to decrease the need for narcotics in acute renal colic.

○ **What is the risk for stone recurrence after an initial symptomatic episode of urolithiasis?**

The stone recurrence rate is 50% within 5 years from the first stone episode.

○ **Can stone disease be ruled out in the absence of hematuria?**

No, approximately 15% of patients with ureteral stones have no RBC/hpf on microscopic urinalysis.

○ **What diagnostic imaging should be used if there is clinical suspicion of urolithiasis?**

Unenhanced helical CT scan without contrast has been shown to be the most sensitive and specific imaging study available for stones and can also assist in diagnosing other nonrenal causes of flank pain.

○ **Should a KUB be performed when the CT scan has already identified a stone? Why or why not?**

Yes, a KUB should be immediately performed when the CT scan has demonstrated a stone for several reasons. First, it provides a baseline study to easily track progress of the stone. Next, it separates radiopaque from radiolucent stones. Finally, it provides a clear idea of the shape and size of the stone as well as its surgical orientation.

○ **Compare modalities of imaging as diagnostic tests for urolithiasis.**

Ultrasound detects 50% to 60% of stones.
KUB detects 60% to 70%.
IVU detects 70% to 90%.
Noncontrast CT scan detects 90% to 100%.

○ **What differential diagnoses with urolithiasis may be evaluated using noncontrast CT?**

Pyelonephritis	Tumor with urinary retention	Pancreatitis
Diverticulitis	Renal mass or tumor	Ileus
Appendicitis	Duodenal ulcer with perforation	Benign stenosis of the ureter
Aortic aneurysm	Renal pelvis tumor	Pancreatic tumor

○ **What are some of the limitations of CT imaging of renal stones?**

CT cannot identify pure indinavir stones. It also cannot differentiate between radiolucent and radiopaque stones, and it does not always give an accurate rendering of the exact size or shape of some stones. It is also expensive and has significant radiation exposure so it cannot be used in pregnancy.

○ **How accurate is CT in diagnosing urolithiasis?**

98% sensitivity, 95% specificity, 98% positive predictive value, and 95% negative predictive value.

○ **Is MRI a useful imaging study in urolithiasis?**

MRI does not visualize stones and should not be used to make the diagnosis of urolithiasis. MR urography may have a role in the evaluation of flank pain in pregnancy, although ultrasound is the usual first choice in imaging.

○ **Are forced fluids helpful in the management of acute renal colic?**

A recent randomized trial demonstrated that fluid bolus in the emergency department did not impact pain or stone passage. As such, forceful hydration may not help with stone expulsion although many patients with acute renal colic will be dehydrated and may need IV fluid replenishment for other reasons.

○ **What fluids and drinks should generally be avoided in stone formers?**

Phosphoric acid in soda drinks will acidify the urine and increase the risk of kidney stones. Performance drinks are often high in sodium content and will increase the risk of stones.

○ **How does dietary sodium impact the risk of stone formation?**

Every teaspoon of salt increases urinary calcium by 23 mg. It leads to higher rates of bone resorption and fluid retention while decreasing urinary citrate levels by 20%.

○ **Is significant oral calcium restriction recommended for calcium stone formers?**

Aggressive calcium restriction increases the risk of stone formation. Calcium is important for bone homeostasis and to bind oxalate in the bowel. A moderate limitation of calcium intake is reasonable.

○ **What complementary approaches are available for patients with hypercalciuria?**

Fish oil supplementation (Eicosapentanoic acid, n-3 fatty acid) competes with arachidonic acid (n-6) resulting in a decrease in prostaglandin E2. This leads to a decrease in renal calcium excretion, increase of renal calcium reabsorption, and decreased bone resorption. It has been demonstrated to decrease urinary supersaturations for both calcium phosphate and calcium oxalate.

○ **In what percentage of patients can at least one metabolic abnormality predisposing to urolithiasis be identified?**

A probable metabolic etiology for nephrolithiasis is found in 97% of patients who are properly evaluated.

○ **What is the most common type of stone formed?**

Calcium oxalate stones make up approximately 70% of all renal calculi.

○   **What type of crystal is depicted in this urine sample?**

Figure A.

Figure B.

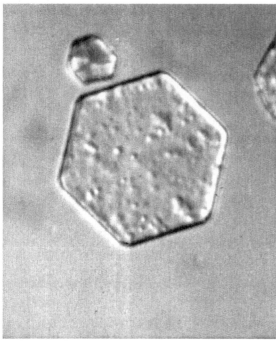

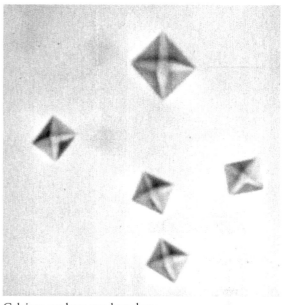

Calcium oxalate: star-box shape.

Cystine: hexagonal shape.

Figure C.

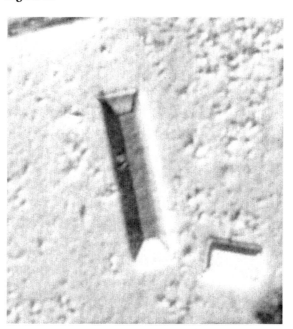

Calcium phosphate: coffin shape.

○ **What are the five most important urinary chemical abnormalities found in stone formers?**

Hypercalciuria, hypocitraturia, hyperuricosuria, hyperoxaluria, and low urinary volume.

○ **Citrate is an important inhibitor of stone formation. What drink is highest in citrate content?**

Grapefruit juice (14,500 mg/L of citrate). However, grapefruit juice is also high in oxalate content. The most effective means to obtain dietary citrate is 4 oz of concentrated lemon juice per day, usually as lemonade.

○ **How does citrate supplementation affect citrate levels in the urine?**

Citrate absorbed from the intestines is converted to bicarbonate in the liver. This increased alkali load stimulates renal excretion of citrate, raises the urinary pH, and increases urinary citrate levels.

○ **In what ways does citrate inhibit calcium stone formation?**

Citrate binds calcium, forming a soluble complex in urine and competing with its binding with oxalate or phosphate. Citrate also may alkalinize the urine, thereby inhibiting the formation of both calcium oxalate and uric acid crystals.

○ **What is the optimal level of oral citrate supplementation and how can this be determined clinically?**

An optimal concentration of 320 to 340 mg of citrate/L of urine and 24-hour urine levels ≥600 to 650 mg of citrate have been suggested as long as the urinary pH remains at or below 7. While a 24-hour urine test for citrate would be optimal, it is impractical to perform this test too often. Another method is to maximize the potassium citrate supplementation until the patient reaches maximum tolerance or the pH exceeds 7. FDA-approved urinary dipsticks to specifically monitor urinary pH are now available commercially. (www.uridynamics.com)

○ **What is the most important chemical mediator of intestinal absorption of calcium?**

The most important chemical mediator of calcium absorption is calcitriol (1,25-dihydroxyvitamin D_3), which increases calcium transport across the intestinal lumen. The conversion of precursors to calcitriol is initiated by hypophosphatemia and parathyroid hormone (PTH).

○ **What additional effects does PTH have on calcium homeostasis?**

PTH is a polypeptide that stimulates the osteoclasts to resorb bone, releasing calcium and phosphate into the bloodstream. PTH also acts upon the kidney to resorb calcium from the urine into the blood.

○ **PTH increases calcium resorption in the kidney, so explain why we find hypercalciuria in patients with hyperparathyroidism.**

The calcium resorption effect of PTH is overcome in hyperparathyroidism by the extremely high serum calcium levels.

○ **True or False: The incidence of stone formation in hyperparathyroid patients is unrelated to the degree of serum calcium or PTH elevations.**

True.

○ **What percentage of hyperparathyroid patients will have nephrolithiasis as their presenting or initial symptom?**

Twenty-two percent.

○ **In what ways are hyperparathyoid stone formers different from hyperparathyroid patients without nephrolithiasis?**

Hyperparathyroid stone formers are more likely to be younger and have hypercalciuria. Their hyperparathyroidism is almost always caused by parathyroid adenomas as opposed to hyperplasia.

○ **How much dietary calcium is absorbed on a daily basis?**

Approximately 33% of the total dietary calcium (600–1200 mg or 15 mg/kg) is absorbed and 100 to 200 mg is secreted into the intestinal tract for a net absorption of approximately 100 to 300 mg. Calcium ions that are complexed in the GI tract to phosphate, oxalate, citrate, and sulfate are not absorbed.

○ **How is hypercalciuria defined? (Give at least three definitions.)**

The excretion of greater than 200 mg/24 h on a diet of 400 mg calcium and 100 mEq sodium for a week. On an unrestricted diet, hypercalciuria can be defined as >275 mg calcium/d for men, >250 mg/d for women. Another definition is more than 4 mg of calcium/kg body weight/d.

○ **What is the estimated percentage of patients with calcium oxalate stones who will demonstrate hypercalciuria?**

Approximately 35%.

○ **What are the three basic types of hypercalciuria?**

1. Absorptive hypercalciuria caused by increased intestinal absorption of calcium.
2. Renal leak hypercalciuria caused by an abnormality in renal absorption of calcium.
3. Resorptive hypercalciuria caused by augmented bone demineralization.

○ **How important is the differentiation of the type of hypercalciuria in clinical practice?**

Not very, except for research purposes and for the identification of hyperparathyroidism. What is more important is the patient's response and compliance with therapy.

○ **What is the "simplified" approach to hypercalciuria?**

First, exclude hyperparathyroidism by checking a serum calcium and parathyroid hormone level. Dietary measures, such as limitations on oral calcium intake, can be used initially. If these measures fail and the hypercalciuria persists, then a thiazide diuretic should be used.

○ **When should a calcium loading test be performed?**

There is virtually no current role for a calcium loading test outside of a research or investigative protocol.

○ **Describe the pathophysiology, diagnosis, and treatment of type 3 absorptive hypercalciuria?**

Type 3 absorptive hypercalciuria or renal phosphate leak hypercalciuria is caused by a defect in renal phosphate reabsorption. This leads to high urinary phosphate levels and hypophosphatemia that stimulates vitamin D activation to increase intestinal phosphate absorption to correct the low serum phosphate. The increased vitamin D levels will also inadvertently increase intestinal calcium absorption, where the excess calcium is eventually excreted in the urine as hypercalciuria. The diagnosis is made by the concurrent finding of hypercalciuria, relative hypophosphatemia, high urinary phosphate, and increased serum vitamin D levels. Treatment is by oral phosphate that suppresses the vitamin D activation. Thiazides are relatively ineffective in this particular form of hypercalciuria.

○ **Is an elevated serum calcium an effective screening test for absorptive hypercalciuria?**

No. The increased absorption of calcium secondarily increases the filtered calcium presented to the kidney, thereby suppressing parathyroid function and subsequently decreasing renal resorption of calcium. The hypercalciuria offsets the increased intestinal absorption, thereby keeping serum calcium in the normal range.

○ **Is an elevated serum calcium an effective screening test for renal hypercalciuria?**

No. Renal leak of calcium results in lowering of serum calcium that stimulates PTH and 1,25-dihydroxy-vitamin D_3. This results in an increase in intestinal absorption of calcium, which normalizes the serum calcium levels.

○ **What is the medication of choice for renal hypercalciuria?**

Thiazides specifically correct the renal leak of calcium by augmenting calcium reabsorption in the distal and proximal tubules.

○ **How effective is thiazide in reducing hypercalciuria and preventing kidney stone recurrences in these patients?**

Thiazides reduce urinary calcium excretion by approximately 30% and can reduce stone recurrences by up to 80%.

○ **What other medication besides thiazide can also reduce renal excretion of calcium?**

Indapamide (Lozol) acts similarly but is technically not a thiazide.

○ **What should one consider if thiazide is not effective in preventing stone recurrences or controlling hypercalciuria?**

Look for an increase in dietary sodium or calcium as well as a decrease in potassium leading to intracellular acidosis and hypocitraturia. Also consider optimizing other aspects of metabolic stone disease such as uric acid, urinary oxalate, and total volume.

○ **Thiazides are contraindicated or ineffective in a subset of hypercalciuric patients. What other treatment modalities can be used to help control hypercalciuria?**

Amiloride, sodium cellulose phosphate, and orthophosphates as well as reasonable dietary calcium limitations.

○ **Is an elevated PTH diagnostic of resorptive hypercalciuria?**

No. PTH is secondarily increased in renal hypercalciuria. An oral calcium load will suppress the hypersecretion of PTH in renal hypercalciuria. This can help differentiate this entity from primary hyperparathyroidism.

○ **How does sodium cellulose phosphate work to inhibit stone formation and what are the potential side effects?**

Sodium cellulose phosphate is a nonabsorbable ion exchange resin that binds calcium and inhibits calcium absorption in the intestine. Side effects include hypomagnesemia via binding of intestinal magnesium. Patients also get secondary hyperoxaluria since more divalent cations are bound in the gut leaving more oxalate available for absorption. Lastly, there can be a negative calcium balance with consequent stimulation of PTH. Supplementation of magnesium and limitation of dietary oxalate are important adjuncts with the use of this agent.

○ **How do orthophosphates work and what are their side effects?**

Orthophosphates exert their hypocalciuric effect by inhibiting $1,25\text{-OH}_2\text{-D}_3$ synthesis. Side effects include secondary PTH stimulation and soft tissue calcification. Orthophosphates are indicated in vitamin D–dependant absorptive hypercalciuria and in cases of hypophosphatemia. They are also the drugs of choice for renal phosphate leak hypercalciuria (absorptive hypercalciuria type 3).

○ **What is the drug of choice for absorptive hypercalciuria type 1 in patients at risk for osteoporosis?**

Thiazides. They act by causing diuresis and increasing renal absorption of calcium. The main side effects include hypokalemia and hypocitraturia. These can be overcome by the addition of potassium citrate supplements.

○ **Why is it important to limit sodium intake when taking thiazides for stone disease?**

Thiazides inhibit sodium reabsorption in the ascending limb of the Loop of Henle, causing contraction of the extracellular volume. This leads to increased sodium and calcium reabsorption in the proximal convoluted tubule. Excess sodium intake would inhibit the ability of thiazides to contract the extracellular volume and limit their hypocalciuric response.

○ **Is the hypocalciuric response to thiazides routinely permanent?**

No. If the response to thiazides is lost, a 6-month "drug holiday," during which time sodium cellulose phosphate therapy or orthophosphates can be utilized, will often reinstate responsiveness to thiazides.

○ **When are thiazides contraindicated with hypercalciuria?**

Hyperparathyroidism and patients with severe sulfa allergies.

○ **Why are thiazides contraindicated in these patients?**

Resorption of calcium from bone and from the kidney in hyperparathyroidism causes hypercalcemia which would be further increased after thiazide therapy. Thiazides contain sulfa molecules and so should be used cautiously in those with a documented sulfa allergy.

○ **What is the most common cause of hypercalcemia in the outpatient setting?**

Hyperparathyroidism. It should be suspected in all patients with high or high-normal serum calcium and calcium urinary lithiasis.

○ **How does one diagnose hyperparathyroidism?**

Assays that measure the intact molecule or the carboxy-terminal portion of PTH are approximately 90% sensitive in detecting elevations in blood levels of PTH. PTH also causes an increase in cAMP, which can be measured in the urine.

○ **What is "subtle" or "subclinical" hyperparathyroidism and how is it diagnosed?**

"Subtle" or "subclinical" hyperparathyroidism is defined as a condition where the serum calcium and PTH levels are both elevated or high normal but are not diagnostic of overt hyperparathyroidism. A temporary course of thiazides with increased oral calcium intake (a thiazide challenge test) should decrease serum PTH levels except in cases of true hyperparathyroidism. Even if negative, repeat testing should be done periodically to rule out true or clinical hyperparathyroidism that might develop later.

○ **What are alternative treatments for primary hyperparathyroidism if the patient cannot undergo parathyroidectomy?**

Orthophosphates, bisphosphonates, and potassium citrate can be used if surgery is contraindicated. Estrogen supplements can be tried in postmenopausal women.

○ **What is the most common cause of hypercalcemia in the inpatient setting?**

Malignancy. Less than 1% of patients with urinary lithiasis have a malignancy. The most common tumors in descending order of occurrence are lung, breast, renal cell, head and neck, and hematologic.

○ **Why does malignancy cause hypercalcemia?**

The mechanism for most hypercalcemia-related malignancy is osteoclastic bone resorption stimulated by cytokines and other substances released by the tumor, such as PTH-related polypeptide, prostaglandins, tumor necrosis factors, and transforming growth factors.

○ **What are other causes of hypercalcemia?**

Hyperthyroidism, glucocorticoid excess, pheochromocytoma, prolonged immobilization, familial hypocalciuric hypercalcemia, thiazides, lithium, milk-alkali syndrome, vitamin A toxicity, and granulomatous diseases such as sarcoidosis, histoplasmosis, tuberculosis, leprosy, silicosis, and coccidiomycosis. Sarcoid granulomas may produce calcitriol.

○ **How is hypercalcemia treated?**

Hypercalcemia is treated by addressing the underlying cause, hydration, bisphosphonates, calcitonin, and mithramycin.

○ **What calculi are radiolucent?**

Uric acid, sodium urate, ammonium urate, xanthine, silica, protease medication, and 2,8-dihydroxyadenine calculi.

○ **How does hyperuricosuria lead to stone formation?**

Stones secondary to hyperuricosuria are a result of the precipitation of sodium-urate crystals in the urine. These crystals can initiate both urate and calcium oxalate stones. They also remove certain inhibitors of stone formation and lower urinary pH.

○ **Why would a person on a high-protein, low-carbohydrate diet (such as the Atkins diet) be more likely to form renal stones?**

High purine content of meat may lead to the formation of uric acid stones and hyperuricosuria. Patients on the Atkins diet have been shown to have more acidic urine, higher urinary calcium and uric acid, and low urinary citrate levels.

○ **What evidence supports the causal relationship between increased protein intake and nephrolithiasis?**

Population studies show that the increase in societal consumption of protein is associated with increased incidence of stone disease. Protein intake increases urinary calcium, uric acid, and oxalate. Protein moderation is recommended—aggressive protein restriction can increase the risk of stones. Patients should target a dietary protein intake of 0.8 to 1 g/kg/d.

○ **Why are humans and dalmatians the only mammals prone to uric acid urolithiasis?**

We both lack uricase, a hepatic enzyme that converts uric acid to soluble allantoin.

○ **What causes hyperuricosuria?**

Hypersecretion of urate can be caused by increased dietary purines, gout, or states of overproduction of purines such as malignancy, myeloproliferative diseases, and glycogen storage diseases. Urate stones may also be found in states of chronic diarrhea such as Crohn's disease, ulcerative colitis, or jejuno-ileal bypass, which produce a state of acidosis via bicarbonate loss and dehydration.

○ **What is another effect of systemic acidosis that promotes stone formation?**

Systemic acidosis is the most important etiologic factor for the development of hypocitraturia.

○ **What foods are highest in purine content?**

Beef, poultry, pork, peanuts, and fish.

○ **What is the strongest urinary chemical promoter of kidney stone production?**

Oxalate is the strongest chemical promoter, approximately 15 times stronger than calcium.

○ **Does urinary oxalate come primarily from dietary sources?**

No. Approximately half of the enteric oxalate is degraded by luminal bacteria. Most (80%) of the urinary oxalate comes from hepatic conversion.

○ **Name two common GI bacteria that degrade intestinal oxalate?**

Oxalobacter formigenes and *Pseudomonas oxaliticus.*

○ **What are the characteristics of *Oxalobacter formigenes*?**

It is a gram-negative rod and obligate anaerobe that has a nutritional requirement for oxalate, degrading 70 to 100 mg of oxalate daily in a normal person with normal anatomy, bowel function, and diet. It usually prevents excessive absorption of oxalate, which may impact hyperoxaluria and stone formation.

○ **In what conditions would one see decreased colonization of *Oxalobacter formigenes* in the gut?**

Oxalobacter colony counts have been demonstrated to be decreased in stone formers. There is evidence that patients who have undergone bariatric surgery have fewer colonies of oxalobacter present in the GI tract, however, studies are ongoing to evaluate the effects of modern day bariatric surgery. Oxalobacter is sensitive to antibiotic therapy and may be decreased or absent in those receiving antibiotics.

○ **Besides hyperoxaluria, what other disorder is found in patients after bariatric surgery that would increase their overall risk of kidney stones?**

Hypocitraturia.

○ **In what conditions does dietary oxalate contribute significantly to urinary oxalate?**

Secondary hyperoxaluria (enteric hyperoxaluria) occurs in patients with short bowel syndrome, inflammatory bowel disease, jejunoileal bypass, or intestinal malabsorption. Intestinal fat malabsorption characteristic of ileal disease results in saponification of calcium and magnesium. This decreases the amount of calcium available to complex with oxalate in the intestinal lumen, raising the free oxalate pool available for intestinal absorption.

○ **What other conditions can lead to hyperoxaluria?**

Pyridoxine deficiency, excess ascorbic acid ingestion, ethylene glycol ingestion, and methoxyflurane anesthesia.

○ **What is type 1 primary hyperoxaluria and what causes it?**

Primary hyperoxaluria type 1 is an extremely rare autosomal recessive disorder resulting in increased hepatic production of oxalate. It typically presents in childhood. It is caused by a deficiency of the enzyme alanine-glyoxylate aminotransferase that converts glyoxylate to glycine. Without this enzyme, oxalate levels increase substantially; 50% of patients develop end-stage renal disease by age 15 and 80% by age 30.

○ **How is type 1 primary hyperoxaluria treated?**

Pyridoxine (vitamin B6) supplementation is a cofactor in the glyoxylate pathway and may be helpful. Early liver transplantation can avoid renal failure and other problems if the disease can be diagnosed early. If not, then a combined liver–kidney transplant is the only curative treatment available.

○ **What dietary restrictions would you recommend for hyperoxaluria?**

Leafy green vegetables, rhubarb, spinach, cocoa, okra, potatoes, peanuts, turnips, chocolate, pecans, carrots, berries, tea, powdered coffee, nuts, broccoli are known to be generally high in oxalate content.

○ **What are some medical therapies for hyperoxaluria?**

High doses of oral calcium 0.25 to 1.00 g/d or more are recommended especially in cases of enteric hyperoxaluria. This complexes with the free oxalate in the intestinal tract. Large doses of pyridoxine 100 to 200 mg/d are beneficial in primary hyperoxaluria. Side effects of pyridoxine include hypomagnesuria. Doses higher than 200 mg/d can be associated with peripheral neuropathy. Cholestyramine helps in enteric hyperoxaluria by binding free intestinal oxalate where calcium cannot be used. Iron supplements can also do this and may be helpful in controlling hyperoxaluria.

○ **What other stone disease is characterized by autosomal recessive inheritance?**

Cystinuria is a rare autosomal recessive disorder characterized by >250 mg/d urinary excretion of cystine and flat hexagonal crystals in the urinary sediment, which increase in solubility with the increase in pH (especially pH >7.5).

○ **Can cystinuria be ruled out on the basis of patient age at presentation?**

No. Some patients do not present until the fifth or sixth decade.

○ **What other dicarboxylic amino acids are affected by the inheritance of the above renal tubular absorption abnormality?**

Cystine, **O**rnithine, **L**ysine, and **A**rginine. COLA is a useful mnemonic. These amino acids are more soluble than cystine, so they do not form calculi.

○ **What specific gene is responsible for cystinuria?**

The dibasic amino acid transporter gene SLC3A1.

○ **What is a characteristic radiographic appearance of cystine stones?**

Ground glass appearance. Less opaque than calcium stones.

○ **What is the first line of medical therapy for cystine stones?**

Aggressive hydration (aiming for 3–4 L of urine per day) and alkalinization to a pH of 7 to 7.5.

○ **What is a potential side effect of alkalinization beyond a pH of 7.5?**

Calcium phosphate crystallization.

○ **What are the advantages of potassium citrate over sodium bicarbonate as an alkalinizing agent?**

Limits sodium intake, which is of special importance in patients with congestive heart failure and hypertension. It does not promote calcium oxalate crystallization to the same degree and it tends to last longer.

○ **What other medications may be used to treat cystine stones?**

Drugs that contain a disulfide structure can reduce cystine to form soluble cysteine. These include D-penicillamine, α-mercaptopropionylglycine, and captopril. Penicillamine has been associated with frequent side effects including nephrotic syndrome, exfoliative dermatitis, and pancytopenia. α-mercaptopropionylglycine has a more favorable safety profile, making it the drug of choice. Tiopronin can be used in patients who manifest adverse effects to the above-mentioned drugs. Dietary restriction of methionine should be instituted, but is usually of limited benefit due to tolerance and lack of compliance.

○ **What vitamin should be supplemented if D-penicillamine is utilized?**

Pyridoxine (vitamin B6). Deficiency of vitamin B6 leads to gastrointestinal upset, glossitis, dermatitis, and seizures.

○ **What is the sodium nitroprusside test?**

Examination of a spot urine sample for cystine can be performed by the nitroprusside test. The cyanide-nitroprusside colorimeter test gives a magenta ring at urinary cystine levels of greater than 75 mg/L.

○ **What is the chemical composition of struvite stones (infection stones)?**

Struvite or infection stones consist of magnesium, ammonium, phosphate, and carbonate-apatite (calcium).

○ **What types of bacteria are associated with struvite stones?**

Urinary tract infection caused by urease-producing organisms leads to the formation of struvite stones. The most common culprits include *Proteus, Pseudomonas, Klebsiella,* and *Staphylococcus. Escherichia coli* does not produce urease.

○ **Why is urease important?**

Urease splits urea in the urine to ammonia (contributes to ammonium in struvite stones) and bicarbonate. Bicarbonate creates alkaline urine, promoting the crystallization of struvite stones. Struvite does not precipitate unless the pH is >7.

○ **What is a staghorn calculus?**

Staghorn calculus describes the appearance of a calculus that has formed on a matrix cast of the pyelocalyceal system of the kidney. It is most commonly a struvite calculus, however, cystine and uric acid calculi may form staghorn configurations.

○ **What is the goal of medical therapy for struvite stones?**

Antibiotics are used to maintain sterile urine. Antibiotic suppression after clearance of the offending organism is useful, but complete elimination of the stone is the ultimate goal of therapy. Urine culture results should direct the selection of the most appropriate antibiotic.

○ **What adjunctive medical therapies are useful for struvite stones?**

Urease inhibitors such as acetohydroxamic acid are useful. Acetohydroxamic acid reduces the urinary saturation of struvite and retards calculus formation. The recommended dosage is 250 mg three times per day. Limiting side effects include gastrointestinal upset, headaches, anxiety, and hallucination.

○ **What potentially serious complication is associated with the use of acetohydroxamic acid?**

Deep venous thrombosis is a rare but potentially serious complication associated with this medication.

○ **Which Renal Tubular Acidosis type is associated with nephrolithiasis?**

Renal tubular acidosis (RTA) describes several conditions (types 1, 2, and 4) where defects in renal/urinary acidification lead to metabolic acidosis. Only type 1 RTA is characterized by nephrolithiasis, hypokalemia, hyperchloremia, and nonanion gap metabolic acidosis. Approximately 70% of adults with distal RTA (type 1) have renal calculi.

○ **What is the metabolic defect in RTA type 1 and what urinary abnormalities does it produce?**

Defective excretion of hydrogen ions by the distal tubule results in a high urinary pH. The urine remains relatively alkaline (pH >6.0) despite systemic acidosis caused by the inability of the distal tubule to maintain a proton gradient. Systemic acidosis results in hypercalciuria due to decreased renal reabsorption, increased bone resorption, and hypocitraturia.

○ **When should you suspect RTA type 1?**

Clinical suspicion is raised by hypocitraturia, hypokalemia, systemic acidosis (serum bicarbonate <23 mEq/L), nephrocalcinosis on radiographs, recurrent calcium phosphate stones (>30% of total stone burden), and urine pH >6.

○ **How do you diagnose RTA type 1 and how is it treated?**

Ammonium chloride load test. Diagnostic if urine pH >5.5 after taking 100 mg NH_4Cl/kg body weight the day prior. However, since the therapy for RTA type 1 and severe hypocitraturia is essentially the same (potassium citrate supplementation), there is little need for this particular test in clinical practice.

○ **What medications may promote stone formation and should be elicited in the medication history? (Identify at least five by name.)**

Indinavir and other protease inhibitors used for HIV as well as triamterene can form stones from the medication. Carbonic anhydrase inhibitors like acetazolamide can cause overly alkaline urine and calcium phosphate stones. Excess vitamin C can be metabolized to oxalate. Excess vitamin D can cause absorptive hypercalciuia. Uricosuric agents like probenecid lead to hyperuricosuria. Topiramate (Topamax), a migraine prevention medication, can cause metabolic acidosis that can lead to stones. Other agents that can promote stone formation include antacids, calcium supplements, chemotherapeutics, theophylline, and furosemide.

○ **When is allopurinol used and how does it work?**

Allopurinol (300 mg/d) is used for hyperuricosuric calcium oxalate nephrolithiasis and uric acid nephrolithiasis. It decreases urate synthesis by inhibiting hepatic xanthine oxidase and lowers blood and urinary urate. Allopurinol should be given with a moderate sodium restriction. Allopurinol dosage should be adjusted in hyperuricemic (gout) patients to maintain a serum uric acid level at or below 6.

○ **What type of stone may form as a result of allopurinol therapy?**

Xanthine, although this is quite uncommon.

○ **What new drug may be used as a nonpurine analogue inhibitor of xanthine oxidase?**

Febuxostat is a newer, orally administered drug. Dosing is 80 to 120 mg/d. It is metabolized by the liver. It has not been studied specifically in stone disease at this time.

○ **What medications are associated with the formation of ammonium urate calculi?**

Laxatives, acetazolamide, allopurinol, triamterene, and sulfonamides. Of these, laxative abuse is by far the most common.

○ **How is urine pH helpful in predicting the stone chemical composition?**

Low urine pH (<5.5) suggests the presence of uric acid or cystine calculi while an alkaline pH (>7.5) suggests the presence of struvite or calcium phosphate stones.

○ **What is gouty diathesis and how is it treated?**

Gouty diathesis is defined as calcium nephrolithiasis associated with hyperuricemia or gout. Patients typically are aggressive stone formers. The mainstay of treatment is to alkalinize the urinary pH to approximately 6.5. Potassium citrate has been demonstrated to provide adequate alkalinization with minimal side effects. Potassium citrate 30 to 60 mg/d is given in two or more divided doses. Sodium bicarbonate is a less expensive option; however, it should be used with caution in patients with hypertension or congestive heart failure. Elevation of the urinary pH above 7 should be avoided to prevent precipitation of calcium phosphate.

○   **When should allopurinol be used in the prophylaxis of kidney stones and what is the dosage?**

Allopurinol is recommended in all active stone patients with gout or hyperuricemia, especially if they also have uric acid stones or hyperuricosuria. Uric acid stones that are not adequately controlled with alkalinization therapy alone and patients who cannot take sufficient alkalinizing medication to obtain an optimal pH may also be candidates for allopurinol therapy. While the standard dose is 300 mg/d, the dosage should be titrated in hyperuricemic patients to obtain a serum uric acid level of 6 or less. No more than 300 mg should be taken at one time. Initial dosing should begin at 100 mg/d to avoid stimulating a gout attack and then increased weekly. Maximum dosage is 800 mg/d.

○   **Allopurinol has been associated with skin rashes and peripheral neuropathy. What treatments are used as prophylaxis for these complications?**

Allopurinol should be stopped for a skin rash as it represents a potentially serious allergic response. No prophylaxis is available. However, vitamin B6 can be helpful in minimizing the potential neuropathy from allopurinol use.

○   **What is an intravenous alternative for alkalinization?**

Sodium lactate (1/6 M). Infuse 500 mL every 8 hours. Sodium lactate is completely converted to bicarbonate within 1 to 2 hours.

○   **When should the liquid version of potassium citrate be used instead of tablets?**

In any case where there is more rapid intestinal transit time, patients have difficulty swallowing the tablets, or urinary citrate levels fail to increase on tablet therapy alone.

○   **How should potassium citrate therapy be titrated?**

Adjust the dosage based on keeping the pH at or below 7.0 while maximizing the 24-hour urine citrate level. A bedtime dose helps supplement the normal nocturnal "alkaline tide."

○   **What diseases are calcium phosphate stones associated with?**

Primary hyperparathyroidism, renal tubular acidosis, sodium alkali therapy.

○   **Who should be offered prophylactic testing with a 24-hour urine study?**

All kidney stone patients who are children should definitely be tested as well as those with kidney transplants, solitary kidneys ureteral reimplantations, and renal failure. Patients with multiple stones or frequent recurrences should be encouraged to have the testing. Ultimately, any kidney stone patient who is motivated to follow long-term preventive treatment suggestions is potentially a candidate for 24-hour urine testing. Patients need to understand that kidney stones are a lifelong problem and even the best preventive treatment plan may occasionally fail.

○   **What are the critical elements of a successful kidney stone preventive testing program?**

Correct urine collection procedures are very important. But even more important is making sure that interested patients understand that stone preventive therapy is ongoing and lifelong. Those without the motivation and discipline to follow a reasonable treatment plan indefinitely should not receive the testing. The most critical elements of 24-hour urine testing are total volume, calcium, uric acid, sodium, oxalate, and citrate. Phosphate, magnesium, and sulfate are also recommended as well as blood testing for uric acid, calcium, and CO_2.

○ **What general advice should be given to kidney stone formers who do not elect to perform 24-hour urine testing?**

Increase water intake. Moderate your diet, particularly purines and high-oxalate foods. Limit salt intake. For calcium oxalate stone formers, ask them to consider at least a nightly potassium citrate supplement.

○ **What is the recommended daily water intake for kidney stone formers?**

While eight separate 8 oz glasses of water daily is often quoted, the better answer is whatever is necessary for that patient to generate 2000 mL or more of urine per day. This is roughly just a little more than half gallon.

○ **Is it necessary or recommended to have patients wake up during the night to drink extra water?**

This is almost never necessary, with the possible exception of cystine stone formers where a 3000 mL daily urinary volume is sometimes necessary.

○ **What are the statistical odds for other family members of stone formers to eventually develop stones?**

Approximately 25% for male children of stone formers. Female children approximately 8%. The highest risk ratio would be between brothers where the lifetime risk is approximately 50% if one brother is a stone former.

○ **Medullary sponge kidney is associated with what three urinary abnormalities associated with kidney stones?**

Medullary sponge kidney is associated with an increased risk of urinary tract infections, renal leak hypercalciuria, and hypocitraturia.

○ **What tests should be obtained prior to percutaneous chemolysis of calculi?**

Stone composition should be known. Urinary tract infection should be excluded by urine culture. Urinary extravasation should be excluded by antegrade contrast study.

○ **What is the solution of choice for chemolysis of uric acid calculi?**

Sodium bicarbonate (50 mEq in 1 L of 0.45% NaCl, pH 8).

○ **What is the solution of choice for chemolysis of cystine calculi?**

Acetylcysteine (0.3 M) in tromethamine E (Tham E, pH 10).

○ **What are the main ingredients in Suby G's solution and hemiacidrin solution, utilized for struvite calculi dissolution?**

Citric acid and magnesium citrate. Both these solutions maintain a pH of 4.

○ **What was a potentially lethal complication of irrigation with hemiacidrin?**

Hypermagnesemia. Magnesium is added to the solution to decrease uroepithelial irritability. With high intrapelvic pressures (>25 cm H_2O), hypermagnesemia can occur, leading to respiratory depression.

○ **What laboratory studies should be monitored during hemiacidrin irrigation?**

Daily magnesium levels, creatinine and phosphorus levels. Urine culture every 3 days.

○   **What is a finding on physical examination suggestive of a high magnesium level?**

Depressed deep tendon reflexes.

○   **How would hypermagnesemia be treated?**

Intravenous calcium, furosemide, and saline.

○   **What are some changes during pregnancy that could alter stone formation?**

Placental production of 1,25-(OH)$_2$ vitamin D can stimulate hypercalciuria through increased intestinal absorption. This may be offset by increased renal excretion of citrate and nephrocalcin.

○   **True or False: Pentosan polysulfate (Elmiron) can be used to treat otherwise intractable recurrent stone disease.**

True. Reports indicate that Elmiron coats urinary crystals with a synthetic GAG layer reducing crystal aggregation and subsequent stone formation.

○   **What are the two most common metabolic problems in pediatric stone formers?**

Hyproctiraturia and hypercalciuria are the most common.

○   **Pyridoxine (vitamin B$_6$) may decrease hepatic oxalate production by facilitating what chemical reaction?**

Pyridoxine helps convert glyoxalate to glycine.

○   **Randall's plaques are always of what chemical composition?**

Calcium phosphate (hydroxyapatite).

○   **Hypermagnesemia is a potential complication of irrigation with Renacidin (magnesium carbonate) or Suby's solution. What are the symptoms and treatment for hypermagnesemia?**

Hypermagnesemia is characterized by confusion, lethargy, paralysis, and possibly coma.
    Treatment involves saline infusion with Lasix diuresis. In severe cases, IV calcium gluconate can be used. Hemodialysis is the preferred treatment in patients with renal failure.

○   **What percentage of bladder stones are 100% uric acid?**

Approximately 50%.

○   **What four medical problems are associated with abnormally elevated vitamin D levels?**

Hyperparathyroidism, sarcoidosis, malignant tumors, and granulomatous disease.

○   **When should orthophosphate therapy for calcium nephrolithiasis should not be used?**

In renal failure with a GFR of 30 mL/s or less.

○   **Do obese patients actually have more kidney stones, or does it just seem that way?**

Obese patients actually do make more stones.

○ **True or False: Oxadrop, a freeze-dried product containing five different lactic acid bacteria, has been shown to significantly reduce urinary oxalate excretion in idiopathic hyperoxaluria.**

False. A randomized, placebo-controlled trial by Goldfarb et al. (2007) failed to show any benefit.

○ **Should patients with struvite (infection) stones have 24-hour urine metabolic testing?**

Yes, just like other stone formers.

○ **What is the most common urinary metabolic problem found in struvite stone formers other than infection?**

Hypercalciuria.

○ **At what 24-hour urine excretion of cystine should specific therapy be initiated?**

Usually at 250 mg of cystine per 24 hours.

○ **What is the optimal pH for most cystine stone formers and for calcium stone formers?**

Usually a pH of 7.5 is suggested even though this may increase the risk of calcium phosphate stones. The feeling is that the increased solubility of cystine at this pH level justifies the risk. Calcium stone formers are generally optimized at a pH of approximately 6.5.

○ **What is the formula for estimating the total 24-hour urinary creatinine excretion in men and women and why is it important?**

Women: 17 × body weight (kg)

Men: 22 × body weight (kg)

This is useful in determining the reliability of a 24-hour urine collection.

○ **What diagnosis is suggested by urolithiasis with hypercalciuria, hypercalcemia, and hyperuricemia together with parathyroid suppression and azotemia? What specifically causes the calcium abnormalities?**

Sarcoidosis. Overproduction of $1,25\text{-}(OH)_2$ vitamin D by pulmonary macrophages causes the calcium metabolism abnormalities.

○ **What additional study is recommended in calcium stone forming hypercalciuric children besides blood and 24-hour urine testing?**

Bone mineral density testing for osteoporosis and osteopenia.

○ **What are the three acceptable surgical treatments for symptomatic ureteral stones in pregnancy?**

Percutaneous nephrostomy, double J stents, and ureteroscopic stone extraction.

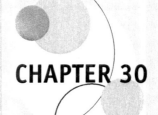

CHAPTER 30 **Genitourinary Trauma**

James M. Cummings, MD

○ **What percentage of all hospital trauma admissions involve renal trauma?**
Approximately 3%.

○ **What percentage of all abdominal trauma involves the kidneys?**
Approximately 10%.

○ **True or False: The presence or absence of hematuria is not a good indicator of traumatic injury.**
True. In one study, 13% of proven renal gun shot victims had no hematuria.

○ **What are the indications for imaging of the kidneys following blunt trauma?**
Gross hematuria or microhematuria combined with shock defined as systolic BP <90 at any time following the injury are absolute indications for GU tract imaging.

○ **In children, what are the indications for imaging of the kidneys following blunt trauma?**
All children who sustain blunt trauma and have greater than five RBC per high-power field on a microscopic urinalysis or a positive dipstick should undergo radiographic assessment of the kidneys.

○ **Staging of renal trauma is best accomplished with what radiographic test?**
CT scanning of the kidneys provides detailed images of the kidneys that allow for a clear delineation of most renal injuries and their severity.

○ **What are the advantages, if any, of an IVP over CT scans in the evaluation of GU trauma?**
It allows a functional assessment of the kidneys. Also, it can be done in the OR or ER. However, CT gives a better assessment of the renal anatomy and permits diagnosis of concurrent injuries. Therefore, CT scans are the standard for trauma imaging of the kidneys.

○ **The kidney is rich in tissue factor. What does this do and why is this important?**
Tissue factor activates the extrinsic coagulation cascade that promotes hemostasis after an injury.

○ **A small cortical laceration in the kidney with a small perirenal hematoma would be classified as what grade injury?**

Grade II.

○ **What are the absolute indications for renal exploration following blunt trauma and how is it done?**

An expanding or pulsatile retroperitoneal hematoma must be explored. Initial control of the involved renal pedicle prior to opening of the hematoma must be achieved by means of a retroperitoneal incision medial to the inferior mesenteric vein and anterior to the aorta. The dissection is carried cephalad until the involved renal pedicle is encountered. Vascular control is achieved and the hematoma can now be entered.

○ **An attempt to repair a traumatic injury to the main renal artery should be pursued under what circumstances?**

Repair of the main renal artery should be attempted only in a hemodynamically stable patient who has no other associated major organ system injuries, an ischemia time of less than 8 to 10 hours, and/or bilateral renal injuries or injury to a solitary kidney.

○ **What is the treatment of choice for a renal arteriovenous fistula?**

Angiographic arterial embolization.

○ **The parents of a 12-year-old child with a solitary kidney wants to know the risk of the child losing the remaining kidney in contact sports. What are the risk statistics you should tell them?**

It has been estimated that six kidneys per 1 million children will be injured per year with only one kidney lost per 2.67 million children per year.

○ **Hypertension following renal trauma can result from what two mechanisms?**

1. Renal vascular injury leading to stenosis or occlusion of the renal artery or one of its branches.
2. Compression of the renal parenchyma from extravasated blood and urine (Page kidney).

○ **A 1-cm segment of the left ureter is damaged during an elective left colectomy. The injury is recognized intraoperatively. The best choice for management at that time is?**

Debridement of any devitalized tissue, mobilization of the two ends of the ureter, and a spatulated ureteroureterostomy over a stent. The area must be adequately drained postoperatively.

○ **You are called to the OR to consult on a patient with a massive gunshot injury to the left abdomen. The trauma team has identified a 5-cm defect in the middle left ureter. The patient has become unstable and the trauma team wants to close and move the patient to the ICU for further resuscitation. What is your best option?**

Ligate the proximal ureter and have a percutaneous nephrostomy placed when the patient has stabilized. Perform operative reconstruction at a later date when the patient is better prepared.

○ **Does a ureteral injury sustained during an aortobifemoral grafting procedure require a nephrectomy?**

No. In the past it was felt that with a 50% risk of mortality from graft infection, a nephrectomy was a safer option than reconstruction. However, with better stenting and diversion techniques, newer antibiotics, and improved graft materials, ureteral reconstruction can be performed as long as adequate diversion and drainage is done. The risk is also lowered if omentum or some other tissue barrier is placed between the graft and the ureter.

○ **Which portion of the ureter is most likely to be injured during a hysterectomy?**

At the level of the broad ligament where the ureter passes beneath the uterine vascular pedicle in close proximity to the cervix.

○ **Following a ureteral reimplant with a psoas hitch, a patient complains of anterior thigh numbness. What is the most likely etiology for this complaint?**

The genitofemoral nerve lies on the anterior aspect of the ileopsoas muscle. Injury to this nerve can occur during suturing of the bladder to the tendon of the psoas minor muscle.

○ **What are the options for closing a large gap between the proximal end of a damaged ureter and the bladder when a psoas hitch will not reach?**

Initially, the bladder should be mobilized on the contralateral side to the injury. This often involves division of vascular structures (superior vesical artery, obliterated umbilical artery, etc.). A Boari bladder flap can gain considerable length. Another option is to do a caudal nephropexy that can gain additional length to allow for closure of the defect. When these maneuvers are unsuccessful, a transureteroureterostomy can be performed in the patient with unprepared bowel, otherwise an ileal interposition graft may need to be employed.

○ **Where should you anastomse the distal end of the ileal interposition graft?**

Directly to the bladder. This allows freer passage of mucus than an anastomosis to the distal ureter.

○ **Contraindications to the use of an ileal ureter for ureteral repair include?**

Impaired renal function (Cr >2 mg/dL), untreated bladder outlet obstruction, or poor bladder emptying for other reasons.

○ **The arterial vascular supply of the ureter comes most commonly from what sources?**

- Upper ureter—renal artery.
- Middle ureter—iliac artery.
- Lower ureter—superior vesical artery.

○ **A retrograde pyelogram done at the end of a difficult ureteroscopic stone extraction shows moderate extravasation at the previous location of the stone. Visual inspection reveals a perforation of the ureter and a wire placed initially is still in place in the renal pelvis. Appropriate management at this time is?**

Placement of a ureteral stent along with a Foley catheter to maximally drain the system and allow for healing of the ureter. A follow-up retrograde pyelogram should be performed at approximately 6 weeks postoperatively to assess healing of the involved area.

○ **Avulsion of the ureter during ureteroscopy occurs under what circumstances?**

The most common cause is a basket engaging a stone and trapping ureteral mucosa simultaneously. A basket can also cut directly into the ureter and trap the mucosa. Finally, the ureteroscope alone can cause avulsion if it fits tightly in the ureter and intussuscepts when withdrawn.

○ **A woman presents with continuous urinary leakage 2 weeks following an abdominal hysterectomy. On physical examination, urine is identified in the vaginal vault. A cystogram is normal. What is the diagnosis and what test should be done next?**

An IVP should be performed to rule out ureterovaginal fistula.

○ **In an adult suspected of having bladder trauma, what volume of contrast should be instilled into the bladder and how many films are required?**

The bladder should be filled under gravity pressure with up to 400 mL of contrast, or until a bladder contraction occurs. Following adequate AP filling views, oblique views need to be obtained as well as drainage views of the anatomic pelvis.

○ **What is the major pitfall of CT cystography in the evaluation of a bladder injury?**

If done with IV contrast only, the bladder may not be sufficiently distended to reveal the injury and thus gives a false-negative result.

○ **Extraperitoneal bladder ruptures may be managed nonoperatively under what circumstances?**

If adequate bladder drainage via a large Foley catheter or suprapubic catheter can be achieved, there is no perforating bony fragment in the bladder wall, and the injury does not involve the bladder neck, nonoperative management can be successful. Close clinical follow-up is mandatory in this situation.

○ **What is the correct management of an intraperitoneal bladder rupture?**

Intraperitoneal bladder ruptures should be managed with surgical exploration, a multilayered closure, adequate bladder drainage, and possible drainage of the space of Retzius.

○ **You are called to the OR during a cesarean section for a bladder injury. On inspection, there is a 2-cm laceration of the anterior bladder. Your next step should be?**

Open the bladder sufficiently to be able to inspect the entire bladder for other possible bladder injuries and to ensure that the ureteral orifices are intact. Only after ensuring the integrity of the bladder and ureters should a bladder closure be performed.

○ **In the United States, what is the most common event leading to a vesicovaginal fistula?**

Iatrogenic injury during gynecologic surgery (particularly hysterectomy) is the most common etiology of fistulas. Fistulas from childbirth are more common in underdeveloped countries.

○ **Vesicovaginal fistulas following hysterectomy are a result of what etiologic event?**

An unrecognized bladder injury during hysterectomy with subsequent urinary extravasation into the surgical field and drainage via the vaginal cuff suture line leads to formation of the fistula.

○ **What is the best time to repair a vesicovaginal fistula following an uncomplicated hysterectomy?**

Timing of the repair depends largely on the time interval to the diagnosis of the injury as well as the clinical condition of the patient. Although 3 to 6 months have been recommended in the past, early intervention can be successful if there is minimal inflammation in the tissues and there are no other complicating factors.

○ **Tissues commonly used for interposition grafts in surgical repair of vesicovaginal fistulas include?**

Labial fat pad (Martius graft), gracilis muscle, peritoneum, and omentum.

○ **When used for interposition for vesicovaginal fistula repair, the omentum is mobilized on which vessel?**

The omentum is mobilized off the greater curvature of the stomach and the right gastroepiploic arterial supply is preserved. This is usually the dominant vessel supplying the omentum, and mobilization in this manner often allows the omentum to reach the deep pelvis.

○ **What are the most common causes of spontaneous rupture of an augmented bladder?**

Mucus plugging, chronic distension, or poor patient compliance with catheterization schedules.

○ **What are the two major classifications of pelvic fractures?**

The Tile classification and the Young classification.

○ **Physical findings of a posterior urethral injury include?**

Blood at the meatus, a distended bladder, and a high-riding prostate gland on rectal examination are all consistent with a posterior urethral injury.

○ **How does one diagnose a posterior urethral injury?**

Retrograde urethrography with the patient in a semioblique position is an effective method of diagnosing this injury. Extravasation of contrast is diagnostic. Attempted catheterization is controversial and can convert a partial urethral disruption into a complete disruption.

○ **A 32-year-old male victim of a motor vehicle accident suffers a pelvic fracture. Retrograde urethrography shows extravasation at the level of the membranous urethra. He is otherwise stable and no other immediate management is planned by the trauma team or orthopedics. What is the best urological management at this point?**

Management of a posterior urethral injury is controversial. In an otherwise stable patient, options include immediate realignment and delayed repair. Primary realignment may be possible in patients with limited pelvic bleeding. In this scenario, every attempt is made to avoid the pelvic hematoma and a urethral Foley catheter as well as a suprapubic catheter is placed. In a delayed repair, a suprapubic catheter is placed and plans are made for a possible urethroplasty after convalescence from the other injuries.

○ **What steps can be taken to gain length for an end-to-end bulboprostatic urethral anastomosis for repair of a stricture from a membranous urethral injury?**

- Mobilization of the urethra up to the penoscrotal junction.
- Division of the intercavernosal septum.
- Inferior pubectomy.
- Routing of the urethra over one of the cavernosal crura.

○ **What are the causes of erectile dysfunction (ED) following a pelvic fracture?**

Arteriogenic problems may occur as a result of injury to the internal pudendal artery. Venogenic impotence may ensue if there is direct injury to the corpus cavernosum. Neurogenic impotence can result from injury to the cavernous nerves, pelvic plexus, or sacral nerve roots. Most believe that impotence after pelvic fracture is a result of the injury itself and not the subsequent urethroplasty needed to repair the urethra.

○ **The best candidates for penile revascularization for traumatic impotence have what characteristics?**

- Demonstration of a focal arterial obstruction without diffuse atherosclerosis.
- Young patients and otherwise healthy patients.
- Patient has strong sexual desire and is highly motivated.

○ **A man presents with priapism. He gives a history of falling on a ladder and straddling one of the rungs 2 months ago. What type of priapism does the patient have, what are the likely characteristics of the blood aspirated from the penis, and how should the patient be treated?**

Blood gas determinations will show high oxygen levels since the likely etiology is arteriovenous fistula from the straddle injury. Arteriography with selective embolization of the fistula is the recommended treatment.

○ **True or False: A Winter shunt is a useful adjunct to the management of traumatic (high-flow) priapism.**

False. Surgical drainage of the corpus cavernosum is usually not required with high-flow priapism.

○ **A 24-year-old male suffers a gunshot wound to the penis. On examination, there is an entrance wound in the lateral midshaft with an exit wound at the ventral penoscrotal angle. The next step should be?**

Performance of a urethrogram to check for urethral injury is mandatory prior to any planned surgical intervention.

○ **A urethrogram in a male with a gunshot wound to the penis demonstrates stretching and elongation of the urethra in the penile urethra but no extravasation. The best management for this injury is?**

The best management for this patient is careful placement of a small urethral catheter. It should be left indwelling for 10 to 14 days, followed by a voiding cystourethrogram.

○ **A urethrogram in a male with a gunshot to the penis shows extravasation in the midpenile urethra. There is minimal swelling on physical examination. The patient is stable without other significant injuries. How should the injury be managed?**

Exploration, debridement, and primary repair if the defect is small.

○ **In penile amputation injuries, how should the amputated portion of the penis be optimally preserved for transport?**

Wrapped in saline soaked gauze and placed within a plastic bag, which is then immersed in a cooler with ice slush surrounding the bag.

○ **What are the clinical signs reported by the patient with a penile fracture?**

A "cracking" sound or "pop" followed by pain, rapid detumescence, and pronounced swelling.

○ **What is the single diagnostic test recommended for patients presenting with an obvious penile fracture?**

Retrograde urethrogram.

○ **What percentage of penile fractures will also have a urethral injury?**

Approximately 10% of these patients will have an associated urethral injury.

○ **What is the best management of penile fractures?**

Surgical exploration, identification of the tunica injury, and primary closure of the defect.

○ **A male presents with the skin of the penis dark from ischemia from a constricting ring left on at the base of the penis for 24 hours. Management should be?**

Excision of the ischemic penile skin is the first step. Following resolution of the inflammatory process, split-thickness, unmeshed skin grafts can be applied to cover the penis.

○ **The flap of choice for penile or phallic reconstruction is?**

The free forearm flap based on the radial artery.

○ **How should testis ruptures from blunt trauma be managed?**

Exploration, debridement of nonviable tissue, and reconstruction of the tunica defect.

○ **Describe the recommended immediate management of the testes after a major scrotal skin loss.**

Place the testes in thigh pouches to preserve them for future reconstruction.

○ **How should major scrotal skin loss be repaired?**

Meshed split-thickness skin grafts covering the testes and sutured to the remaining skin at the groin and perineum.

○ **Emergency reversal of clopidrogel (Plavix) is required to control bleeding in a trauma patient. How is this done?**

Platelet transfusion.

○ **What is the incidence of ED following traumatic injuries to the posterior urethra and how is it best treated?**

The incidence is more than 90%. PDE5 inhibitors are relatively ineffective. Intracavernosal injection is the most effective and successful medical therapy in this group with an 82% success rate reported in previously potent patients.

○ **True or False: The best way to manage a paraphimosis that cannot be easily reduced manually is immediate surgery.**

False. Usually the problem is distal edema. This can often be managed with simple manual compression for 5 minutes. If this is not successful, a moist gauze pad and an elastic compression wrap can be applied. This will almost always reduce the swelling and edema of the distal penis and allows for manual reduction of the paraphimosis. Surgery is a last resort.

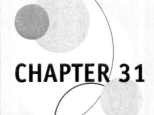

CHAPTER 31 Adrenal Physiology

Daniel A. Barocas, MD

○ **What is the weight of a normal adult adrenal gland?**

Five grams.

○ **Embryologically, does the adrenal arise from a single structure?**

No, the adrenal cortex and medulla are derived from embryologically distinct structures. The cortex develops from embryonic mesoderm and the medulla from embryonic neurectoderm. The hormonal secretions of each have different actions. Regulation of cortical and medullary secretions are independent of each other. Despite their anatomic proximity, there is virtually no functional relationship between the adrenal cortex and medulla.

○ **In patients with renal ectopia or agenesis, where does the ipsilateral adrenal gland lie?**

It lies in its normal orthotopic position. Since the adrenal gland and the kidney are of different embryologic origins, their migrations to their final anatomic positions take place independently.

○ **What percentage of the adrenal gland is made up of the adrenal cortex?**

The cortex constitutes 90% of the gland.

○ **What are the three zones of the adrenal cortex?**

Zona glomerulosa lies immediately beneath the capsule of the gland, the zona fasciculata is the middle zone and is the largest portion of the cortex, and the zona reticularis is the innermost zone.

○ **Is there a functional significance between the anatomic zonations of the adrenal gland?**

Yes, each anatomic zone is also a functional zone with aldosterone being produced exclusively in the zona glomerulosa, cortisol is produced in the two inner zones, zona fasciculata and the zona reticularis, adrenal androgens are produced in the inner cortical zone, the zona reticularis.

○ **What are the building blocks of adrenal hormones?**

Adrenal cells are capable of synthesizing cholesterol de novo, but most of the adrenal cholesterol used for steroidogenesis is derived from circulating lipoproteins and in particular from low-density lipoproteins (LDL).

○   **What is the first step in the production of adrenal steroid hormones?**

The first step is the production of pregnenolone from cholesterol via two hydroxylations followed by cleavage of the cholesterol side chain. Pregnenolone has no known biologic activity, but it is an intermediate in the production of all the biologically active steroid hormones.

○   **How are adrenal hormones stored?**

Adrenal hormones are steroid hormones, and as all biologic steroid hormones, adrenal hormones are not stored but are secreted immediately upon synthesis. The rate of steroid hormone secretion can be controlled by regulation of synthesis.

○   **Are active forms of adrenal hormones free or bound in serum?**

Only the free hormone is biologically active; however, all steroid hormones are largely protein-bound when they circulate in plasma. Because of the limited solubility of steroid hormones in water, protein binding acts to increase the amount of hormone that can circulate in the blood. Since the protein-bound fraction of hormone is relatively resistant to metabolism, protein binding also increases the plasma half-life of steroid hormones.

○   **Adrenal androgen production is limited by what factors?**

Many steroid compounds can be synthesized by the adrenal cortex, however, the enzymes required for the production of testosterone and estrogen are found in low concentration in the cortical cells. Consequently, androgens are normally produced in only very small quantities.

○   **Does the androgen precursor dehydroepiandrosterone (DHEA) have any androgenic activity in males?**

Only minimal; DHEA is secreted in large quantities by the adrenal cortex in males. DHEA has much less activity than testosterone, and in males, the overall effect of DHEA as an androgen is negligible. In females, both DHEA and androstenedione may be converted to testosterone at extra-adrenal sites, thus it has more androgenic activity in females.

○   **What stimulates adrenal androgen production?**

ACTH influences adrenal androgen production and seems to be the primary stimulus. However, it is clearly not the only factor, as evidenced by dissociation of ACTH and adrenal androgen production during events such as puberty and stress. Other regulators are not completely delineated, but it appears to be independent of gonadotropins.

○   **What are the principal androgens produced by the adrenal glands?**

Dehydroepiandrosterone (DHEA), dehydroepiandrosterone sulfate (DHEAS), and androstenedione are the principal androgens produced by the adrenals.

○   **How substantial is adrenal androgen production compared to total androgen production?**

The major androgen products of the adrenals are weak in their androgen effect. They are converted to more potent androgens, testosterone, and dihydrotestosterone in peripheral tissues. Even so, adrenal androgens contribute 5% to 10% of the production rate of testosterone in an adult male, making a negligible contribution compared to testicular production. The proportion of adrenal androgen production is substantially higher in females (40%–60%). However, overall adrenal androgen production is rarely physiologically important in the natural state and is only clinically apparent in disease states of overproduction, such as congenital adrenal hyperplasia.

○   **How does ketoconazole affect adrenal androgen production?**

It inhibits the cytochrome P-450–dependent enzymes important for steroidogenesis. Therefore, the conversion of cholesterol to pregnenolone is shut down, inhibiting production of testicular and adrenal androgens, as well as cortisol.

○   **There are five enzymes involved in the conversion of cholesterol to cortisol. What are the consequences of deficiencies of these enzymes?**

This family of disorders is known as congenital adrenal hyperplasia. In general, steroidogenesis is shunted to increased production of androgens in favor of cortisol and mineralocorticoid. The characteristic manifestations depend upon the enzyme affected, but typically include virilization of females and can include life-threatening salt-wasting due to lack of mineralocorticoid.

○   **What tests are used to distinguish adrenal tumors in women with hirsutism?**

Serum testosterone and DHEA.

○   **What is the most important mineralocorticoid produced by the adrenal cortex?**

Aldosterone, although produced in small quantities is the most physiologically important mineralocorticoid. Other mineralocorticoids such as 11-deoxycorticosterone (DOC) have both glucocorticoid and mineralocorticoid properties but are secreted in such small quantities that they are physiologically unimportant.

○   **What is the half-life of plasma aldosterone?**

Twenty to thirty minutes.

○   **What is the most significant regulator of aldosterone secretion?**

Angiotensin II is the primary physiologic control of aldosterone secretion. Angiotensin II directly stimulates production of aldosterone by the zona glomerulosa. A second less important stimulus is an elevated serum potassium level. Hypokalemia blunts the adrenal gland's ability to synthesize aldosterone thus causing a decrease in production and secretion.

○   **What is the basis of aldosterone production and its role in the renin-angiotensin-aldosterone system (RAAS)?**

In response to multiple stimuli, but primarily hypovolemia and decreased renal perfusion, renin is released from the juxtaglomerular apparatus (JGA) of the afferent arteriole. Renin cleaves angiotensin I (AI) from angiotensinogen. Angiotensin-converting enzyme converts AI to angiotensin II (AII) primarily in the pulmonary vasculature. Secretion of aldosterone results from direct stimulation of the adrenal gland by AII. The actions of aldosterone include a) increased renal conservation of sodium, b) increased glomerular filtration fraction by increasing efferent arteriole tone, c) increased peripheral vasomotor tone, and d) increased thirst. The overall effect is an increase in plasma volume and renal perfusion.

○   **What are the main physiologic functions of aldosterone?**

To regulate sodium resorption in the kidney, gut, salivary gland, and sweat glands.

○   **What is the site of action of aldosterone within the kidney?**

The principle site of aldosterone action is the distal tubule of the nephron.

○ **What is the mechanism of action of aldosterone within the kidney?**

Aldosterone stimulates transcription of the gene that encodes for a sodium–potassium ATPase, leading to increased numbers of sodium–potassium exchange pumps in the basolateral membrane of distal tubule epithelial cells. This conserves sodium in the nephron and water follows the sodium. The same mechanism is at play in the gut, salivary glands, and sweat glands.

○ **What is Conn's syndrome?**

Conn's syndrome is primary hyperaldosteronism.

○ **What are the clinical features of Conn's syndrome?**

The clinical features of Conn's syndrome include hypertension, hypokalemia, hypernatremia, alkalosis, and periodic paralysis.

○ **What laboratory abnormalities are typical of Conn's syndrome?**

The laboratory abnormalities of Conn's syndrome include hypokalemia, hypernatremia, alkalosis, decreased plasma renin activity (PRA <2 ng/mL), and high urine and plasma aldosterone (>15 ng/dL). Aldosterone-to-PRA ratio is >20:1.

○ **What is the phenomenon of renal escape?**

In primary aldosteronism after a gain of 1.5 kg of extracellular fluid, there is a decrease in absorption of sodium at the proximal tubules. Escape is associated with an increase in renal artery pressure and an increase in atrial natriuretic factor (ANF). Renal escape limits the clinical hypertensive response in patients with primary hyperaldosteronism.

○ **What is the most common cause of primary hyperaldosteronism?**

The most common cause is an aldosterone-producing adenoma of the adrenal gland.

○ **What is the most common cause of secondary hyperaldosteronism?**

The most common cause is renal arterial disease or renal parenchymal disease. This disease is a disorder with oversecretion of aldosterone secondary to excess production of angiotensin II and the renin-aldosterone-angiotensin system (RAAS).

○ **In treatment of an aldosterone-producing adrenal adenoma, adrenalectomy should be preceded by what preoperative measure?**

Adequate clinical treatment of hypertension and correction of hyperkalemia or other metabolic abnormalities.

○ **What is the treatment of primary aldosteronism caused by bilateral hyperplasia?**

The treatment is medication with the drug spironolactone, which is a competitive antagonist of the aldosterone receptor.

○ **What are the three endocrine glands required for regulation of cortisol synthesis and release?**

The hypothalamus, pituitary, and adrenal glands.

○ **Where is corticotropin-releasing hormone (CRH) produced and what is its function?**

CRH is synthesized in the hypothalamus and is carried to the anterior pituitary via the portal blood. CRH stimulates ACTH release.

○ **What are secondary stimulants of ACTH?**

Vasopressin, oxytocin, epinephrine, angiotensin II, vasoactive intestinal peptide, gastrin-releasing peptide, atrial natriuretic factor, and γ-aminobutyric acid are all secondary stimulants.

○ **What complex is ACTH derived from?**

ACTH is a 39-amino acid polypeptide produced from the protein proopiomelanocortin (POMC). Other POMC derivatives include β-lipotropin, α-melanocyte-stimulating hormone, β-melanocyte-stimulating hormone, β-endorphin, methionine, and enkephalin.

○ **Is ACTH produced constantly throughout the day?**

No, ACTH secretion is characterized by an intermittent diurnal rhythm leading to parallel changes with cortisol and ACTH.

○ **With respect to the normal diurnal variation with circulating cortisol levels, is the level higher in the morning or evening?**

Healthy subjects have a peak of cortisol levels in the morning with a fall throughout the day and into the evening. Patients with Cushing's syndrome lose the diurnal variation of circulating cortisol.

○ **What is the relationship between ACTH and circulating cortisol?**

ACTH and circulating cortisol are reciprocally related.

○ **What effects do glucocorticoids have on cellular metabolism?**

Glucocorticoids are essential for life and affect a wide spectrum of cellular metabolism including increased glycogen synthesis, increased gluconeogenesis, decreased peripheral glucose utilization, protein catabolism, and decreased immune-mediated inflammation. In disease states and stress, hypertension, muscle wasting, myopathy, osteopenia, and glucose dysregulation are seen.

○ **What is Cushing's syndrome?**

A symptom complex caused by excess glucocorticoid production. Manifestations include obesity, hypertension, diabetes, weakness, muscle atrophy, hirsutism, skin striae, moon facies, easy bruising, acne, and psychologic changes.

○ **What is the primary laboratory test to identify Cushing's syndrome if it is clinically suspected?**

The key to diagnosing Cushing's syndrome is establishing the presence of excess glucocorticoid. Therefore, a 24-hour urine to measure cortisol and creatinine is the primary laboratory test. The 24-hour urine collection commences following the first morning void and continues throughout a 24-hour period until completion of the next morning void. The urine should remain refrigerated in an opaque container until transported to the laboratory. Creatinine helps to confirm a complete collection.

○ **How accurate is urinary free cortisol as a screening test for Cushing's syndrome?**

Although 3.3% of individuals without Cushing's syndrome will have elevated values, this test is 95% specific for Cushing's syndrome.

○ **What test may be used if urinary free cortisol is equivocal?**

A low-dose dexamethasone test; 1 mg of dexamethasone is given at 11 PM and the cortisol is checked at 8 AM the following morning. A normal person's cortisol will be suppressed to <2 ng/mL by negative feedback on ACTH and CRH production. If plasma cortisol is not suppressed, Cushing's syndrome is present.

○ **How is the dexamethasone suppression test performed?**

1 mg of oral dexamethasone is ingested at bedtime. Serum cortisol is measured the next morning. Serum cortisol should be less than 2 μg/dL in normal individuals.

○ **False-positive may occur in what conditions?**

Obesity, alcoholism, renal failure, anorexia, and bulimia. Exercise and acute illness will also raise serum cortisol levels. Phenobarbital, phenytoin, and rifampin increase dexamethasone metabolism and may also cause false-positive results.

○ **What steps can be taken to identify the etiology of excess glucocorticoids?**

After the excess of glucocorticoids has been established by urinary free cortisol and/or a low-dose dexamethasone suppression test, the next step is to determine whether the hypercortisolism is ACTH-dependent or ACTH-independent. This can be accomplished by measuring late-afternoon ACTH with concurrent serum cortisol. A high ACTH value (>50 pg/mL) suggests ACTH dependence, whereas a low value (<5 pg/mL) suggests ACTH-independent Cushing's syndrome.

○ **What are the etiologies of ACTH-independent Cushing's syndrome?**

ACTH-independent causes of Cushing's syndrome account for approximately 18% of cases of Cushing's syndrome. Specific etiologies include adrenal adenoma, adrenal carcinoma, and bilateral adrenal hyperplasia.

○ **What are the etiologies of ACTH-dependent Cushing's syndrome?**

ACTH-dependent causes of Cushing's syndrome account for the majority of cases of Cushing's syndrome. Specific etiologies include pituitary hypersecretion and ectopic ACTH production.

○ **What is Cushing's disease?**

Pituitary hypersecretion of ACTH, usually secondary to a pituitary adenoma, which results in increased production and secretion of glucocorticoids.

○ **What percentage of patients with Cushing's syndrome actually has Cushing's disease?**

Seventy-five to eighty-five percent of Cushing's syndrome is due to Cushing's disease. Other causes of Cushing's syndrome include adrenal adenomas, adrenal carcinomas, and ectopic secretion of either CRH or ACTH.

○ **What are the treatments of Cushing's disease?**

Treatments for Cushing's disease include transphenoidal hypophysial microsurgery to remove the pituitary adenoma. This treatment is effective in 85% to 95% of patients. Other treatments include pituitary external beam radiation and heavy particle proton beam therapy.

○ **If Cushing's syndrome is diagnosed during pregnancy, is immediate treatment warranted or should it wait until the postpartum period?**

Both maternal and fetal morbidity have been reduced with treatment of Cushing's syndrome during pregnancy, either by surgical removal of an adrenal adenoma during the second trimester or by transphenoidal adenomectomy or with medications such as metyrapone.

○ **What is the most common cause of ectopic or exogenous glucocorticoid excess causing Cushing's syndrome?**

Exogenous steroid administration.

○ **ACTH may be produced ectopically by which tumors?**

Oat cell, small cell lung tumors, and carcinoid tumors.

○ **What is Nelson's syndrome?**

Ten to twenty percent of individuals undergoing bilateral adrenalectomy for severe Cushing's syndrome will suffer from growth of a pituitary adenoma (usually a chromophobe adenoma). Growth of the space-occupying lesion is attributed to the lack of hypothalamic/pituitary feedback and high levels of ACTH. Increased production of ACTH and melanocyte-stimulating hormone (a derivative of POMC) cause typical signs and symptoms of muscle weakness and skin hyperpigmentation. Mass effect can cause headaches, visual disturbances, and cranial nerve compression. With the development of treatments for Cushing's disease other than bilateral adrenalectomy, Nelson's syndrome is rarely encountered today.

○ **What is Addison's disease?**

Addison's disease is an inadequate production of corticosteroids by the adrenal cortex caused by a defect within the adrenal cortex rendering them unable to synthesize normal amounts of steroid hormones. Radiation therapy involving the adrenals can also cause Addison's disease.

○ **What is the most common cause of adrenal insufficiency?**

The most common cause of Addison's disease is withdrawal of exogenous steroid therapy. Additional causes include adrenal tuberculosis or lymphocytic adenitis with adrenal fibrosis, malignant infiltration of the adrenal, sarcoidosis, histoplasmosis, blastomycosis, and coccidioidomycosis. Additionally, Addison's disease may occur with administration of aminoglutethimide, ketoconazole, mitotane, or suramin.

○ **What is the classic triad of Addison's disease?**

Hyponatremia, hyperkalemia, and azotemia is the classic triad, however, the entire triad is present in only 50% to 60% of cases. Other disorders associated with Addison's disease may include hypercalcemia, hyperthyroidism, hypothyroidism, and diabetes.

○ **What symptoms are associated with Addison's disease?**

Symptoms associated with Addison's disease are weakness, prostration, dehydration, and coma.

○ **How does one diagnose adrenal insufficiency?**

The clinical test for Addison's disease is failure to increase plasma or urinary corticosteroid levels in response to an ACTH infusion. The screening test involves administration of ACTH or cosyntropin 0.25 mg IV. Cortisol is checked 60 minutes after administration and should be at least 18 μg/dL if normal.

○ **What can cause acute adrenal insufficiency?**

Acute adrenal insufficiency can be caused by withdrawal of exogenous steroids, sepsis, bilateral adrenal hemorrhage, surgical bilateral adrenalectomy, or surgical removal of a functional adenoma in a patient with an atrophic contralateral adrenal.

○ **What is the treatment of acute adrenal insufficiency?**

The treatment is administration of glucocorticoids along with replacement of saline.

○ **What is the treatment of chronic Addison's disease?**

Maintenance with chronic glucocorticoids and mineralocorticoids.

○ **What are the major catecholamines secreted by the adrenal medulla?**

Epinephrine, norepinephrine, and dopamine.

○ **Why is epinephrine secretion localized to the adrenal medulla?**

The enzyme phenylethanolamine-*N*-methyltransferase (PNMT) is located exclusively in the adrenal medulla, and catalyzes the methylation of norepinephrine to epinephrine. This can be clinically significant in patients with extra-adrenal pheochromocytoma, in which case only norepinephrine is produced because of the absence of PNMT at the extra-adrenal site.

○ **Are glucocorticoid and epinephrine production related?**

Yes, high levels of glucocorticoids are necessary to maintain levels of PNMT and thus epinephrine production. This may explain the proximity of the adrenal medulla to the venous drainage system within the adrenal gland.

○ **What are the substrates of epinephrine and norepinephrine?**

Dietary tyrosine and phenylalanine.

○ **What is the major regulation of catecholamine biosynthesis?**

Activation of tyrosine hydroxylase activity, which combines phenylalanine and tyrosine to form dopa as a precursor to norepinephrine. Tyrosine hydroxylase activity may be regulated by the adrenal cortex.

○ **How are catecholamines stored?**

They are stored in separate vesicles within nerve terminals.

○ **What causes preganglionic sympathetic nerves to release catecholamines?**

In general, catecholamine release is stimulated by sympathetic stimulation. Stress, pain, cold, heat, asphyxia, hypotension, hypoglycemia, and sodium depletion, all cause catecholamine release.

○ **What is the serum half-life of catecholamines?**

Less than 20 seconds.

○ **How are catecholamines degraded?**

They are degraded by the action of catechol-O-methyltransferase (COMT) and monoamine oxidase (MAO), following reuptake by nerve terminals.

○ **How are catecholamine breakdown products measured?**

The primary metabolite of catecholamine breakdown is urinary vanillylmandelic acid (VMA) with metanephrine and normetanephrine being secondary breakdown products. These are best measured by means of a 24-hour urine collection.

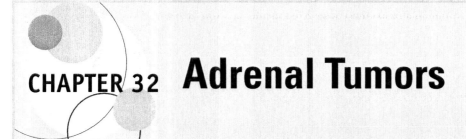

CHAPTER 32 **Adrenal Tumors**

Paul L. Crispen, MD, and
Matthew T. Gettman, MD

○ **How often are adrenal masses incidentally detected on CT scans?**

Five percent of the time.

○ **What radiographic criterion is utilized when distinguishing benign from malignant adrenal masses detected on noncontrast-enhanced CT scans?**

Radiographic density measured by hounsfield units. Adrenal lesions <10 hounsfield units are considered benign.

○ **What is the contrast washout test and how is it used?**

This is a test to determine if an adrenal mass is benign or malignant. An intravenous contrast agent is given and a CT scan is done after an 80-second delay. Another scan is done 10 minutes later and the two scans are compared. A washout or decrease in contrast enhancement of 50% or more is indicative of benign disease, less than 50% is specific for malignancy.

○ **What are the two general questions one needs to answer when working up an adrenal mass?**

1. Whether it is functional or nonfunctional.
2. Whether it is benign or malignant.

○ **What is the differential diagnosis of a benign, incidental adrenal mass?**

The more common adrenal lesions are adrenal adenomas, myelolipomas, and adrenal cysts. Less commonly one encounters ectopic tissue, pheochromocytoma, hyperplasia, aldosteronomas, and adrenal hemorrhage.

○ **How does adrenal hemorrhage occur and which side is affected most?**

Adrenal hemorrhage can occur following difficult childbirth and more often affects the right side. This phenomenon has been attributed to an increase in intra-abdominal pressure that is transmitted through the short right adrenal vein and into the parenchyma resulting in hemorrhage.

○ **What are the two most common adrenal lesions detected incidentally?**

Adenomas (75%) and myelolipomas (6%).

○ **What is the differential diagnosis of a malignant adrenal mass?**

Adrenocortical carcinoma, pheochromocytoma, neuroblastoma, and metastatic disease.

○ **What is the difference between Cushing's disease and Cushing's syndrome?**

Cushing's syndrome refers to the group of signs and symptoms that result from excessive glucocorticoids. Cushing's disease refers to Cushing's syndrome caused by the hypersecretion of ACTH from the pituitary gland.

○ **What is the most common cause of Cushing's syndrome?**

Use of exogenous steroids.

○ **What percentage of patients with endogenous Cushing's syndrome will have Cushing's disease?**

Approximately 75% to 85%.

○ **What is the most direct and reliable index of glucocorticoid function?**

The 24-hour excretion of cortisol in the urine. Patients with Cushing's syndrome often lose the diurnal variation or show higher basal levels than healthy subjects.

○ **In the dexamethasone suppression test, what serum and urine endpoints should change?**

There should be a fall in 17-hydroxycorticosteroid, urinary free cortisol, or plasma cortisol.

○ **How does one determine if a patient has ACTH-dependent or ACTH-independent hypercortisolism?**

The simultaneous measurement of both plasma ACTH (corticotropin) and cortisol by 2-site immunoradiometric assay.

○ **When using the metyrapone-stimulation test to differentiate between pituitary Cushing's and ectopic ACTH secretion, what result does one look for?**

Metyrapone blocks the conversion of 11-desoxycortisol to cortisol. As plasma cortisol concentrations fall, the pituitary gland secretes more ACTH, thus increasing urinary 17-hydroxy corticosteroid levels. Patients with Cushing's disease have a normal or supranormal increase in 17-hydroxy corticosteroid urinary excretion. Patients with ectopic ACTH-secreting tumors will have little or no increase in urinary 17-hydroxy corticosteroid levels, since ectopic ACTH production will not be influenced by plasma cortisol feedback on the pituitary gland.

○ **What is the radiographic appearance of a solitary adrenal adenoma?**

Adrenal adenomas are usually larger than 2 cm, associated with atrophy of the opposite gland, and are of low density because of the high lipid concentration.

○ **Name three agents used to reduce the secretion of functional steroids in patients with Cushing's syndrome.**

1. Aminoglutethimide blocks the conversion of cholesterol to pregnenolone. Patients given aminoglutethimide must be observed for adrenocortical insufficiency, since aldosterone production is also impaired.

2. Metyrapone blocks the conversion of 11-desoxycortisol to cortisone.

3. Ketoconazole blocks cytochrome P-450–mediated side-chain cleavage and hydroxylation at both the early and late steps in steroid biosynthesis.

○ **What is Nelson's syndrome and when has it been seen in the treatment of Cushing's disease?**

Historically, patients with Cushing's disease often were treated with bilateral adrenalectomy. Ten to twenty percent of these patients subsequently developed pituitary tumors, usually chromophobe adenomas, secondary to the lack of hypothalamic/pituitary feedback and high ACTH production. This could occur years after bilateral adrenalectomy and can be treated by prophylactic pituitary radiation.

○ **What is the currently accepted treatment of choice for Cushing's disease and what are the cure rates?**

Presently, transphenoidal hypophysial microsurgery for the removal of pituitary adenomas results in cure rates of approximately 90%.

○ **Why is the size cutoff for an adrenal carcinoma reported to be both 5 and 6 cm?**

Studies have shown that tumors <6 cm in size pathologically are unlikely to be adrenal carcinomas. However, CT scanning underestimates the size of the adrenal glands, so a 5-cm cutoff is used radiographically as the equivalent of the 6-cm pathologic size.

○ **What percentage of adrenal carcinomas are functional?**

Of the adrenal carcinomas, 62% to 79% are functional.

○ **How do functional adrenal carcinomas present?**

Functional adrenal lesions typically present as Cushing's syndrome (40%), Cushing's syndrome and virilization (24%) and virilization alone (20%) (virilization in females with either increased DHEA-17 ketosteroid or increased testosterone, feminizing syndrome in the male), hyperaldosteronism (2.5%), or a combination of the above.

○ **What is the sensitivity and specificity of the contrast washout test?**

Sensitivity, 98%; specificity, 100%.

○ **What is a collision tumor?**

A metastatic adrenal lesion located in or adjacent to an adrenal adenoma.

○ **What can one do to further work up an incidentally discovered nonfunctional adrenal mass, measuring between 3 cm and 6 cm in size?**

One can perform a fine-needle aspirate of the mass under ultrasound or CT scan guidance. Studies have supported a 96% incidence of obtaining significant cytologic material and an 86% incidence of accurately differentiating benign from malignant disease processes. Additionally, one can perform an MRI, and a high signal–intensity ratio on T2 images is suggestive of a malignant lesion.

○ **What is the reported complication rate for percutaneous needle biopsy of the adrenal gland and what complications are most likely?**

3%. Pneumothorax and hemorrhage are most common. Pancreatitis can develop following the biopsy of left-sided lesions, especially if an anterior approach is used.

○ **What primary cancers metastasize to the adrenal gland?**

The most common metastatic lesions to the adrenal gland include melanoma and carcinoma of the breast and lung. Additionally, carcinomas of the kidney, contralateral adrenal gland, bladder, colon, esophagus, gallbladder, liver, pancreas, prostate, stomach, and uterus can metastasize the adrenal gland.

○ **Virilization in the absence of elevated urinary 17-ketosteroids in a female patient should raise the suspicion of what other lesion?**

In addition to adrenocortical tumors that secrete testosterone, one should also consider testosterone-secreting ovarian tumors.

○ **A male patient with a functional adrenocortical tumor presents with gynecomastia, testicular atrophy, and impotence. What is the presumed diagnosis, likelihood of malignancy, and prognosis?**

This patient likely has an estrogen-secreting adrenocortical tumor that secretes androstenedione, which is converted peripherally to estrogens. Eighty percent of these lesions are malignant, with the 3-year survival being <20%.

○ **Can primary hyperaldosteronism be due to adrenal carcinoma?**

Yes. While primary hyperaldosteronism is usually due to small, benign, solitary adenomas, in Conn's syndrome or bilateral adrenal hyperplasia, it also can be caused by adrenocortical carcinoma.

○ **How does the presentation of adrenocortical carcinoma in children differ from that in adults?**

The majority of these tumors are hormonally active, usually presenting with Cushing's syndrome, virilization in the female, and isosexual precocious puberty in males.

○ **What syndromes can be associated with adrenocortical carcinoma in children?**

Beckwith–Wiedemann syndrome (exomphalos, macroglossia, gigantism, and neonatal hypoglycemia), isolated hemihypertrophy, and Li-Fraumeni syndrome.

○ **What is the differential diagnosis in the pediatric age group?**

In children younger than 5 years, neuroblastoma and Wilm's tumor are likely.

○ **What is the 5-year survival of adrenocortical carcinoma?**

Approximately 45%, with the most common metastatic sites being lung, liver, and lymph nodes.

○ **What pathologic criteria are utilized when classify adrenocortical carcinomas?**

The Weiss criteria based upon mitotic rate, atypical mitoses, venous invasion, nuclear grade, presence of clear cytoplasm, growth pattern, necrosis, sinusoidal, and capsular invasion.

○ **Describe the staging criteria utilized for adrenocortical carcinomas?**

T1: tumor ≤5 cm, invasion absent.
T2: tumor >5 cm, invasion absent.
T3: tumor involves adrenal fat.
T4: tumor invades adjacent organs.

○ **What is the standard recommended management of adrenocortical carcinoma?**

Surgical removal of the primary tumor, with an attempt to remove the entire lesion with contiguous organs (spleen, kidney) en bloc if necessary, and a regional lymphadenectomy.

○ **How often does adrenal carcinoma present with metastases and how often is the inferior vena cava (IVC) involved?**

Approximately 32% of the time; 19% will have IVC involvement.

○ **What drugs are available for the medical management of advanced adrenocortical carcinoma?**

Mitotane, a DDT-derivative, has been shown to induce a tumor response in 35% of patients. Ketoconazole has an adrenolytic effect. However, these compounds, in addition to metyrapone, have not been shown to improve long-term survival.

○ **Do calcifications in adrenal cysts suggest that these are actually malignant?**

No. Fifteen percent of adrenal cysts contain calcifications and this does not imply malignancy.

○ **What findings constitute the diagnosis of primary hyperaldosteronism?**

Hypokalemia with metabolic alkalosis, suppressed peripheral renin activity together with elevated urinary and plasma aldosterone levels in hypertensive patients.

○ **What factors can limit the evaluation of serum potassium and urinary aldosterone levels in patients with hyperaldosteronism?**

Hyponateremia can limit the evaluation of serum potassium and hypokalemia can limit the evaluation of urinary aldosterone.

○ **What is the most sensitive diagnostic test for hyperaldosteronism?**

Urinary excretion tests are more sensitive than serum studies. A 24-hour urine for aldosterone and sodium under conditions of prolonged sodium loading (>10 g/d diet for 5–7 days) with urinary aldosterone >14 μg and urinary sodium >250 mEq confirms the diagnosis.

○ **Name two causes of hyperaldosteronism.**

Solitary adenoma and bilateral adrenal hyperplasia.

○ **What test can help to differentiate the source of a hyperaldosteroma and how accurate is it?**

Postural aldosterone stimulation test. Patients with solitary adenomas may have a decrease or stabilization of aldosterone. The use of postural aldosterone stimulation testing is limited by an accuracy of only 70%.

○ **What plasma aldosterone-to-renin ratio is suggestive of primary aldosteronism?**

A plasma aldosterone-to-renin ratio >50 (aldosterone ng/dL to PRA ng/mL/h) is more common in primary aldosteronism than either essential hypertension or renal vascular disease.

○ **What is the best test to lateralize functional aldosterone-producing adenomas?**

Adrenal vein sampling of aldosterone is very sensitive in lateralizing these lesions.

○   **At the time of renal vein sampling to measure aldosterone, what else should be measured and why?**

Cortisol, in order to confirm correct positioning of the catheter during sampling.

○   **What is the management of a solitary unilateral adrenal mass identified on CT scan with biochemical criteria consistent with primary aldosteronism?**

After confirming functional status of the lesion, surgical extirpation would be appropriate. Adrenal vein sampling is not essential to lateralize the tumor, but can be helpful.

○   **What measures should be taken prior to surgical removal of a solitary adenoma associated with hyperaldosteronism?**

Treatment of hypertension with spironolactone or a calcium channel blocker and correction of potassium depletion.

○   **In patients with primary aldosteronism secondary to bilateral adrenal hyperplasia, what is the medical management of choice and how does it work?**

Medical therapy consisting of spironolactone, which is a competitive antagonist of the aldosterone receptor, is sufficient for many patients.

○   **Is the pattern of hypertension with pheochromocytomas sustained or paroxysmal?**

Sustained hypertension is found in 37% of patients with pheochromocytomas, and is a more common finding in children and patients with multiple endocrine adenoma type-2 (MEA-2). Paroxysmal hypertension affects approximately 47% of patients, females > males. A third pattern, sustained hypertension with superimposed paroxysms, is found in 50% to 65% of patients.

○   **Is it possible to have a pheochromocytoma in a normotensive patient?**

Yes. Approximately 10% of pheochromocytomas are found in normotensive patients. It is important not to eliminate pheochromocytomas from your differential diagnosis in a normotensive patient with an adrenal mass.

○   **Pheochromocytomas may be the part of what familial syndrome?**

Pheochromocytomas occur in MEA-2, which is a triad including pheochromocytoma, medullary carcinoma of the thyroid, and parathyroid adenomas. In addition, pheochromocytomas are part of the MEA-3, which includes medullary carcinoma of the thyroid, mucosal neuromas, thickened corneal nerves, alimentary tract ganglioneuromatosis, and frequently a marfanoid habitus. Pheochromocytomas may also be the component of MEA-2a or von Hippel-Lindau disease. Finally, pheochromocytomas may be associated with neuroectodermal dysplasias, including Von Recklinghausen's disease (neurofibromatosis), tuberous sclerosis, and Sturge–Weber syndrome.

○   **When is a partial adrenalectomy indicated?**

In patients with bilateral and hereditary adrenal tumors.

○   **How do the manifestations of pheochromocytoma in children vary from those in adults?**

Children manifest a higher incidence of familial pheochromocytomas (10%) and bilaterality (25%). Additionally, there is a 15% to 30% incidence of multiple pheochromocytomas in children and a 15% to 30% incidence of extra-adrenal location as well.

○ **What are the most common locations for extra-adrenal pheochromocytomas?**

The organ of Zuckerkandl (close to the origin of the inferior mesenteric artery), bladder wall, heart, mediastinum, carotid, and glomus jugulare bodies.

○ **What symptom is classically associated with extra-adrenal pheochromcytoma involving the urinary bladder?**

Micturition syncope.

○ **What laboratory tests confirm the diagnosis of pheochromocytoma?**

Elevated levels of catecholemines in the blood or urine occurs in 95% to 100% patients with pheochromocytomas. Specifically, plasma norepinephrine, epinephrine, and dopamine levels and urinary catecholemines should be used as an initial test.

○ **What is the utility of CT scanning for detecting pheochromocytomas?**

CT scanning detects >90% of pheochromocytomas of adrenal origin, and approximately 75% of extra-adrenal pheochromocytomas. Computed tomography alone cannot differentiate between pheochromocytomas and other adrenal lesions nor can one delineate malignant potential based upon the CT scanning alone.

○ **What clinical, biochemical, and histologic features distinguish malignant from benign pheochromocytomas?**

None. Malignancy is suggested by large tumor size, DNA ploidy pattern, local invasion, and the presence of metastases.

○ **What is the characteristic appearance of pheochromocytoma on MRI scanning?**

They appear as a characteristically bright image on T2-weighted studies. MRI is considered the best scanning procedure for patients with biochemical findings suggestive of pheochromocytoma.

○ **What is an MIBG scan and how is it useful?**

The metaiodobenzylguanidine (MIBG) scan images adrenal medullary tissue and is particularly useful for identifying pheochromocytomas of extra-adrenal origin or multiple pheochromocytomas. The MIBG scan has an overall sensitivity and specificity of 87% and 99%, respectively. False-negative rate is 10%.

○ **What is the preoperative medical preparation for patients with pheochromocytomas?**

All patients must be vigorously hydrated in preparation for surgery since elevated catecholamines levels lead to significant dehydration. Additionally, patients are started on an α-adrenergic blocker such as phenoxybenzamine, with an initial divided dose of 20 to 30 mg orally, increasing to 40 to 100 mg as needed. Secondly, β-adrenergic blockers can be added to the α-blockers to protect against arrhythmias and permit reduction in the α-blocker requirement. β-Blockers are usually only added when cardiac arrhythmias are identified. Labetalol (Normodyne) is a nonselective β-blocker and a selective α-adrenergic blocker that has been shown to control hypertension associated with pheochromocytoma.

○ **What problem can arise if β-blockers are initiated prior to α-blockers?**

There can be a marked rise in the total peripheral vascular resistance secondary to unopposed α-adrenergic activity that can lead to circulatory collapse.

○   **What additional drug might be used in the preoperative preparation of patients with pheochromocytomas who have cardiomyopathies, multiple catecholamine-secreting paragangliomas, or resistance to α-blockers?**

α-Methylparatyrosine (metyrosine) decreases the rate of catecholemine synthesis (the conversion of tyrosine to dopa).

○   **How should the surgeon and anesthesiologist be prepared for fluctuations in blood pressure at the onset of anesthetic induction in surgery?**

The patient must be volume-expanded with several liters of intravenous crystalloid prior to induction of anesthesia. In addition, α- and β-adrenergic blocking agents should be readily available for IV use. Phentolamine, a short-acting α-blocker (50 mg per 500 mL of ringers lactate), or sodium nitroprusside (50 mg per 250 mL of 5% dextrose in H_2O) should be on hand. Esmolol or propranolol should be available for persistent tachycardias or arrhythmias.

○   **What are the indications, advantages, and disadvantages for using a modified posterior incision for adrenal tumors?**

A modified posterior lumbotomy may be utilized in patients with right-sided adrenal aldosterone-secreting tumors or benign adenomas <5 cm. The main advantage over a flank or transabdominal incision is the excellent exposure of the vena cava in the region of the short right adrenal vein. The disadvantages include a limited visual field and compression of the abdominal contents and thoracic cavity that may impair respirations in the jack-knife position. This approach is not recommended for pheochromocytomas or malignant adrenal tumors.

○   **Following surgical exposure of a pheochromocytoma, what anatomic structure must be initially addressed?**

The adrenal vein should be divided initially to avoid systemic release of catecholemines during manipulation of the adrenal gland.

○   **What other therapy can be used in patients with hypertensive pheochromocytoma crisis that is refractory to sodium nitroprusside, α-blockers, and β-blockers?**

Magnesium sulfate. It lowers catecholamine release and acts as a very effective α-adrenergic antagonist and arterial dilator. It is also an excellent cardiac antiarrhythmic in the presence of high epinephrine levels. The use of magnesium sulfate has reportedly been lifesaving in a number of cases of refractory pheochromocytoma crisis.

○   **What is the 10% rule?**

10% of pheochromocytomas are malignant, 10% are bilateral, 10% are found in the pediatric age group, 10% will be extra-adrenal, and 10% are associated with multiple endocrine neoplasia (MEN) syndrome.

○   **Why is it important in cases of pheochromocytoma to start medical therapy with α-blocker treatment before using any β-blockers?**

This prevents paradoxical hypertensive crises. Ideally, a 4-week course of α-blocker therapy with phenoxybenzamine is suggested. Many patients are also volume-depleted and may require vigorous fluid resuscitation just before and/or just after their extirpative surgery.

○   **What medical problem needs to be carefully monitored postoperatively after pheochromocytoma surgery and how should it be treated?**

Hypotension due to lack of catecholamine vasoconstriction is the most common medical problem encountered postoperatively, although hypoglycemia may also appear. The hypotension is best treated with volume replacement. Vasoconstricting medications should be avoided if possible.

○   **When, if ever, is a bilateral adrenalectomy indicated?**

In patients who are surgical candidates but fail medical therapy. Also, in bilateral adrenal disease such as macronodular adrenal hyperplasia.

CHAPTER 33 Renal Physiology

Mary Ann Lim, MD, and
Ernie L. Esquivel, MD

○ **What are the three major functions of the kidneys?**

1) First, the kidneys control the composition and volume of body fluids and maintain acid–base balance.

2) Second, blood is filtered in the glomerulus, forming a protein-free ultrafiltrate.

3) Third, the kidneys act as endocrine organs, producing hormones such as renin and erythropoietin, and produce active vitamin D_3.

○ **What is the nephron and what are the different segments that comprise each one?**

The kidney is composed of more than 1 million functional units called nephrons. Each nephron consists of the glomerulus contained within Bowman's capsule, the proximal tubule, the loop of Henle, and the distal tubule, which ultimately drain into the collecting duct.

○ **What are the cells that comprise the glomerulus?**

The glomerulus is composed of a capillary network lined by endothelial cells, a central region of smooth muscle-like mesangial cells, which provide structural support, and an outer layer of epithelial cells called podocytes.

○ **What are the components of the glomerular filtration barrier?**

Blood in the capillary lumen is filtered through the fenestrated endothelial cells, an intervening glomerular basement membrane, and the interdigitated foot processes of the podocytes separated by slit diaphragms, producing a cell- and protein-free ultrafiltrate within the lumen of Bowman's capsule.

○ **What prevents albumin from normally appearing in the urine?**

Filtration of albumin is hindered by its size, which is restricted by the filtration barrier to molecules less than 42 Å, and by its negative charge, which is repelled by sialoglycoproteins on the glomerular basement membrane.

○ **What percentage of total body weight is comprised by water and how is it distributed into different compartments?**

Total body water (TBW) comprises 60% of total body weight, of which 40% is intracellular fluid and 20% is extracellular fluid (includes plasma and interstitial fluid).

○ **Which electrolyte in the body regulates the volume of extracellular fluid (ECF)?**

Sodium is the major extracellular solute; hence the retention or excretion of Na^+ by the kidney is critical for the regulation of ECF volume. Sodium retention or increased oral intake leads to ECF volume expansion and Na^+ loss leads to ECF volume depletion.

○ **How does the kidney handle Na^+ in the setting of congestive heart failure?**

Congestive heart failure is a volume-excess state characterized by pulmonary and interstitial edema. However, the effective circulating volume in the body is decreased due to poor cardiac output and leads to low renal perfusion. This activates the renin–angiotensin system and the sympathetic nervous system, causing sodium retention; thus, further perpetuating the edema. Urine sodium levels are less than 10 mEq/dL. Sodium avidity is also seen in edematous states due to cirrhosis and nephrotic syndrome.

○ **What is the kidney's response to an increase in salt intake?**

Increased Na^+ intake leads to an increase in extracellular fluid volume. The renin–angiotensin system is inhibited and sympathetic tone is diminished. Atrial natriuretic peptide levels are elevated. These lead to decreased Na^+ reabsorption and increased urinary Na^+ loss or natriuresis.

○ **What is the juxtaglomerular apparatus and what are its functions?**

The thick ascending limb of Henle's loop comes into contact with the vascular pole (afferent and efferent arterioles) of its own glomerulus, forming the juxtaglomerular apparatus (JGA). The juxtaglomerular apparatus is important in the autoregulation of renal blood flow and of the glomerular filtration rate. It also controls renin secretion.

○ **What are the three cells types that make up the juxtaglomerular apparatus and which ones control renin secretion?**

Granular cells (also called juxtaglomerular cells), extraglomerular mesangial cells, and the macula densa cells. The macula densa cells of the juxtaglomerular apparatus secrete renin.

○ **How does the kidney maintain a relatively constant renal blood flow (RBF) and GFR?**

The two mechanisms of autoregulation are the myogenic reflex and tubuloglomerular feedback. An increase in renal blood flow will lead to vasoconstriction of the afferent arteriole caused by vascular smooth muscle contraction; thus decreasing flow. An increase in renal blood flow will also enhance delivery of Na and Cl to the distal tubule. This is sensed by the macula densa, which will activate mechanisms that constrict the afferent arteriole.

○ **What are the effects of activation of the renin-angiotensin-aldosterone system?**

Renin stimulates angiotensin I (AI) production in the liver from angiotensinogen. Angiotensin-converting enzyme (ACE) converts AI to angiotensin II (AII). AII binds to AT_1 and AT_2 receptors, leading to systemic and efferent arteriolar vasoconstriction, increased Na^+ reabsorption by the proximal tubule, and production of aldosterone by the zona glomerulosa cells of the adrenal cortex. Aldosterone leads to Na^+ retention and K^+ loss and metabolic alkalosis as a result of H^+ secretion.

○ **What are the effects of ACE inhibitors and angiotensin receptor blockers (ARBs)?**

These drugs will decrease the glomerular filtration rate, decrease proteinuria, and lower systemic blood pressure. Hyperkalemia may result from decreased K^+ loss caused by hypoaldosteronism.

○ **How do nonsteroidal anti-inflammatory agents (NSAIDs) affect the kidney?**

NSAIDs inhibit cyclooxygenase, an enzyme important for the synthesis of vasodilatory prostaglandin E_2 and I_2 in the kidney. Low prostaglandin levels will lead to vasoconstriction of the afferent arteriole, hence decreasing GFR, and to Na^+ retention.

○ **What are the effects of norepinephrine and dopamine on renal blood flow?**

Both afferent and efferent arterioles are innervated by sympathetic neurons. Norepinephrine constricts both and decreases RBF. Dopamine at low doses (up to 5 μg/kg/min when delivered exogenously) leads to vasodilation and increases RBF. At higher doses, it vasoconstricts the arterioles.

○ **How good are serum urea and creatinine levels as surrogate measures of an individual's GFR?**

Urea is reabsorbed in the kidney and creatinine is secreted by tubules. As a consequence, urea levels underestimate the GFR, whereas creatinine levels overestimate it. Tubular secretion of creatinine increases with worsening kidney function.

○ **What factors are important to consider when using the serum creatinine levels to calculate creatinine clearance?**

Two commonly used formulas are the Cockroft-Gault and MDRD equations. The Cockroft-Gault formula takes gender, weight, and age into account. The MDRD equation has race as an added variable.

$$\textbf{Cockcroft-Gault: } C_{Cr} \text{ (mL/min)} = \frac{(140 - \text{age in years}) \times (\text{weight in kg})}{72 \times \text{serum creatinine (mg/dL)}}$$

Multiply by 0.85, if female.

$$\textbf{MDRD: } \text{eGFR (mL/min/1.73 m}^2) = 186 \times (S_{Cr})^{-1.154} \times (\text{age})^{-0.203}$$
$$\times (0.742 \text{ if female}) \times (1.210 \text{ if African American})$$

○ **Calculate the serum osmolality of a patient whose [Na] = 142 mEq/L, glucose = 180 mg/dL, and urea nitrogen = 12 mg/dL.**

$$\text{Osmolality (mOsm/kg H}_2\text{O)} = 2[\text{Na}] + \frac{\text{glucose}}{18} + \frac{\text{BUN}}{2.8} = 2(142) + \frac{180}{18} + \frac{12}{2.8} \approx 303$$

This patient has a serum osmolality of 303 mOsm/kg H_2O. The normal serum osmolality ranges between 280 and 295 mOsm/kg H_2O; hence, this person has hyperosmolal serum due to hyperglycemia.

○ **Where are osmoreceptors located and what do they control?**

Thirst is controlled by osmoreceptor cells in the anterolateral hypothalamus. A second set of osmoreceptors located in the wall of the third ventricle controls the secretion of antidiuretic hormone (ADH) from the supraoptic and paraventricular nuclei of the hypothalamus.

○ **What stimuli lead to ADH release?**

ADH is secreted in response to an increase in plasma osmolality more than 295 mOsm/kg H_2O as well as to volume contraction and hypotension.

○ **What are the effects of ADH on the kidney?**

ADH binds to V_2 receptors in the collecting duct, activating a G-protein that increases cyclic AMP levels. This stimulates the insertion of aquaporin-2 water channels in the apical membrane, permitting water entry into the cell. Exit of water into the interstitium occurs via aquaporin-3 and aquaporin-4 water channels in the basolateral membrane.

○ **Distinguish central from nephrogenic diabetes insipidus.**

Diabetes insipidus (DI) is characterized by polyuria. Hypernatremia and volume contraction may develop if the patient is unable to keep up with water loss. Central DI results from absence of ADH caused by damage to neurons in the hypothalamus or posterior pituitary. In nephrogenic DI, there is resistance to circulating ADH caused by genetic defects in aquaporin-2 or V_2 receptor or to acquired conditions, such as hypercalcemia, hypokalemia, or lithium therapy.

○ **What is Fanconi syndrome?**

Proximal tubular reabsorption of amino acids, glucose, urate, phosphate, K^+, and HCO_3^- is defective in the Fanconi syndrome, leading to excess urinary excretion. These patients develop hypokalemia, hypophosphatemia, and metabolic acidosis due to type 2 or proximal renal tubular acidosis.

○ **How is Fanconi syndrome treated?**

Treatment is with replacement of fluids and lost electrolytes, usually phosphates, sodium bicarbonate, and potassium.

○ **What are the five classes of diuretics and where do they act to increase Na^+ excretion?**

1) Osmotic diuretics (mannitol) inhibit tubular reabsorption of Na^+ and water by the proximal tubule.

2) Carbonic anhydrase inhibitors (acetazolamide) inhibit proximal HCO_3^- reabsorption in the proximal tubule.

3) Loop diuretics (furosemide, bumetanide) inhibit the Na-K-2Cl cotransporter in the thick ascending limb of Henle's loop.

4) Thiazide diuretics (hydrochlorothiazide, metolazone) inhibit the Na-Cl cotransporter in the early distal tubule.

5) Potassium-sparing diuretics include spironolactone, a competitive inhibitor of aldosterone action in the cortical collecting duct, and amiloride and triamterene, which inhibit the Na^+ channel in the collecting duct.

○ **Why does hyponatremia develop with thiazide diuretics and not with loop diuretics?**

Volume contraction stimulates antidiuretic hormone to increase water reabsorption. In patients taking thiazides, this increase in body water dilutes the serum Na concentration. However, loop diuretics wipe out the hypertonicity in the renal medulla; hence, increased water reabsorption is not possible.

○ **How do thiazides and loop diuretics affect urinary calcium excretion?**

Thiazides increase Ca^{2+} reabsorption in the distal tubule; thus decreasing urinary calcium excretion and potentially leading to hypercalcemia. Loop diuretics increase urinary calcium loss. Hypocalcemia does not occur, since chronic use leads to increased proximal tubule Ca^{2+} reabsorption.

○ **How does one treat hyperkalemia?**

To increase K^+ uptake by cells, administer one ampule of $NaHCO_3$, 10 to 20 U of insulin and 50 g glucose, and nebulized albuterol. Intravenous 10% calcium gluconate is administered to counteract the membrane effects of hyperkalemia. Oral or rectal Kayexalate removes K^+ via the gut. If all else fails, hemodialysis is employed.

○ **What are the manifestations of hyperaldosteronism?**

Hyperaldosteronism leads to hypertension due to Na^+ retention, hypokalemia, and metabolic alkalosis.

○ **How does one calculate the anion gap?**

Anion gap $(AG) = Na^+ - (Cl^- + HCO_3^-)$

The normal anion gap ranges between 8 and 12.

○ **What are the causes of an anion gap metabolic acidosis?**

Methanol, uremia, diabetic ketoacidosis, paraldehyde, isoniazid, isopropyl alcohol, lactic acidosis, ethylene glycol, ethanol, salicylates, starvation ketosis.

○ **What are the causes of a nonanion gap metabolic acidosis?**

Hyperalimentation, acetazolamide, renal tubular acidosis, diarrhea, ureteral diversion, posthypocapnia, spironolactone.

○ **Which of the renal tubular acidoses (RTA) is associated with stone formation?**

Type 1 (distal) RTA is associated with hypercalciuria, hyperphosphaturia, and nephrolithiasis, usually with calcium phosphate stones (although struvite stones are also seen). Several mechanisms are responsible for this. (1) hypercalciuria and hyperphosphaturia, both from bone buffering of acidosis and decreased tubular reabsorption; (2) high urine pH, thus promoting formation of calcium phosphate stones (as opposed to calcium oxalate stones); and (3) low urinary citrate from increased citrate reabsorption as a result of acidosis (citrate is a potent inhibitor of stone formation).

○ **What is type 4 renal tubular acidosis?**

Type 4 RTA refers to metabolic acidosis caused by aldosterone deficiency or resistance. Hyperkalemia develops as a result of decreased K^+ secretion and the metabolic acidosis is often mild. It is commonly seen in patients with chronic kidney disease. Fludrocortisone (Florinef) may be used to treat it, but it leads to Na^+ retention and edema.

○ **What are the metabolic abnormalities seen after prolonged vomiting?**

Loss of gastric acid (HCl) leads to metabolic alkalosis. The resulting volume contraction and Cl^- depletion increases renal HCO_3^- reabsorption. In addition, hypokalemia ensues and this further enhances HCO_3^- reabsorption.

○ **What mechanisms lead to contraction alkalosis?**

Volume contraction leads to metabolic alkalosis (increase in serum HCO_3^-) and several mechanisms are involved. The compensatory increase in Na^+ reabsorption enhances HCO_3^- reabsorption, and the increase in aldosterone stimulates urinary H^+ loss. In patients taking diuretics, hypokalemia will stimulate HCO_3^- reabsorption.

○ **What other electrolyte abnormalities are frequently seen in patients with hypomagnesemia?**

Hypomagnesemia impairs the secretion of parathyroid hormone (PTH) and leads to skeletal resistance to the action of PTH. Thus, patients may manifest positive Chvostek's and Trousseau's signs due to hypocalcemia. For unclear reasons, hypomagnesemia also leads to increased urinary K^+ loss; hence, hypokalemia often ensues.

○ **What are the mechanisms by which parathyroid hormone (PTH) increases serum calcium?**

PTH increases serum calcium by

- stimulating bone resorption by activating osteoclasts;
- increasing the synthesis of active vitamin D_3 by enhancing 25-OH cholecalciferol-1α-hydroxylase activity, thereby increasing intestinal Ca^{2+} absorption; and
- by increasing Ca^{2+} reabsorption in the distal tubule.

○ **What mechanisms lead to secondary hyperparathyroidism in chronic kidney disease?**

- Phosphate retention due to decreased urinary excretion of phosphorus.
- Decreased renal production of active vitamin D_3.
- Hypocalcemia.

○ **Why do patients with chronic kidney disease develop anemia?**

Peritubular interstitial cells in the kidney produce erythropoietin (EPO) in response to hypoxia. EPO stimulates the formation of red blood cells. In chronic renal failure, EPO levels are decreased.

CHAPTER 34
Renovascular Hypertension

Jay Laurence Bloch, MD

○ **Renovascular hypertension is caused by hypoperfusion leading to renin release, renin converts angiotensinogen to angiotensin, which is subsequently converted to angiotensin II by angiotensin-converting enzyme (ACE). List three physiologic effects of angiotensin II.**

1. Direct systemic vasoconstriction.

2. Stimulation of aldosterone secretion resulting in extracellular volume expansion.

3. Preferential glomerular efferent arteriolar vasoconstriction, thus maintaining glomerular filtration despite renal artery hypoperfusion.

4. Recent studies have also revealed additional mechanisms including sympathetic nervous system activation and formation of reactive oxygen species (Garovic and Textor, 2005).

○ **What percentage of renovascular disease is due to atherosclerosis?**

It is estimated that 70% to 90% of renal arterial lesions are due to atherosclerosis. These lesions more often affect the ostium and proximal third of the renal artery. The adjacent aorta is also affected. Fibromuscular dysplasia frequently involves the distal two-thirds of the main renal artery as well as its branches (Kim et al., 2007).

○ **True or False: Pulmonary edema is not a clinical feature of atherosclerotic renal artery stenosis.**

False. Clinical features of atherosclerotic renal artery stenosis include sudden onset of hypertension after age 50, malignant hypertension or hypertension difficult to manage with three or more medications, peripheral vascular disease, severe retinopathy, azotemia (particularly in patients utilizing an ACE inhibitor or angiotensin II receptor antagonist), hypokalemia, renal atrophy, abdominal bruit, and pulmonary edema.

○ **True or False: An abdominal bruit is highly specific for renal artery stenosis.**

True. In patients with angiographically proven renal artery stenosis, abdominal bruits were audible with a sensitivity range of 39% to 63% and a specificity range of 90% to 99%. Thus, the presence of an abdominal bruit is highly indicative of renal artery stenosis, but the absence of an abdominal bruit should not rule it out (Kim et al., 2007).

○ **True or False: Endovascular stent placement is more often utilized in the elderly with at least grade 3 chronic kidney disease (QFR 45.5 mL/min/1.73 m^2) versus younger patients or those with lesser degrees of chronic kidney disease.**

True. In one study of 258 patients undergoing endovascular stenting, the mean age was 71 years and 85% of these patients had at least grade 3 chronic renal disease. These patients typically have additional cardiovascular problems and require additional risk-intervention strategies (reduction of cholesterol, discontinuation of smoking, intensive hypertension control with medications) both before and after revascularization (Garovic and Textor, 2005).

○ **Which two classes of antihypertensive medications precisely manage renovascular hypertension?**

ACE inhibitors and angiotensin II receptor antagonists. Most renovascular hypertension can be managed with these and other antihypertensive medications introduced over the past two decades. Previously, less than half of the patients with renovascular hypertension were adequately controlled by medications available at that time. It is arguable whether individuals with well-controlled blood pressure benefit much from revascularization (Garovic and Textor, 2005).

○ **True or False: Renal failure is a side effect of ACE inhibitors.**

True. Insofar as ACE inhibitors cause dilation of the glomerular efferent arteriole, there may be a decrease in glomerular filtration rate (GFR). In unilateral renal artery stenosis, the change in total GFR is usually minimal due to compensatory increase in GFR by the contralateral kidney. However, vascular stenoses that involve both kidneys or a solitary kidney are more likely to be affected by ACE inhibitors resulting in acute renal failure. In one study, this occurred in 8 of 136 patients (6%) within 1 month of therapy. Discontinuation of the ACE inhibitor resulted in reversal of the acute renal failure in all but one patient (Garovic and Textor, 2005).

○ **True or False: Restenosis is common following endovascular stenting.**

False. Endovascular stents have greatly improved the patency rates compared with angioplasty alone. Current studies report restenosis following endovascular stent placement as occurring in the range of 12% to 14% (complication rate 7%–9%). Endovascular procedures to restore patency to the renal arteries have increased quite remarkably since the mid-1990s, One reason maybe the number of "drive-by" renal angiographies performed during another catheterization, especially coronary angiography (Garovic and Textor, 2005).

○ **True or False: Randomized controlled prospective studies have clearly demonstrated the benefit of endovascular stents over medication alone.**

False. Currently, there is a lack of consensus regarding intervention with endovascular stents. Many nephrologists advocate the use of medication only, whereas interventional subspecialties, especially cardiologists, argue the potential benefits of stent placement. Cardiovascular outcomes in renal atherosclerotic lesions (CORAL) is an ongoing NIH-multicenter clinical trial that will follow these two groups of patients—one treated by medication only, the other with medications and an endovascular stent. Hopefully, through such prospective trials, the true value of endovascular stenting will be determined (Garovic and Textor, 2005).

○ **How often is a clear abdominal bruit heard in renal artery stenosis (RAS)?**

Forty-six percent of patients.

○ **Do nonsteroidal antiinflammatory drugs (NSAIDs) have any effect on plasma renin levels?**

Yes, they cause a decrease.

○ **True or False: Gadolinium-DTPA–enhanced magnetic resonance angiography will not detect accessory renal arteries any better than nonenhanced images.**

False. Contrast images allow better visualization of accessory renal arteries. Studies are highly accurate in detecting RAS >50%, with a sensitivity of 93% and specificity of 98%. MRA is particularly useful in patients with impaired renal function who are at increased risk for contrast-induced nephropathy.

○ **Given a group of hypertensive patients on at least three antihypertensive medications with a diastolic BP ≥95 mm Hg, what is the prevalence of RAS?**

It is 25%. This may be a simple but useful set of criteria to select patients for diagnostic studies. Renovascular hypertension accounts for approximately 5% of all hypertensive patients, yet it is the most common cause of secondary hypertension. Not only can RAS cause hypertension, but it may also lead to progressive renal failure. Modern, less invasive diagnostic techniques, combined with percutaneous transluminal angioplasty and renal stenting, have stimulated a renewed interest in this subject.

○ **True or False: Ischemic nephropathy accounts for ≤5% of patients with ESRD on dialysis.**

False. Seventeen percent of patients are dialysis-dependent because of ischemic nephropathy. Significant RAS has been demonstrated in >50% of patients with a creatinine clearance <50 mL/min. Particularly at risk are patients with DM, hypertension, and generalized atherosclerosis. Median survival of patients on dialysis due to ischemic nephropathy is 27 months versus 56 months for other etiologies.

○ **True or False: Fibromuscular dysplasia progresses to occlusion in 15% of patients.**

False. Nonatheromatous causes of RAS do not commonly progress to occlusion; conversely, 15% of atherosclerotic RAS cases progress to occlusion. The time to occlusion is brief (13 months) in patients presenting with >75% occlusion.

○ **True or False: Atherosclerotic RAS progresses from less than 60% to greater than 60% within 1 year in 30% of patients.**

True. The lumen narrows most rapidly from <60% to >60%; 44% of patients progress by 2 years and by 3 years 48% progress. The progression occurs bilaterally in 20% to 50% of these patients.

○ **In patients undergoing cardiac catheterization, risk factors for RAS include each of the following except which one: extent of CAD, female sex, smoking, or hypertension?**

Hypertension. Both multivariate and univariate analysis of patients undergoing cardiac catheterization failed to identify hypertension as a risk factor for significant RAS Other risk factors that were identified include increasing age, CHF, PVD, and creatinine >1.06 mg/dL.

○ **True or False: Renal angiography is the gold standard for screening for RAS**

False. Although angiography remains the gold standard for identifying RAS, risks include nephrotoxicity and possible complications of arterial puncture (hematoma, cholesterol embolization). Digital subtraction angiography may preclude the need for arterial puncture, but in so doing, requires a larger dose of contrast. CO_2 angiography obviates the need for iodinated contrast but is not readily available and is more operator-dependent. Lastly, conventional angiography may miss stenoses en face, requiring oblique imaging to project stenoses (as opposed to CT or MRI imaging).

○ **True or False: A decrease in renal length of >1 cm is seen in most patients with RAS >60%.**

False. Renal dimensional changes of this magnitude are seen in only 26% of such patients. More important is Doppler interrogation of the extrarenal and intrarenal (segmental, interlobar) arteries. Extrarenal Doppler parameters include peak systolic velocity >200 cm/s, renal aortic ratio >3.3 to 3.5, end-diastolic velocity >150 cm/s. Intrarenal Doppler parameters include a resistive index <0.45 to 0.59, difference of resistive index with contralateral kidney >0.05 to 0.08, pulsatility index <0.93 (difference of PI with contralateral kidney >0.14), acceleration time >60 to 120 milliseconds, and acceleration >7.4 m/s².

○ **True or False: Doppler renal sonography is highly accurate in screening for RAS**

True. Five independent studies evaluating a total of 597 patients demonstrated a sensitivity of 89% to 93% and a specificity of 92% to 98%. Positive predictive value of 88% to 98% and negative predictive values of 92% to 98% were reported. The lumbar approach to evaluating the intraparenchymal arteries is unaffected by the number of accessory arteries, bowel gas, or obesity. DRS is operator-dependent and may not yield accurate results regarding multiple renal arteries or branch occlusions. A galactose microbubble-based agent may enhance the Doppler signal but is generally not necessary.

○ **True or False: Spiral CT angiography no longer requires contrast since predictions regarding RAS can be made by evaluating renal arterial calcifications.**

False. Seventeen percent of patients with no calcification, 30% of patients with <3 mm calcification, and 44% of patients with >3 mm calcification had ≥75% RAS However, the data do not preclude the use of contrast for accurate diagnostic information. Contrast-enhanced CT studies may visualize vessels as small as 1 mm.

○ **True or False: Captopril challenge tests and renal vein sampling are poor screening tools for ischemic nephropathy.**

True. These tests are most useful in differentiating renovascular hypertension from other etiologies. Ischemic nephropathy is often secondary to atherosclerotic RAS The tests are less sensitive in the situation of bilateral disease and renal compromise.

○ **True or False: Surgical revascularization for ischemic nephropathy virtually always results in substantial improvement in serum creatinine.**

False. Fifty-five percent of patients improved (i.e., 20% decrease in serum creatinine), 32% of patients revascularized remained stable,14% of patients worsened, and 6% died perioperatively (accumulated data from eight studies involving 352 patients from 1983 to 1992).

○ **List three preoperative criteria indicative of renal improvement following revascularization for total occlusion of the renal artery.**

Any of the following—collateral vessels with nephrogram on angiography, swift preop deterioration of GFR, patent vessels distal-to-proximal occlusion (back bleeding during revascularization surgery), viable nephrons on biopsy, renal length >9 cm, lateralization of renin secretion, and differential urinary concentration on split-function tests. The criteria need to be used together as a guide as individual parameters lack predictive value.

○ **True or False: Overall, 10% of renovascular operations for hypertension and renal insufficiency fail.**

True. Postoperative management following revascularization should include routine evaluation of blood pressure, serum creatinine, and periodic noninvasive radiologic assessment of renal blood flow (e.g., Doppler renal sonogram, nuclear renography, MRA). Approximately 10% of patients following revascularization will demonstrate recurrent hypertension or a diminution of renal function. This may be caused by restenosis of the operated vessel, stenosis of the contralateral renal artery, or progressive nephrosclerosis.

○ **Is PTA more successful with atherosclerotic or fibromuscular disease?**

Results are better with fibromuscular disease.

○ **What is eplerenone?**

It is a selective aldosterone inhibitor used for an antihypertensive. ACE inhibitor medications are still the preferred agents for medical treatment of RAS hypertension.

○ **What about angiotensin receptor blockers?**

They appear to be equally effective as ACE inhibitors.

○ **Serum creatinine may increase after therapy with ACE inhibitors. How much of an increase is acceptable?**

Usually up to about 35% above baseline.

○ **True or False: Splenorenal bypass is an ideal operation following a failed left aortorenal bypass.**

True. The success of the operation depends on the celiac trunk, which is visualized on the lateral aortic film of conventional angiogram, or by less invasive means. The splenic artery is divided proximally to avoid distal splenic atherosclerosis, and anastomosed end-to-end to the left renal artery. The spleen will remain viable, as collateral blood flow is derived from the gastroepiploic and short gastric vessels.

○ **True or False: Hepatorenal bypass is an ideal operation following a failed right aortorenal bypass.**

True. Patency of the celiac axis needs to be ascertained preoperatively. A saphenous vein graft is interpositioned between the common hepatic artery (where it divides into the main hepatic artery and gastroduodenal artery, thus forming a trifurcation) and the renal artery. The proximal anastomosis is performed end-to-side and the hepatic artery is not divided because of ischemic risk to the gallbladder (ischemic risk to the liver is minimal due to portal venous circulation). An end-to-end anastomosis is performed to the kidney to reduce turbulent flow.

○ **True or False: Iliorenal bypass or supraceliac aortorenal bypass are the operations of choice following a failed aortorenal bypass.**

False. If the celiac axis is involved by advanced disease or is inaccessible due to prior surgery, the operations above are indicated. Iliorenal bypass is limited by possible progressive disease involving the iliac vessel and requires a long graft (saphenous vein or synthetic) directed cephalad. Supraceliac aortorenal bypass often requires a thoracic as well as an abdominal incision and is much more difficult to tunnel to the right renal artery.

○ **True or False: Renovascular surgery patients are commonly hypertensive postoperatively.**

True. Postoperatively these patients are hypertensive due to hypervolemia, hypothermic vasoconstriction, or pain despite a patent arterial anastomosis. Management is with nitroprusside infusion to maintain the diastolic BP at approximately 90 mm Hg to insure adequate renal perfusion (avoiding graft thrombosis) yet, not so high to prevent anastomotic hemorrhage.

○ **True or False: Risk of hemorrhage following reoperation for renovascular disease is no different than that following the primary operation.**

False. Because of dense retroperitoneal fibrosis from the primary operation, hemorrhage is more likely to occur, as embedded lumbar vessels are more difficult to secure and the anastamosis itself is more arduous. Other likely sources of hemorrhage include the ipsilateral adenal and an untied branch of a saphenous vein graft. Extra-aortic techniques during secondary operations avoid the potential complication of aortic hemorrhage requiring aortic clamping.

○ **Renal artery thrombosis postoperatively following renovascular surgery occurs because of what problems? (List at least two, try to get all four.)**

Hypotension, hypovolemia, arteriolar nephrosclerosis, or a hypercoagulable state may result in thrombosis. Kidneys with severe nephrosclerosis are best managed by nephrectomy. Technical problems are the most likely cause of postoperative thrombosis (mishandling, kinking, distortion, or angulation of the bypass graft, or atheromatous emboli).

○ **True or False: Secondary revascularization results in cure or improvement in BP in 97% of patients.**

True. The operative mortality in one series was 1.4% with the incidence of nephrectomy being approximately 40% at reoperation. Nephrectomy will control BP as well as revascularization, and is indicated for the nonsalvageable kidney producing renin.

○ **True or False: Renal arterial bypass grafting (RABG) is more likely to normalize serum creatinine in patients with renovascular hypertension versus percutaneous transluminal renal angioplasty (PTRA) or percutaneous transluminal stent placement (PTSP).**

False. Actually all three failed to substantially alter creatinine in a study involving 130 patients. In comparing these modalities, the results are as follows:

	PTRA	PTSP	RABG
Technical success	91%	98%	92%
Complications	13%	16%	38%
Decrease in mean arterial BP at 12 months following procedure	21 mm Hg	20 mm Hg	20 mm Hg
Initial treatment costs	$1400	$2600	$15,000

○ **True or False: Percutaneous transluminal stent placement is highly successful in preventing congestive heart failure and pulmonary edema in patients with bilateral renal artery stenosis or stenosis in a solitary functioning kidney.**

True. In this study, 23 of 56 patients (41%) had a history of the above-referenced comorbidity prior to PTSP of one or both arteries. Following the procedure, 77% of these patients remained free of congestive heart failure and pulmonary edema (mean follow-up 18.4 months). In contradistinction, only 4 of 34 subjects (12%) with unilateral stenosis and a normal contralateral kidney had a history of congestive heart failure or pulmonary edema, and only 1 of 3 (33%) subjects were free of CHF and pulmonary edema following PTSP.

○ **Percutaneous transluminal renal angioplasty (PTRA) for ostial atherosclerotic renal artery stenosis yields results similar to percutaneous transluminal stent placement (PTSP).**

False.

	PTRA	PTSP
Primary success rate (<50% residual stenosis)	57%	88%
Secondary patency rate at 6 months	29%	75%
Restenosis following initial success	48%	14%

Secondary stent placement following early or late failure of PTRA resulted in success rates similar to patients undergoing primary PTSP. Despite the potential cost savings in stents using PTRA, the need for reintervention is greater. Therefore, PTSP is currently a better approach for ostial atherosclerotic stenosis.

○ **True or False: Renovascular hypertension is rare in children.**

False. It is relatively common. Hypertension in children is most often secondary hypertension (70%–80%). The other common surgically correctable cause of secondary hypertension in children is coarctation of the aorta.

○ **What is the "nutcracker syndrome," where does it occur, how does it cause gross hematuria, how is it treated, and what other medical problem is associated with it?**

Nutcracker syndrome describes the uncommon situation where the left renal vein is compressed between the aorta and the superior mesenteric artery. This results in left renal venous hypertension, which over time leads to the development of collateral veins and varices. If any of these thin-walled varices should rupture into the collecting system, left-sided hematuria results. Usual symptoms are hypertension that may be uncontrollable, left-sided hematuria, and sometimes flank pain. Standard testing for hematuria such as urinary red blood cell morphology, IVP, cystoscopy, and even ureteroscopy are usually unrewarding except for identification of left-sided hematuria. If suspected, magnetic resonance angiography or CT scans looking for compression of the left renal vein are useful. Treatment with angioplasty and stenting is usually successful. Other treatment options include vein graft interposition, nephropexy, and renal autotransplantation.

CHAPTER 35 Renal Transplantation

Christian S. Kuhr, MD, FACS

○ **What is the average waiting time for a deceased donor kidney transplant?**

Variable depending on the region of the United States, but ranges between 2 and 10 years.

○ **What are the two leading causes of end-stage renal disease in the United States?**

Diabetes (31%), chronic glomerulonephritis (28%). Other causes include polycystic kidney disease (12%), hypertensive nephrosclerosis (9%), systemic lupus (3%), and interstitial nephritis (3%).

○ **Nephrectomy of the native kidneys is indicated for what clinical situations?**

- Large polycystic kidneys with pain or early satiety.
- Chronic severe reflux.
- Significant proteinuria.

○ **Do blood transfusions confer a survival advantage for the transplanted kidney?**

Before calcineurin inhibitors (e.g., cyclosporine and tacrolimus) were routinely used there was a benefit. Currently, the risk of sensitization outweighs any advantage and this practice is not used.

○ **What causes hyperacute rejection and what is the treatment for it?**

This is caused by preformed antibodies and no treatment is effective.

○ **How is acute rejection treated and how successful is it?**

Anti-T-cell antibodies (ATG and OKT3) and steroids allow rescue of more than 50% of cases.

○ **What is the frequency of acute cellular rejection and how is it diagnosed?**

The incidence is 20% to 25% and it occurs most frequently 1 to 3 months posttransplant. Diagnosis is made with a renal biopsy.

○ **Where do urine leaks typically occur?**

The ureterovesical junction is the most common site for a urine leak. A urine leak early after transplantation is most frequently caused by ischemia of the tip of the ureter. Symptoms include lowered urine output, azotemia, and lower abdominal or suprapubic pain.

○ **What is the overall graft survival for deceased donor and living donor transplanted kidneys?**

Deceased donor		Living donor
87%	1 y	93%
76%	3 y	86%
10 y	half-life	13 y

○ **How often are vascular complications encountered after transplantations?**

Approximately 3% of the time.

○ **What fluid collections may appear around a transplanted kidney and when are they most likely to appear?**

In order of the usual presentation:

- 1 to 3 weeks posttransplant—urinoma or hematoma.
- 2 to 10 weeks posttransplant—lymphocele.
- 4 to 5 weeks posttransplant—abscess.

○ **36-year-old female underwent a deceased donor renal transplant 2 days ago. Her donor was a 57-year-old male hypertensive who died of a stroke. Cold ischemia time was 26 hours. Her most recent creatinine is 7.8 mg/dL. Her current immunosuppressive agents include antithymocyte globulin (ATG) at 10 mg/kg, mycophenolate mofetil 1 g bid, and prednisone 50 mg bid. Her urine output has been ranging from 5 to 10 mL/h. A renal scan was obtained. Figure 1 demonstrates the transplant kidney 30 minutes after injection of isotope. What is the diagnosis?**

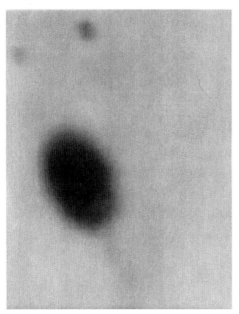

Figure 1.

The history is suggestive of delayed graft function or acute tubular necrosis (ATN). Factors that contribute include deceased donor, donor age, prolonged cold ischemia, unwitnessed cardiac arrest, pressor agents in the management of the donor, and poor perfusion of the kidney (low blood pressure). The renal scan demonstrates uptake of isotope but no excretion. This may also be seen in acute rejection and cyclosporine toxicity, however, rejection 2 days postoperatively is rare as immunosuppression is often maximized early on.

○ **18-year-old female with a history of reflux nephropathy and neurogenic bladder receives a living related kidney transplant from her mother. Her creatinine has come down from 10.8 mg/dL to 4.7 mg/dL on postoperative day 2. She develops some mild lower abdominal pain over the incision and a temperature of 38.1°C. A renal scan is obtained. Figure 2a shows the transplant kidney 4 minutes after injection of isotope, and Figure 2b is the same study 24 minutes after injection. What is the diagnosis?**

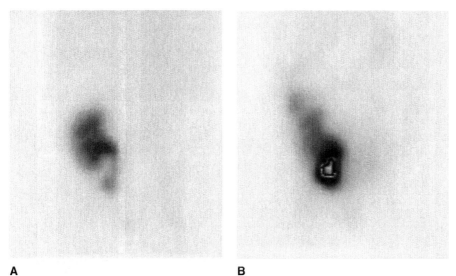

A

B

Figure 2.

The scan demonstrates extravasation of isotope confirming the diagnosis of a urine leak. If present, urine leaks are usually identified early in the postoperative course and often within the first week since surgery. Early clinical findings include wound drainage, pain, fever, and elevated serum creatinine. The most common etiologies include ureteral injury, ischemic ureter, surgical technique, and urinary retention.

○   A 40-year-old diabetic male received a deceased donor renal transplant 6 weeks ago. He presents in clinic with right leg edema and an elevated creatinine from 1.5 mg/dL to 2.2 mg/dL. Tacrolimus level is therapeutic. A renal ultrasound and CT scan were obtained (Fig. 3a, 3b). Diagnosis?

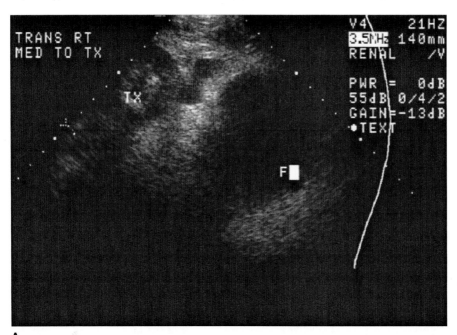

A

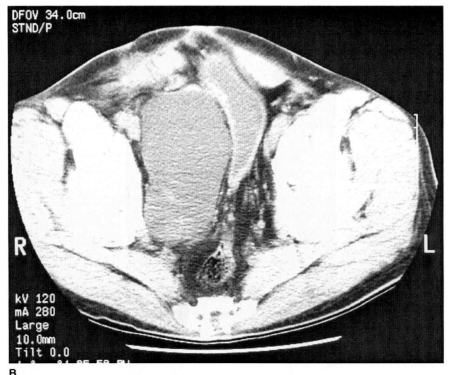

B

Figure 3.

The ultrasound demonstrates a fluid collection with mild hydronephrosis confirmed by findings on the CT scan. Fluid was aspirated and found to have a creatinine of 2.6 mg/dL supporting a diagnosis of a postoperative lymphocele. The source of the lymph is from the recipient lymphatics overlying the iliac vessels disrupted during vascular mobilization or from the donor kidney. Treatment is surgical marsupialization into the peritoneal cavity.

○ **A patient received a renal transplant 10 days ago. The postoperative course was complicated by wound drainage and a urine leak was diagnosed. He is taken to the operating room to repair the leak and upon exposing the ureterovesical anastomosis site, the distal one-third of the ureter is found to be ischemic. What is the best management option?**

Pyelovesicostomy offers the best option for a successful outcome. Ischemic necrosis of the ureter is caused by damage to the arterial supply usually during the kidney procurement. The arterial supply to the transplanted ureter originates from the renal hilar vessels. Other options include pyeloureterostomy to the patient's ipsilateral native ureter.

○ **An 18-year-old female with end-stage renal disease secondary to vesicoureteral reflux presents for evaluation for a possible renal transplant. She makes approximately 1 L of urine a day. A urinalysis demonstrates bacteriuria and 5 to 10 WBCs per HPF. She is asymptomatic. What should be the next step in her evaluation and should you perform a nephrectomy of her native kidney prior to any transplant?**

A urine culture to confirm an infection and a voiding cystourethrogram to evaluate her lower urinary tract. High-grade reflux, if present with recurrent pyelonephritis, should be addressed with native nephrectomy prior to transplant.

○ **A 35-year-old male with a T6-7 cord injury from an MVA 19 years ago presents for renal transplant evaluation. He has developed end-stage renal disease secondary to vesicoureteral reflux. He is on intermittent catheterization, but despite q2h caths, he is still incontinent. His pretransplant management would include?**

Urodynamics with a leak point pressure confirm the presence of a small-volume, high-pressure bladder. Therapy includes a trial of anticholinergics, and if this is not successful, then bladder augmentation prior to transplantation should be undertaken.

○ **A 45-year-old farmer presents for a kidney transplant. He has end-stage renal disease secondary to diabetes. During your evaluation you discover that he was recently treated for a squamous cell carcinoma on the back of his neck, which was completely excised. No nodal disease is present on examination. Assuming the rest of his evaluation is normal, can he be considered for transplantation?**

Yes. Nonmelanotic skin lesions are not a contraindication to transplantation. Recurrences of those tumors can be effectively followed clinically and treated as they arise. Prophylaxis with sunscreen after transplantation should also be recommended. Contraindications would include untreated malignancies or recent treatment (less than 2 years) of other nonskin (except melanoma) cancers.

○ **A 48-year-old mother is willing to donate one of her kidneys to her daughter with end-stage renal disease. During her evaluation, a renal angiogram of her kidney is obtained. She is found to have two left renal arteries and one right renal artery. The right renal artery is also found to have evidence of mild fibromuscular dysplasia. The best choice is?**

She would not be considered suitable as a donor. Angioplasty or vascular reconstruction can be considered but only after thorough discussion with all involved. Loss of a renal unit could jeopardize the donor's health in the future.

○ **A patient with rising creatinine undergoes a transplant renal biopsy. The histology shows proliferative endarteritis, interstitial fibrosis, and tubular atrophy. This is consistent with?**

Chronic allograft nephropathy (also known as chronic rejection), an immune-mediated process resulting in renal damage. It is associated with gradual dysfunction and eventual graft loss and does not respond to current antirejection therapies.

○ **T-cell activation and proliferation underlies the initiation of acute rejection. T-cell proliferation occurs after what two events occur at the cellular level between T cells and antigen presenting cells?**

T-cell activation requires the interaction of the T-cell receptor and the antigen bound to MHC. This is termed signal 1. A second signal mediated through a costimulatory receptor (e.g., CD28) is necessary for T-cell activation and proliferation. Without this second signal, anergy (T-cell unresponsiveness) occurs.

○ **A 48-year-old male underwent deceased donor renal transplant 7 months ago. His maintenance immunosuppression consists of prednisone, mycophenolate mofetil, and tacrolimus. His posttransplant course had been unremarkable until 1 week ago when he developed lethargy, lack of energy, and a temperature of 38.1°C. Laboratory tests revealed a WBC of 3.1 thou/mm^3, platelet count of 103 thou/mm^3, and a hemoglobin of 12.9 g/L. His evaluation should include?**

Serum testing for cytomegalovirus (CMV). CMV is a common infection of transplant recipients and can present with lethargy, leukopenia, thrombocytopenia, hepatitis, gastrointestinal ulceration or inflammation, chorioretinitis, and pneumonia. The diagnosis can be confirmed by culture of the buffy coat, PCR analysis, or inferred by changes in CMV IgG or IgM titers. Treatment consists of decreasing immunosuppressive medications, antivirals (Ganciclovir), and γ-globulin.

○ **A recipient of a renal transplant develops fever, rising creatinine, and peripheral adenopathy. A transplant renal biopsy demonstrates a lymphocytic infiltrate and node biopsy reveals a B-cell lymphoma. This condition is seen in patients with which risk factors?**

Posttransplant lymphoproliferative disorder (PTLD) is associated with primary Epstein-Barr virus (EBV) infection, excessive immunosuppression, and preceding symptomatic CMV infection. Level of EBV replication appears to have predictive value in assessing the risk of the disease.

○ **A 75-kg patient is diagnosed with posttransplant lymphoproliferative disorder (PTLD). He was transplanted 7 months prior to the diagnosis and his immunosuppression consists of cyclosporine, mycophenolate, and prednisone. Management of this problem should include?**

Decrease or even withdrawal of immunosuppression is an important part of curing this condition. PTLD is often the result of excessive immunosuppression associated with a positive EBV serology. Other possible treatments include antiviral therapy, chemotherapy, and/or radiation therapy.

○ **A 28-year-old, 65-kg female with a stable renal graft for 3 years wishes to become pregnant. Her creatinine is 1.9 mg/dL and her immunosuppressive medications include cyclosporine, mycophenolate, and prednisone. What should be your advice to her on whether to proceed with a pregnancy?**

Successful pregnancies in renal transplant recipients have been extensively reported. Mycophenolate may be teratogenic and should be discontinued. The incidence of birth defects in neonates from mothers on immunosuppressive medication is no different than in the nontransplanted population. Patients on cyclosporine may see higher rates of hypertension (20%–60%) and preeclampsia (30%), and approximately 50% of babies are born prematurely or of low birth weight.

○ **Organ preservation solutions are designed to mimic what type of fluid?**

Intracellular fluid. This prevents cellular edema and the loss of intracellular potassium.

○ **A 47-year-old female is diagnosed with allograft failure and has been placed back on dialysis. She is still on cyclosporine, azathioprine, and prednisone. Her nephrologist starts to decrease her immunosuppression by stopping her azathioprine and cyclosporine and tapering her prednisone over 2 weeks. After 10 days, the patient presents with pain over her graft, fever, and microhematuria. Management should include?**

This patient is experiencing an acute rejection of her kidney from immunosuppression withdrawl. Azathioprine can be stopped immediately. Cyclosporine can be reduced by 50% and discontinued after 2 months. Prednisone should be tapered gradually over 2 to 3 months. This patient should be treated with a steroid bolus to reverse the rejection and then placed on a longer taper. If the symptoms cannot be reversed, then a transplant nephrectomy is indicated.

○ **A 12-year-old girl underwent a deceased donor renal transplant. She received antithymocyte globulin induction therapy and then was started on steroids and azathioprine. Her postoperative course was unremarkable and her creatinine decreased to 2.8 mg/dL on day 3 after surgery. She should now be started on what additional medication?**

A calcineurin inhibitor should be added at this point. Her renal function is satisfactory and should tolerate it. The choice is between cyclosporine and tacrolimus. Although the experience with tacrolimus is limited in pediatric patients, it may be a better choice than cyclosporine because of its side-effect profile. Tacrolimus has no hypertrichosis and minimal gingival hyperplasia, and, because of this improved cosmetic side-effect profile, it may be a better choice in the adolescent age group.

○ **A 6-year-old boy has end-stage renal disease secondary to chronic obstruction from recurrent renal calculi. A metabolic work up for his stones reveals high serum and urinary oxalate levels consistent with type 1 primary hyperoxaluria. He has no evidence for urinary tract infection. What is your recommendation regarding his candidacy for a renal transplant?**

Type 1 primary hyperoxaluria has been considered a contraindication to renal transplantation because of the deleterious effect of oxalate deposition in the graft. However, a combined kidney and liver transplant would provide the deficient enzyme and thus prevent further stone formation. Intensive hemodialysis to reduce plasma oxalate prior to surgery and postoperative diuresis will also decrease the risk of oxalate deposition in the new kidney.

○ **A 34-year-old diabetic patient undergoes kidney–pancreas transplantation with bladder drainage. Three months postoperatively he presents with frequency, urgency, dysuria, and hematuria. Urinalysis shows a pH of 5.5, mild proteinuria, numerous RBCs and WBCs. Urine culture is negative. The cause and management of this condition is?**

Urinary drainage of the exocrine function of the pancreas can lead to activation of the enzyme trypsinogen. This can be brought on by acid urine, volume depletion, or bladder dysfunction and can result in a chemical cystitis, urethritis, or balanitis. Treatment involves analgesics, hydration, alkalinization of the urine, and Foley catheter drainage. Antibiotics are useful if concomitant infection is present. If symptoms are refractory to treatment, conversion to enteric drainage of the pancreas is indicated.

○   **A 27-year-old male with an ileal conduit and renal failure secondary to neurogenic bladder presents for transplant evaluation. He has had his conduit for 18 years, and his bladder is still in place. During his evaluation, you order a urodynamic assessment of his bladder and find his bladder volume to be 250 mL, no hyperreflexia, and a urine flow rate of 9 mL/min with a postvoid residual of 175 mL. His best option for drainage is?**

Although he has a low flow rate and poor emptying of his bladder, he will likely do better with undiversion to his bladder. He will likely need to do intermittent catheterizations, but this is associated with a lower infection rate than conduit drainage. He will need to have this reviewed with him prior to transplantation, and if the patient is motivated, he can start to learn the procedure prior to his surgery. His low bladder volume may also improve with time once a normal urine flow returns to the bladder.

○   **A 46-year-old, 75-kg female receives a deceased donor renal transplant. She has end-stage renal disease secondary to diabetes. Postoperatively her urine output is >100 mL/h and her creatinine has dropped from a preop value of 7.6 mg/dL to 3.8 mg/dL over 2 days. Her medications at this point include basiliximab 20 mg IV on day 1 postsurgery, cyclosporine 250 mg bid, mycophenolate mofetil 1 g bid, and prednisone 50 mg bid on a taper. Her cyclosporine level is 395 ng/mL. Her serum potassium is 6.5 mEq/L. She receives kayexalate, sodium bicarbonate, and insulin with IV dextrose, but her potassium only drops to 6.2 mEq/L. Another management option should include?**

Cyclosporine is known to produce hyperkalemia in the face of improving renal function. She did not respond to standard treatment in this case and her cyclosporine level is high (normal 200–250). Reduction of her cyclosporine dose may improve her potassium or at least make it more responsive to treatment. This should be combined with a decrease in her dietary potassium plus discontinuation of any potential potassium sparing diuretics.

○   **A renal biopsy is obtained from a renal transplant patient with a rising creatinine. The histology is read out as interstitial lymphocytic invasion, mild tubulitis with normal glomeruli and vessels. The diagnosis is?**

This biopsy demonstrates mild acute rejection. The cellular infiltrate and tubular changes are characteristic for rejection. In more severe cases, lymphocytic infiltration of vessels and a larger interstitial inflammatory response is seen.

○   **A 31-year-old renal transplant recipient develops a persistent cough and low-grade fever. She sees her local physician who diagnoses mycoplasma pneumonia and starts her on erythromycin 500 mg tid. Her renal function is normal (creatinine = 1.7 mg/dL) and she is on cyclosporine, mycophenolate mofetil, and prednisone. Five days later she presents with hypertension (BP 180/110), tremors, and an elevation of her creatinine to 2.3 mg/dL. The best method to resolve these abnormalities is?**

This patient is demonstrating signs of cyclosporine toxicity. The best way to confirm this is to obtain a cyclosporine level. The likely cause of this sudden elevation is the erythromycin. Erythromycin will inhibit the elimination of cyclosporine through the P450 enzyme system. The best course of action here is to lower her cyclosporine dose and monitor her cyclosporine levels. Once she stops erythromycin, she can return to her normal cyclosporine dose.

○   **A renal transplant recipient presents with new-onset hypertension. He is 1 year out from his transplant and his medications include tacrolimus, mycophenolate mofetil, and prednisone. His tacrolimus level is normal; his most recent creatinine level is 1.8 mg/dL. On examination, his blood pressure is 192/105, pulse 86. Abdominal examination reveals no masses, no tenderness, normal bowel sounds, and a bruit over the right lower quadrant. Pulses are normal to palpation. Diagnostic options for the hypertension include?**

Transplant renal artery stenosis usually presents between 3 and 24 months after surgery. Hypertension is the usual mode of presentation, but this can also be seen with graft dysfunction. This diagnosis is made more difficult in patients with existing hypertension and/or marginal renal function. Deterioration of renal function after being placed on angiotensin-converting enzyme inhibitors may suggest the diagnosis, but to confirm its presence, Doppler ultrasound and/or angiography are required.

○ **The same patient from the previous question undergoes angiography and confirms renal artery stenosis in the transplant kidney. Treatment options include?**

There are three options available for treatment. First is medical management. If he can be controlled with a reasonable level of medications and his creatinine remains stable, then no further treatment is required. The second option is angioplasty with stent placement. This can often be done at the time of angiography but is associated with a recurrence rate as high as 16% and response rates are variable. In general, lesions 1 cm away from the anastomosis respond better than lesions located at the site of anastomosis. The latter have a higher chance of rupture at the time of angioplasty. Finally, surgical repair can be done but should be approached cautiously, as the degree of fibrosis around the vessels and kidney makes this a very difficult undertaking.

○ **A patient undergoes deceased donor renal transplantation and is treated initially with antithymocyte globulin, prednisone, and azathioprine. Once his renal function drops below 4.0 mg/dL, he is started on cyclosporine. One week after his transplant, he experiences a rise in his creatinine and a diagnosis of acute rejection is made by biopsy. He responds to pulse steroids with normalization of his creatinine. Two weeks later he returns again with an elevation of his creatinine, and an ultrasound demonstrates a large fluid collection in the pelvis with hydronephrosis. What is the diagnosis and what treatment should he receive?**

Pelvic fluid collections in a transplant patient can be either lymphatic or urine. This can be confirmed by needle aspiration of the fluid and sending a sample for creatinine level. This patient was found to have a urine leak, as the creatinine level of the fluid was 64 mg/dL. Urine leaks can present late, especially when associated with a history of rejection or other conditions that can affect its blood supply. Management this far out from transplantation is best carried out percutaneously, as surgical treatment is more difficult. Percutaneous nephrostomy tube insertion and nephrostogram will confirm the site of leakage and also allow for antegrade stent placement. Percutaneous drain placement is also required and this will usually allow the leak to resolve. If it fails to repair itself, then surgical intervention is required.

○ **A 39-year-old female with a living related renal transplant done 2 years previously presents with a rising creatinine. An ultrasound study demonstrated hydronephrosis of the transplant kidney and a 2-cm stone in the renal pelvis. No other abnormalities are detected. What are the treatment options in this patient?**

Calculus disease in a transplant kidney can be treated in the same fashion as stones in nontransplant kidneys. Percutaneous nephrolithotomy is easily performed in transplant kidneys because of their superficial location and is probably the best option in this case. Other options include ESWL in the prone position and ureteroscopy. Ureteroscopy is often the most difficult option because of the position of the transplant ureter. Flexible ureteroscopy is a better choice to gain endoscopic access to the ureter if needed. A 24-hour urine metabolic panel for kidney stone prevention is required in renal transplant patients with nephrolithiasis.

○ **A 52-year-old obese male with ESRD secondary to HTN undergoes deceased donor renal transplantation. Postoperatively, he is placed on prednisone, tacrolimus, and mycophenolate mofetil. During his hospital stay hyperglycemia develops. What is the likely etiology?**

Steroids at high dose effect insulin resistance, and tacrolimus is known to cause insulin resistance in transplant patients. Lowering the dose of this drug or even stopping it in favor of cyclosporine may make his glucose levels easier to control since there is a lower incidence of steroid-induced diabetes with cyclosporine.

○ **A 51-year-old, 80-kg male receives a deceased donor renal transplant. He is placed on cyclosporine, azathioprine, and prednisone. His postoperative course is unremarkable. Three months after his transplant, his creatinine is noted to rise and a biopsy confirms acute rejection. His medications at this point include prednisone 10 mg/d, cyclosporine 225 mg bid, and azathioprine 100 mg/d. His cyclosporine level was 235 ng/mL at the time of diagnosis. His rejection responds to 3 days of IV solumedrol 500 mg. Appropriate management of his immunosuppression at this point should include?**

This patient developed a rejection episode on what appears to be adequate immunosuppression. A normal cyclosporine level and appropriate doses for his weight confirm this. Now that his rejection is treated, he should not be placed on the same regimen that brought on the rejection. An appropriate alternative would be switching cyclosporine to tacrolimus and changing azathioprine to mycophenolate mofetil. This should decrease his risk of future rejections.

○ **A kidney transplant recipient is diagnosed with acute rejection. He is initially treated with steroids but fails to respond. He then is started on OKT3 5 mg/d for treatment of steroid-resistant rejection. On the first day of his treatment he develops fevers, hypotension, and shortness of breath. The most likely cause for this is?**

OKT3 is a monoclonal antibody directed at the CD3 complex on T cells. It depletes circulating T cells and modulates or removes the CD3 molecule from the cell surface, making the cell nonfunctional. A side effect of OKT3 is cytokinerelease syndrome seen usually within the first 30 to 60 minutes of the first or second dose. It presents with fevers, chills, nausea, vomiting, diarrhea, weakness, myalgia, bronchial spasm, or hypotension. It is believed to be mediated through cytokine release, mainly TNF and INF-γ. Premedication with antihistamines, steroids, and nonsteroidal anti-inflammatory drugs will reduce the symptoms.

○ **Daclizumab, a novel immunosuppressive agent, is approved for use in transplant recipients. What is its mechanism of action?**

Daclizumab is a humanized murine monoclonal antibody directed toward CD25, the IL-2 receptor. It competitively inhibits IL-2 from binding to its receptor on the T cell and has been shown to be a useful agent when used with other immunosuppressive drugs for induction therapy.

○ **A renal transplant recipient elects to undergo surgical drainage for a recurrent pelvic lymphocele. During the procedure, while opening the lymphocele sac, the transplant ureter is transected. The best method of repair is?**

A new ureteroneocystostomy is the procedure of choice. If the ureteral length would not allow this, then a psoas hitch or Boari flap would be required. The blood supply of the transplant ureter comes from the renal artery. Therefore, only the proximal portion is viable. Attempts at ureteroureterostomy will fail due to the now ischemic distal portion.

○ **A patient is preparing to receive a deceased donor renal transplant from a 27-year-old MVA donor that has recently become available. During the evaluation you get a phone call saying the crossmatch is positive. This means?**

A crossmatch is performed by mixing donor lymphocytes with recipient serum. A positive result means that the donor cells were lysed, and thus indicates that the recipient serum had preformed antidonor-HLA antibodies. Anti-HLA antibodies are developed through exposure to foreign HLA. This can occur through previous transplants, blood transfusions, and pregnancy. Transplantation in this setting will result in hyperacute rejection and therefore, the next available candidate should be substituted.

○ **A 47-year-old diabetic female has undergone two previous renal transplants. Both failed due to rejection, one after 2 years and the most recent one after 4 years. She wishes to be placed on the waiting list for a third kidney and during her evaluation her PRA (panel reactive antibody) is found to be 99%. What does this result mean?**

A PRA is obtained by testing a recipient's serum against a panel of lymphocytes from different volunteers. Volunteers are selected based on their HLA type so that as many HLA antigens as possible are present in the panel. If someone has a PRA of 99%, it means that they reacted (lysed the cells) with 99% of the panel and therefore have numerous anti-HLA antibodies and a high probability of a positive crossmatch to any future donor. This has prognostic significance in that the chance of finding a donor for her that will yield a negative crossmatch is approximately 1%.

○ **An example of a xenograft would be?**

A xenograft is a tissue graft from one species to another. Examples would include pig-to-monkey or baboon-to-human transplants. An allograft is the transplantation of tissues within the same species but to genetically nonidentical individuals (e.g., standard renal transplant). An autograft would be a transplant of tissue from the same person or animal to a different site (e.g., skin graft, saphenous vein graft).

○ **A father wants to donate his kidney to his dialysis-dependent son. Both he and his son complete the evaluation and are found to be healthy for the proposed living related kidney transplant. As an aside, the father asks how close a match between he is with his son. What can you tell him without laboratory information?**

The transplant "match" refers to the HLA identity shared between a recipient and the donor. The genes that encode the HLA proteins are located on the short arm of chromosome 6 and one allele comes from each parent. We routinely type for HLA-A, HLA-B, and HLA-DR antigens; therefore, the son in this example will match three antigens. Simply put offspring and parents share 50% identity. Additional matches would be coincidental and relate to the frequency of alleles in the population.

○ **Acute anuria in a patient immediately following a living donor transplant suggests what diagnoses?**

Venous or arterial thrombosis or severe hypovolemia with hypotension (i.e., shock). This clinical development demands emergent treatment and consideration of reexploration if thrombosis or surgical bleeding are to be treated and the allograft salvaged. Urgent ultrasound imaging can confirm or rule out a vascular catastrophe though may unnecessarily delay treatment.

○ **What are the options for treating a contracted, noncompliant bladder in an anuric patient being prepared for a renal transplant?**

Bladder augmentation surgery using an intestinal segment is the standard recommended treatment. The bladder can be used as a reservoir with the patient performing intermittent self-catheterization. This has been shown to be preferable to urinary diversion in patient satisfaction and has fewer complications. Bladder rehabilitation, using progressively larger amounts of fluid to gradually stretch the bladder, is another option and may be worth trying before resorting to more aggressive therapies. Urinary diversion is used as a last resort.

○ **What are the three most common causes of end-stage renal failure in children?**

Glomerulonephritis is the most common followed in order by congenital or inheritable diseases, collagen vascular disease, and obstructive uropathy. In adults, diabetes is the most common cause, followed by hypertensive disease and glomerulonephritis.

○ **What is the overall mortality rate for end-stage renal disease patients in the United States?**

Approximately 24% per year, but this varies according to age, cause of renal failure, and other factors. Diabetic patients generally have poorer outcomes.

○ **What are the two most common causes of death in end-stage renal disease patients?**

Cardiovascular disease is the most common followed by infections and infectious complications.

○ **At what level of renal failure do symptoms of uremia typically appear?**

Usually, uremic symptoms only appear when 90% of the original renal function has been lost. This corresponds to a creatinine clearance of 10 to 15 mL/min.

○ **Is end-stage renal disease associated with ED or infertility?**

Yes, both and decreased libido as well.

○ **What is the difference in 5-year survival for a transplant patient who received a live donor kidney compared to a deceased donor kidney?**

The live donor kidney recipient has approximately a 10%-survival advantage overall and a 15%-allograft survival advantage compared to the deceased donor donor.

○ **Is anticoagulation always required during kidney transplantation?**

No, it is generally not necessary, although antiplatelet medications are commonly used.

○ **How does cytomegalovirus infection affect outcomes after renal transplantation?**

CMV infection can be life-threatening so demands early intervention. Patients who develop a CMV infection have an increased incidence of developing acute rejection and, in turn, patients in whom acute rejection is diagnosed have poorer graft survival.

○ **What is the most prevalent cause of late kidney graft loss in surviving renal transplant recipients and what are its characteristics?**

Chronic allograft nephropathy or interstitial fibrosis and tubular atrophy. It is characterized by a relatively slow but variable decrease in renal function. This is often accompanied by hypertension and proteinuria. The process often begins approximately 3 months after transplantion. Calcineurin inhibitor (cyclosporine, tacrolimus) nephrotoxicity is a common cause and contributing factor. Switching to sirolimus may be useful clinically in this situation.

○ **What percentage of renal transplant patients on long-term mTOR inhibitor immunosuppressives are likely to need statin drugs to regulate dyslipidemia?**

Approximately 60%.

CHAPTER 36
Benign Renal Cystic Disease

John Chandler William, MD

○ **Describe the radiographic characteristics of a simple renal cortical cyst on intravenous pyelography and CT scan images.**

On intravenous pyelography, a simple cyst is a well-circumscribed lucent mass that may distort the contour of the kidney and may show a "beak sign" with normal parenchyma. Computed tomography demonstrates a mass with water density (-10 to $+20$ HU) with an imperceptible wall, sharp margins with the renal parenchyma, and no enhancement after intravenous contrast administration.

○ **Describe the radiographic characteristics of a simple renal cortical cyst on MRI scans and ultrasound.**

On T1-weighted MRI, the mass is homogenous with low signal intensity (less than liver or renal cortex), and on T2-weighted images the lesion is homogenously hyperdense. There is no enhancement following intravenous administration of Gadolinium-DTPA. On ultrasound, cysts are well demarcated with no internal echoes. They are usually spherical in shape and demonstrate an increase in through-transmission with acoustic enhancement within the cyst.

○ **Describe the radiographic characteristics of a complicated cyst.**

A complicated cyst has an unusual contour, internal septations, calcifications, and/or evidence of enhancement on a contrasted CT scan.

○ **What is the Bosniak criteria for cyst classification?**

Delineates cysts into five categorizes of renal cysts. The categorizations have management implications associated with the potential risk of malignancy.

○ **What is Bosniak I?**

Bosniak I cysts are solitary and fulfill the sonographic and CT criteria for simple cysts. Sharp, thin, smooth-walled, spherical, or ovoid water density lesions (-10 to $+20$ Hounsfield units), with no internal echoes and no enhancement after intravenous contrast administration on CT.

○ **What is Bosniak II?**

Considered benign 90% of the time, these cysts can have thin central septations, thin peripheral calcifications, or they can be hyperdense nonenhancing lesions with Hounsfield units between 50 and 100. They are less than 3 cm in size.

○ **What is Bosniak IIF?**

These cysts can have several thin central septations, thickened peripheral calcifications, or they can be hyperdense minimally enhancing lesions. They are greater than or equal to 3 cm in size.

○ **What is Bosniak III?**

These are complicated cysts with extensive calcifications, thickened walls (greater than or equal to 1 mm thick), and irregular borders. They have irregularly enhancing walls. There should be a high level of suspicion for malignancy in these lesions.

○ **What is Bosniak IV?**

A complex cystic renal mass with thick septa and/or thick walls, thickened calcifications that can be central or peripheral, and/or an enhancing component on contrasted images. These lesions can be found in association with solid tumor.

○ **What is the current classification of cysts based upon?**

Several classifications have been proposed upon microscopic findings, clinical presentation, or radiographic appearance. Most recent publications in the urologic literature follow the 1987 classification given by the Committee on Classification, Nomenclature and Terminology suggestions of the American Academy of Pediatrics, Section on Urology. The primary distinctions are genetic and nongenetic.

○ **What are genetic renal cystic diseases?**

- Autosomal dominant (adult) polycystic kidney disease.
- Autosomal recessive (infantile) polycystic kidney disease.
- Juvenile nephronophthisis—medullary cystic disease complex.
- Juvenile nephronophthisis (autosomal recessive).
- Medullary cystic disease (autosomal dominant).
- Congenital nephrosis (familial nephritic syndrome) autosomal recessive.
- Familial hypoplastic glomerulocystic disease (autosomal dominant).
- Rare multisystemic disorders (von Hippel-Lindau disease, tuberous sclerosis, etc.).

○ **What are the nongenetic renal cystic diseases?**

- Multiscystic dysplastic kidney.
- Benign multilocular cyst.
- Simple cysts.
- Medullary sponge kidney.
- Sporadic glomerulocystic kidney disease.
- Acquired renal cystic disease.
- Calceal diverticulum.

○ **What is autosomal dominant polycystic disease (ADPKD)?**

Also known as adult polycystic kidney disease, this is an important cause of renal failure and accounts for almost 10% of all dialysis patients. The incidence is approximately 1 in 500 to 1 in 1000. While this condition typically presents in the third to fifth decades of life, it has been identified in newborns. Large irregular cysts of varying sizes appear diffusely throughout the renal cortex and the medulla. Renal function is impaired and hypertension and microscopic hematuria are common.

○ **What is autosomal recessive polycystic kidney disease (ARPKD)?**

RPK is typically diagnosed during infancy and carries a 50% mortality rate in the first few hours to days of life. This disease has a spectrum of severity with the most severe form being diagnosed at birth and the less severe forms are diagnosed later in infancy/childhood. The affected newborn has massively enlarged kidneys that are hyperdense on sonography due to the presence of multiple subcapsular cysts. All patients have some degree of hepatic fibrosis with lesions in the periportal region of the liver. This pathologic entity can be readily diagnosed by the gross appearance of the kidneys.

○ **What is juvenile nephronophthisis?**

Both juvenile nephronophthisis and medullary cystic disease cause polydipsia and polyuria in more than 80 % of cases. The cysts are medullary in position. There is severe renal tubular defect associated with the inability to conserve sodium. The polyuria is refractory to vasopressin and a large salt-intake diet is required to maintain sodium balance. There is associated growth retardation in juvenile nephronophthisis.

○ **Describe the renal cysts associated with tuberous sclerosis.**

The renal cysts of tuberous sclerosis are unique in that they have a lining of hypertrophic, hyperplastic eosinophilic cells.

○ **Describe the renal cysts associated with von Hippel-Lindau Disease?**

The cysts usually resemble simple benign cysts with flattened epithelium that some investigators consider precancerous.

○ **What is the sonographic appearance of autosomal recessive polycystic kidney disease (ARPKD) in the newborn?**

Bilateral, symmetrically enlarged, homogenously hyperechoic kidneys, usually without evidence of large discrete cysts.

○ **In what polycystic kidney disease (autosomal dominant or recessive) would you suspect liver pathology?**

Both. Autosomal dominant polycystic kidney disease is associated with hepatic cysts that become evident in adulthood and increase in incidence with age. Autosomal recessive polycystic kidney disease is associated with congenital hepatic fibrosis in all affected individuals.

○ **What is the essential histopathologic finding to diagnosis of dysplasia?**

Primitive ducts.

○ **In what renal cystic diseases is there a high incidence of renal cell carcinoma?**

The highest incidence, 35%, is in von Hippel-Lindau disease. Tuberous sclerosis has a 2% incidence of associated renal malignancy. All others carry the same incidence of renal cell carcinoma as the general population.

○ **How do patients with medullary sponge kidney present?**

Renal colic, gross hematuria, and urinary tract infections.

○ **Can UPJ obstruction be different from multicystic kidney disease based only on sonographic findings?**

Yes, it is possible. In multicystic kidney disease, the cysts are arranged in a random fashion. In UPJ obstruction, the largest cyst-like structure is medial or central, representing the renal pelvis, and communications can be demonstrated between the central "cyst" or renal pelvis and the "peripheral cysts" which are actually the calyces.

○ **In unilateral multicystic kidney disease, what is the typical contralateral urologic finding?**

Twenty to forty percent of patients have contralateral vesicoureteral reflux. Three to ten percent of patients will have a contralateral UPJ obstruction.

○ **What is acquired renal cystic disease (ARCD)?**

Acquired renal cystic disease is a feature of end-stage renal disease rather than a response to dialysis. The cysts are predominately in the cortex, generally less than 1 cm in diameter, and are associated with a sixfold increased risk of renal cell carcinoma.

○ **What is the most common presentation of acquired renal cystic disease?**

Loin pain, hematuria, or both.

○ **What is the incidence of renal cell carcinoma in acquired renal cystic disease?**

Three to six times higher than the general population.

○ **What is the incidence of autosomal recessive polycystic kidney disease (ARPKD)?**

Incidence is 1 in 40,000 births.

○ **What is the typical clinical presentation of ARPKD?**

Large kidneys or flank mass. Other findings include oligohydramnios, oliguria, cysts of the renal tubules, and congenital hepatic fibrosis of varying degrees.

○ **What specific genetic abnormality is associated with autosomal dominant polycystic kidney disease (ADPKD)?**

In ADPKD, 95% are caused by a gene located on the short arm of chromosome 16; 50% of the patient's offspring will be affected; and 5% are caused by a defect on chromosome 4. Usually have symptoms later in life.

○ **What is the usual age and typical clinical presentation of ADPKD?**

ADPKD usually presents between the ages of 30 and 50 years. It occurs uncommonly in newborns. The clinical presentation is with hypertension, flank pain, hematuria, and urinary tract infection.

○ **What other systemic anomalies are associated with ADPKD?**

Aneurysm of the circle of Willis (10%–40%). Cysts in the liver, spleen, pancreas, and lung. Diverticula of the colon. Mitral valve prolapse.

○ **What is the different diagnosis for a neonate with bilateral renal enlargement and homogenous hyperechoic kidneys?**

- Autosomal recessive polycystic kidney disease (ARPKD).
- Autosomal dominant polycystic kidney disease (ADPKD).
- Sporadic glomerulocystic kidney disease.
- Contrast nephropathy.
- Renal vein thrombosis.

○ **On what chromosome do we find the genetic defect for ARPKD?**

Chromosome 6.

○ **What is the histology of ARPKD?**

The kidney retains fetal lobulation, with small cysts and no normal renal parenchyma. The renal vessels and ureter appear normal. Collecting duct ectasia is present.

○ **In ARPDK, the cysts develop from which specific part of the nephron?**

The cysts are derived principally from the collecting duct.

○ **What is the histology of ADPKD?**

Cyst sizes range from a few millimeters to several centimeters. Focal tubular dilatation, epithelial hyperplasia, or adenoma of cyst wall. The vessels show atherosclerosis and interstitial fibrosis in advanced stages.

○ **In ADPKD, the cysts develop from which specific part of the nephron?**

Microcysts and macrocysts are derived from the entire nephron.

○ **What percentage of renal failure in children is caused by juvenile nephronophthisis?**

Ten to twenty percent.

○ **Which chromosome contains the genetic defect for juvenile nephronophthisis?**

Chromosome 2.

○ **What is the inheritance pattern for juvenile nephronophthisis and for medullary cystic disease?**

Juvenille nephronophthisis is autosomal recessive on chromosome 2. Medullary cystic disease is autosomal dominant with an unidentified chromosomal abnormality.

○ **What are the manifestations of von Hippel-Lindau (VHL) disease?**

VHL is an autosomal dominant condition manifested by cerebellar hemangioblastomas; retinal angiomas; cysts of the pancreas, kidney, and epididymis. It is also associated with pheochromocytomas in approximately 20% of patients and renal cell carcinomas.

○ **What are the clinical manifestations of tuberous sclerosis?**

Tuberous sclerosis is part of a triad of epilepsy, mental retardation, and adenoma sebaceum. The hallmark lesion is a superficial cortical hamartoma of the cerebrum. Although renal cysts have been associated with tuberous sclerosis, angiomyolipomas are more common than cysts.

○ **What is a multicystic kidney and how common is it?**

Multicystic kidney (multicystic dysplastic kidney) is a severe form of dysplasia in which there is no functioning renal parenchyma. The kidney does not have a reniform shape and calyceal drainage is not present. A "bunch of grapes" has been used to describe the gross appearance of the kidney. Renal size is variable. Multicystic kidney is the most common type of renal cystic disease and one of the most common causes of an abdominal mass in infants.

○ **What are the characteristics of medullary sponge kidney?**

Medullary sponge kidney is characterized by the dilatation of the distal portion of the collecting ducts, which may be associated with cysts and diverticula. The dilated collecting tubules have a distinct appearance on pyelography and look as if they were brushed on with the "bristles of a paint brush." One-third of patients have hypercalcemia that tends to be the "renal calcium leak" type. Patients with medullary sponge kidney tend to have a relatively high incidence of renal calculi, urinary tract infections, and hypocitraturia.

CHAPTER 37 **Renal Tumors, Adults**

Paul L. Crispen, MD, and
Matthew T. Gettman, MD

○ **How quickly is the incidence of renal cell cancer increasing?**

Two percent annually. Although renal cancer is more common in men, the incidence in women is rising faster (2.2% vs. 1.7%).

○ **What is the most common benign solid renal tumor?**

Renal cortical adenoma. These tumors are seen in up to 35% of autopsies and frequently cause no symptoms. Symptomatic lesions occur more commonly in females and are best treated with partial nephrectomy. Most of these lesions are less than 1 cm in diameter and 50% of these tumors occur bilaterally.

○ **Can information from a percutaneous needle biopsy of a renal mass be considered reliable?**

Analysis of biopsies on permanent section is significantly more reliable than frozen-section analysis. With experienced pathologists and radiologists, the expected sensitivity and specificity of a percutaneous needle biopsy is 97% and 100%, respectively.

○ **What are the indications for a biopsy of a renal mass?**

Percutaneous biopsy is advocated only when clinical or radiologic evidence suggests a diagnosis other than renal cell carcinoma (such as lymphoma), or when a definite diagnosis is absolutely necessary.

○ **What is the incidence of renal cell carcinoma (RCC)?**

Renal cell cancer accounts for 3% of adult malignancies. Approximately 54,000 new cases of RCC are expected to be diagnosed in 2008, with approximately 13,000 RCC-related deaths. RCC accounts for up to 90% of all kidney tumors.

○   **How is renal cancer staged?**

By TNM staging system.

T1a: confined to the kidney <4 cm.

T1b: confined to the kidney >4 cm and <7 cm.

T2: confined to the kidney >7 cm.

T3a: perinephric fat and/or ipsilateral adrenal gland involvement.

T3b: tumor extension into the renal vein but not extending above the diaphragm.

T3c: tumor extension into the renal vein extending above the diaphragm or invasion into the wall of the vena cava.

T4: tumor extension beyond Gerota's fascia, involvement of adjacent organs other than the ipsilateral adrenal gland.

○   **What is the standard of care in the treatment of renal tumors clinically localized to the kidney?**

Nephrectomy—partial or radical.

○   **What are additional treatment options for patients with T1a tumors?**

Observation, cryoablation, and radiofrequency ablation.

○   **Synchronous metastases occur in what percentage of RCC patients?**

Up to one-third of patients will have synchronous metastases. Metachronous metastases occur in 10% to 20% of patients at 5-year follow-up. The prognosis is much worse for patients with synchronous metastasis.

○   **How frequently does RCC invade adjacent organs?**

RCC invades adjacent organs in approximately 10% of cases. Invasion of adjacent organs is associated with a very poor prognosis with reported 5-year survival rates of less than 5%. In many cases, surgical intervention can require partial resection of contiguous structures including colon, pancreas, liver, or spleen. Preoperative imaging often overstates the possibility of direct liver invasion.

○   **A patient undergoes a partial nephrectomy for organ-confined RCC. What recurrence rates would be expected in the ipsilateral kidney and the contralateral kidney?**

Recurrence in the ipsilateral kidney would be 1% to 5% and 1% to 3% in the contralateral kidney.

○   **What percentage of RCCs occur bilaterally?**

One to five percent of RCC patients have tumors present in both kidneys simultaneously.

○   **What is the incidence of the different histologic types of RCC?**

Clear cell (80%) followed by papillary (15%), chromophobe (5%), collecting duct cancer (1%), and renal medullary carcinoma (<1%).

○   **What is the prognosis for cystic clear cell RCC?**

Excellent. Cystic clear cell RCC is associated with a low rate of systemic progression following complete surgical excision.

○ **True or False: At least 50% of renal cell carcinomas are vimentin-positive on immunohistochemical analysis.**

True. In addition, high-grade tumors, clear cell cancers, and those with sarcomatoid differentiation are more commonly vimentin-positive. Almost all renal cell carcinomas stain positively for keratin 8 and 18 and the majority stains positively for epithelial membrane antigen. This is useful in diagnosing metastases.

○ **What cystic renal diseases are associated with an increased incidence of RCC?**

Acquired renal cystic disease is associated with a four- to sixfold increased risk of RCC over the general population. von Hippel-Lindau disease has a known incidence of bilateral renal cysts in 76% of affected individuals with a 35% to 38% incidence of RCC in affected individuals. Tuberous sclerosis is associated with a 2% increased risk of RCC over the general population.

○ **Which types of RCC are more aggressive?**

Renal medullary carcinoma and collecting duct carcinoma are more aggressive subtypes. The behavior of clear cell, papillary, and chromophobe types are best predicted by stage and grade.

○ **Which type of RCC is associated with multifocality?**

Papillary RCC is associated with a 15% incidence of multifocality within the affected kidney.

○ **What is the predominant group of patients in whom the renal medullary type of RCC appears?**

Renal medullary carcinomas occur almost exclusively in association with sickle cell trait or hemoglobin SC disease. These are very aggressive tumors and tend to occur in younger patients.

○ **What is the renal cell type of origin of most RCCs?**

Proximal convoluted tubule.

○ **What is the renal cell type of origin of Bellini tumors?**

The origin of the Bellini tumors is the collecting duct. Renal medullary carcinomas are thought to arise from the calyceal epithelium.

○ **What are the risk factors for RCC?**

Tobacco use, male gender, and urban dwellers. The majority of RCC occur in the fifth to seventh decade of life, however, a recent trend suggests a higher incidence in younger females and adolescents. RCC is more commonly seen in patients with von Hippel-Lindau disease, horseshoe kidneys, acquired renal cystic disease, and obesity.

○ **List the hereditary forms of RCC?**

von Hippel-Lindau (VHL) disease, Birt-Hogg-Dube, hereditary papillary RCC, and hereditary leiomyomatosis and RCC syndrome

○ **What are the specific genetic abnormalities associated with each of the hereditary forms of RCC?**
- VHL: VHL gene on chromosome 3p.
- Birt-Hogg-Dube: BHD1 gene on chromosome 17p.
- Hereditary papillary RCC: c-met protooncogene on chromosome 7q.
- Hereditary leiomyomatosis and RCC: fumarate hydratase on chromosome 1q.

○   **What is von Hippel-Lindau disease?**

A rare, autosomal dominant, multiorgan syndrome associated with a 50% incidence of RCC; 75% incidence of renal, epididymal, and pancreatic cysts; cerebellar hemangioblastomas; retinal angiomas; and pheochromocytoma. Typically, RCC in this instance tends to be multiple and bilateral (80%). Historically, one-third of patients die from RCC.

○   **What is the most common cause of hereditary pheochromocytoma?**

VHL syndrome.

○   **Can the size or appearance of renal lesions in VHL disease predict the presence of RCC?**

No. No correlation exists between the size of a lesion and the diagnosis of RCC. Twenty-five to thirty-five percent of RCC in VHL occur in cystic lesions.

○   **A patient with VHL has small bilateral renal tumors. At what point is surgical intervention indicated?**

The balance between oncologic control and preservation of renal function is crucial in patients with small renal tumors. In VHL patients, tumors less than 3 cm have been associated with a low rate of progression to metastatic disease. For this reason, close surveillance with surgical intervention when a tumor reaches 3 cm in size can be employed in this population.

○   **A patient with VHL has diffuse, high-volume, bilateral renal lesions. What treatment is best?**

The best treatment in this case would be bilateral nephrectomy with subsequent transplantation. Nephron-sparing surgery, while technically feasible in many cases, is best reserved for patients with cystic and low-volume, nondiffuse solid lesions.

○   **What is the function of the VHL gene?**

The VHL gene is a tumor suppressor gene. The VHL protein complex helps to maintain appropriate levels of HIF-1, depending on oxygen availability. When VHL is mutated, HIF-1 levels increase, leading to the activation of angiogenesis pathways.

○   **Do sporadic clear cell RCC have mutations of the VHL gene?**

Yes, 50% to 60% of clear cell RCC have mutations of the VHL gene. Another 15% to 20% have hypermethylation of the VHL gene.

○   **Describe Birt-Hogg-Dube syndrome (BHD).**

Autosomal dominant disorder characterized by cutaneous fibrofolliculomas, lung cysts, and renal tumors. Renal tumors are noted in approximately 30% of patients with BHD syndrome. The most common renal tumors are oncocytomas and chromophobe RCC; these tumors are often multifocal and bilateral.

○   **Describe hereditary papillary RCC syndrome (HPRCC).**

Autosomal dominant disorder characterized by bilateral multifocal type 1 papillary tumors.

○ **Describe hereditary leiomyomatosis and RCC syndrome (HLRCC).**

Autosomal dominant disorder characterized by type 2 papillary tumors and cutaneous and uterine leiomyomas. Although only 20% of patients with HLRCC syndrome develop renal tumors, the tumors have been noted to be very aggressive.

○ **True or False: Renal cell carcinomas typically have a true histologic capsule.**

False. Most RCCs are surrounded by a pseudocapsule.

○ **What accounts for the yellowish gross appearance of many clear cell renal cell carcinomas?**

The presence of cholesterol causes the gross yellow appearance of these tumors. The lipid substances tend to dissolve during histologic preparation, creating the microscopic appearance of clear cells.

○ **True or False: Nuclear grade is a predictor of survival that is independent of pathologic stage.**

True. Nuclear grade has a significant impact on survival for all stages of RCC.

○ **What is the typical clinical presentation for most RCC cases and how does it differ from the classic triad?**

Incidental in the modern era. Hematuria (gross or microscopic), mass, and flank pain are not uncommon. The classic triad of pain, hematuria, and flank mass occurs in only 10% to 15% of patients. Presenting symptoms can often be attributed to metastasis or paraneoplastic syndromes.

○ **What is responsible for the increased detection of incidental renal tumors?**

The routine use of cross-sectional imaging (CT scans) to evaluate abdominal symptomatology.

○ **What must be considered prior to the administration of IV contrast in the evaluation of renal mass?**

Renal function. Impaired renal function places patients at risk for complications following the administration of iodine and gadolinium-based contrast agents. Iodine-based contrast is associated with the risk of acute nephrotoxicity and worsening renal function. Gadolinium has been associated with nephrogenic systemic fibrosis.

○ **What are housfield units and how do they help to differentiate renal tumors on computed tomography?**

Hounsfield units are a measure of radiodensity on CT scans. Enhancement of 15 or more Hounsfield units following the administration of contrast are suggestive of a malignancy, however, benign lesions such as oncocytoma will also enhance. Whereas, tumors containing areas with negative Hounsfield units, suggestive of fat, are likely angiomyolipomas.

○ **Differentiate between the Bosniak classification of renal cysts and their relationship to malignancy.**

- Category I: A simple cyst with through transmission on ultrasound and a clearly defined wall. There are no internal septa, echoes, or calcifications. This portends a remote chance for cancer.
- Category II: A septated, nonenhancing cyst that can have thin peripheral calcifications and minimally thickened wall. This lesion carries roughly a 15% chance of malignancy.
- Category III: A complex cyst with a thickened wall, a hyperdense cyst that shows no enhancement with contrast administration, can have thick calcifications, or thickened septa that carry roughly a 50% cancer.
- Category IV: An enhancing, thick-walled cyst with irregular borders, thick calcifications that may be central, and carries roughly a 95% chance of malignancy.

○ **What is the likelihood of missing a small RCC (<3 cm diameter) on intravenous urography?**

30%.

○ **What are the indications for a partial nephrectomy?**

Solitary kidney, bilateral renal masses, renal insufficiency, or anticipated renal insufficiency secondary to a comorbid disease process are imperative indications. However, partial nephrectomy has been shown to offer equivalent oncologic efficacy in small renal tumors compared to radical nephrectomy in small renal tumors (≤4 cm). With the additional benefit of preserving renal function, the "elective" application of partial nephrectomy has greatly expanded and is now considered the gold standard for the treatment of small renal tumors.

○ **Intraoperatively, what maneuver is imperative prior to proceeding with a partial nephrectomy?**

Complete exposure of the kidney to exclude multifocality. Ipsilateral multifocal disease is noted in up to 5% of patients at the time of nephrectomy. Intraoperative ultrasound is a valuable adjunct in this regard.

○ **How commonly are paraneoplastic syndromes associated with RCC?**

Paraneoplastic syndromes are seen concurrently with or develop in 30% of patients with RCC and are more common in patients with advanced disease.

○ **Describe Stauffer syndrome.**

Reversible hepatic dysfunction in the absence of metastatic disease. Patients have abnormal liver function tests, fever, and hepatic necrosis, which typically resolve after nephrectomy. Persistence or recurrence of disease is a poor prognostic sign.

○ **What other disease is associated with Stauffer syndrome?**

Xanthogranulomatous pyelonephritis.

○ **Which type of RCC is frequently observed in patients with Stauffer syndrome?**

Clear cell type.

○ **What is the etiology of hypercalcemia in patients with RCC?**

Hypercalcemia has been noted in approximately 15% of patients with RCC. Osteolytic bone metastasis or paraneoplastic syndrome frequently cause hypercalcemia. Stromal cells of RCC are thought to produce a parathyroid hormone-like peptide responsible for the paraneoplastic syndrome.

○ **List the levels of tumor thrombus associated with RCC.**

- Level 0: limited to the renal vein.
- Level 1: extending into the IVC, <2 cm above the renal vein.
- Level 2: extending >2 cm above renal vein, but below the hepatic veins.
- Level 3: extending to the hepatic veins, but below the diaphragm.
- Level 4: extending above the diaphragm.

○ **What is the incidence of venous involvement by a tumor thrombus in RCC?**

Renal vein only, up to 25%; inferior vena cava, 5% to 10%; atrial, 1%.

○ **What clinical findings are suggestive of an increased risk for venous involvement by RCC?**

The presence of a varicocele, leg edema, deep vein thrombosis, recurrent pulmonary emboli, and caput medusae are reported manifestations but are found infrequently. A high index of suspicion for patients with larger, centrally located tumors is an important finding.

○ **What is the blood supply of the vena cava tumor associated with RCC?**

When vascularized, parasitized vessels from the renal artery typically feed the tumor thrombus.

○ **Describe the collateral venous circulation in cases where the IVC is occluded secondary to tumor thrombus.**

IVC occlusion at the level of renal veins leads to dilatation and increased venous return via the retroperitoneal (hemiazygous system, lumbar veins, and Batson's plexus), gonadal, mesenteric, and pelvic plexus.

○ **What is the differential diagnosis and incidence of a vena cava tumor thrombus?**

Wilms' tumor, transitional cell carcinoma, sarcoma, lymphomas, primitive neuroectodermal tumors, adrenal cortical carcinoma, testis tumors, and pheochromocytoma. Five percent of RCC cases have vena cava involvement.

○ **Where are the most common sites of metastasis from RCC?**

The most common sites are the lung, bone, lymph nodes, liver, adrenal glands, brain, heart, spleen, and skin.

○ **Describe general 5-year survival for RCC with tumor confined to the kidney, with perinephric fat involvement, with vena cava thrombus, with node-positive disease, or metastasis.**

The 5-year survival for organ-confined RCC is 85% to 90%, 70% to 75% for perinephric fat involvement, 40% to 60% for vena cava thrombus, 10% to 20% with node involvement, and 0% to 5% for metastatic disease.

○ **What is the role, if any, of cytoreductive nephrectomy for patients with metastatic RCC?**

Cytoreductive nephrectomy can be completed prior to the systemic therapy, for palliation, or in conjunction with resection of select solitary metastasis. In fact, randomized series have demonstrated a significant increase in survival in patients undergoing cytoreductive nephrectomy prior to systemic therapy compared to patients not undergoing nephrectomy. In addition, nephrectomy in conjunction with resection of a solitary pulmonary metastasis has yielded 5-year survival rates of 30% to 35%. Patients with CNS metastasis represent a special case in which they are treated preferentially prior to cytoreductive nephrectomy.

○ **Should solitary metastases in RCC be surgically resected if possible?**

Yes. Metastatectomy has been associated with increased long-term survival.

○ **List the various forms of systemic therapy for metastatic RCC.**

Immunotherapy and targeted therapy. Since the introduction of targeted therapy, the use of immunotherapy has decreased significantly. However, immunotherapy is the only form of therapy for metastatic RCC that has been associated with the potential for a complete treatment response.

○ **List the various forms of immunotherapy for metastatic RCC.**

- *Active specific immunotherapy:* stimulation of T cell by immunization of patient with inactivated autologous tumor cells, limited proven benefit.
- *Adoptive immunotherapy:* typically involves either in vitro or in vivo interleukin stimulation (usually IL-2) of peripheral lymphocytes (lymphocyte-activated killer cells or LAK cells), reported response rates up to 20%.
- *Cytokines:* typically α-interferon or IL-2 therapy with direct or indirect cytotoxic effects on the tumor, response rates of 5% to 25%.
- Vaccines and stem cell transplantation techniques are being developed.

○ **List the various forms of targeted therapy for metastatic RCC.**

Tyrosine kinase inhibitors, mTOR inhibitors, and VEGF monoclonal antibodies

○ **List the benefits of targeted therapy compared to immunotheray.**

Decreased toxicity, oral administration (tyrosine kinase and mTOR inhibitors), increased partial response rate, and disease stabilization compared to cytokine therapy.

○ **What are common side effects of the oral tyrosine kinase inhibitors?**

Hand-and-foot syndrome, rash, mucositis/stomatitis, hypertension, neutropenia, hypophosphatemia, anemia, fatigue, hypothyroidism, and diarrhea.

○ **What is the most common renal sarcoma in adults?**

Leiomyosarcoma accounts for 60% of renal sarcomas and is best treated with surgical removal. Other less common tumors include osteogenic sarcoma, liposarcoma, carcinosarcoma, fibrosarcoma, rhabdomyosarcoma of adults, and malignant fibrous histiocytoma.

○ **What is the characteristic substance secreted by juxtaglomerular cell tumors?**

Renin. These are extremely rare, profusely vascular benign tumors that not uncommonly are difficult to locate because of the small size. They occur in young adults and adolescents. Patients typically present with sever hypertension, polydipsia, polyuria, myalgia, and headaches. A partial nephrectomy should be considered if the diagnosis is made preoperatively.

○ **True or False: Patients with juxtaglomerular cell tumors typically have hyperkalemia.**

False. The hyperreninemia causes a secondary hyperaldosteronism followed by hypokalemia.

○ **At autopsy, what percentage of leukemia cases will have renal involvement?**

Up to 50%. Usually malignancies of the lymphoid type appear in the kidney as part of the systemic disease process. Non-Hodgkin's lymphoma is more common than Hodgkin's disease. Multiple, bilateral renal masses are common. The treatment is systemic for the most part. Lymphoid malignancies are the most common secondary tumors of the kidney.

○ **Besides lymphoid malignancies, where are the sites of primary tumors that metastasize to the kidney?**

Virtually any solid neoplasm can metastasize to the kidney. Lung cancer (squamous cell) frequently metastasizes to the kidney as well as breast cancer and uterine cancer. Up to 20% of patients with lung cancer have occult renal metastases. Malignant melanoma is also frequently noted in the kidneys at autopsy.

○ **What renal tumors contain fat?**

Angiomyolipomas are the most common. Less common tumors that contain fat include lipomas, liposarcoma, some Wilms' tumors, an occasional oncocytoma, and very rarely renal cell carcinoma.

○ **What syndrome is associated with angiomyolipomas?**

Tuberous sclerosis. This is an autosomal dominant inherited disease associated typically with multiple and bilateral AML, mental retardation, and adenoma sebaceum. AML in these patients develop frequently in late childhood. Although AML occur in 80% of patients with tuberous sclerosis, less than 40% of patients with AML have features of tuberous sclerosis.

○ **What is another name for angiomyolipoma (AML)?**

Renal hamartoma. These tumors contain fat, smooth muscle, and blood vessels. The incidence is 0.3% to 2%. Isolated AML are commonly seen in middle-aged women. The majority of AML appear as single asymptomatic lesions and are not associated with tuberous sclerosis.

○ **Does AML occur in other locations besides the kidney?**

Angiomyolipoma (hamartoma) have been reported to occur in the bone, heart, lung, brain, and eye.

○ **What is the name of the pulmonary condition that can be seen concurrently with AML?**

Pulmonary lymphangiomyomatosis.

○ **What is Wunderlich's syndrome?**

Spontaneous retroperitoneal hemorrhage associated with an AML.

○ **Are any other renal tumors associated with tuberous sclerosis?**

Renal cell carcinoma has been observed concurrently with angiomyolipoma in patients with tuberous sclerosis.

○ **What percentage of renal cancers result in spontaneous perinephric hemorrhage?**

Up to 60% of cases of spontaneous perinephric hemorrhage are caused by renal cancers; however, this association has significantly decreased due to the increased incidental detection of small renal tumors.

○ **How do patients with AML typically present?**

Tumor size correlates well with symptoms. Most small lesions are asymptomatic. Lesions larger than 4 cm are at increased risk for hematuria, spontaneous rupture, retroperitoneal bleeding, pain, and possibly fever. At least 10% of patients with AML develop acute hemorrhage requiring intervention.

○ **What hormone receptors are associated with AML?**

AMLs have been noted to express androgen, estrogen (α and β subtypes), and progesterone receptors.

○ **What chromosomal abnormalities are associated with angiomyolipomas?**

Loss of heterozygosity at chromosome 16p13 has been observed in 50% of AML occurring in association with tuberous sclerosis and 10% of sporadic AML. Changes in chromosome 9q have also been linked to tuberous sclerosis.

○ **What are the treatment options for AML?**

Observation, angioinfarction, and partial nephrectomy. Asymptomatic patients with small tumors are often followed with serial imaging unless renal function decreases or tumor diameter increases. It has been suggested that asymptomatic tumors larger than 4 cm be treated. All symptomatic tumors should be treated.

○ **What features are rarely seen with oncocytoma?**

Hemorrhage, cystic degeneration, and necrosis.

○ **What is the characteristic organelle seen in oncocytomas on electron microscopy?**

Mitochondria. The abundant mitochondria are responsible for the eosinophilic cytoplasm seen in the polygonal, uniform cells of oncocytomas. Mitotic figures are rare.

○ **What is the incidence of multifocal or bilateral oncocytomas?**

Oncocytomas are multifocal in 3% to 5% of cases. Bilateral oncocytomas can occur in approximately 3% to 5% of cases.

○ **Do oncocytomas ever occur concurrently with renal cell carcinoma?**

Yes. Ten percent of oncocytomas occur concurrently with a renal cell carcinoma in either the ipsilateral or contralateral kidney.

○ **What chromosomal changes are associated with oncocytoma?**

Oncocytomas are characterized by loss of the Y chromosome and translocations involving the long arm of chromosome 1. Abnormalities of chromosomes 3, 7, and 17 are rare in oncocytomas.

○ **What are the classic radiographic signs associated with the appearance of oncocytomas?**

Oncocytomas can have a "spoke wheel" appearance on angiography created by the vessels, whereas on CT, the presence of a stellate scar has been reported. Oncocytomas are also sharply demarcated, with no calcification, and isodense with a homogeneous pattern of enhancement.

○ **Can oncocytomas be reliably differentiated from RCC on imaging alone?**

No.

○ **True or False: Oncocytomas occur exclusively in the kidney.**

False. Oncocytomas have also been reported in the parathyroid and thyroid glands, salivary glands, and the adrenal glands.

○ **How common are renal oncocytomas?**

They account for 10% of all renal tumors. They are more common in men with a peak incidence in the sixth to eighth decade. Paraneoplastic syndromes and spontaneous rupture are uncommon. The radiographic differentiation from RCC is difficult.

○ **What is the renal cell type of origin for oncocytomas?**

Intercalated cells of the renal collecting tubules.

○ **True or False: Wilms' tumor in adults is typically associated with a better prognosis than presence of Wilms' tumor in children.**

False. The prognosis is generally not as good in adults compared to children. Furthermore, adults typically present with a more advanced stage compared to children.

○ **What is the most common malignant tumor observed in a horseshoe kidney?**

RCC followed by Wilms' tumor. The incidence of Wilm's tumor in horseshoe kidneys, however, is much higher than normal kidneys.

○ **What are classic features for cystic nephroma?**

An uncommon multicystic tumor that is solitary, unilateral, and multilobular. Predilection for middle-aged women, frequently in the upper pole.

○ **Can a cystic nephroma and a cystic RCC be differentiated radiographically?**

No. For this reason, all complex cysts (Bosniak III–IV) should be surgically explored in appropriate surgical candidates.

○ **What is the best way to predict postoperative renal insufficiency in patients undergoing nephrectomy for renal cell carcinoma?**

Probably a combination of creatinine clearance and Technetium-99m-mercaptoacetyltriglycine (Tc-MAG3) renal scintigraphy. A preoperative Tc-MAG3 clearance rate of 130 mL/min/1.73 m^2 has been suggested as a cutoff point in predicting significant renal insufficiency postop.

○ **When is a bone scan clearly indicated in the metastatic workup of patients with renal cell carcinoma?**

In patients with unexplained bone pain or elevated serum alkaline phosphatase levels.

○ **How often are metastases found at the time of initial presentation of renal cell carcinoma?**

Approximately one-third will have metastatic disease when their cancer is first diagnosed. Ten to twenty percent will develop metastases over the subsequent 5 years.

○   **How can you distinguish clinically between a small renal cell carcinoma and a renal cortical adenoma?**

You cannot.

○   **What is the incidence and significance of adrenal metastases in renal cell carcinoma and how does adrenalectomy affect the outcome?**

The incidence of adrenal metastases at the time of nephrectomy for renal cell cancer is just under 4%. Reports indicate that the prognosis for these cases is generally poor regardless of whether or not an adrenalectomy is done. This suggests that there may be little therapeutic benefit in performing a simultaneous adrenalectomy.

○   **During a laparoscopic nephrectomy, the patient develops sudden hypotension and a new "mill-wheel" cardiac murmer is detected. What is the diagnosis and recommended treatment of this condition?**

The patient has developed a gas embolism. The earliest sign of this entity is an extremely rapid and sudden decrease in end-tidal carbon dioxide, which literally happens in a matter of seconds. This is due to the gas embolism blocking the pulmonary outflow from the heart. This is why all laparoscopic cases should be appropriately monitored for carbon dioxide. Severe hypotension, development of the typical mill-wheel cardiac murmer and a rapid decline in oxygen saturation occur somewhat later and are associated with a poorer prognosis. Treatment involves immediate removal of carbon dioxide gas from the abdomen and placing the patient in a steep left lateral decubitus/Trendelenburg position to minimize any right ventricular outlet obstruction. Central venous catheter aspiration of the gas embolism may be necessary.

○   **Following a partial nephrectomy, a patient develops increased output from their flank drain after their Foley catheter was removed. Analysis of the drain fluid is consistent with urine. How should the patient be managed?**

Urine leak following partial nephrectomy is best managed with Foley catheter drainage. Occasionally, a ureteral stent will also need to be placed to maximize drainage. However, the vast majority of urine leaks heal with these conservative measures. Repeat surgical exploration should not be performed and is associated with the risk of completion nephrectomy.

○   **If renal ischemia is required during a partial nephrectomy, what measure can be performed to decrease renal injury?**

Limit ischemic time, utilization of cold ischemia, adequate hydration, and IV administration of mannitol and furosemide prior to vascular clamping.

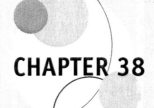

CHAPTER 38 Renal Tumors, Children

Jonathan C. Routh, MD, and
Matthew T. Gettman, MD

○ **What is the incidence of Wilms' tumor in children in North America?**

Roughly 500 cases of Wilms' tumor occur in North America per year, giving an incidence of roughly 8 per 1,000,000. Wilms' tumor is the most common malignant pediatric renal tumor, and accounts for 7% of all childhood cancers.

○ **How often are congenital anomalies associated with Wilms' tumor?**

Fifteen percent of cases. Congenital anomalies are much more common in patients with bilateral or simultaneous multifocal tumors.

○ **What is the relationship of aniridia to Wilms' tumor?**

Aniridia is found in 1% of patients with Wilms' tumors and 40% of patients with aniridia will develop Wilms' tumor, but only if they lack WT1.

○ **What genitourinary abnormalities are associated with Wilms' tumor?**

Horseshoe kidney and other renal fusion anomalies, renal ectopia, Mullerian duct anomalies, hypospadias, and cryptorchidism have been reported in 5% of cases.

○ **How frequently does hemihypertrophy occur with Wilms' tumor?**

Three percent of cases. Hemihypertrophy can be complete, partial, unilateral, or crossed. It is more common in females than males. This is also associated with 11p abnormalities.

○ **What skin lesions are associated with Wilms' tumor?**

Hemangiomas, cafe au lait spots, neurofibromas, and nevi are seen in 3% of cases.

○ **What is Beckwith–Wiedemann syndrome?**

A rare congenital syndrome associated with exomphalos, splenomegaly, hepatomegaly, macroglossia, hyperinsulinemic hypoglycemia, hemihypertrophy, and gigantism. Most cases are sporadic; 15% have autosomal dominant inheritance. Beckwith–Wiedemann syndrome is associated with WT2 abnormalities.

○ **What is the incidence of Wilms' tumor in patients with Beckwith–Wiedemann syndrome?**

It is 5% to 10%. Patients with Beckwith–Wiedemann syndrome and nephromegaly are at an increased risk of Wilms' tumor.

○ **What other syndromes are associated with an increased incidence of Wilms' tumor?**

Microcephaly, Perlman, Soto, and Simpson–Golabi–Behmel syndromes, developmental delay, spina bifida, intersex, trisomy 18, mixed gonadal dysgenesis, and nephrotic syndrome.

○ **Has a familial basis for Wilms' tumor been described?**

Yes, approximately 1% of patients have a positive family history for Wilms' tumor. This is thought to be inherited in an autosomal dominant manner.

○ **What chromosomal abnormalities have been associated with Wilms' tumor?**

Deletions in chromosome 11p13 are most commonly reported. The gene at this locus has been cloned and designated the WT1 tumor suppressor gene. A second Wilms' tumor locus, WT2, has been also identified on chromosome 11p15. 20% of Wilms' tumor patients have loss of heterozygosity on chromosome 16q and 11% of Wilms' tumor patients have loss of heterozygosity on chromosome1p.

○ **What is WAGR syndrome?**

The WAGR syndrome is seen in children with **W**ilms' tumor, **A**niridia, **G**enitourinary malformation, and mental **R**etardation. Most children with WAGR syndrome have a chromosomal deletion on chromosome 11p13. WAGR patients are at high risk of renal failure and of bilateral tumors.

○ **What is Denys–Drash syndrome?**

A syndrome of male pseudohermaphroditism, renal mesangial sclerosis leading to renal failure, and Wilms tumor. It is associated with mutations of WT1 on chromosome 11p13.

○ **What is the incidence of bilateral Wilms' tumors?**

Bilateral disease occurs in 5% of patients (4% synchronous, 1% metachronous).

○ **Do sporadic, heritable, and bilateral cases of Wilms' tumor have varying mean ages of presentation?**

Yes. Bilateral and heritable cases of Wilms' tumors present with a mean age of 2.5 years, whereas sporadic cases have a mean age of presentation of 3.5 years.

○ **How common is Wilms' tumor in neonates?**

Wilms' tumor is very rare in the newborn. The more likely solid renal tumor in this age group is congenital mesoblastic nephroma or neuroblastoma.

○ **True or False: Wilms' tumor occurs most commonly after the age of 6 years.**

False. Fifty percent of patients are 1 to 3 years old, 75% are younger than 5 years, and 98% are younger than 10 years at diagnosis. The peak incidence occurs between 1 and 3 years.

○ **What is the prognostic significance of Wilms' tumors occurring in older children?**

Patients presenting at an older age typically have a more advanced tumor that is less responsive to treatment.

○ **What are the common presenting symptoms for patients with Wilms' tumors?**

Abdominal mass is most common (90%) followed by hypertension (0%–60%), pain (20%–30%), nausea and vomiting (15%), fever (10%–20%), and gross hematuria (5%–10%).

○ **An acquired von Willebrand's disease is observed in what percentage of newly diagnosed Wilms' tumor patients?**

In 5% to 10% of patients. All newly diagnosed patients should undergo a coagulation screen with platelet count, bleeding time, prothrombin time, and activated partial thromboplastin time prior to surgery.

○ **What percentage of Wilms' tumors have a tumor diameter greater than 5 cm?**

Ninety percent.

○ **How frequently does Wilms' tumor have venous extension into the inferior vena cava?**

Four percent of patients have a tumor thrombus in the vena cava.

○ **What are the common sites of metastasis for Wilms' tumor?**

The most common site of distant metastasis is the lungs. Pulmonary metastases are present at diagnosis in 8% of patients. The other common site of metastasis is the liver.

○ **What histopathologic features are classically seen with Wilms' tumor?**

The gross appearance of the tumor is a fleshy ("brain-like") tan tumor with a pseudocapsule. Hemorrhage or cysts may be present. Microscopically, one will typically see blastemal, stromal, and epithelial elements. Sixty percent of cases will have a predominant component.

○ **What is the most important prognostic indicator in Wilms' tumor?**

Unfavorable or anaplastic histology. Unfavorable histology has the most significant prognostic impact when the tumor extends beyond the kidney, i.e., in higher-stage tumors.

○ **True or False: Unfavorable histology is most commonly seen in Wilms' tumors of patients younger than 2 years of age.**

False. Unfavorable histology (anaplasia) is rare in Wilms' tumors presenting in the first 2 years of life. Anaplastic features are not commonly encountered in infants.

○ **What is the incidence of unfavorable histology among Wilms' tumor patients?**

Unfavorable histology accounts for 5% to 10% of Wilms' tumor cases, but is responsible for 50% of Wilms' tumor deaths.

○ **What possible precursor lesions have been implicated in Wilms' tumor?**

Nephrogenic rests. Precursors to Wilms' tumor are found in 25% to 40% of cases. Presence of precursor lesions in one kidney is highly suggestive of precursor lesions in another kidney and, therefore, helps in identifying patients at risk for tumor in the contralateral kidney.

○ **What are nephrogenic rests?**

Clusters of abnormally persistent nephrogenic cells; microscopically, these are not easily distinguished from Wilms' tumor. These are thought to be premalignant lesions, although most do not develop into Wilms' tumor. They may be classified as perilobar or intralobar.

○ **What is nephroblastomatosis?**

Bilateral, symmetrical enlargement of kidneys characterized by diffuse proliferation of nephrogenic rests.

○ **True or False: A 3-year-old child's CT scan demonstrates a large Wilms' tumor in the left kidney with a normal right kidney. Proper management includes left nephrectomy with right renal exploration to exclude occult metastasis or nephroblastomatosis.**

False. Under current guidelines, it is no longer necessary to explore the contralateral kidney if a preoperative fine-cut CT or MRI shows no abnormality.

○ **What clinical scenarios preclude primary surgical excision for Wilms' tumor?**

Most patients with bilateral disease, extensive intravascular tumor extension, or tumors that require resection of adjacent organs to complete excision should undergo neoadjuvant chemotherapy, then surgery.

○ **Is open biopsy necessary to confirm the diagnosis in patients with suspected bilateral Wilms' tumor?**

No. Percutaneous biopsy is an alternative, and in some cases, it is reasonable to begin chemotherapy without histologic confirmation of Wilms' tumor. However, in European trials, 5% of patients who underwent chemotherapy without biopsy were found to not have Wilms' tumor at nephrectomy, including some patients with benign renal tumors.

○ **What effect does tumor spillage at the time of surgery have on the local abdominal relapse rate?**

Tumor spillage results in a sixfold increase in local abdominal relapses.

○ **What is the staging system used for Wilms' tumors?**

Stage I—tumor completely confined to kidney and completely excised.
Stage II—tumor beyond kidney but completely removed without spillage.
Stage III—residual abdominal disease: nodes involved, diffuse spillage, peritoneal implants, positive margin, incomplete resection.
Stage IV—hematogenous metastasis.
Stage V—bilateral disease (each side should also be staged).

O   **True or False: The treatment protocol for patients with unfavorable (focal anaplasia) stage I disease is the same as patients with favorable stage II disease.**

True. Both groups of patients should receive 18 weeks of adjuvant actinomycin D and vincristine, without radiotherapy.

O   **Do primary Wilms' tumors appear exclusively in the kidneys?**

No. Extrarenal Wilms' tumors have been reported in the retroperitoneum, sacrococcyx, cervix, groin, and gonads. The prognosis of patients with extrarenal Wilms' tumors is comparable to patients with intrarenal Wilms' tumors.

O   **What chemotherapeutic agents are currently used for Wilms' tumor?**

For stage I and II favorable histology tumors, actinomycin and vincristine are used. For stage III and IV favorable histology tumors, doxorubicin is added, along with radiation. For high-stage unfavorable histology tumors, patients will usually receive five drugs and radiation: actinomycin, vincristine, doxorubicin, cyclophosphamide, and etoposide.

O   **Are any chemotherapy drugs used for Wilms' tumor associated with the development of long-term side effects?**

Doxorubicin is associated with long-term risk of cardiotoxicity. This risk is directly proportional to the dose of doxorubicin used. Roughly 20% of children with Wilms' tumor who receive doxorubicin will develop congestive heart failure.

O   **True or False: Second malignancies have not occurred in patients with Wilms' tumor.**

False. Sarcomas, adenocarcinomas, lymphomas, and leukemias have all been reported. The incidence of second malignancies at 15 years posttreatment is 1.6% in the National Wilms' Tumor Study Group.

O   **What factors place patients at an increased risk for second malignancy?**

Prior treatment for relapse, the amount of abdominal radiotherapy, and use of doxorubicin place patients at increased risk for a second malignancy.

O   **Do horseshoe or fused kidneys predispose patients for Wilms' tumor?**

Wilms' tumor is two to eight times more common in patients with horseshoe or fused kidneys.

O   **True or False: All pediatric renal tumors have a better prognosis when diagnosed at a younger age.**

False. Although the predominant renal tumors of childhood, Wilms' tumor and neuroblastoma, do have a better prognosis when diagnosed at a younger age, this is not true of all tumors. Rhabdoid tumor of the kidney, for example, is associated with a much poorer prognosis when diagnosed in infants.

O   **What pediatric renal tumor is associated with polyhydramnios?**

Congenital mesoblastic nephroma is associated with a maternal history of polyhydramnios; 15% of patients will have other associated congenital abnormalities.

○ **What are the most common urologic abnormalities seen with multicystic dysplastic kidney? What test should be obtained for these patients?**

Contralateral vesicoureteral reflux (~30%) and ureteropelvic junction obstruction (~10%) can be seen in MCDK patients; VCUG should therefore be obtained.

○ **What are the most common cystic renal tumors in children?**

Multicystic dysplastic kidney, cystic Wilms' tumor, multilocular cystic nephroma.

○ **What cystic renal tumor commonly occurs in both young males and middle-aged females?**

Multilocular cystic nephroma. In women older than 40 years, cystic nephroma will often present with pain or hematuria.

○ **A 12-year-old boy presents with diastolic hypertension and hypokalemia. He has a 3.0-cm renal mass on CT scan. What laboratory tests should be obtained?**

Serum renin level. The suspected diagnosis is a juxtaglomerular tumor and serum renin levels would be elevated.

○ **True or False: By definition, patients with juxtaglomerular tumors have primary hyperaldosteronism.**

False. Juxtaglomerular tumors secrete renin which causes profound hypertension and *secondary* hyperaldosteronism.

○ **A 16-year-old girl with Klippel–Trenaunay syndrome presents with hematuria. What diagnosis should especially be considered?**

Renal hemangioma. Renal hemangiomas have been reported in the cortex, medulla, or renal pelvis. Most are small, single lesions and 50% are below the limits of radiologic detection. Symptomatic lesions appear more commonly in adults often with hematuria, which may become massive.

○ **A 9-year-old girl has microscopic hematuria and a honeycombed peripelvic renal mass noted on abdominal CT. What is the most likely diagnosis?**

The appearance of a honeycombed mass in a peripelvic location is most consistent with a lymphangioma. About one-third of lymphangiomas have been reported to occur in children.

○ **What tumor is referred to as the bone-metastasizing renal tumor of childhood?**

Clear cell sarcomas. The other tumor to consider in the setting of a child with a bony metastasis and a primary renal tumor is renal cell carcinoma.

○ **What are the most common solid renal tumors at the following ages: 1 month, 3 years, 10 years, and 18 years?**

At 1 month, congenital mesoblastic nephroma; at 3 years, favorable histology Wilms' tumor; at 10 years, Wilms' tumor and renal cell carcinoma are equally likely; and at 18 years, renal cell carcinoma.

○ **How do clear cell sarcomas differ from Wilms' tumors?**

These tumors have a significant component of clear cells, predilection for bone and brain involvement, and a poor prognosis. They represent 5% of all pediatric renal tumors and 50% present before 2 years of life.

○   **True or False: The majority of clear cell sarcomas have bone metastases.**

False. Despite its nickname, clear cell sarcoma has bone metastasis in only 15% to 20% of cases.

○   **Have rhabdoid tumors of the kidney been reported in conjunction with brain tumors?**

Yes, rhabdoid tumors have coexisted with medulloblastoma and other intracranial neoplasms and have been known to metastasize to the brain. The other renal tumor with propensity for brain metastasis is clear cell sarcoma. Patients with either diagnosis should have a brain MRI or CT performed in the early postoperative period.

○   **What are typical survival rates for patients with favorable and unfavorable Wilms' tumor, clear cell sarcoma, and rhabdoid tumor of the kidney?**

Four-year survival rates for these tumors are 90%, 70%, 75%, and 25%, respectively.

○   **A 2-month-old boy has a unilateral renal mass. What renal tumor is most commonly the cause?**

Congenital mesoblastic nephroma. More common in boys, it is effectively treated with nephrectomy.

○   **Microscopically, congenital mesoblastic nephroma resembles what other types of tumors?**

Congenital mesoblastic nephroma has a spindle-cell pattern that is very similar to leiomyoma or leiomyosarcoma.

○   **What are the typical characteristics of RCC in children?**

RCC accounts for only 3% to 5% of renal tumors in children. The tumors typically present above 10 years of age, most commonly with an abdominal mass. No sex predilection exists. Survival for RCC in children is worse than Wilms' tumor survival.

○   **What is a translocation carcinoma?**

A solid renal mass found in preteen children, often following treatment for neuroblastoma or Wilms' tumor. Histologically, this appears similar to papillary renal cell carcinoma but has a distinct genetic abnormality: translocation of chromosome 17 to chromosome X. Lymph node involvement by translocation carcinoma appears to have a fair prognosis, although hematogenous metastasis remains prognostically grim.

○   **A 13-year-old boy with sickle cell trait is found to have a renal mass with multiple pulmonary nodules. What is the likely diagnosis?**

Medullary renal cell carcinoma is found in patients with sickle cell hemoglobinopathy and is highly lethal. Mean age at diagnosis is 13 years.

○   **True or False: All cases of angiomyolipoma reported in children have been associated with tuberous sclerosis.**

False. While angiomyolipoma is a very rare tumor in children, cases have been reported without features of tuberous sclerosis.

○   **Who is Wilms' tumor named after and when was it first characterized?**

It was named for Max Wilms who first described it in 1899.

○ **What are the distinctive pathological features of Wilms tumor?**

Pathologically, Wilms' tumor is characterized as a triphasic tumor with three distinct patterns. There is an epithelial component, a stromal element, and a blastemal component.

○ **What is the significance of elevated urinary catecholamines in the evaluation of childhood neoplasms?**

Urinary homovanillic acid (HMA) or vanillylmandelic acid (VMA) is elevated in over 90% of patients with neuroblastoma. There is an inverse relationship between the VMA/HMA ratio and survival in disseminated disease.

○ **What is the most common extracranial tumor in children?**

Neuroblastoma, which accounts for 10% of all childhood cancers.

○ **What molecular and genetic markers are important in neuroblastoma?**

N-*myc* amplification is associated with a less favorable prognosis, as are elevated levels of neuron-specific enolase, ferritin, and chromosome 1p deletion. Tumor DNA aneuploidy is associated with a more favorable prognosis.

○ **At what age is Wilms tumor more common than neuroblastoma?**

Wilms tumor is more common in children older than 2 years of age. Younger children are more likely to have neuroblastoma.

○ **Bright blue nodules are found subcutaneously in a newborn. What problem does this suggest?**

Possible disseminated neuroblastoma. Particularly in a newborn, this may represent Stage IV-S neuroblastoma, which carries a good prognosis.

○ **What is the significance of stippled calcifications noted in a solid retroperitoneal mass?**

Approximately 50% of neuroblastomas have such stippling.

○ **A newborn presents with an abdominal mass and hematuria. What diagnosis does this suggest, what causes it, and how is it treated?**

Renal vein thrombosis. This is usually due to a hypercoagulable state or reduced intravascular volume such as from dehydration or infection. Renal vein thrombosis is usually unilateral and treatment generally involves only supportive measures. Thrombolytic therapy and/or anticoagulants are generally used only when there is vena caval or bilateral involvement.

○ **Are the kidneys usually palpable in normal neonates?**

Yes, both kidneys can usually be palpated.

○ **Turner's syndrome is associated with what urologic abnormality?**

Horseshoe kidney is more common in patients with Turner's syndrome.

CHAPTER 39
Renal/Ureteral Stone Surgery

Andrew I. Fishman, MD, and
Michael Grasso III, MD

○ **What are the most common renal stones in North America?**

Calcium stones (calcium oxalate, calcium phosphate, mixed) account for approximately 70% of stones in the United States, while infection stones account for 15% to 20%. Uric acid stones make up 5% to 10% and cystine stones 1% to 5% of stones diagnosed in this country.

○ **What are the ingredients of "triple phosphate" stones?**

Triple phosphate stones are composed of calcium, magnesium, and ammonium phosphate.

○ **Which stones are most dense on plain radiograph?**

Calcium hydrogen phosphate stones (Brushite), followed by calcium oxalate monohydrate.

○ **Which stones are radiolucent on plain radiography?**

Uric acid, sodium urate, ammonium urate, xanthine stones, 2,8-dihydroxyadenine (rare), matrix, and indinavir stones are all radiolucent on plain radiography.

○ **Which of these stones cannot be seen on CT scan without IV contrast?**

Indinavir (Crixivan) is a protease inhibitor used for treatment in HIV patients that cause stone formation. Indinavir can obstruct the ureter as a precipitate or as a pasty sludge. This type of stone is most commonly diagnosed endoscopically. If there is suspicion of a kidney stone and the patient is taking protease inhibitor drugs such as indinavir, an IVP would be a better choice for a confirmatory imaging study.

○ **Do all cystinuric patients produce kidney stones?**

No. Cystinuria is an inherited disorder of renal tubular reabsorption of cystine, ornithine, lysine, and arginine. These four amino acids can be remembered by the mnemonic COLA. Of these four, only cystine is relatively insoluble in urine and will precipitate to form stones. Patients with 24-hour urine cystine levels less than 400 mg/d rarely produce stones, while those with elevated levels over 1000 mg/d will produce large stone fragments unless treated medically.

○ **What are the most common complications of medical therapy for cystinuria?**

Thiola and D-penicillamine are the two agents that are used commonly to treat cystinuria. Both agents act on the disulfide bond creating a more soluble compound. Patients on these agents require 24-hour urine protein collections to rule out nephrotic syndrome, which is often reversible when the medications are stopped.

○ **Which gas is produced by Holmium:YAG laser lithotripsy of cystine stones?**

A malodorous sulfur dioxide gas is given off during laser lithotripsy of cystine stones.

○ **Which geometric principle is the basis for most ESWL generators?**

The first ESWL generator employed clinically was the Dornier HM#3. This device employed a sparking electrode placed at the F1 position of a brass semi-ellipsoid. The firing of this electrode created shock waves that were focused by the ellipsoid to the site of the kidney stone at the F2 position.

○ **What are the factors that limit success with ESWL therapy?**

Large stone burdens (size and number), stone composition, stone location, and clinical features such as body habitus and obesity are all factors that limit the stone clearance rate. A slower ESWL rate and good contact between the treatment head and the patient also help improve the efficiency of the shock wave therapy.

○ **Which stones are most resistant to ESWL therapy?**

Cystine stones are most resistant, followed by brushite stones, and then calcium oxalate monohydrate stones. Calcium oxalate dehydrate are the most brittle.

○ **Stones in which position are the most difficult to fragment with ESWL—proximal, mid, or distal ureteral stones?**

Midureteral calculi, especially those located between the level of the inferior and superior margin of the sacroiliac joint are hardest to approach with ESWL. The patient is positioned prone and the stone may be difficult to visualize/localize against the background of the pelvic bones with current imaging.

○ **What are the two absolute contraindications to ESWL?**

Pregnancy and uncorrected coagulopathy.

○ **What is "steinstrasse"?**

Steinstrasse, meaning "stone street" in German, refers to a column of stone fragments that may line up in the ureter following ESWL. This may lead to symptoms of obstruction.

○ **How is steinstrasse treated?**

In mild cases, observation alone may be enough. Double pigtail catheters, ESWL, and ureteroscopy are other available options.

○ **Which medications have been shown to help facilitate stone passage rates?**

Tamsulosin (Flomax) and nifedipine improve stone passage from the distal ureter by approximately 30%. Other α-blockers also increase spontaneous passage.

○ **What is the most important factor in predicting spontaneous stone passage?**

Stone size. If 4 mm or less, 90% will pass spontaneously.

○ **What are the three areas of functional narrowing of the ureter?**

The ureteropelvic junction is the proximal site of narrowing, followed by the level at which the ureter traverses the iliac vessels, and finally the ureterovesical junction.

○ **Which of these areas is most often the narrowest point in the ureter?**

The intramural segment at the ureterovesical junction.

○ **What are the two major complications associated with ureteropyeloscopy?**

The two major complications are acute, intraoperative ureteral wall perforation or avulsion and postoperative ureteral strictures. In the largest series, this complication rate occurred less than 0.5%.

○ **Which portion of the ureter is the most common location for ureteral avulsion during ureteroscopy?**

The proximal ureter is the most common site for ureteral avulsion.

○ **What is the next step in treatment if a ureteral avulsion is encountered?**

Prompt proximal drainage, most often performed with a percutaneous nephrostomy tube, with subsequent staged repair.

○ **What are the indications for hospitalization in a patient with a ureteral calculus?**

The following are indications for hospitalization and/or treatment: Intractable pain requiring parenteral analgesics, severe colic and/or intractable nausea and vomiting with dehydration, fever, leukocytosis, or bacteriuria, a stone in a solitary kidney, simultaneous bilateral ureteral stones with obstruction, complete obstruction of the kidney which is not transient and azotemia.

○ **What are the different types of endoscopic lithotriptors?**

Electrohydraulic, ultrasonic, laser, and ballistic.

○ **What endoscopic instrument is required for retrograde treatment of a lower pole calculus?**

Actively deflectable, flexible ureteropyeloscopes are essential in treating intrarenal stones, particularly those in the lower pole. Active endoscopic tip deflection facilitates placement of laser fibers and extractors (e.g., baskets and graspers). The application of a semirigid ureteroscope in treating intrarenal stones is limited.

○ **Laser lithotripsy of uric acid stones produces which toxin?**

Cyanide.

○ **True or False: Blind basketing of ureteral calculi is an acceptable method of extracting ureteral stones.**

False. With the advent of ureteroscopic lithotripsy, blind basketing has been completely abandoned. Stone extraction with force using this method often results in severe tissue trauma, and a stone could occasionally be engaged within a basket that subsequently could not be safely extracted from the ureter resulting in an adverse situation.

○ **What is the potential consequence of a submucosal stone?**

A stone granuloma may form; this may lead to a ureteral stricture.

○ **What is the incidence of symptomatic urinary calculi in pregnancy?**

The incidence has been estimated at 1 in 1500 pregnancies.

○ **True or False: The incidence of urinary stone formation is higher among pregnant women.**

False. Elevated urinary citrate levels are a protective mechanism correcting for the significant hypercalciuria associated with pregnancy.

○ **True or False: An IVP is contraindicated in pregnancy.**

False, although every effort should be made to reduce unnecessary radiation exposure.

○ **Which side and in what trimesters does physiologic hydronephrosis occur in pregnancy?**

It occurs more commonly on the right side and in the first and third trimester of pregnancy.

○ **What are the indications for urologic intervention of symptomatic ureteral calculi in the pregnant woman?**

Severe intractable pain, urosepsis, and obstruction of a solitary kidney with azotemia are all well-established indications for intervention.

○ **What factors affect the success of endoincision for ureteral strictures?**

Long stricture length >2 cm, periureteral fibrosis (e.g., secondary to endometrioma, idiopathic retroperitoneal fibrosis, etc.), and a history of prior abdominal radiation are all factors that negatively affect the success of endoincision of a ureteral stricture.

○ **What is Dietl's crisis?**

Flank pain that occurs or is exacerbated by increased fluid intake or a diuretic effect from ingestion of fluids such as alcohol. This is often associated with ureteropelvic junction obstruction.

○ **What is a struvite stone?**

A struvite stone is an infectious stone caused by urea-splitting bacteria (*Proteus, Pseudomonas,* and *Klebsiella* are common examples). A struvite stone comprises a mixture of magnesium ammonium phosphate and carbonate apatite.

○ **Can struvite stones form in acidic urine?**

No, they cannot. An alkaline urine of pH >7.0 is necessary.

○ **What is the consequence of an untreated staghorn struvite calculus?**

Over time, an untreated staghorn calculus has a significant chance of causing death (∼28%) due to renal failure or sepsis. As such, the American Urological Association Nephrolithiasis Clinical Guidelines panel recommends that newly diagnosed struvite staghorn calculi be treated actively rather than be followed conservatively and observed.

○ **How are staghorn calculi removed?**

Anatrophic nephrolithotomy is effective but rarely performed today. Percutaneous endoscopic stone removal (PCNL) is considered the standard of care. Other modalities, including shock wave lithotripsy, can be used adjunctively.

○ **What is the indication for treating large intrarenal stones ureteroscopically?**

Metabolic noninfectious stones can be treated successfully using retrograde ureteroscopic techniques. When stone burdens exceed 2.5 cm, staged therapy is commonly necessary. In patients where PCNL is contraindicated such as certain ectopic kidneys, ureteroscopy offers an alternative treatment modality.

○ **True or False: Percutaneous nephrostomy tracts should always be placed through anterior calyces.**

False. The posterior approach is preferred except in special circumstances. The anterior approach has a higher risk of bowel injury.

○ **Why should one avoid placing a percutaneous nephrostomy tube directly into the renal pelvis?**

A direct approach to the renal pelvis may injure the renal hilar vessels. Additionally, a pyelotomy tract closes slower than a nephrostomy tract, and is associated with greater urinary leakage postoperatively.

○ **What is the transfusion rate following percutaneous nephrostomy?**

Approximately 5% for simple stones and 10% for complete staghorn therapy.

○ **What are the risk factors for pneumothorax with PCNL?**

Supracostal access has a higher risk of pneumothorax and hydrothorax. It is approximately 10% over the 12th rib, but can approach approximately 50% over the 11th rib. Treatment is based on thoracentesis and/or placement of a small caliber thoracostomy tube.

○ **What are the different methods available to dilate a nephrostomy tract?**

Balloon dilatation (employed with a hydronephrotic system), Amplatz dilators (employed commonly with a branching stone), or metal telescoping dilators (employed when there is significant retroperitoneal fibrosis from prior renal surgery) are the commonly used methods.

○ **What are the common causes of delayed bleeding following Percutaneous Nephrolithotomy?**

This complication, which occurs in less than 1% of patients, is usually secondary to pseudoaneurysm formation or an arteriovenous fistula.

○ **What is the most common postoperative complication following percutaneous nephrolithotomy for a staghorn calculus?**

Fever from urinary extravasation and/or atelectasis.

○ **Which calculi are the least amenable to chemolysis?**

Calcium oxalate stones, the most common of all renal calculi, are the least amenable to chemolysis.

○ **Which electrolyte must be monitored closely when using Renacidin chemolysis?**

Magnesium levels. Hypermagnesemia, although occurring mainly in those with severe renal impairment, may also occur in those with normal renal function. Mucosal erosions, urinary tract infections, and elevated intrarenal irrigation pressures may contribute to elevated serum magnesium levels.

○ **Exactly how big is 3 French?**

3 French = 1 mm = 0.038 inch.

○ **How does one differentiate between a calyceal diverticulum and a hydrocalyx?**

Calyceal diverticula are considered to be congenital in origin and arise from a fornix of a minor calyx. A hydrocalyx is considered to be an acquired condition secondary to infundibular stenosis caused by various conditions (TB, stones, prior surgery, inflammation). Renal papillae are present within and diagnostic of a hydrocalyx. A calyceal diverticulum will not have a renal papilla inside it but will be lined only by transitional epithelium.

○ **What is the optimal recommended treatment for a severely septic patient with pyonephrosis?**

Prompt percutaneous nephrostomy drainage, which can usually be done with only a local anesthetic. Depending on the consistency of the infected fluid, a larger-caliber catheter may be required. A retrograde catheter can also be placed but usually requires anesthesia and is more difficult to irrigate if it becomes obstructed by thick inspissated material.

○ **What nonkinking flexible metal is the preferred component of guidewires and baskets?**

Nitinol (nickel–titanium alloy) is a strong but flexible metal that is the preferred component for ureteroscopic access guidewires. The Terumo guidewire is the premier ureteral access wire. This lubricious and flexible guidewire is commonly employed with ureteral strictures and impacted stones.

For flexible ureteroscopic access, the Teflon-jacketed nitinol-based zebra wire is commonly employed by many urologists. Stainless steel Segura baskets have been replaced for stone extraction by tipless nitinol designs.

○ **What are the standard stone basket types along with their relative individual strengths and weaknesses?**

The Dormia basket is the standard, symmetrical, spiral wire design. It is effective but usually requires a twisting motion to encompass the stone. A double wire design is also available that increases the radial, spreading force while keeping the space between wires relatively open.

The Segura type basket uses four flat wires arranged in a symmetrical fashion. It cannot be twisted or safely turned, but has good radial spreading force that is useful in narrowed ureters or in tight quarters.

The Leslie type baskets use an asymmetrical design that works something like a net. Two distal base pillars split into a 4- or 8-wire net. The open "front" allows for easy entry of stones while the "back" prevents distal migration of the stone. Essentially the basket works like a net. These designs work best when the proximal ureter is somewhat dilated so they can fully deploy. They also work well as a backstop when using intracorporeal lithotripsy to prevent proximal migration of larger stone fragments. To do this, the basket is opened above the stone before starting lithotripsy. The stainless steel "parachute" and the popular nitinol "escape" baskets are examples of this design.

○ **Which patients should undergo metabolic testing after passing a first stone?**

In general, patients who have their first episode of renal colic and pass their first stone do not require metabolic workup. There are exceptions that include; any child with a metabolic stone, patients with rare stone compositions (e.g., cystine), and patients who require significant surgical intervention for complex stone burden.

○ **Is ureteral dilation always required for ureteroscopic access?**

No, with less than 8-French semirigid and flexible ureteroscopes, the need to dilate the intramural tunnel for access is low (<5%). As a general rule, dilators up to 12-French are preferred in this setting and cause the least ureteral trauma.

○ **When is open surgery indicated for intrarenal calculi?**

In cases with large intrarenal stones and/or multiple infundibular stenosis, where an excessive number of access tracts would be required, anatrophic nephrolithotomy is indicated. This open procedure also facilitates infundibuloplasty that is key to intrarenal drainage.

○ **What are the indications for laparoscopic pyelolithotomy or ureteral lithotomy?**

Patients who failed prior endoscopic treatments can be treated laparoscopically. In addition, those patients who have renal or ureteral stones and are going to undergo lapararoscopic reconstruction such as pyeloplasty can have them both treated simultaneously.

○ **What is the indication for a laparoscopic or open nephrectomy in a patient with a large staghorn calculus?**

Xanthogranulomatous pyelonephritis (XGP) is defined by a large infectious renal stone burden and no functional renal parenchyma on nuclear renal scan. Laparoscopic or open nephrectomy is indicated in this setting.

CHAPTER 40

TCC of the Upper Urinary Tracts

Thomas W. Jarrett, MD

○ **What is the mean age of occurrence of transitional cell cancer of the upper urinary tracts?**

65 years.

○ **What is Balkan nephropathy?**

A degenerative interstitial nephropathy common to certain rural Balkan areas. Affected individuals are 100 to 200 times more susceptible to upper tract TCC. Tumors tend to be low grade, multiple, and bilateral.

○ **What is the most common presenting sign of upper tract urothelial tumors?**

Hematuria is seen in 75% of cases followed by flank pain in 30% of cases. Rarely do upper tract tumors remain asymptomatic.

○ **Primary urothelial cancers can be located in the bladder and/or upper urinary tracts. What percentage of urothelial tumors are located in the upper urinary tract?**

Approximately 5% to 8% of all urothelial tumors are located in the ureter and/or renal collecting system.

○ **What percentage of primary renal tumors will be of urothelial origin?**

Five percent of primary renal tumors will be of urothelial origin.

○ **What histology is most commonly found with urothelial tumors of the upper urinary tract?**

Transitional cell carcinoma (TCC) accounts for more then 90% of upper tract urothelial tumors. Squamous cell and adenocarcinoma make up the majority of the remaining tumors.

○ **What are some of the tumor markers reported for upper tract tumors?**

These include cyclooxygenase 2, EP4 receptors, oncoprotein p53, proliferation marker ki67, and tissue inhibitor of metalloproteinase I. p53 over expression tends to correlate with tumor progression.

○   **What are acceptable ways of making the diagnosis of upper urinary tract TCC?**

Diagnosis was traditionally made by the characteristic radiolucent filling defect of the upper urinary tract as well as cytologic evaluation of the urine. In some cases, sonography or cross sectional imaging may be necessary to rule out a radiolucent stone as the cause of a filling defect. With improvements in upper urinary tract endoscopy, ureteroscopy with biopsy should be strongly considered in all patients to confirm the diagnosis.

○   **What other histologic patterns are found with upper tract tumors?**

Squamous cell carcinoma and adenocarcinoma are less commonly seen and are usually associated with chronic inflammation from kidney stones, obstruction, and/or infection.

○   **What is the most common risk factor contributing to the development of upper urinary tract TCC?**

Cigarette smoking is the risk factor most strongly associated with transitional cell carcinoma of the bladder and upper urinary tracts. The risk increases threefold in a patient with a history of significant tobacco abuse when compared to the general population.

○   **What are some other risk factors for upper tract TCC?**

Exposure to cyclophosphamide, phenacetin, arsenic, and various aromatic amines and amides.

○   **What is Acrolein?**

A metabolic breakdown product of cyclophosphamide. It is thought to be the causative agent in the development of TCC.

○   **True or False: Tumors linked to chemotherapy use tend to be high grade.**

True.

○   **What is Lynch syndrome II?**

A hereditary syndrome involving upper urinary tract tumors and early colon tumors.

○   **What is the incidence of a bilateral upper tract involvement (either synchronous or metachronous)?**

Approximately 2% to 5% of patients with upper tract TCC will have involvement of the contralateral system at some point in their lives. The percentage may be higher in patients with associated carcinoma in situ.

○   **How is bilateral disease treated?**

Renal sparing surgeries are recommended when possible. These techniques include ureteroscopic, percutaneous, and segmental resections. Rarely, autotransplantation and pyeloneocystostomy may be necessary.

○   **What percentage of patients who initially present with TCC of the bladder will subsequently develop a tumor of the upper urinary tract?**

Upper urinary tract cancer occurs in 2% to 4% of patients with bladder cancer.

○ **What percentage of patients who initially present with TCC of the upper urinary tract will subsequently develop a bladder tumor?**

Approximately 50% of upper urinary tract TCC patients will develop bladder tumors at some point in their lives. This necessitates vigilant lifetime bladder surveillance in all patients with upper urinary tract tumors.

○ **What are the two most clinically important prognostic variables?**

Tumor grade and stage are the most important prognostic indicators. All studies have shown the prognosis significantly worsens with higher grade and stage lesions.

○ **What is the incidence of multifocality with upper tract TCC?**

Multifocality is seen in approximately one-third of patients and is directly related to tumor grade.

○ **Are tumor grade and stage related?**

Tumor grade and stage are matched in the vast majority of cases. It is quite rare for a low-grade lesion to show potential for invasion and/or metastasis. The opposite is true for high-grade lesions.

○ **What is the pattern of spread for upper tract TCC?**

TCC of the upper urinary tract can spread by direct extension, lymphatic invasion, and/or vascular invasion.

○ **What is the traditional treatment of organ-confined TCC of the upper urinary tract?**

The propensity of upper tract TCC toward multifocality and ipsilateral recurrence has led to ipsilateral nephroureterectomy with a bladder cuff as the best treatment for reducing the risks of disease recurrence and progression. Distal ureterectomy with ureteroneocystostomy may be considered for solitary low-grade lesions of the distal ureter. Exceptions to this rule are patients who may be at risk for renal failure and hemodialysis following removal of a renal unit. Examples include patients with solitary kidneys, bilateral disease, chronic renal insufficiency, and/or other risk factors for renal failure. In such cases, the risks of long-term hemodialysis may be greater than the risks of the disease itself and an organ-sparing approach should be considered.

○ **What surgical approaches may be used for total nephroureterectomy?**

Nephroureterectomy requires surgical exposure of the kidney and bladder. This requires either a single midline or thoraco-abdominal incision or a two-incision approach, flank and lower abdomen. Laparoscopic techniques have recently been incorporated to reduce the morbidity of the procedure. Both total laparoscopic and laparoscopic assisted procedures have been reported with decreased morbidity and equivalent cancer outcomes.

○ **What is the role of lymphadenectomy?**

Lymphadenectomy should be considered in all patients with high-grade and/or invasive lesions. It traditionally was done for staging purposes, although there may be some therapeutic value based on studies with bladder TCC.

○ **What organ-sparing alternatives to nephroureterectomy are available in the treatment of localized TCC of the upper urinary tract?**

Open local excision and endoscopic resection are established alternatives to nephroureterectomy.

O   **What endoscopic techniques are acceptable for the treatment of upper urinary tract TCC?**

Endoscopic therapy can be performed in a retrograde ureteroscopic fashion or an antegrade percutaneous fashion. Rarely, a combined approach is necessary.

O   **Are patients with a normal contralateral kidney candidates for organ-sparing therapy?**

This is a controversial area of urologic oncology; however, it is generally accepted that patients with low-grade and low-stage TCC are at low risk for disease progression. Organ-sparing therapy is acceptable provided the patient is compliant and committed to life long follow-up of the ipsilateral collecting system with ureteroscopy.

O   **With patients treated with organ-sparing therapy, is there any evidence that ipsilateral recurrence compromises patient survival?**

Especially when dealing with low-grade disease, there is little evidence to suggest that survival is compromised by ipsilateral recurrences. Recurrences can be addressed with repeat endoscopic treatment, surgical excision, or nephroureterectomy.

O   **What are the benefits of the retrograde ureteroscopic approach over the antegrade percutaneous method?**

The retrograde ureteroscopic approach has two distinct advantages: (1) ureteroscopy can generally be performed on an out-patient basis with minimal risk of complications, (2) ureteroscopic techniques maintain a closed system and thus have a lower theoretical risk of tumor seeding of nonurinary tract surfaces. The ureteroscopic approach works well for low-volume and low-grade tumors.

O   **What are the limitations of the ureteroscopic approach?**

Limitations of this approach include (1) inability to treat a large volume of tumor, (2) limitations of ureteroscopes to reach all portions of the kidney (i.e., lower pole system), and (3) limitations of biopsy specimens. Specimens obtained ureteroscopically are generally sufficient to establish tumor grade but are of inadequate depth to establish stage by assessing depth of invasion.

O   **When is the percutaneous approach generally favored?**

The percutaneous approach is generally indicated for larger tumors and/or those that are not easily accessible through the ureteroscopic approach (i.e., lower pole lesions). Unlike ureteroscopy, larger caliber instruments can be used for removal of larger tumor burdens. In addition, deep tissue specimens can be obtained for staging purposes.

O   **What is the best follow-up study for transitional cell carcinoma of the upper urinary tract treated with conservative management?**

Ureteroscopic evaluation is the most effective way of screening for ipsilateral tumor recurrences. Simple radiographic evaluation is not sufficient, as it has been shown that up to 75% of early tumor recurrences were visible endoscopically and not radiographically.

O   **With endoscopic management, what are the risks of tumor seeding of noninvolved urothelial surfaces or the nephrostomy tract?**

A significant concern of endoscopic therapy has been the theoretical possibility of tumor seeding of the normal urothelial surfaces and/or nephrostomy tract. Although there are individual case reports describing such problems, the majority of the literature has not supported this concern.

○ **Topical immuno or chemotherapy has been effective adjuvant therapy for bladder TCC. Have any studies shown significant improvement with regard to tumor recurrence or prevention of disease progression when this therapy is used for the upper urinary tract?**

Adjuvant topical therapy via nephrostomy tubes and ureteral catheters has been described. To date, no study has shown a statistically significant benefit with regard to recurrence and disease progression. This may be due to low patient numbers or possibly due to inadequate contact time with the urothelial surfaces of the upper urinary tract.

○ **What systemic chemotherapy regimens are available for the treatment of metastatic upper tract TCC?**

Available chemotherapeutic protocols for TCC of the upper urinary tract are identical to their bladder counterparts. Because of the rarity of the disease, no large studies have been performed that show significant benefit. However, these tumors are similar to their bladder counterparts and should respond in the same fashion.

○ **Is there a role for radiation therapy in the treatment of TCC of the upper tracts?**

Limited. It can be used for hemostasis in patients where other therapies cannot be used. Radiation may also be helpful as an adjunct to chemotherapy in patients with advanced disease.

○ **True or False: Patients with upper tract TCC tend to have a worse prognosis if they had a previous history of bladder cancer?**

True.

○ **How often will TCC of the upper tracts develop in patients with carcinoma-in-situ (CIS) of the bladder?**

Approximately 25% of the time.

○ **Does endoscopic resection of upper tract TCC offer equivalent overall survival to standard definitive surgical extirpation?**

In appropriate patients, yes. Patients with clinically localized upper tract TCC can be offered an endoscopic approach initially while allowing for more aggressive surgery at a later date if necessary. Also, there is a higher rate of recurrence with endourological treatment.

○ **What is Aristolichia fangchi and why is it important urologically?**

It's a Chinese herb used for weight loss. Its use has been associated with TCC of the upper tracts.

Howard J. Korman, MD, FACS, and
Damon Dyche, MD

○ **What is the incidence and treatment for bladder adenocarcinomas?**

The incidence is less than 2% of all bladder cancers. They are associated with exstrophy and are relatively resistant to radiation and chemotherapy. Radical cystectomy is the recommended treatment.

○ **What kind of cancer is associated with long-term catheterization and stones?**

Squamous cell cancer of the bladder.

○ **Which groups tend to have a worse prognosis?**

African American women.

○ **What specific agents in cigarette smoke are thought to be the most carcinogenic?**

Nitrosamine, 2-naphthylamine, and 4-aminobiphenyl.

○ **What is the most common kind of bladder cancer?**

Transitional cell carcinoma (TCC) accounts for more than 90% of all bladder cancers. Squamous cell carcinoma accounts for 3% to 7%, with adenocarcinoma and metastatic carcinomas uncommon.

○ **Other than smoking, what are the risk factors for bladder cancer?**

Analgesic abuse (phenacetin), exposure to chemicals in the workplace such as 2-naphthylamine, paints, oils, gasoline, zinc, and chromium as well as pelvic irradiation, chronic cystitis, and treatment with cyclophosphamide.

○ **Does coffee consumption increase the risk of bladder cancer?**

No.

○ **On which chromosome is the tumor suppressor gene p53 found?**

Chromosome 17.

○ **What is the most common presentation of bladder cancer?**

Gross, painless hematuria. Frequency, urgency, and dysuria can be linked to carcinoma in situ (CIS).

○ **Which method of urinary cytology has the best diagnostic yield: voided or bladder wash?**

It has been estimated that the sensitivity of a single barbotage specimen is equivalent to that of three voided specimens (Matzkin et al., 1992).

○ **What does FISH stand for and how should the test be used?**

Fluorescence **I**n-**S**itu **H**ybridization. It is primarily used for assessing the response to intravesical therapy such as BCG in patients with superficial bladder cancer and to help determine whether or not to use BCG in borderline cases. A positive response after treatment indicates a high risk for recurrence. It is best used as a yearly screen.

○ **What exactly is the FISH detecting and on which chromosomes?**

Aneuploidy of chromosomes 3, 7, and 17, as well as the 9p21 locus.

○ **Of patients who have a positive urovision FISH with a negative cystoscopy and imaging, how many will eventually develop a urothelial tumor?**

Approximately one-third of these cases will lead to an eventual diagnosis of cancer. Instead of a cancer being missed on the diagnostic workup, the likely explanation is that FISH detects precancer DNA mutations that promote tumor development in the future.

○ **How often do synchronous upper tract urothelial tumors coexist when a bladder tumor is diagnosed?**

2.4% of the time.

○ **If a person has a known upper tract disease, what is the risk of developing a bladder tumor?**

30% to 75%.

○ **What are the most predictive factors of disease progression for superficial TCC of the bladder?**

Tumor grade, stage, and the presence of CIS are the most significant prognostic factors. Other risk factors include lymphovascular invasion, tumor size, architecture, multifocality, and frequency of prior tumor recurrences.

○ **What are the most predictive factors of lymph node metastasis for invasive TCC of the bladder?**

Tumor grade and depth of tumor invasion.

○ **What is the current TNM staging system for cancer of the urinary bladder?**

- Ta: Noninvasive papillary carcinoma.
- Tis: Carcinoma in situ.
- T1: Tumor invades lamina propria.
- T2: Tumor invades muscle.
    - T2a: Superficial muscle (inner half).
    - T2b: Deep muscle (outer half).

- T3: Tumor invades perivesical fat.
    T3a: Microscopic invasion.
    T3b: Macroscopic invasion
- T4: Tumor invades adjacent organs.
    T4a: prostate, rectum, uterus, or vagina.
    T4b: pelvic or abdominal wall.

○ **What are the main indications for intravesical therapy after transurethral resection of a bladder tumor?**

High-grade tumor, multiplicity, CIS, positive urinary cytology after resection, and unresectable tumor.

○ **What are the risk factors for systemic side effects from intravesical therapy?**

Anything that increases drug absorption may lead to systemic toxicity. These factors include low molecular weight of the intravesical agent (thiotepa), extensive area of resection, bladder perforation, gross hematuria, urinary tract infection, and instillation close to the time of resection.

○ **What side effects are common to most forms of intravesical therapy?**

Hematuria, cystitis, and irritative voiding symptoms.

○ **Which intravesical agent is most commonly associated with the side effect of myelosuppression?**

Thiotepa, because of its low molecular weight, is easily absorbed and can be associated with myelosuppression.

○ **Which intravesical agent is most often associated with the side effect of contact dermatitis?**

Mitomycin C is caustic to the skin when direct contact is made.

○ **What are common side effects associated with bacillus Calmette–Guerin (BCG)?**

Cystitis, hematuria, fever, sepsis, granulomatous prostatitis, pneumonitis, or hepatitis. Deaths have also been reported from systemic BCGosis.

○ **What is the mechanism of action of BCG?**

The bacillus organism binds to the cell surface through fibronectin binding sites, which activates the immune system.

○ **What is the expected, disease-specific, survival rate for patient with high-grade superficial TCC or CIS at 10 and 15 years?**

70% and 63%, respectively. Overall, in the Herr study, 27% died of other causes, 34% died of bladder cancer, and 37% were alive at 15 years. Only 25% were alive with an intact bladder (Herr et al., 1992).

○ **What is the effect of anticoagulants on BCG therapy?**

Anticlotting drugs inhibit the binding of BCG to fibronectin, thus patients should be off anticoagulants when receiving BCG if at all possible.

○ **What drugs are used to treat BCG infection or overtreatment?**

Isoniazid (INH), rifampin, and ethambutol are the primary therapies. Streptomycin may also be used.

○   **What is the treatment for systemic BCG sepsis?**

Patients with severe voiding symptoms/hematuria and a fever >38.5°C should be hospitalized and started on oral isoniazid 300 mg and rifampin 600 mg a day until symptoms resolve. Patients with hemodynamic changes and persistent high-grade temperature should also receive ethambutol 15 mg/kg/d and possibly prednisone 40 mg/d in addition to isoniazid and rifampin. Isoniazid, rifampin, and ethambutol should be continued for 3 to 6 months. Cycloserine inhibits growth of the bacillus within 24 hours. It is usually used in combination with isoniazid, rifampin, and ethambutol. The major side effect of cycloserine is a lowering of the seizure threshold.

○   **How can the risk of BCG complications be diminished?**

BCG therapy should not be initiated until 2 to 4 weeks after transurethral resection of the bladder tumor (TURBT). If gross hematuria is present or catheterization is traumatic, BCG should be withheld.

○   **What are other immunotherapeutic agents that have been used?**

Keyhole–Limpet hemocyanin (KLH), oral bropirimine, and interferon have also been studied but are not currently first line therapies.

○   **What is the reported response rate to valrubicin in patients who do not respond to BCG?**

21%.

○   **What is the optimal course of intravesical therapy?**

The optimal duration, dosage, and timing of intravesical therapy has yet to be determined and remains under investigation. Patients usually receive a 6-week induction course. Maintenance doses after induction are now more commonly used: 3 weekly instillations at 3 months, 6 months, and every 6 months thereafter.

○   **What are possible indications for partial cystectomy?**

Tumor in a diverticulum or a small (<2 cm) isolated invasive tumor away from the trigone. Total radical cystectomy remains the treatment of choice for most invasive bladder cancers due to high recurrence rates reported following partial cystectomy in patients with muscle invasive disease.

○   **What are the indications for radical cystectomy for superficial disease?**

Recurrent or persistent high-grade disease, carcinoma in situ (CIS), failure of intravesical therapy, refractory hematuria from a large volume tumor, unresectable tumor, or a strong clinical suspicion of understaging.

○   **What degree of clinical understaging is associated with T1 disease?**

Understaging as high as 33% has been reported.

○   **What is the most accepted treatment for muscle invasive bladder cancer?**

Radical cystectomy. Bladder preservation with radiation and chemotherapy can be used for select patients but has not been shown to be better than surgical extirpation.

○   **What are local recurrence rates after radical cystectomy for invasive bladder cancer?**

Ten percent of patients have a local recurrence after radical cystectomy (Soloway et al., 1994).

○ **What are the expected 5-year survival rates for T2, T3, and N1 disease?**

Estimated 5-year survival is 65%, 30%, and 20%, respectively.

○ **What is the urethral recurrence rate following cystoprostatectomy if tumor was present in the prostatic urethra on final pathology? (Stein et al., 2005)**

Urethral recurrence following radical cystoprostatectomy is 5% (urothelium), 12% (ducts), and 18% (stroma) if urethrectomy is not performed.

○ **What is the risk of a urethral recurrence after cystectomy?**

Approximately 10%.

○ **In what percentage of patients is incidental adenocarcinoma of the prostate found at the time of radical cystoprostatectomy?**

Reports in the literature indicate that approximately 28% of patients undergoing radical cystoprostatectomy have incidental adenocarcinoma found in the pathological specimen.

○ **List the common complications associated with ileal conduit urinary diversions.**

Pyelonephritis, stomal stenosis, parastomal hernias, ureterointestinal anastomotic strictures, anastomotic leaks, hyperchloremic metabolic acidosis, and stone formation.

○ **List the common complications associated with orthotopic urinary diversions.**

Pyelonephritis, stomal stenosis, ureterointestinal anastomotic strictures, metabolic abnormalities, reservoir and renal stones, mucous retention, and nocturnal incontinence.

○ **What is the cut-off for renal function for performing orthotopic diversions and why?**

Patients with a serum creatinine greater than 2.5 mg/dL are usually excluded due to the high likelihood of metabolic complications (Korman et al., 1996).

○ **What percentage of patients undergoing continent urinary diversion suffer from metabolic acidosis?**

Metabolic acidosis can occur in up to 50% of patients, often requiring life-long oral alkalinization therapy.

○ **Why is the distal 15 to 20 cm of the ileum commonly spared with the various diversion techniques?**

Vitamin B_{12} (cobalamin) is absorbed in the distal ileum. A B_{12} deficiency can lead to megaloblastic anemia with a mean red blood cell volume (MCV) >100 fL and hypersegmented neutrophils. This type of a deficiency usually takes about 5 years to develop from the time of surgery and results in demyelination injury to the dorsal and lateral columns of the spinal cord.

○ **What is the traditional systemic chemotherapy regimen for metastatic bladder cancer?**

Methotrexate, vinblastine, Adriamycin, and cisplatin (MVAC) is the most commonly used chemotherapeutic regimen for metastatic bladder cancer if the patient is healthy enough to tolerate the side effects of treatment with 50% to 70% response rates reported in the literature. 2-year survival is only 15% to 20%. Taxol-based regimens are currently being studied as a means of decreasing toxicity while hopefully maintaining efficacy and are now being evaluated as second-line chemotherapy.

○ **How has the standard of care changed for the use of systemic chemotherapy for metastatic bladder cancer?**

The combination of gemcitabine (Gemzar) and cisplatin has been shown to have a similar survival outcome with lower toxicity compared to MVAC (Von der Masse et al., 2000). Although the newer treatment regimen is not without side effects (50% neutropenia/thrombocytopenia), its lower toxicity profile has made it the treatment of choice for most centers (Aparico et al., 2005).

○ **What is the most common hematogenous site of bladder cancer metastasis?**

Liver (38%), lung (36%), bone (27%), adrenal (21%), and bowel (13%).

○ **What is the most common site of metastasis overall for bladder cancer?**

Lymph node metastases are the most common (78%), and most frequently involve the obturator lymph nodes (64%).

○ **What is the most common side effect associated with high-dose interferon used as intravesical treatment for refractory superficial TCC?**

A flu-like syndrome occurs in up to 20% of patients. Local symptoms are rare. The expense of high dose intravesical interferon has limited its use as a primary therapy. Complete response rates of 25% to 43% have been reported.

○ **What is the reported 5-year survival rate after treatment with external beam radiation therapy in stage T2-T3 disease?**

20% to 40%.

○ **Which vitamins may have a secondary preventative effect against bladder cancer?**

High doses of vitamins A, B_6, C, and E have been shown to decrease the 5-year recurrence rate of noninvasive urothelial carcinomas by 40%, as compared to a group taking only the recommended daily allowances.

○ **Carcinoma in situ frequently has alterations of what molecular markers?**

P53 and RB.

○ **What is the 3-year mortality rate of untreated muscle invasive transitional cell carcinoma of the bladder?**

Eighty to ninety percent by 3 years.

○ **True or False: The presence of hemorrhagic cystitis correlates with the later development of bladder cancer.**

False. No such correlation exists.

○ **What is MESNA and what is it used for?**

MESNA stands for 2-mercaptoethane sulfonate. It is a chemoprotective agent that is administered during cyclophosphamide or ifosfamide therapy to help reduce the incidence of hemorrhagic cystitis.

○ **What is acrolein?**

Acrolein is the most significant carcinogenic metabolite of cyclophosphamide.

○ **What are the differences between Brunn's nests, cystitis cystica, and cystitis glandularis?**

Brunn's nests are essentially benign urothelial growths in the submucosal layer of the bladder. They are caused by an invagination or invasive growth of the basal layer and are usually considered a normal urothelial variant. Cystitis cystica and cystitis glandularis are variations of von Brunn's nests. Cystitis cystica has a cyst-like appearance with a liquid filling the center of the lesion. Cystitis glandularis occurs when additional glandular metaplasia has occurred and the cells become more columnar.

○ **Is cystitis glandularis considered benign or malignant and what other entities is it associated with?**

It is generally considered benign but may be associated with pelvic lipomatosis and can develop into adenocarcinoma.

○ **What is the most effective intravesical chemotherapy agent for transitional cell carcinoma of the bladder?**

Mitomycin C is the most active intravesical chemotherapy agent. (BCG is technically considered immunotherapy.)

○ **What is the effect of a single intravesical application of chemotherapy after TUR of a Ta T1 bladder tumor?**

With solitary tumors, the reduction in recurrence rate was 39% compared to similar patients who did not get the instillation. Patients with multiple tumors did not see as much benefit.

○ **What is the preferred management of an inadvertent bladder perforation during TUR of a bladder tumor?**

Open repair is associated with a very high rate of extravesical tumor recurrence and should be avoided. Catheterization and/or percutaneous drainage should be employed when possible. Animal studies have suggested that a single immediate low dose (>0.3125 mg/m^2) intraperitoneal instillation of mitomycin C can be helpful.

○ **Does brachytherapy for prostate cancer increase the subsequent risk for bladder cancer and, if so, by how much?**

Radioactive seed implantation (brachytherapy) alone for prostate cancer or with an external radiation therapy boost does not appear to significantly increase the risk of subsequent bladder cancer beyond age matched controls.

○ **How is a Hautmann ileal neobladder created and why is the shape important?**

The Hautmann neobladder is created from a "W" of ileum with each limb approximately 15 cm in length and a 5-cm tail. The bowel is opened on its antimesenteric border and the edges sewn together to create a sphere. The shape is important because a sphere has the largest possible volume with the lowest luminal pressure. For a given vesicle radius and internal pressure, a spherical vessel will have half of the wall pressure of a cylinder (law of Laplace).

○ **What is the purpose of the tail on a Studer neobladder?**

The Studer neobladder has a 15- to 20-cm isoperistaltic limb that acts to carry urine toward the reservoir and theoretically prevent reflux.

○ **What are the risks and benefits of a nonrefluxing anastomosis?**

A nonrefluxing anastomosis is designed to prevent reflux of urine that could lead to high upper tract pressures and pyelonephritis (neither of which is actually prevented). A nonrefluxing type of anastomosis is prone to stricture.

○ **What is fluorescent cystoscopy and how can it improve standard cystoscopy?**

A photoactive porphyrin such as 5-aminolevulinic acid (5-ALA) or hexaminolevulinate (HAL) is instilled into the bladder. The porphyrins accumulate preferentially in neoplastic tissues. A blue light illuminates the areas of high porphyin concentrations, emitting a red fluorescence. Preliminary studies have shown that 25% to 35% more cases of small papillary tumors and CIS are identified as compared to standard cystoscopy. Prospective studies are needed to see if there actually is a lower "recurrence rate" with fluorescence screening because fewer tumors and margins are missed on the initial resection.

○ **At least how many lymph nodes should you remove during a cystoprostatectomy with pelvic lymph node dissection? (Stein et al., 2005)**

More than 15. With lymph node-positive disease, patients who had more than 15 lymph nodes removed, during dissection had 11% 10-year recurrence-free survival advantage compared to patients who had fewer than 15 node resected.

○ **What is the significance of the number of positive lymph nodes on recurrence rate? (Stein et al., 2005)**

<8 positive nodes: 40% 10-year recurrence-free survival versus 10% if less than 8 nodes were positive.

○ **What survival advantage can be gained by the administration of neoadjuvant chemotherapy?**

Fourteen percent survival advantage at 5 years. The South West Oncology Group compared cystectomy alone versus neoadjuvant MVAC and cystectomy, and found a 14% survival advantage at 5 years (Grossman et al., 2003).

○ **Do childhood cancer survivors (non-Hodgkin's lymphoma, retinoblastoma, leukemia, and soft tissue sarcomas) have an increased risk of bladder cancer as adults?**

Yes. Their risk is five times greater than the general population.

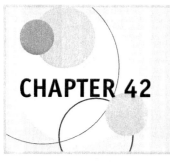

CHAPTER 42

Squamous Cell Carcinoma and Adenocarcinoma of the Bladder

A. Ari Hakimi, MD, and
Reza Ghavamian, MD

○ **Non-transitional cell carcinoma (non-TCC) makes up what percentage of bladder cancers in developed nations?**

Less than 10% of all bladder cancers in developed nations are non-TCC.

○ **Are non-TCCs considered more aggressive or less aggressive than TCC of the bladder?**

Non-TCCs of the bladder typically present at a more advanced stage and setting than TCC and are almost always invasive. The 5-year relative survival of squamous cell carcinoma (SCC) patients is less than half the figure for TCC, while the survival for adenocarcinoma is roughly 25% lower than TCC.

○ **Why is squamous cell carcinoma of the bladder an important public health problem in Egypt?**

In Egypt, where schistosomiasis is endemic, about 80% of squamous cell carcinoma of the bladder are caused by *Schistosoma haematobium.*

○ **Is schistosomiasis only associated with squamous cell carcinoma?**

No, schistosomiasis also increases the incidence of transitional cell carcinoma of the bladder.

○ **Can squamous cell carcinoma coexist with transitional cell carcinoma?**

Yes, transitional epithelium has tremendous metaplastic potential and therefore squamous cell carcinoma elements are also frequently seen with invasive transitional cell carcinoma.

○ **How does SCC of the bladder typically present?**

Most patients have irritative voiding symptoms with or without gross hematuria.

○ **What are the cystoscopic and histological characteristics of SCC of the bladder?**

SCCs of the bladder are almost always solitary lesions and tend to be sessile and ulcerated. They are well differentiated and have a low incidence of lymph node and distant metastases. Bilharzial lesions are less likely to be stage T4 and are usually bulky, nodular, and located in the upper hemisphere of the bladder.

383

○   **What are the proposed risk factors nonbilharzial squamous cell cancers?**

Reported risk factors include African American race, cigarettes smoking, chronic irritation of the bladder mucosa from bladder calculi or long-term indwelling Foley catheters, chronic urinary infectious, bladder diverticula, cyclophosphamide exposure, and intravesical bacillus Calmette–Guerin (BCG).

○   **What is the proposed carcinogenic mechanism?**

This is not completely understood, but could be the result of formation of nitrite and *N*-nitroso compounds that result from parasitic and bacterial metabolism.

○   **What other patients are found to have squamous epithelium in their bladder?**

Vaginal type nonkeratinizing stratified squamous epithelium is commonly found in the trigone of many women and in men receiving estrogen for prostate cancer. These patients should not be diagnosed with squamous metaplasia.

○   **What patient populations are at greatest risk for the development of squamous metaplasia?**

Eighty percent of paraplegic patients are found to have squamous metaplasia of the bladder.

○   **In squamous metaplasia, is keratinization considered a good or bad prognostic sign?**

Keratinization is somewhat ominous because it is more closely associated with carcinoma; 21% progress to malignancy.

○   **What is the name of the above condition?**

Leukoplakia.

○   **How should these patients be followed?**

Patients with biopsy-proven keratinizing squamous metaplasia of the bladder should have periodic (at least yearly) cystoscopy and urine cytology examinations.

○   **What percentage of paraplegic patients with squamous metaplasia will go on to develop squamous cell carcinoma?**

Approximately 5% of paraplegics with squamous metaplasia will go on to develop squamous cell carcinoma and 21% if keratinization is present.

○   **What other patient populations are at risk for squamous cell carcinoma of the bladder?**

These tumors account for approximately 20% of bladder cancers arising within bladder diverticula, 50% occur in patients with nonfunctioning bladders and also account for 15% of bladder cancers in patients who have had renal transplants.

○   **How does nonbilharzial squamous cell carcinoma differ from bilharzial squamous cell carcinoma of the bladder?**

In bilharzial squamous cell carcinoma, the tumors are usually well differentiated with a low incidence of lymph node or distant metastases. In nonbilharzial squamous cell carcinoma of the bladder seen in the United States, the tumors tend to be poorly differentiated and advanced at diagnosis so the patients tend to have a poorer prognosis.

○ **What is the role of chemotherapy and radiation in the treatment of squamous cell carcinoma of the bladder?**

Chemotherapy has not been very effective in the treatment of squamous cell carcinoma of the bladder. In addition, transurethral resection, partial cystectomy, and radiation therapy alone have not been effective.

○ **What has been shown to be the most effective treatment against squamous cell carcinoma of the bladder?**

The most effective treatment at this time is radical cystectomy with pelvic lymph node dissection. The role of preoperative radiation is not well defined and there are currently no large studies to prove its survival advantage.

○ **What percentage of patients with squamous cell carcinoma of the bladder are found to have involvement of their urethra?**

Approximately 50% of patients are found to have urethral involvement; therefore, it has been suggested that urethrectomy should be routinely performed in all patients undergoing a cystectomy.

○ **What is the prognosis of squamous cell carcinoma of the bladder?**

Stage for staging the prognosis is equivalent to transitional cell carcinoma of the bladder. A recent study from Egypt placed the 5-year survival at 50% for bilharzial cancers compared to 39% for nonbilharzial tumors.

○ **What percent of primary bladder cancers are adenocarcinomas?**

Adenocarcinoma of the bladder accounts for less than 2% of primary bladder cancers in Western countries but up to 10% of bladder cancers in nations with endemic schistosomiasis.

○ **What are the different classifications of bladder adenocarcinoma?**

Bladder adenocarcinomas can be classified as primary vesical, urachal, and metastatic. Urachal carcinomas represent approximately one-third of primary bladder adenocarcinomas.

○ **What are the different cell types of primary vesical adenocarcinoma?**

In one large series, vesical adenocarcinomas were mucinous (23.6%), enteric (19.4%), signet-ring cell (16.7%), mixed (12.5%), or not otherwise specified (27.8%).

○ **What are the histologic features?**

There is a predominantly glandular pattern, but in poorly differentiated tumors, areas of solid growth are evident. The glands resemble intestinal adenocarcinoma of typical or colloid type. The epithelial lining can have a mucinous character. Eight percent of the tumors can have papillary features.

○ **What is linitis plastica of the bladder?**

This is primary vesical adenocarcinoma of the signet-ring cell type. It accounts for 3% to 5% of primary adenocarcinomas of the bladder. It can present with a diffusely thickened bladder wall on imaging studies, especially computed tomography or ultrasonography. Sheets of tumor cells, fibrosis, and mural thickening typical of linitis plastica of the stomach is characteristic of these tumors and they are generally associated with a worse prognosis.

○ **Which patient populations are at increased risk for bladder adenocarcinomas?**

Patients with intestinal urinary conduits, augmentations, pouches, and ureterosigmoidostomies are at increased risk. Adenocarcinoma is also the most common type of cancer in bladder extrophy.

○   **With what premalignant lesion in the bladder is adenocarcinoma associated?**

Adenocarcinomas of the bladder are most often associated with cystitis glandularis.

○   **What treatment offers the best chance for cure in patients with primary adenocarcinoma of the bladder?**

Radical cystectomy with a bilateral pelvic lymph node dissection offers the best chance of cure for localized adenocarcinoma of the bladder. Retrospective analysis of bilharzial adenocarcinoma indicates that adjuvant radiation may improve survival, but no such data exist in the nonbilharzial setting.

○   **What is the prognosis for bladder adenocarcinomas?**

There is no concrete evidence to suggest that adenocarcinoma of the bladder carries a worse prognosis stage for stage than transitional cell carcinoma. However, they are generally thought to be associated with a poor prognosis because 60% to 65% are stage T3-4 at diagnosis. Of the different cell types, signet-ring cell carcinoma is more undifferentiated and hence carries the worst prognosis.

○   **What is the incidence of urachal carcinoma?**

0.35% to 0.7%, with predilection for males (72%–80% of the cases).

○   **The majority of urachal tumors are of which cell type?**

Urachal tumors are usually adenocarcinomas; however, primary squamous cell carcinoma, transitional cell carcinoma, and even rarely sarcomas of the urachus have been described.

○   **How do urachal tumors present?**

Urachal tumors may present with a bloody or mucoid discharge from the umbilicus. Urachal tumors may also produce a mucocele, which occurs as a midline infraumbilical palpable abdominal mass. Fifteen percent of urachal tumors do not produce mucin.

○   **What are the other presenting symptoms?**

Tumors invading the bladder lumen can produce mucus in the urine. This happens in only 15% to 33% of cases. Tumors that complicate extrophy are remarkable primarily for their presence on the anterior abdominal wall. Other symptoms include dysuria and frequency, lower abdominal pain.

○   **What is the most common finding on radiography?**

Sixty percent of urachal tumors have areas of low attenuation on CT, which is reflective of the tumor's high mucin content.

○   **What is essential in the diagnosis of urachal carcinomas?**

Cystoscopy and transurethral biopsy is essential for tumor location assessment and tissue diagnosis. Usually cystitis, cystica/glandularis, and dysplasia are absent.

○   **What other neoplastic processes can mimic urachal carcinoma?**

Metastatic prostate, colonic, ovarian, and endometrial carcinoma all have the potential to locally invade the bladder. Therefore, tissue diagnosis is important.

○ **What is the prognosis of primary urachal adenocarcinomas?**

These tumors usually portend a worse prognosis than primary vesical adenocarcinomas. Patients with predominantly mucin histology have a 79% 5-year survival. Patients with papillary, tubular, or signet-ring cells had a 33% 5-year survival based on one study.

○ **What is the overall 5-year survival?**

43% to 50%.

○ **How should urachal tumors be treated?**

Radical cystectomy with an en-bloc excision of the urachus is the treatment of choice in patients with large tumors as histologically these tumors exhibit wider and deeper infiltration of the bladder wall. However, for small localized tumors at the bladder dome, partial cystectomy with complete removal of the urachal ligament and umbilicus is acceptable. Extended partial cystectomy has been shown to be the treatment of choice as survival is related to the stage at presentation rather than extent of surgical resection.

○ **Are urachal tumors sensitive to radiation or chemotherapy therapy?**

Urachal tumors are usually unresponsive to chemotherapy, and radiation therapy is also ineffective. However, the MD Anderson group reported a 33% response rate using 5-fluorouracil, leucovorin, and cisplatin, with or without gemcitabine.

○ **Where are the common metastatic sites for urachal adenocarcinomas?**

Urachal tumors can metastasize to the iliac and inguinal nodes as well as the omentum, liver, lung, and bones.

○ **What are the more common primary sites for adenocarcinomas metastatic to the bladder?**

Rectum, stomach, endometrium, breast, prostate, and ovary.

○ **Are any additional investigations necessary once a diagnosis of adenocarcinoma of the bladder is established?**

Patients should be evaluated for a possible source of a primary adenocarcinoma site. This includes computed tomography of the abdomen and pelvis, barium enema, and colonoscopy when the index of suspicion is high and in patients in whom linitis plastica of the bladder is diagnosed, upper endoscopy to rule out a stomach primary is indicated.

CHAPTER 43 Urethral Lesions

Benjamin N. Breyer, MD, and
Badrinath Konety, MD, MBA, FACS

○ **From distal to proximal, what are the anatomic names of the urethral segments?**

- Fossa navicularis-granular urethra.
- Penile-pendulous urethra.
- Bulbous urethra.
- Membranous urethra.
- Prostatic urethra.

○ **Describe the different types of epithelia lining the male urethra.**

The prostatic and membranous urethra are lined with transitional epithelium, the bulbar urethra is lined with squamous epithelium, and the glanular portion of the urethra is lined by stratified squamous epithelium.

○ **What is the average length of the male urethra?**

The average length of the male urethra is 21 cm.

○ **What is the lacuna magna?**

The dorsal expansion of the fossa navicularis in the glans penis is called the lacuna magna.

○ **What portion of the urethra do Cowper's glands and the glands of Littre open into?**

Cowper's glands open into the membranous urethra, while the glands of Littre open into the dorsal urethra.

○ **What is the specific feature of the male urethral blood supply which is advantageous in planning urethral reconstructive surgery?**

The male urethra has a dual blood supply—proximally from the bulbar artery, a branch of the internal pudendal artery, and distally from the dorsal artery of the penis, which is a terminal branch of the pudendal artery. This fact allows for complete excision of diseased segments of the urethra during urethral reconstruction.

○   **What is the name of the deep penile fascia and its attachments?**

Buck's fascia surrounds the corpus spongiosum and corpora cavernosa. Distally, Buck's fascia is connected to the undersurface of the glans at the corona. Proximally, Buck's fascia encloses each crus of the corpora cavernosa and the bulb of the corpus spongiosum.

○   **When Buck's fascia remains intact after injury to the anterior urethra, what is the expected appearance?**

Typically, if Buck's fascia remains intact, bruising, hematoma, and swelling will be confined to the penis.

○   **What is the name of the superficial penile fascia and its attachments?**

Colles' fascia of the perineum attaches laterally to the fascia lata of the thigh, the ischia, and the inferior rami of the pubis. Anteriorly, Colles' fascia is continuous with the Dartos layer of the scrotum and Scarpa's fascia on the anterior abdominal wall.

○   **How do injuries that violate Buck's fascia and leave Colles' fascia intact appear?**

A butterfly or saddle perineal appearance of a hematoma may be present. In addition, a scrotal hematoma and bruising on the anterior abdominal wall to the level of the clavicles is possible.

○   **What are the most common sites of iatrogenic urethral injury?**

The penoscrotal junction and the external urethral meatus are the most common sites of iatrogenic urethral injury.

○   **What is the incidence of urethral injury following pelvic fractures?**

Approximately 10% of pelvic fractures are accompanied by urethral injury, whereas a majority of patients with urethral injury will have pelvic fractures. Approximately 10% of patients with posterior urethral injury will also have an accompanying bladder rupture.

○   **What is the most common cause of external urethral meatal stenosis requiring surgical repair?**

Balanitis xerotica obliterans is the most common cause of meatal stenosis requiring surgical repair.

○   **What is the proper technique for obtaining a retrograde urethrogram (RUG)?**

A retrograde urethrogram is obtained by positioning the patient obliquely at 45 degrees, with the bottom leg flexed 90 degrees at the knee and the top leg kept straight. A 12F Foley catheter is introduced into the fossa navicularis, the balloon inflated with 2 mL saline to prevent dislodgement, the penis placed on gentle traction, and 20 to 30 mL of undiluted water-soluble contrast material is injected with the film exposed while injecting.

○   **How do blunt injuries to the urethra occur?**

Blunt urethral injuries typically result from straddle-type trauma incurred after forceful contact of the perineum with a blunt object. Any focused external force, as encountered in falls and vehicular accidents, can crush the immobile bulbous urethra against the inferior pubic symphysis.

○ **A 40-year-old male presents after a motorcycle crash with blood at his meatus. What is the next step in his urinary tract evaluation?**

Blood at the meatus is seen in at least 75% of patients after external anterior urethral trauma. No urethral instrumentation should be undertaken until a proper retrograde urethrogram is obtained if meatal blood is present or suspicion of urethral injury exists. If the urethra is in continuity or only partially disrupted, an attempt at placing a well-lubricated Foley catheter should be made.

○ **What other radiologic methods other than a retrograde urethrogram can be employed in evaluating urethral injuries?**

Urethral strictures resulting from urethral trauma can also be evaluated by a sonographic urethrogram. A sonographic urethrogram allows determination of the extent of periurethral fibrosis, spongiofibrosis, and luminal size. This is important because in the case of most urethral strictures, subepithelial spongiofibrosis extends well beyond the grossly identifiable stricture area. MRI can be useful in the evaluation of posterior urethral disruptions.

○ **What is the main continence mechanism in men with complete urethral disruption?**

The bladder neck constitutes the main continence mechanism in men with complete urethral disruption.

○ **What are the two main principles to be kept in mind during the excision and reanastomosis of urethral strictures?**

Excision and reanastomosis should be avoided in pendulous urethral strictures because it can result in shortening of the penile urethra and chordee. A similar situation can result if >2 cm of bulbar urethra is excised.

○ **What are the most common indications for two-stage urethral reconstruction?**

The most common indications prompting a two-stage urethral reconstruction are: an extremely long or full-length urethral stricture, multiple strictures, presence of urethrocutaneous fistula, periurethral inflammation, or extensive local scarring.

○ **What are the principal advantages and disadvantages of immediate primary urethral reanastomosis versus delayed primary reanastomosis?**

Immediate primary urethral reanastomosis results in a low rate of urethral stricture formation but is accompanied by a high rate of complications such as impotence and incontinence. Delayed primary repair results in higher urethral stricture rates but the impotence and incontinence rates are considerably lower. Early endoscopic realignment with delayed primary repair combines the two approaches and has been found to yield lower stricture rates while reducing complication rates in small series of patients.

○ **A 38-year-old male accidentally discharges his handgun while carrying it under his belt. He has a large gash in his penile urethra. How should this be managed?**

Immediate repair is indicated. A tension-free, watertight closure with absorbable sutures should be employed over a Foley catheter.

○ **Which is the only genitourinary malignancy more common in women?**

Urethral carcinoma is the only genitourinary malignancy more common in women. Squamous cell carcinoma is the most common histologic type in both sexes, followed by transitional cell carcinoma.

○   **What are the most common risk factors for urethral carcinoma in men and women?**

The risk factors are as follows: urethral strictures, venereal disease, transitional cell carcinoma of the bladder, human papilloma virus (HPV) subtypes 16 and 18 infections. In women, urethral diverticula can also constitute a risk factor for urethral carcinoma. Biopsies should be done on all unusual appearing strictures, especially if they appear erythematous.

○   **What are some common symptoms of urethral carcinoma?**

Frequently similar to those of benign voiding dysfunction. The onset is typically insidious. General lower urinary tract symptoms such as frequency, hesitancy, and nocturia, obstructive voiding symptoms such as straining and weakened stream incontinence secondary to retention and urinary overflow, hematuria, purulent, necrotic watery discharge, urethral or perineal pain, and swelling.

○   **What are some common physical examination findings of urethral carcinoma?**

Palpable mass on the ventral surface of penis or the perineum, periurethral abscess, urethral diverticula, and urethral-cutaneous and urethral-vaginal fistulas.

○   **What is the key pathologic feature that determines the need for a urethrectomy along with a radical cystoprostatectomy in patients with transitional cell carcinoma of the bladder?**

Presence of transitional cell carcinoma invading the prostatic stroma on urethral biopsy necessitates a urethrectomy along with cystoprostatectomy in cases of transitional cell carcinoma of the bladder. Urethrectomy is not considered mandatory in cases with carcinoma in situ of the urethra or tumor invasion into the prostatic ducts and acini without stromal encroachment. In cases where urethrectomy is not deemed necessary, involvement of the prostatic urethral margin dictates the need for urethrectomy which is usually performed within 2 months following the cystoprostatectomy.

○   **How is male urethral cancer treated?**

Surgery is the main treatment. Low-stage urethral carcinoma, especially if located in the anterior urethra, is treated with local resection or Nd:YAG laser fulguration. More extensive disease requires wider resection with partial penectomy, total penectomy, or en-bloc resection. There is no demonstrated benefit to prophylactic lymphadenectomy in these patients. Radiation and chemotherapy can be useful additions in advanced cases for palliation.

○   **What is the most common site of malignant melanoma in the genitourinary tract?**

The urethra is the most common site of malignant melanoma in the urinary tract. It is most often located at the fossa navicularis in men. It most often occurs in individuals in their sixties to eighties, survival is poor and dissemination can occur by direct extension, lymphatic, or hematogenous spread.

○   **What is commonly believed to be the site of origin of urethral adenocarcinoma in men?**

Cowper's glands are commonly believed to be the site of origin of urethral adenocarcinoma in men.

○   **What is the most common histologic type of cancer occurring in a urethral diverticulum in women?**

Adenocarcinomas are the most common histologic type of tumor that occur in urethral diverticula in women.

○ **What is the Grabstald classification of urethral tumors in women?**

According to the Grabstald classification, female urethral tumors are classified as involving the anterior (external meatus and distal one-third) or entire (posterior two-thirds may extend to anterior) urethra. However, survival from urethral carcinoma is only dependent upon stage at diagnosis and tumor size with location having no impact.

○ **What is the American Joint Committee on Cancer Tumor Node Metastasis (TMN) staging system for urethral cancer?**
 • Primary tumor (T) (men and women):
   Tx: Primary tumor cannot be assessed.
   T0: No evidence of primary tumor.
   Ta: Noninvasive papillary, polypoid, or verrucous carcinoma.
   Tis: Carcinoma in situ.
   T1: Tumor invading subepithelial connective tissue.
   T2: Tumor invading any of the following: corpus spongiosum, prostate, periurethral muscle.
   T3: Tumor invading any of the following: corpus cavernosum, beyond prostate capsule, anterior vagina, bladder neck.
   T4: Tumor invades other adjacent organs.
 • Regional lymph nodes (N):
   Nx: Regional nodes cannot be assessed.
   N0: No regional lymph node metastasis.
   N1: Metastasis in a single lymph node, 2 cm or less in greatest dimension.
   N2: Metastasis in a single lymph node, larger than 2 cm in greatest dimension, or in multiple lymph nodes.
 • Distant metastases (M):
   Mx: Distant metastasis cannot be assessed.
   M0: No distant metastasis.
   M1: Distant metastasis.

○ **What is the prognosis for urethral cancer?**

Anterior lesions have a better prognosis, probably because penectomy offers a better opportunity for a wide surgical margin. Five-year survival for anterior urethral cancer is approximately 50%, while posterior cancers have only a 10% to 15% 5-year survival rate.

○ **What are the principles of management of female urethral carcinoma?**

Early-stage female urethral carcinoma can be managed with laser fulguration or radiation. Invasive tumors require local resection with or without neoadjuvant radiation therapy. Combined external beam and interstitial radiation therapy have been used for palliation.

○ **How many female patients with urethral cancer present with metastases at presentation?**
Approximately 14%.

○ **What are the demographic patterns of gonococcal and non-gonococcal urethritis (NGU)?**

Gonococcal urethritis caused by the gram-negative diplococcus *Neisseria gonorrhoeae* occurs more commonly in adolescent inner city males with a large incidence in African Americans. NGU, one of the major causes of which is *Chlamydia trachomatis*, is commonly found in educated Caucasians of higher socioeconomic class including students.

○ **Who are the carriers of *N. gonorrhoeae*?**

Both sexes can be asymptomatic carriers of *N. gonorrhoeae* and symptomatic infections can also occur in both sexes. Humans are the sole host for this organism.

○ **What are the criteria for diagnosing NGU?**

The presence of inflammatory cells on a urethral smear in the absence of *N. gonorrhoeae* suggests a diagnosis of NGU. Presence of significant inflammation is indicated by the presence of >4 neutrophils/oil immersion field (400×).

○ **What is the optimal means of documenting infection by *C. trachomatis*?**

C. trachomatis infection is best confirmed by culturing the organism from urethral swabs or staining with fluorescein conjugated antichlamydial monoclonal antibodies.

○ **What associations between gonococcal urethritis and NGU should be considered when evaluating patients with gonococcal urethritis?**

Forty-five percent of patients with gonococcal urethritis will have concomitant infection with *C. trachomatis*. Hence, all such patients should be treated for both infections simultaneously.

○ **What are the standard therapeutic antibiotic regimens used to treat gonococcal urethritis and NGU?**

- Gonococcal urethritis—single dose ofloxacin (400 mg po), ciprofloxacin (500 mg po), cefixime (400 mg po), or ceftriaxone (250 mg IM). Spectinomycin 2 g IM can also be used.
- NGU—Azithromycin single dose (2 g po), doxycycline 7 days (100 mg po bid), erythromycin or tetracycline 7 days (500 mg po qid), ofloxacin 7 days (300 mg po bid). Ciprofloxacin is not effective in treating *C. trachomatis* infections. Partners though asymptomatic should be treated since 33% of them will be carriers.

○ **What are other organisms commonly implicated in NGU?**

Ureaplasma urealyticum, Trichomonas vaginalis, Herpes simplex virus (HSV) types I and II, and Human papilloma virus (HPV) are other commonly implicated organisms.

○ **What are the best methods to establish infection with HSV and HPV?**

HSV infection can be established by viral culture, while HPV infection can best be established by testing for the presence of viral DNA.

○ **What are the standard therapeutic regimens used in the management of NGU caused by organisms other than *C. trachomatis*?**

Ureaplasma urealyticum responds to treatment with erythromycin and tetracycline (500 mg po q.i.d. for 7 days). *Trichomonas* is treated with metronidazole (250 mg po t.i.d. for 7 days). Partners though asymptomatic should also be treated since they could be carriers. HSV infections can respond to topical or oral acyclovir (for primary or recurrent episodes). HPV infections are treated with topical podophyllin, 5-Fluorouracil, cryotherapy, laser fulguration, electrocautery, or surgical excision.

○ **What are the common complications ensuing from urethritis?**

Epididymitis—*C. trachomatis* is the most common organism responsible for epididymitis in younger men. Urethral strictures can occur as a consequence of both gonococcal urethritis and NGU. Disseminated gonococcal infections with septic arthritis, tenosynovitis occur more commonly in pregnant women. NGU is associated with Reiter's syndrome of uveitis and arthritis. It is the most common cause of peripheral arthritis in young men.

○ **What is the incidence of gonococcal resistance to tetracycline?**

Five to fifteen percent and increasing.

○ **Can probenecid and penicillin still be used for gonorrhea?**

Currently, resistance to this combination therapy from the past is too high, so other regimens are preferred.

○ **What is the recommended therapy for recurrent chlamydial urethritis?**

Prolonged 14- to 28-day course of erythromycin.

○ **Urethral prolapse most frequently occurs in which patient population?**

Urethral prolapse occurs almost exclusively in African American girls between ages 1 and 9 years.

○ **What is believed to be the pathophysiology of urethral prolapse?**

Urethral prolapse is thought to occur during episodes of increased abdominal pressure in a urethra, where there is poor attachment of the smooth muscle layers. The cleavage plane is usually between the inner circular and outer longitudinal muscle layers.

○ **What is the standard therapeutic management of urethral prolapse?**

Standard therapy for urethral prolapse entails topical application of estrogen cream and sitz baths. Formal surgical excision may be required if the prolapse is persistent.

○ **What is the pathophysiologic mechanism resulting in acquired urethral diverticula?**

Acquired urethral diverticula result from infected and obstructed periurethral glands that rupture into the urethral lumen.

○ **What are the tumors that have been found in urethral diverticula?**

Urethral adenocarcinoma, transitional cell carcinoma, squamous cell carcinoma, and nephrogenic adenoma are the tumors that have been found in urethral diverticula. Of these, adenocarcinoma is the most common.

○ **What are the three Ds of symptoms that are characteristic of urethral diverticula?**

Dysuria, postvoid **D**ribbling, and **D**yspareunia are the symptoms characteristic of urethral diverticula.

○ **What is the diagnostic study to demonstrate the presence of a urethral diverticulum?**

Many believe MRI is the imaging modality of choice. While 100% sensitive, an MRI is expensive. A retrograde urethrogram with a double balloon catheter or voiding cystourethrogram can also be employed.

○   **What are the surgical principles employed to treat a urethral diverticulum?**

In the setting of small distal diverticulum, some may be simply marsupialized. For more proximal or larger lesions, complete excision is required. The urethral defect should be closed without tension with multiple layers utilizing the periurethral fascia and vaginal wall flaps. A Martius flap of labial fat maybe interspersed between suture lines to help prevent fistula formation.

○   **What is circinate balanitis?**

Circinate balanitis manifests as a shallow ulcer on the glans penis. It is painless, has gray borders, and is typically associated with Reiter's syndrome.

○   **What is the difference between senile urethritis and a urethral caruncle?**

Both are benign conditions occurring in postmenopausal women, with the former being more common. Senile urethritis results in eversion of the external urethral meatus due to shortening of the vagina. It can be mistaken for a urethral caruncle and responds to estrogen replacement therapy. Urethral caruncle is a red, friable mass located on the posterior lip of the external urethral meatus. It is composed of connective tissue, blood vessels, and inflammatory cells. It may require local excision.

○   **What is commonly believed to be the cause of congenital urethral strictures?**

Incomplete rupture of the cloacal membrane is believed to result in congenital urethral strictures.

CHAPTER 44

Diagnosis and Staging of Prostate Cancer

David A. Levy, MD

○ **What are the current recommendations for screening for prostate cancer in American men?**

To date, there is no consensus on screening for prostate cancer in American men. The American Urological Association currently recommends initiating screening at age 50 for white men with no family history of prostate cancer and age 45 for black men with no family history of the disease. In men with a first-degree relative with the disease, initiation of screening should begin at age 45 for whites and at age 40 for blacks.

○ **What is considered a "normal" PSA?**

Normal PSA ranges have been determined to be 0 to 4 ng/mL. Age-specific normal reference ranges and acceptable rates of change in the PSA value over time (PSA velocity) have been delineated and may enhance the identification of individuals at risk for the disease.

○ **What are the age-specific normal reference ranges for PSA?**

- For men aged 40 to 49 years, the normal reference range is 0 to 2.5 ng/mL.
- For men aged 50 to 59 years, the normal reference range is 0 to 3.5 ng/mL.
- For men aged 60 to 69 years, the normal reference range is 0 to 4-5 ng/mL.
- For men aged 70 to 79 years, the normal reference range is 0 to 6.5 ng/mL.

○ **So which is better, the normal range or the age-specific range?**

It isn't yet clear exactly what the optimal range should be. If the criteria are too strict, curable cancers will not be detected. If too liberal, too many unnecessary biopsies will be done. While the 0 to 4.0 range has proved very effective, age-related adjustments seem reasonable. For age 65 and above, a PSA range of 0 to 4.0 can be used, and for age 64 and younger, a PSA range of 0 to 2.5 has been suggested.

○ **What is the current suggested PSA cutoff level for men aging 65 years and younger being screened for prostate cancer?**

2.5 is the current threshold level for men 65 years of age and younger.

○ **What percentage of the cancers detected in prostate screenings are estimated to be clinically insignificant?**

Less than 7%.

○ **At what point should routine prostate cancer screenings (digital rectal examinations and PSA determinations) be stopped?**

The consensus opinion is that there is a declining benefit of treatment of screening detected prostate cancer with advancing age and that men with less than a 10-year life expectancy, usually age 75, should probably not undergo routine prostate cancer or PSA screenings.

○ **What is the normal function of PSA?**

PSA is a protease whose normal function is to help liquify the semen. It has no other known function.

○ **When was PSA approved for prostate cancer screening by the FDA?**

1986.

○ **What percentage of prostate cancers are found in men with "normal" PSA levels?**

Approximately 20%.

○ **What is PSA velocity?**

PSA velocity is the rate of change of serum PSA over time. Studies have indicated that the acceptable rate of change in PSA over 12 months is <0.75 ng/mL or approximately 25%. Changes that exceed this rate are considered abnormal and should be carefully considered by the interpreting physician. An individual should have several PSA determinations over time intervals to provide for correct interpretation.

○ **What types of events can adversely affect PSA results?**

A number of factors will affect the accuracy of PSA results. A vigorous digital rectal examination, urinary retention, passage of a Foley catheter, acute prostatitis, recent prostate biopsy, and any maneuver that "manipulates" the gland will falsely elevate the PSA. Interpretation of serum PSA results following any of these events should be delayed for 21 days to allow sufficient time for resolution of the false elevation of the PSA.

○ **What is the serum half-life of PSA?**

Published reports have documented the serum half-life of PSA to be 2.2 ± 0.8 days and 3.3 ± 0.1 days depending upon the testing method used. Based on these data, one should wait at least 21 days following manipulation of the gland to allow for a sufficient number of half-lives to yield a reliable result before drawing a serum PSA.

○ **What is free PSA and what is the significance of free PSA?**

PSA is a glycoprotein produced by the prostatic epithelial cells and once in the serum approximately 40% is bound to α_2-macroglobulin and is unmeasureable. The remaining fraction of PSA is bound to α_1-antichymotrypsin or circulates free in the serum and both are measurable by commercial techniques. Conclusive studies have indicated that individuals with prostate cancer tend to have a lower percent free PSA, and cut off limits have been assigned to this value. A free PSA less than 25% is considered to be a prognostic factor for prostate cancer. Levels of 10% or less are associated with a 50% incidence of prostate cancer.

○ **Can free PSA be used to assess the relative risk for carcinoma of the prostate in all men?**

No. The utility of free PSA is restricted to men with a total PSA between 4 and 10 ng/mL. There have been no definitive studies that indicate an application of free PSA to individuals with a total PSA less than 4 ng/mL. If the total PSA is less than 4.0 ng/mL, one may employ the age-specific reference ranges for PSA and PSA velocity to better assess an individual's risk for disease.

○ **Can the serum PSA level reliably predict pathological stage?**

No. The serum PSA level alone cannot be used to reliably predict the pathological stage of disease. Approximately 70% to 80% of patients with locally advanced prostate cancer have a serum PSA levels >10 ng/mL. The Gleason biopsy score may have more predictive value in predicting the extent of disease.

○ **You are sent an individual with an elevated PSA for evaluation. He has no symptoms or clinical findings suggesting BPH, LUTS, or prostatitis. What should be your next step?**

Rather than rush directly into a prostate biopsy, consider the patients age, general state of health, medications, and state of mind. If he is anxious about prostate cancer and demands a biopsy, it may be best to do so for his anxiety. For most patients, it is often best to repeat the PSA level after a 30-day course of antibiotics. A decision about a possible biopsy can be made at that time. In many cases, the PSA returns to baseline avoiding a potentially painful biopsy.

○ **A 54-year-old man with an enlarged prostate on rectal examination has a serum PSA of 3.6 ng/mL and a free PSA of 45%. There is no family history of prostate cancer. How would you counsel him about his risk for prostate cancer?**

Autopsy studies from 1954 indicate that the overall risk for prostate cancer in 50-year-old men is 30%. This individual has BPH by examination and although his free PSA is over 25%, which is consistent with the diagnosis of BPH, his total PSA is less than 4.0 ng/mL and therefore the free PSA may not have much bearing. This patient's current risk for indolent disease should parallel the age-matched general population. A reasonable course of follow-up may consist of serial PSA measurements to track his PSA velocity.

○ **What is the role for digital rectal examination (DRE) in assessing patients at risk for prostate cancer?**

Data reported in the literature indicate that DRE alone detects less than 1.7% of all diagnosed prostate cancers even when there is a high index of suspicion of glandular abnormalities. However, DRE does provide useful information about the size and potential resectability of the prostate in individuals with prostate pathology. It may also detect asymmetry that could suggest a tumor.

○ **What is the accuracy of clinical staging based on DRE?**

The accuracy of DRE alone in men with palpable lesions approximates 50% and of those individuals diagnosed by this modality alone more than 70% will be upstaged at the time of pathological examination.

○ **What is the best role for DRE in assessing patients at risk for prostate cancer?**

DRE is utilized best in combination with PSA determination and transrectal ultrasound-guided biopsies. This combination provides for the most efficient means of evaluating men at risk for prostate cancer.

○ **Can ultrasound reliably diagnose prostate cancer?**

No. Numerous published studies have indicated the absence of a pathognomonic appearance of prostate cancer on ultrasound. Although a higher percentage of cancers are hypoechoic, prostate cancer can also be hyperechoic or isoechoic on transrectal ultrasound imaging.

○ **What is the role for ultrasound in diagnosing prostate cancer?**

Ultrasound is a very useful adjunct in diagnosing prostate cancer and has its greatest utility in directing the biopsy needle to particular areas of the prostate gland.

○ **When performing transrectal needle biopsy of the prostate, how many biopsies should be done?**

Historically, six cores were thought to represent a reasonable sampling of the gland with the cores including left- and right-sided biopsies from the base, mid, and apical portions of the gland. Reports in the literature over the years have indicated that six cores may be insufficient and performing 12 biopsies has now become the norm with the biopsies being more laterally located and adding medial apical biopsies in lieu of transitional zone biopsies. Recent publications indicate the lack of sufficient benefit and efficacy of saturation biopsy at the initial biopsy setting although this may be useful as a secondary measure in select cases.

○ **Is the biopsy result indicative of overall disease burden?**

Yes. There have been a number of studies that indicate that the biopsy result has prognostic information about overall disease burden. The Gleason score of the biopsy specimen is the most important prognostic factor for capsular extension of disease. Additionally, the percent of core involved and the number of cores involved can give predictive information for capsular extension and lymph node involvement.

○ **What is the strongest prognostic factor for prostate cancer–related death?**

The biopsy Gleason score has consistently been shown to be a significant prognostic factor for cancer-related death in individuals diagnosed with the disease. To date, there have been no reliable prognostic data reported for preoperative PSA results or free PSA results.

○ **What agents are being studied for their potential use in the prevention of prostate cancer and their proposed mechanisms?**

- Dutasteride (Avodart) inhibits both type 1 and type 2 forms of 5-alpha-reductase.
- Vitamin D induces cell-cycle arrest and has an antiproliferative effect on prostate cancer cells.
- Cox-2 inhibitors selectively block prostaglandin production and may reduce expression of several androgen-inducible genes.
- Lycopenes are antioxidants that may inhibit prostate cancer cell growth.
- Green tea–derived polyphenols induce apoptosis, inhibit cell growth, and dysregulate the cell cycle.
- Selenium inhibits cell proliferation and induces apoptosis. Vitamin E has shown direct antiandrogen activity.

○ **A 64-year-old man with a normal digital rectal examination undergoes a transrectal needle biopsy of the prostate for a PSA of 4.9 ng/mL. One out of eight cores, the left base, is positive for Gleason's 3 + 3 adenocarcinoma. What is his clinical stage?**

One of the more commonly used staging systems is that outlined by the American Joint Commission on Cancer (AJCC). Based on this staging system, this individual would be classified as having T1c disease, i.e., tumor identified by needle biopsy.

○ **The patient in the previous question underwent a radical retropubic prostatectomy. The pathology report revealed disease involving the entire left side of the gland with no capsular penetration. The lymph nodes were negative. What is his pathologic stage?**

Using AJCC criteria, disease confined by the capsule and involving more than one half of the lobe but not more than one lobe with negative lymph nodes is classified as pT2b, N0, M0 disease.

○ **A 58-year-old man underwent a radical perineal prostatectomy for unilateral Gleason's 3 + 4 in 1 out of 8 core biopsies. His PSA was 4.3 ng/mL. The pathology specimen showed disease involving both sides of the gland with capsular penetration at the left apex. What is his stage?**

AJCC criteria support a diagnosis of pT3a, Nx, M0 in this individual. A pelvic lymph node dissection was not done and therefore one cannot assess the status of the lymph nodes.

○ **A 69-year-old man underwent a radical retropubic prostatectomy and the pathology report revealed disease on both sides of the gland with extension through the capsule bilaterally and 0 out of 13 lymph nodes involved. What is his pathologic stage?**

Based on the AJCC criteria, the correct diagnosis is pT3a, N0, M0 disease.

○ **A 63-year-old man whose father had prostate cancer has a total PSA of 11.8 ng/mL and a free PSA of 11%. A transrectal ultrasound-guided needle biopsy of his prostate revealed no evidence of cancer in eight cores. What is a reasonable approach to his management?**

This individual certainly is at high risk for having prostate cancer and probably warrants a repeat biopsy. One could consider doing more extensive biopsies including biopsies of the transitional zone and far lateral peripheral zone biopsies. Mapping biopsies done under anesthesia and often numbering as high as 15 or more cores in which the gland is more thoroughly sampled may be helpful.

○ **A 78-year-old healthy asymptomatic man presents with a PSA of 8 ng/mL and a free PSA of 20%. He has no voiding symptoms, minimal nocturia, and no history of past GU problems. On physical examination, his prostate is enlarged, asymmetric but not clinically suspicious. What is the next best course of action?**

This individual has a minimally elevated PSA when one considers the age-specific reference ranges. He is asymptomatic from a GU standpoint. A conservative approach with serial PSA determinations is not unreasonable in this situation. In a younger man, a biopsy would be recommended.

○ **A 54-year-old man with no comorbid disease underwent a transrectal needle biopsy of the prostate for a PSA of 18 ng/mL and a free PSA of 8%. The pathology showed Gleason 4 + 5 in all six cores and there was evidence of perineural invasion. What is your next course of action?**

This individual has a very poor chance of being cured of his disease. The overwhelming majority (approximately 80%) of patients with this Gleason pattern will suffer a biochemical failure within 5 years of monotherapeutic intervention. Furthermore, the likelihood of his having positive lymph nodes based on his biopsy results must be considered. Brachytherapy alone would be a poor choice, since it does not effectively treat disease in the extracapsular space. Radical prostatectomy for maximal local control of the disease with an option for early adjuvant radiation therapy to sterilize the field may be an option depending upon the lymph node status, but this will likely only extend his time period of biochemical freedom of disease rather than result in cure. A multimodality approach in this young individual with no comorbid disease will be required to maximize his outcome. A ProstaScint scan would be useful to see if he has localized or disseminated disease. If localized, cryotherapy would be another option.

○ **A 57-year-old healthy man presents with a PSA of 3.2 ng/mL. His previous PSA 6 months ago was 2.3 ng/mL and 6 months prior to that his PSA was 1.5 ng/mL. What is your next course of action?**

Although this man has a PSA within the age-specific reference range (0–3.5 ng/mL), his PSA velocity is out of the accepted range of normal. He has a sufficient PSA history to make this determination and his most recent findings warrant further investigation. A TRUS-guided biopsy of the prostate would not be unreasonable. Alternatively, a 30-day course of antibiotics can be given and then the PSA level repeated. Further therapy would depend on the second PSA level.

○ **A 69-year-old, obese, insulin-dependent diabetic man with a history of hypertension, coronary artery disease, s/p CABG, and a 70 pack per year smoking history presents with a PSA of 5.4 ng/mL. What is the next best course of action?**

This individual has significant comorbid disease and his PSA is minimally elevated. He is asymptomatic from a GU standpoint. A careful assessment of his overall condition reveals that he is not a good candidate for anesthesia. One must determine how aggressive they should be in evaluating patients at risk for disease, and whether the risk benefit ratio warrants further evaluation/intervention. Close observation with repeat PSA measurements may not be unreasonable for this individual. If a biopsy is done and is positive for prostate cancer, watchful waiting, external beam radiation, and hormonal therapy are all possible treatments.

○ **Is there a role for MRI in the routine evaluation for prostate cancer?**

The role of MRI in diagnosing and staging prostate cancer has been studied extensively. Endorectal coil and newer body surface coil MRI of the prostate have shown utility in staging select patients with prostate cancer. However, the lack of sensitivity and specificity of MRI in differentiating benign from malignant prostate tissue preclude the use of MRI as a reliable means to diagnose the disease. Extracapsular extension and seminal vesicle involvement have been identified with MRI and correlated with pathologic findings, but the associated costs and the availability of the equipment are factors that preclude the use of MRI as a first-line imaging modality for patients with prostate cancer. MRI is used by a number of institutions for assessment of metastatic disease and confirmation of bony involvement as well as for Prostascint determinations.

○ **A 64-year-old man presents with a PSA of 52 ng/mL and a free PSA of 8%. He complains of back pain and left hip pain. What is the next best course of action?**

This individual likely has bony metastases from his disease. He requires prompt diagnosis with a prostate biopsy as well as a serum alkaline phosphatase level and a radiologic evaluation of his bones. If he has metastatic disease, initiation of hormonal deprivation therapy is reasonable. Radiation therapy to the bones should be considered.

○ **What are the risks of starting LHRH therapy alone in a patient with metastatic prostate cancer?**

Initiation of LHRH therapy is associated with a testosterone flare that usually lasts about 14 days, after which castrate levels of testosterone are achieved. During the flare period, individuals can suffer from exacerbation of obstructive voiding symptoms and increased bone pain, and if there is vertebral involvement with bony metastases, they can develop spinal cord compromise or even paralysis. Additionally, compression fractures of the spine or any other involved bone may occur during the flare period depending upon the degree of bony involvement. Therefore, it is wise to begin antiandrogen therapy at the time of initiation of LHRH therapy in an effort to minimize potential morbidity in these select patients. The duration of antiandrogen administration should be a minimum of 2 weeks. Orchiectomy avoids this flare phenomenon, as does LHRH antagonists.

○ **A thin, 52-year-old man is referred by his internist with complaints of obstructive voiding symptoms, pelvic pain and bilateral lower extremity weakness, and swelling. On physical examination, he has palpable nontender periaortic masses and his prostate is consistent with TIIIc disease. He also has 2+ pitting edema of the lower extremities. A phone call to the internist reveals a PSA was drawn and the result is 914 ng/mL. How would you proceed?**

This patient requires urgent intervention. A CT scan of the abdomen and pelvis reveals massive retroperitoneal adenopathy with compression of the vena cava. There are large iliac lymph nodes identified on the CT scan. There is no evidence of vertebral bony involvement with disease or cord compression. His findings are consistent with advanced prostate cancer as well as vascular compromise from metastatic disease. An urgent orchiectomy is preferred since initiation of LHRH therapy will not result in castrate levels of testosterone for approximately 14 days. Additionally, one should consider CT-guided needle biopsy of the retroperitoneal lymph nodes to confirm the absence of a second primary such as lymphoma. If LHRH therapy is used, antiandrogens should also be used.

○   **Should all patients with prostate cancer have a bone scan as part of the staging evaluation?**

No. Bone scans are often employed to evaluate patients at risk for metastatic prostate cancer. Studies have indicated that the likelihood of a positive bone scan in an individual with a PSA less than 10 ng/mL in the absence of symptoms of bone pain is less than 1%. However, poorly differentiated cancers are known to have diminished PSA production, and therefore, PSA can be misleading in patients with poorly differentiated prostate cancer. If an individual has symptoms of bone pain and/or an elevated alkaline phosphatase, a bone scan is a reasonable staging examination.

○   **Which is more sensitive for the detection of bone metastases, bone scans or plain radiographs?**

Bone scintigraphy is much more sensitive than plain radiography for detection of bony metastases. Plain radiography generally requires a 50% change in the cortical bone density to diagnose a bony metastasis, whereas bone scintigraphy can detect disease with as little as 10% change in the cortical bone density. Ninety-five percent of bone lesions due to prostate cancer are osteoblastic, whereas five percent are osteolytic.

○   **A 73-year-old man presents with a PSA of 23 ng/mL 10 years following 64-Gy external beam radiation therapy for prostate cancer. He has significant bladder outlet obstructive symptoms and a clinical TIIIb prostate. There are no other pertinent findings on history and physical. What is your next course of action?**

This individual should be evaluated with a TRUS biopsy of the prostate to establish the diagnosis of recurrent disease. If the diagnosis of locally recurrent disease is made, LHRH therapy can be initiated cognizant of the fact that he may develop urinary retention due to the testosterone flare. This can usually be presented by using anti-androgen therapy such as Casodex or flutamide. To address his bladder outlet obstruction, one might consider a "channel" TUR of the prostate, but the associated risk of incontinence in a previously radiated patient is as high as 30% in some series. LHRH therapy will not have impact on his voiding function for several months, and alpha blockers are not always effective with a high tumor burden in the prostate. Finally, a metastatic evaluation would be predicated upon abnormal findings on physical examination or blood work. Generally, a PSA of 20 or more is necessary to justify a bone scan.

○   **Is there a role for computed tomography (CT) in the routine staging of prostate cancer?**

No. CT scanning lacks sufficient sensitivity and specificity to reliably increase the accuracy of clinical staging for patients with prostate cancer. Numerous published studies have reported accuracy rates ranging between 15% and 65% for staging individuals with disease. In the absence of bulky disease, CT lacks the resolution necessary to delineate extracapsular extension, and CT cannot differentiate benign from pathologic tissue within the prostate.

○   **Is there a role for CT scanning in assessing the status of the pelvic lymph nodes?**

CT scanning cannot differentiate a suspicious (>1 cm) from an abnormal lymph node (>1.5 cm) with regards to a benign inflammatory condition versus a pathologic process. However, in select individuals with prognostic factors suggestive of lymph node involvement, i.e., significantly elevated PSA, high Gleason score (>7), or bulky clinical disease CT scanning may have a role in staging the patient.

○   **Is there a role for Prostascint in staging patients with prostate cancer?**

Yes. Prostascint uses indium in III capromabpendetide, a radiolabeled monoclonal antibody to prostate-specific membrane antigen to identify soft tissue sites of prostate cancer metastasis. Prostate-specific membrane antigen (PSMA) is selectively expressed in epithelial cells of prostate origin both normal and malignant. Expression is increased in prostate cancer compared to normal epithelium. The scan is best used when correlated with other modalities such as MRI and SPECT.

○ **How is Prostascint most effectively used?**

It is best used in patients with rising PSA to determine if they may still benefit from localized therapy. Purely anatomical tests like CT and MRI cannot demonstrate low volume metastatic disease. It can also be used in higher-risk individuals to help detect extraprostatic disease. This would spare the individuals the complications of local definitive therapy in favor of systemic treatment.

○ **What is the impact of obesity on prostate cancer incidence and aggressiveness?**

Analysis of data from the CaPSURE database of over 10,000 men with prostate cancer showed no correlation between Gleason score and obesity. However, obese patients were more likely to be younger at the time of diagnosis and have more comorbidities. This is thought to be due to more frequent interactions of this group with the medical community which would lead to earlier detection.

○ **What is the risk of fracture in prostate cancer patients receiving androgen ablation therapy?**

According to the SEER database of 50,613 men with prostate cancer, of those surviving at least 5 years after diagnosis, the risk of a fracture was 19.4%.

○ **What is the average amount of bone mass lost in the first 12 months after androgen deprivation therapy is started?**

From 2% to 8%.

○ **What treatments are recommended to reduce osteoporosis in men receiving androgen deprivation therapy?**

Vitamin D and calcium supplementation should be started. Decreasing excessive alcohol intake, stopping smoking, and increasing weight-bearing exercise have been shown to be helpful. If hypercalciuric, a thiazide diuretic may help reduce urinary calcium loss. Oral bisphosphonates have not been shown to increase bone mineral density, but they may reduce the rate of bone loss. Only zoledronic acid (Zometa) has been shown to actually increase bone in men receiving androgen ablation therapy for prostate cancer.

○ **What percentage of men on androgen deprivation therapy for prostate cancer typically receive osteoporosis testing or preventive therapy?**

Less than 15%, with only about 5% receiving bisphosphonate therapy.

○ **What is the most accurate way of measuring bone mineral density?**

Dual energy x-ray absorptiometry (DEXA) is considered the best and most accurate way to measure bone mineral density. Ultrasound is less expensive and more convenient although it is less accurate.

○ **Is a higher free testosterone level associated with an increased risk of prostate cancer?**

Yes, particularly in older men. This suggests that caution should be used in hypogonadal seniors who are considering testosterone replacement therapy which increases free testosterone levels.

○ **Does the presence of hematospermia increase the risk of prostate cancer?**

Yes. Although hematospermia is generally thought of as a benign and self-limiting problem, when it appears in the prostate cancer screening population, it is associated with a significantly higher risk of prostate cancer. This risk is roughly double the risk of the general screened population.

○ **Does a Gleason sum of 4 + 3 = 7 carry a worse prognosis than a Gleason sum of 3 + 4 = 7?**

It isn't clear. We tend to give more weight to the primary Gleason score, but in this case with Gleason 7, the studies are conflicting.

○ **T/F: Bicalutamide (Casodex) 150 mg should no longer be used as monotherapy for prostate cancer?**

True. While there is no problem with the standard approved 50 mg dose, the higher 150 mg daily dose was found to be associated with a higher death rate at 5 years in a large European study.

○ **Over 90% of prostate cancers are adenocarcinomas. What are the other types of prostate cancer that may be found?**

Transitional cell carcinoma and sarcoma are the most common after adenocarcinoma.

○ **What are the histological variations in adenocarcinoma of the prostate?**

Neuroendocrine, endometrioid, small cell, and mucinous are some of the histological variations of prostate cancer.

○ **What are the best nomograms for predicting prostate cancer outcomes and prognosis?**

There are a number of nomograms available but most have not been updated, validated, or had their predictions compared to actual results. Possibly the best and certainly the most well known are the Partin tables. The websites for a few of the most useful nomograms currently available are listed below. They are the Partin tables from Johns Hopkins, nomograms from Dr. Kevin Slawin of Baylor, and the Memorial Sloan Kettering tables.

- Partin Tables: http://urology.jhu.edu/prostate/partintables.php.
- Dr. Kevin Slawin: www.drslawin.com/nomogram.html#.
- Memorial Sloan Kettering: www.mskcc.org/mskcc/html/10088.cfm.

○ **A 57-year-old man with 2-years status postexternal beam radiation therapy for localized prostate cancer presents with a rising PSA. His PSA at the time of diagnosis was 6.07 ng/mL. The PSA has increased from a nadir of 1.02 ng/mL to 2.02 ng/mL to 4.2 ng/mL over the past 12 months. History and physical examination are only revealing a firm radiated prostate. The best course of action is?**

This patient has radiation failure prostate cancer based upon the Phoenix criteria of a PSA nadir + 2 ng/mL. The next best course of action is to obtain pathologic confirmation of recurrent disease. A bone scan would be revealing in a minority of patients in this situation, but may be prudent if salvage therapy is entertained. Imaging to assess extraprostatic disease burden and spread is appropriate after a prostate biopsy has been performed. LHRH therapy is an option, but if the patient proves to have localized recurrent disease curative therapy with salvage radical prostatectomy or cryotherapy may be more appropriate and potentially lifesaving.

○ **A 67-year-old man presents 3-years status postexternal beam radiation therapy with concomitant LHRH analog therapy for localized prostate cancer. His PSA at the time of diagnosis was 13 ng/mL and the Gleason's score was 4 + 3 in 8/14 biopsies. The PSA has increased from a nadir of 0.1 ng/mL to 0.75 ng/mL to 2.24 ng/mL over the past 9 months. Serum testosterone levels are consistently less than 50 ng/dL. What is the next best course of action?**

This patient has hormone-independent radiation failure prostate cancer. His PSA doubling time is less than 9 months, which is a very poor prognostic factor for long-term disease-specific survival. A metastatic evaluation is the best first course of action. Even in the setting of a negative metastatic evaluation, a salvage procedure would be of limited benefit given the following factors: his high primary Gleason score, the rapid doubling time of his PSA, and the hormone-independent progression of his disease. Systemic chemotherapy would usually be reserved until evidence of bony metastases.

○ **A 63-year-old man presents with a PSA of 2.78 ng/mL 6-years status postbrachytherapy for localized Gleason's 3 + 3 prostate cancer. He has biopsy proven localized recurrent disease. A comprehensive history and physical examination reveal no significant findings. The next best course of action is?**

This patient is young with no comorbid factors and salvage therapy is a very reasonable option. Pathologic evidence of recurrent disease and a negative metastatic evaluation allow for options of salvage therapy. CyberKnife radiotherapy is not an option given his history of prior brachytherapy. Salvage prostatectomy is an option but is associated with higher procedure-related morbidity than salvage cryotherapy.

○ **A 64-year-old tile contractor presents with a PSA of 5.17 ng/mL. He has no LUTS and physical examination is revealing only for a mildly enlarged prostate that is asymmetric. The next best course of action is?**

This patient has a single elevated age-specific reference range PSA. Before offering a prostate biopsy it might be prudent to repeat the value to rule out an erratic abnormal result. Cognizant of the greater than 30% risk of indolent disease in this age population, confirmation of an abnormal PSA result is the best choice before proceeding with a biopsy. A 15 to 30 course of antibiotics and a free/total PSA may be helpful in deciding whether or not a biopsy is necessary.

○ **Prior to the implementation of PSA into the physician's armamentarium, what percent of men had nonorgan-confined disease at the time of diagnosis of prostate cancer?**

Prior to widespread use of PSA, 50% to 60% of men had extracapsular extension at the time of surgical extirpation. With the utilization of widespread PSA screening, the incidence of organ-confined disease has increased to 75% to 85% of all prostatectomy specimens.

○ **In 2008, what is the likelihood of a man having metastatic prostate cancer at the time of diagnosis?**

With widespread use of PSA screening, the likelihood of a man having metastatic disease at the time of diagnosis is less than 5%. Additionally, the Partin tables have been revised due to the increased incidence of T1c disease. In the revised nomograms, approximately 77% of all men who underwent surgical extirpation had nonpalpable lesions at the time of diagnosis.

○ **What is uPM3?**

uPM3 was the first urine-based genetic test available to assess an individual's risk for carcinoma of the prostate. This test proved to be highly specific for detection of prostate cancer. uPM3 preliminarily proved to be an independent and specific biomarker that detects prostate cancer. This marker performed similarly to other conventional means of identifying patients at risk for disease. uPM3 is not able to distinguish large or aggressive cancers from more indolent disease.

○ **What is EPCA-2?**

The EPCA-2 is a urine-based test that has been reported on by the Johns Hopkins group and preliminary data are quite convincing that EPCA-2 will provide a more accurate assessment of men with indolent prostate cancer, presence of absence of organ-confined disease, as well as differentiating BPH from carcinoma. The specificity and sensitivity of EPCA-2 surpasses serum PSA testing but further studies are needed prior to clinical implementation.

○ **A 47-year-old man presents with an elevated PSA of 3.7 ng/mL and a nodule on the left base of the prostate gland. Detailed history and physical examination are negative. A TRUS-guided needle biopsy of the prostate is positive for 9/14 cores Gleason 3 + 3 disease. Based upon risk stratification criteria what is this patient's category?**

Favorable factors included in risk stratification include PSA less than 10 ng/mL, Gleason score 6 or less, and clinical T2a disease or less. Therefore, this patient is in the favorable-risk group for 10-year biochemical disease-free survival. A patient without one of the three risk factor criteria would be in the moderate-risk group and the lack of two or more factors place an individual in the high-risk group for 10-year biochemical disease-free survival.

○ **True or False: Black men tend to have higher serum testosterone levels than white men, which might explain their increased risk of prostate cancer.**

False. It's unproven that blacks have higher serum testosterone levels than whites.

○ **True or False: Serum testosterone levels do not affect prostate cancer risk.**

True. In a large collaborative review of 18 studies comprising nearly 4000 prostate cancer patients and 6500 controls, no relationship could be found between the risk of prostate cancer and serum concentrations of any sex hormones including testosterone, dihydrotestosterone, or estradiol. (Endogenous Hormones and Prostate Cancer Collaborative Group, 2008.)

○ **What is the median age for prostate cancer diagnosis?**

Approximately 70.5 years.

○ **What percentage of patients newly diagnosed with prostate cancer are 65 years of age or younger?**

Approximately 20%.

○ **True or False: A negative PSA velocity after a course of antibiotics reasonably eliminates the presence of prostate cancer.**

False. The PSA following the course of antibiotics must still fall below the biopsy threshold level.

○ **What is the significance of "atypical small acinar proliferation" (ASAP) on prostate needle biopsy specimens and how often, if ever, is it associated with prostate cancer?**

Atypical small acinar proliferation is generally considered suspicious for prostate cancer. Approximately 30% of subsequent biopsies demonstrate prostate cancer.

○ **Patients with large prostates (>80 g) are more, less or equally likely to have less aggressive prostate cancers than patients with smaller glands?**

More likely.

○ **In patients with increased PSA levels, a positive rectal examination increases the risk of high-grade prostate cancer by what amount?**

The risk is 2.5 times greater.

○ **What effect does vitamin D have on the development of prostate cancer?**

Vitamin D appears to be protective. Increased sun exposure and growing up in geographic locations with high solar radiation levels can reduce lifetime prostate cancer risk by 50%.

○   **True or False: Studies on doxetaxol-based regimens have shown a survival benefit in all hormone refractory prostate cancer patient groups, including those with asymptomatic disease.**

True.

○   **True or False: Nonfat (skim) milk consumption has been linked to advanced prostate cancer.**

True. Two large studies support such a link. (NIH-American Association of Retired Persons Diet and Health Study of 293,888 men and the Multiethnic Cohort Study of 82,483 men.)

○   **True or False: An MIR of the axial skeleton can show bone metastases earlier than bone scans in patients with hormone refractory prostate cancer.**

True. (Lecouvet, 2007.)

○   **What common drugs have shown activity in reducing biochemical recurrences in high-risk prostate cancer patients receiving high-dose definitive radiation therapy and how? (Hint: it's not an antiandrogen.)**

Statins, presumably through a reduction in antiapoptotic pathways or increased cancer cell sensitivity to radiation. 10-year survival is also increased slightly.

○   **True or False: Diabetic patients have a higher risk of poorly differentiated prostate cancer than nondiabetics.**

True.

○   **A single core from a 12-specimen TRUS-guided prostate biopsy shows Gleason 6 prostate cancer. How often will patients ultimately demonstrate higher Gleason scores, bilaterality, or multifocal disease?**

Slightly less than 50% will develop higher Gleason scores, more than 50% will become bilateral and up to 100% eventually become multifocal.

○   **According to the Baltimore Longitudinal Study of Aging and the National Comprehensive Cancer Network Clinical Practice Guidelines, for men with a total PSA <4 and a benign rectal examination, what PSA velocity should be used as a threshold for a prostate biopsy?**

A PSA velocity of more than 0.35 ng/mL/y has been recommended.

○   **What percentage of cancers detected in patients with a PSA <2.5 are thought to be clinically significant based on pathological features?**

More than 70%.

○   **What secondary malignancies following definitive external beam radiation therapy for prostate cancer have the greatest potential impact on survival and how often do they occur?**

The most dangerous secondary malignancies are bladder, colorectal, and skin (melanoma). The risk is roughly double the risk of nonradiated controls.

○   **The National Comprehensive Cancer Network currently recommends a baseline PSA level starting at what age?**

At 40 years.

○ **What is the most important risk factor for prostate cancer: a positive family history of prostate cancer, race, or baseline PSA level?**

Baseline PSA level is the strongest predictor of prostate cancer risk.

○ **What is the current 10-year cure rate in radiation therapy patients who undergo salvage cryotherapy and what is their disease-specific survival?**

The 10-year cure rate is approximately one-third and disease specific survival is 80%.

○ **What membranous urethral length after radical prostatectomy appears to be a good predictor of postoperative continence?**

>11 mm.

○ **Is PSA significantly influenced by circulating testosterone levels?**

No significant influence is noted in PSA levels across a wide range of testosterone readings.

○ **According to the American Cancer Society, what is the estimated number of new cases of prostate cancer and the number of prostate cancer deaths expected in 2008 in the United States?**

More than 186,000 new prostate cancer cases and 28,000 deaths in the United States are predicted.

CHAPTER 45

Radiation Therapy for Prostate Cancer

Gregory J. Kubicek, MD, and
Richard K. Valicenti, MD, MA

○ **List the most important clinical prognostic factors predicting disease-free survival for prostate cancer?**

- T stage.
- Biopsy Gleason score.
- Pretreatment PSA.

○ **Describe the most important clinical prognostic factors predicting disease-free survival for prostate cancer?**

T stage, biopsy Gleason score, and pretreatment PSA have been the most extensively studied three factors. They provide reproducible outcomes among prostate cancer patients treated with radiation therapy alone. Several investigators (D'Amico) have used a combination of these factors to stratify disease-free survival according to low-, intermediate-, and high-risk groups. Such a strategy is helpful in providing prognostic information for patients and in stratifying patients for prospective trials.

○ **What other clinical prognostic factors can help predict prostate cancer survival?**

PSA doubling time, percent of biopsy scores positive for disease, patient age, comorbidities, and obesity. Race is an unclear prognostic factor with some studies showing a worse clinical outcome for African Americans.

○ **Which of these factors is the strongest predictor of death from prostate cancer?**

Biopsy Gleason score is the clinical prognostic factor that has been consistently shown to best predict death from prostate cancer. While pretreatment PSA has been shown to correlate with biochemical recurrence, no investigator has been able to demonstrate that pretreatment PSA reliably predicts death from prostate cancer.

○ **How would this affect treatment recommendations for radiation therapy?**

In recommending radiation therapy for prostate cancer, more weight should be given to the Gleason score over any other factor. Dose escalation studies have shown more benefit for high-risk and high-grade cancers than for low- or intermediate-risk groups. Also, several prospective randomized trials that have shown that patients with high Gleason score tumors have a survival benefit from the use of long duration adjuvant hormonal therapy.

○ **At what point after beginning hormone therapy should radiation therapy be started?**

There is no clear answer at this point. While most will arbitrarily wait 2 to 3 months, others believe it is best to wait until the PSA nadir is reached. Monthly PSA checks can be used to determine when the PSA nadir has been attained. Depending on initial PSA levels and other factors, this may take 3 to 12 months but averages about 6 months.

○ **A 65-year-old man was recently diagnosed with a Gleason score 4 T1aNxM0 carcinoma of the prostate. His most recent PSA was 30 ng/mL. His prostate gland size is 40 cm³. What is the significance of PSA in this stage of disease?**

Despite his PSA being 30 ng/mL, he has a low risk (<5%) of having prostate cancer extending outside the prostate. Because he has a transition zone cancer, his PSA is not necessarily indicative of the prostate cancer volume, which more strongly correlates with the presence of extracapsular disease.

○ **What is your recommendation for treatment for the above-mentioned patient?**

One may argue that based on his Gleason score and T stage, this patient may be suitable for watchful waiting, but his young age would argue for some form of curative therapy. Despite his PSA having little prognostic significance, his PSA may be too anxiety provoking not to recommend any definitive treatment. Of course, one may consider watchful waiting if he has multiple comorbid conditions that may lead to death in the immediate future. In any event, recommendations should include monotherapy with radiation therapy or surgery since these treatments appear to be equally efficacious for this stage of disease. The use of hormonal therapy is less clear but some would consider it beneficial based on the PSA level.

○ **A 50-year-old has a PSA of 15.0 ng/mL, Gleason 8, and clinical stage T1cNxM0 prostate cancer. How does the PSA influence your treatment decision?**

This patient has high-risk prostate cancer. Whether the patient has monotherapy with standard dose (78–80 Gy) radiation therapy or surgery, his chances of freedom of biochemical failure at 5 years is under 25%. This most likely translates into a 15 year overall survival of 50%. Due to the high-risk category, most oncologists would recommend combined modality therapy with long duration (>2 years) hormonal therapy and radiation therapy. Other therapies that can be considered include radical prostatectomy with adjuvant radiation for pathological high-risk features (extracapsular extension, seminal vesicle invasion, positive margins).

○ **A 61-year-old man undergoes hormonal downsizing (3 months) and has a radical prostatectomy. Pathologically, he is found to have extensive capsular penetration and positive surgical margins. His surgical Gleason score can not be classified by his pathologist. His postoperative PSA at 10 days is 0.4 ng/mL (Chiron assay). What are your recommendations?**

No trials with preoperative hormonal therapy have shown a clinical benefit and thus the hormones that the patient has received are not likely to have any effect on clinical outcome or future treatment recommendations. This patient will likely benefit from salvage external beam radiation to the prostatic bed based on his risk factors including positive margins and capsular extension. The PSA should also be repeated since the biological half-life after a radical prostatectomy is probably no less than 2.2 days. In actuality, his PSA was less than 0.2 ng/mL on repeat measurement a week later.

○ **Same patient as in the previous question and tumor characteristics but the PSA is undetectable. What are your recommendations?**

The recommendations for this patient are still external beam radiation, but in this case it would be termed "adjuvant" rather than "salvage" since there is no evidence of disease at the time of treatment (using PSA as a disease surrogate). Because of the high preoperative PSA value and the presence of capsular penetration and surgical margin positivity, his risk of biochemical failure at 5 years is greater than 50%. There have been two randomized prospective trials (SWOG and ECOG) randomizing patients with postradical prostatectomy risk factors (extracapsular extension, positive margins, seminal vesicle invasion) to observation versus external beam radiation. Both trials showed a benefit in biochemical free survival in the radiation arm.

○ **What radiation dose range is effective adjuvant postoperative radiation therapy and why?**

Radiation doses from 60 to 66.6 Gy in 1.8 to 2 Gy fractions appear safe and effective. The two randomized trials both used 60 to 64 Gy to the prostatic bed. Retrospective evidence shows that a radiation dose >64.8 Gy appears to be more effective than lower doses.

○ **What are the clinical benefits from adjuvant radiation therapy?**

Both of the randomized adjuvant trials have shown that adjuvant post-prostatectomy radiation therapy reduced the risk of biochemical failure and local progression, but a reduction in the risk of dying from prostate cancer was not observed.

○ **Would an isolated local recurrence after a radical prostatectomy require higher radiation doses for biochemical control?**

Larger tumor volumes require more radiation dose than smaller tumors for the same probability of local control. Several authors have reported on radiation dose response for patients with rising PSA after radical prostatectomy and have found that doses higher than 64 Gy are necessary.

○ **What are the important predictors of response to salvage radiation therapy for patients with a rising PSA after a radical prostatectomy?**

A nomogram by Stephenson has shown that preradiation PSA >2.0, Gleason score >8, negative surgical margins, and PSA doubling time >10 months were adverse prognostic factors for biochemical relapse at 6 years. Positive margins as a favorable prognostic factor may appear nonintuitive but is related to the presence of local disease that is thus amenable to cure from radiotherapy.

○ **Which factor is perhaps the strongest predictor?**

The magnitude of the PSA elevation prior to radiation. Several reports have shown that initiating radiotherapy at a lower postradical prostatectomy PSA level is more beneficial, Stephenson has shown that salvage radiotherapy at a PSA <0.4 ng/mL has improved biochemical and disease free survival versus radiotherapy at a PSA >0.4 ng/mL.

○ **What would combined modality treatment provide over monotherapy for an isolated biochemical failure after a radical prostatectomy?**

There has been no completed prospective trial of combined modality therapy for patients with an isolated biochemical failure after a radical prostatectomy. Decisions regarding management thus depend on clinical judgment. Since approximately half of patients fail after salvage radiation therapy, either insufficient radiation therapy is delivered or subclinical distant metastases are already present. If there is still androgen-sensitive prostate cancer clones, there may be a benefit to use hormonal therapy to both potentiate radiation therapy locally and to reduce disseminated disease.

○ **A 70-year-old man has a T1cNxM0 Gleason 8 prostate cancer in 5% of one of six cores. His prebiopsy PSA level was 0.9 ng/mL. Prostate gland size of 30 cm³. Would you expect this patient to have a large tumor burden?**

The patient has findings suggestive of having low volume prostate cancer. A single core biopsy containing 5% or less cancer correlates with low volume of disease and a low risk of capsular penetration.

○ **What is his risk of having lymph nodal metastases?**

He has less than 15% risk of having lymph nodal involvement. Since the risk is relatively low, evaluation of the pelvic lymph nodes with either ProstaScint or pelvic lymph node dissection probably would not provide useful information for guiding therapy.

○ **What are your recommendations and why?**

External beam radiation therapy alone (>78 Gy) to the prostate alone. It is not clear that hormonal therapy would significantly enhance the effect of radiation therapy for this patient due to his low PSA level.

○ **What are the radiation fields used?**

Two prospective randomized trials (RTOG 94-13 and GETUG 01) have addressed the question of radiation to the prostate only or to the whole pelvis followed by a boost to the prostate. Both trials failed to find any improvement with the whole pelvis field although RTOG 94-13 did note an unexpected benefit to the combination of whole pelvis radiation and adjuvant hormone use that warrants further study. However, at this time the data does not support whole pelvis radiation.

○ **A 55-year-old man is diagnosed with T3bN1M0 Gleason 6 prostate cancer, PSA of 29 ng/mL. What is his prognosis with radiation therapy alone?**

Although there appears to be a wide range of estimates made in the literature, nomograms (for example, from Memorial Sloan–Kettering) predict that this patient has approximately a 50% chance of having disease progression at 5 years.

○ **What is his prognosis with combined hormonal therapy and radiation therapy?**

Several retrospective and prospective studies purport 70% to 80% expected survival at 5 years.

○ **Which patients with clinically localized disease are most suitable for prostate seed implantation alone?**

The patient most suited for an implant alone has a tumor with a clinical stage T1–T2a, biopsy Gleason score <7, prostate size <50 cm³, and PSA <10 ng/mL.

○ **What is the incidence of potency after external beam radiation therapy for prostate cancer?**

Depending on patient age, comorbid conditions, use of β-blockers, potent patients undergoing external beam radiation therapy for prostate cancer have 50% to 75% chance of remaining potent after treatment.

○ **What is the incidence of ED after prostate seed implantation (brachytherapy)?**

The incidence is approximately 20% to 25%.

○ **Which form of radiation treatment may lead to a higher incidence of urinary incontinence?**

Prostate seed implantation. The incidence can be as high as 50% if the patient had a prior TURP although such patients infrequently get seed implants due to technical difficulties. External beam radiation therapy causes urinary incontinence in less than 5% of the patients. However, if a TURP is done shortly after external beam radiation therapy, the incontinence rate can be quite high. At least 6 months and preferably a year should elapse between any definitive radiation therapy and a TURP.

○ **What is the mechanism by which radiation therapy causes ED?**

Radiation therapy causes ED primarily through arteriogenic and vascular means as opposed to radical prostatectomy which affects the nerves.

○ **What is the difference between standard, 3D conformal, and intensity modulated radiation therapy (IMRT)?**

These three modalities of radiation therapy planning represent increasingly sophisticated planning techniques that allow the radiation dose to be "sculpted" to minimize exposure to normal tissues (rectum and bladder). Standard radiation therapy is generally limited to about 66 Gy, 3D conformal techniques allow a dose 75 to 76 Gy, and IMRT doses can be in excess of 80 Gy with essentially equivalent side effects.

○ **What is the best way to determine the actual dosing given after brachy therapy?**

A CT scan can be used to calculate the actual dose given by the actual seed placement. The most useful number is the D90, which is the dosage given to 90% of the prostate. Optimal cancer survival results are generally found when the D90 is 140 Gy or more. This dosage can only be achieved with radioactive seed implants either alone or in combination with external beam therapy.

○ **What is the most common side effect of radiation therapy?**

Rectal irritation and GI disturbance.

○ **What is the maximal safe calculated dose to the urethra?**

The urethral dose should be <150% of the maximal dosage.

CHAPTER 46

Surgical Therapy for Prostate Cancer

Daniel M. Hoffman, MD, FACS

Q. What are the treatments for prostate cancer?

There are five general categories of treatment for prostate cancer:

1. The monitoring of the patient without any aggressive therapy. This is sometimes called watchful waiting and consists of a physical examination with serial PSA determinations.

2. Radiation therapy. This can be administered in two ways: external beam radiation therapy and interstitial brachytherapy.

3. Radical prostatectomy either by a retropubic, laparoscopic, or perineal approach.

4. Cryotherapy.

5. Hormonal manipulation.

How effective is orchiectomy?

Orchiectomy results in a reduction of circulating androgens by approximately 97%. Castrate levels of testosterone are achieved within 24 hours of orchiectomy. The hormonal deprivation results in remission of the hormone-dependent prostate tumor growth. Depending upon the Gleason's grade of the cancer, the duration of the remission varies, and biochemical failure/hormone-independent tumor growth will eventually occur.

How do the results of brachytherapy compare with surgical therapy?

In one report comparing brachytherapy and radial retropubic prostatectomy in patients matched for similar pretreatment clinical pathological characteristics, the results showed a mean 7-year disease-free survival rate of 84% for surgical extirpation versus 79% for the iodine brachytherapy series. Although there was a proportionately higher probability of nonprogression for brachytherapy, this was not statistically significant. In most studies, brachytherapy has compared favorably to radical prostatectomy in biopsy-confirmed patients posttreatment.

How are the lymph nodes assessed for metastatic disease?

Although CT scan may be used to evaluate for lymphadenopathy, one cannot differentiate pathologic from nonpathologic nodes if they are <1.5 cm in size. Thus, computed tomography is both nonspecific and nonsensitive. To absolutely rule out metastatic disease of the lymph nodes, a lymphadenectomy is required.

○ **What are the options for pelvic lymphadenectomy?**

If the patient is undergoing radical retropubic prostatectomy, a lymphadenectomy may be performed simultaneously and the lymph nodes can be sent for frozen section analysis to rule out micro metastases. Alternatively, a laparoscopic pelvic lymph node dissection or a minilap lymph node dissection may be performed.

○ **How is a laparoscopic lymph node dissection performed?**

Laparoscopic lymph node dissection can be performed transperitoneally or through a preperitoneal approach. The pelvic lymph nodes are removed and the tissue is sent for analysis.

○ **What are the boundaries for lymph node dissection?**

The distal limit of the dissection is the node of Cloquet located in the femoral canal. The proximal limit of the dissection is the bifurcation of the iliac vessels. The superior limit of the dissection is the external iliac artery, the lateral limit is the pelvic side wall and the inferior limit is the obturator vessels. Thus, all the lymph nodes are dissected off of the external iliac vein, the pelvic side wall laterally, and the obturator nerve and vessels.

○ **Why is laparoscopic pelvic lymph node dissection so infrequently performed now when it was so popular in the early 1990s?**

The surgery was originally intended for patients with a high likelihood of lymphatic metastatic disease where a radical surgery or definitive radiation therapy could be avoided if positive lymph nodes were identified preoperatively. Typical patients would have elevated PSA levels (at least 10 or more) and Gleason sums of 7 or higher. Better understanding of PSA and the use of nomograms like the Partin tables have largely made the laparoscopic pelvic lymph node dissection unnecessary.

○ **What are the complications of pelvic lymph node dissection?**

The most common complication is lymphocele formation. Lymphocele formation can be minimized by clipping or tying feeding lymphatics as coagulation of lymphatics can result in postoperative lymphatic leakage. Damage to the external iliac vein, obturator vessels, and obturator nerve can also occur during pelvic lymphadenectomy.

○ **What are the different methods of radical prostatectomy?**
- Radical retropubic.
- Laparoscopic.
- Perineal.

○ **How is the patient prepared for radical prostatectomy?**

The patient should have adequate cardiac and pulmonary function. If there are any risk factors of cardiopulmonary disease, the patient should be optimized prior to surgery. Screening tests for coagulopathy are mandatory. Preoperative determination should be made of the patient's hemoglobin, hematocrit, and electrolytes. Although the risk of rectal injury is low, patients should undergo bowel prep prior to surgery.

○ **Should the patient donate autologous blood?**

This depends on the surgeon's experience. If the surgeon historically loses more than 500 mL of blood during a radical prostatectomy, it is reasonable to offer the patient the option of donating autologous blood. The blood is commonly donated within the month before surgery. This bears substantial cost, but decreases the risk of a transfusion reaction or a transfusion-associated morbidity.

○ **Are antiembolism precautions necessary for radical prostatectomy/pelvic lymph node dissection?**

Many of the risk factors for deep vein thrombosis and pelvic thrombosis are present: general anesthesia, blood loss, pelvic surgery, and possibly a hypercoagulable state. Lower extremity sequential compression devices and antiembolism stockings are commonly employed to help minimize pooling of blood in the deep veins of the legs. This may be used with or without medical anticoagulation such as subcutaneous heparin or Lovenox.

○ **What is the positioning for the radical retropubic prostatectomy?**

The radical retropubic prostatectomy is performed through a midline infraumbilical incision extending from the umbilicus to the pubic symphysis. The patient is placed supine or in a low lithotomy position with the kidney rest or a rolled towel just above the sacrum with the table slightly hyperextended. During the procedure, reverse Trendelenburg may be helpful in visualizing the apex of the prostate.

○ **Describe the approach to the prostate in a retropubic prostatectomy.**

The radical retropubic prostatectomy is an extraperitoneal procedure. The rectus muscles are split in the midline and the space of Retzius is developed. The bladder is freed from the posterior surface of the pubic symphysis and cleared from the lateral pelvic sidewall. At this time, if so indicated, a bilateral lymph node dissection is performed. After the lymph node dissection is complete and the pathological results obtained, incisions are made in the endopelvic fascia, lateral to the apex of the prostate to gain exposure to the apex of the prostate. If the apex of the prostate is not easily visualized, the puboprostatic ligaments are divided.

○ **Are the puboprostatic ligaments vascular structures?**

No. These are fibrous bands that connect the prostate to the underside of the pubic symphysis. They may be incised without causing excessive bleeding.

○ **What is the structure that is most likely to cause significant bleeding?**

Santorini's plexus, which is a continuation of the dorsal vein of the penis. This is the structure found in the midline that drains between the puboprostatic ligaments and forms the dorsal venous complex which is anterior to the urethra at the apex of the prostate gland.

○ **How is bleeding prevented from the dorsal venous complex?**

A variety of techniques for controlling the dorsal venous complex have been described. In the radical retropubic prostatectomy and laparoscopic prostatectomy, the dorsal venous complex must be transected in order to visualize the apex of the prostate. Bunching sutures paced deeply into the dorsal surface of the prostate from the level of the bladder neck and continuing distally to the apex of the gland are helpful in controlling back bleeding. A right-angle clamp is passed between the dorsal vein complex and the anterior surface of the urethra and the dorsal vein complex is tented up and ligated.

○ **What if these measures do not control bleeding from the dorsal venous complex?**

Direct visualization suture ligation of the transected veins under the pubic symphysis is the best means of stopping the bleeding. Rarely, temporary compression of and possibly suture ligation of the deep dorsal vein of the penis below the level of the pubic symphysis may be helpful in gaining control of bleeding from the dorsal venous complex. Suture ligation will require dissection of the veins at the base of the penis at the dorsal vein.

○   **Aside from the dorsal vein complex, what other important structures are located at the level of the apex of the prostate?**

The external sphincter is located distal to the apex of the prostate. Injury to this muscle can cause permanent urinary incontinence. The neurovascular bundles that supply the erectile function run laterally along the apex of the prostate from 3- and 9-o'clock positions at the level of the external urinary sphincter and 5- and 7-o'clock positions at the base of the gland. If both neurovascular bundles are transected, impotence results.

○   **What is the major blood supply to the prostate?**

The main blood supply to the prostate is from the inferior vesical artery, which is a branch of the hypogastric artery. This penetrates the substance of the prostate at the prostatovesical junction at 8- and 4-o'clock positions posteriorly.

○   **Describe the technique for avoiding injury to the external sphincter and the neurovascular bundles.**

The anterior urethra is incised under direct vision. The Foley catheter is delivered through the urethrotomy and transected while maintaining the fluid in the balloon. The posterior urethra is carefully dissected off of the rectum and is divided. The rectourethralis muscle is divided at apex of the gland in the midline and then the midportion of the dorsal surface of the prostate or Denonvilliers' fascia can be freed in the midline from the rectal surface. Dissection is then carried out along the posterolateral prostate sharply freeing it off of the neurovascular bundles. When vascular branches are identified, they are controlled with fine ligatures or clips. Cautery should be avoided to prevent injury to the neurovascular bundles. As the base of the prostate is reached, the main prostatic pedicle is encountered. The prostatic pedicle at this point should be secured with ligatures or clips. The prostate is then carefully dissected at the level of the prostatovesical junction, starting anteriorly and progressing posteriorly.

○   **What structures are important to preserve at the base of the prostate?**

The bladder neck, trigone, and ureteral orifices.

○   **What can one do to prevent damage to the ureteral orifices?**

Bladder neck preservation is the safest way to preserve the ureteral orifices. Indigo carmine or methylene blue may be administered intravenously to identify the ureteral orifices. If there is any question subsequently whether the ureteral orifices have been violated, placement of ureteral stents prior to the urethrovesical anastomosis should be entertained.

○   **After freeing up the apex of the prostate, the prostatic pedicles and the prostatovesical junction, what structures remain to be dissected free to allow the prostate to be removed?**

The seminal vesicles and ductus differentia. The ductus differentia are identified in the midline and transected. These are then used to delineate the medial side of the seminal vesicles. The seminal vesicles are dissected free from the surrounding tissue and the apical artery identified, controlled, and divided.

○   **What is the blood supply to the seminal vesicle?**

The artery to the seminal vesicle is a division of the hypogastric artery. It penetrates the seminal vesicle at its superior end. These need to be secured before removing the seminal vesicle.

○ **How is continuity of the urinary tract restored?**

The urethrovesical anastomosis is performed in two steps:

1. The bladder neck is reconstructed so that the opening is approximately 1.2 to 1.5 cm. Typically, this is accomplished by closing the bladder neck in a tennis racquet manner anteriorly and/or posteriorly, with care taken to avoid damage to the ureteral orifices. The mucosa is everted using 4-0 absorbable suture to "stomatize" the bladder neck.

2. Sutures are then placed in the urethral stump; once four to six sutures are placed in the urethra, they are sewn through the bladder neck. After all sutures have been placed, a Foley catheter is passed per urethra and directed into the bladder. The sutures are then tied down individually with gentle traction on the Foley catheter to bring the bladder down to the urethra.

○ **What sort of drains are necessary for this surgery?**

The two potential areas of drainage from radical retropubic prostatectomy are urinary drainage from the urethrovesical anastomosis and lymphatic drainage if a lymphadenectomy was performed. Drains (suction or nonsuction) are placed in the left and right side of the pelvis. The incision is then closed in the midline.

○ **How is laparoscopic prostatectomy different from retropubic prostatectomy?**

It is a transperitoneal approach, the dissection is antegrade (starts from the bladder neck and proceeds toward the apex), and the urethrovesical anastomosis is done with a continuous running suture. It avoids the larger low midline incision instead using five or six small incisions for the laparoscopic trocars.

○ **What are the advantages of laparoscopic prostatectomy versus radical retropubic prostatectomy?**

- Shorter hospital stay—usually patients spend only one night in the hospital, i.e., 2 days less than retropubic prostatectomy.
- Less blood loss.
- Faster recovery and quicker return to normal activities.
- Shorter catheter time postop. Generally, the Foley catheter can be removed on postop day 7.

○ **Is there any difference in positive margin, impotence, or incontinence rates between laparoscopic and retropubic prostatectomy?**

None has been described in any current mature series.

○ **What is a DAVINCI or ROBOTIC prostatectomy?**

It is a laparoscopic prostatectomy using the *da vinci* surgical system, which is a surgical tool that uses robotic technology to translate hand movements into precise movements of micro-instruments within the operative site. It allows freedom of movement and accuracy that is not possible with traditional open surgery or unassisted laparoscopic surgery deep in the pelvis.

○ **What are the complications unique to laparoscopic prostatectomy?**

Only those involved with the laparoscopic approach: bowel injury from trocar placement, diaphragmatic irritation from CO_2, and respiratory (ventilatory) difficulty from Trendelenburg and peritoneal insufflation.

○   **What is the optimal positioning for a perineal prostatectomy?**

The patient is placed in the extreme dorsal lithotomy position with a rolled towel or sheet under the sacrum so that the perineum is parallel to the floor. Allen stirrups are used to stabilize the patient's legs.

○   **What incision is used for perineal prostatectomy?**

The incision is made in a convex curvilinear fashion between the ischial tuberosities, anterior to the anus. Prior to the incision, a curved Lowsley tractor is placed per urethra into the bladder.

○   **What are the "pearly gates?"**

The "pearly gates" are also known as Denonvilliers' fascia. When seen, this indicates that the base of the prostate is in view. The rectum is then dissected off of the posterior surface of the prostate by dividing Denonvilliers' fascia using sharp and blunt dissection.

○   **Can the neurovascular bundles be seen and/or preserved in the perineal prostatectomy?**

Yes. Care must be taken to preserve the neurovascular bundles during dissection of the posterolateral portion of the prostate.

○   **How is the prostatovesical junction delineated?**

The prostatovesical junction can be delineated by rotating the wings of the Lowsley tractor in a circumferential manner. Once the junction is well defined, the detrussorotomy is made in the anterior midline at the level of the prostatovesical junction. The wings of the Lowsley tractor can be delivered through this detrusorotomy and dissection is carried circumferentially around the bladder neck using the Lowsley tractor for retraction.

○   **How is the blood supply to the prostate controlled?**

As large vessels are encountered, they may be suture ligated or clipped prior to dividing the apex. The prostate may be rotated anteriorly and the posterior pedicles at the base of the prostate can be visualized and suture ligated before apical dissection.

○   **Describe the technique for seminal vesicle dissections.**

The seminal vesicle dissection is somewhat more problematic with a perineal prostatectomy than a retropubic prostatectomy. Again, the vasa deferentia and ductus deferens are identified in the midline and clipped. Though the dissection down to the apex of the seminal vesicle may sometimes be awkward, with patience the artery to the seminal vesicle may be ligated at the tip of the seminal vesicle and the prostate gland removed.

○   **How is the urethrovesical anastomosis performed in a radical perineal prostatectomy?**

One of the advantages of the perineal prostatectomy compared with the retropubic prostatectomy is that urethrovesical anastomosis is often easier to perform. The bladder neck is tailored to 1.2 to 1.5 cm in diameter, using a tennis racquet approach to avoid damage to the ureteral orifice. Interrupted sutures are used to reanastomose the bladder neck to the urethra, starting in the anterior midline and extending laterally. However, once three-quarters of the anastomosis has been performed, a Foley catheter is placed per urethra and directed into the bladder and the remainder of the anastomosis is completed.

○ **How is a perineal prostatectomy drained?**

A separate perineal stab incision is made and a Penrose drain is placed at the level of the urethrovesical anastomosis. The wound is closed in layers with absorbable sutures.

○ **How long does the patient typically stay in the hospital?**

Patients stay in the hospital until they are tolerating a diet, drainage has tapered off sufficiently, and they are hemodynamically stable. Patients are discharged with their Foley catheter.

○ **How long does the Foley catheter remain?**

The Foley catheter remains in place for 2 to 3 weeks, and then it is removed in the office.

○ **Do any confirmatory tests need to be performed before the Foley catheter is removed?**

Traditionally, a gravity cystogram was performed before removal of the catheter. Due to refinement in technique, this is not uniformly done. If there is any question of urinary leak, a cystogram should be performed prior to removal of the Foley catheter.

○ **If there is excessive drainage from the wound or drainage sites, how can one tell the origin of the fluid?**

The fluid should be sent for creatinine determination. If the creatinine is equivalent to the serum creatinine, a urine leak is ruled out. The drains should be managed conservatively and left in place until the fluid accumulation has subsided. If the drainage persists without evidence of improvement, a lymphatic source is more likely. The patient should be placed on broad-spectrum oral antibiotics and the drains gradually advanced and removed. The lymphatic leak should subside with time, but a lymphocele may accumulate and require internal drainage.

If the fluid has a markedly elevated creatinine, a urine leak is confirmed. Similarly, the patient should be placed on broad-spectrum oral antibiotics and the drains should be taken off of suction and advanced gradually until they are removed. The Foley catheter should be maintained. With adequate drainage, urinary leakage should subside.

○ **What are the intraoperative complications from radical prostatectomy?**

- Hemorrhage.
- Bowel injury.
- Ureteral injury.

○ **How is hemorrhage handled?**

The source must be identified. Generally, this is from the dorsal vein complex or from the prostatic pedicle. The most important step in controlling hemorrhage is to first make sure the patient remains hemodynamically stable. Communication with anesthesia is of major importance. Initially, pressure may be placed on the bleeding area so that anesthesia can maintain or reestablish hemodynamic stability. Dorsal vein complex bleeding was previously described. If the prostatic pedicles are bleeding, then they must be suture ligated. Mass ligatures or widespread electrocautery should not be used because it may damage the surrounding structures. If the urine is grossly bloody in the postoperative period, gentle traction on the Foley catheter can be utilized for short periods of time.

○ **How do rectal injuries occur, what is their frequency, and how are they managed?**

The incidence of rectal injury for patients undergoing a radical perineal prostatectomy is 10%. Injury usually occurs during takedown of the rectum and rectourethralis musculature. If an enterotomy occurs, it is safe to continue with the dissection of the posterior surface of the prostate unless there is fecal soilage. If feces contaminate the wound, the area should be thoroughly irrigated and the operation ended after formation of a diverting colostomy.

The prostatectomy may be continued in the absence of fecal soilage. The rectum should be closed in two layers. Some urologists favor the input of a general surgeon. Assuming that the patient has had preoperative bowel prep, a primary repair should be safe. In addition, a manual dilation or defunctionalization of the anal sphincter should be performed following closure of the incision, and the patient should be kept on a low residue diet for 1 to 2 weeks postoperatively.

Rectal injuries are rare during radical retropubic prostatectomy with an incidence of 5% to 7%. Generally, this occurs during apical dissection in the midline. Following closure of the injury, the anus should be manually dilated and the patient kept on a low residue diet.

○ **What if the patient has fecal drainage from his wound or his drain postoperatively?**

Provided the patient is clinically stable and fit for anesthesia, a diverting colostomy is indicated. The only way to heal a rectal fistula is by complete diversion.

○ **How is ureteral injury handled?**

Ureteral injury is best handled by ureteral reimplantation in the standard fashion.

○ **What are the postoperative complications of radical prostatectomy?**

As with any major pelvic surgery for cancer, deep vein thrombosis of the lower extremity and femoral veins is always a possibility. TED hose and sequential compression devices can be useful intraoperatively. If deep vein thrombosis is clinically suspected, a Doppler ultrasound of the lower extremities and pelvic veins should be ordered immediately.

○ **What are the complications of a deep vein thrombosis (DVT)?**

The catastrophic complication of DVTs is a pulmonary embolus, which is life threatening. Pulmonary embolus causes circulatory collapse and should be suspected when a patient has shortness of breath, tachypnea, tachycardia, and unexplained fever. A confirmatory study is a spiral chest CT. Pulmonary embolism is an emergent situation that should be treated initially with anticoagulation and urgent cardiac or general surgery consultation.

○ **What if the Foley catheter is removed accidentally or falls out prematurely?**

If the catheter falls out, a coudé catheter may be gently passed. If it does not pass easily on the first gentle attempt, the patient should be taken to the cystoscopy suite and under direct visualization a guide wire is placed in the bladder and a council-tipped catheter can be placed into the bladder. This prevents any disruption of the vesicourethral anastomosis.

○ **What if the patient does not void after removal of the Foley catheter?**

If the patient does not void or is uncomfortable, a catheter can be gently passed per urethra. If this does not pass easily, a suprapubic tube can be placed into the patient's bladder, and trials of voiding can be carried out at a later date. Edema at the site of the urethrovesical anastomosis is usually the etiology of failure to void in this situation.

○ **What if the patient develops urinary retention 3 months after surgery?**

A bladder neck contracture is the likely etiology. The urethra may be gradually dilated with filiforms and followers. Alternatively, a direct vision internal urethrotomy may be performed, but this must be done carefully to avoid injury to the sphincter.

○ **What is the major complication risk of a direct vision internal urethrotomy for bladder neck contracture after radical prostatectomy?**

Urinary incontinence. The urethrovesical anastomosis is very close to the external urinary sphincter and when incising an anastomotic stricture, the sphincter may be damaged leading to urinary incontinence.

○ **What if the stricture occurs 3 years after surgery?**

Cystoscopy should be performed to evaluate the stricture. It should be handled with care to avoid incontinence. The surgeon should also be cognizant that this may represent a local recurrence of disease and a PSA should be checked to evaluate this possibility and a biopsy of the stricture may be considered.

○ **What is the incidence of urinary incontinence following radical prostatectomy?**

Depending on the study, continence rates have been reported between 100% and 45% with most studies describing full continence in 85% to 90% of the patients treated with radical prostatectomy. It takes a while to establish continence, and surgeons feel that some stress incontinence between the catheter removal and 6 months postsurgery is not worrisome or negatively prognostic in terms of the patient's overall continence rate postoperatively.

○ **How is incontinence managed?**

For the first year postoperatively, anticholinergics or α-agonists can be used to try to minimize the incontinence. If the incontinence persists, management with an artificial urinary sphincter, a suburethral sling (InVance, AMS), or a trial of submucosal collagen injections at the bladder neck may be indicated.

○ **What is the incidence of impotence following nerve sparing radical prostatectomy?**

Impotence rates for preoperatively potent patients are between 25 and 40%.

○ **Who is the optimal candidate for prostate cryotherapy?**

Patients with localized high-grade prostate cancer, or with recurrent cancer after radiation therapy.

○ **How well does cryotherapy work as a salvage modality?**

Undetectable PSA levels are formed in approximately 65% of patients at 3 years posttherapy.

○ **What is the principle of cryotherapy for prostate cancer?**

Rapid freezing and thawing causes cancer cell death by crystal formation and cell disruption.

○ **What are the theoretical advantages of cryotherapy?**

It is effective even in high Gleason score cancers. It can be used after radiation therapy. If unsuccessful, it can be repeated. It is relatively noninvasive with few complications.

○ **What are the disadvantages of cryotherapy?**

Almost 100% incidence of ED. There is still the possibility of less common complications like incontinence or urethrorectal fistula.

○ **What elements are used for cooling and thawing?**

Liquid Argon is used for cooling and helium for heating/thawing.

○ **What other improvements have made prostate cryotherapy a viable option?**

Temperature probes placed strategically at the apex and rectal wall can automatically stop the freezing at a preset temperature. A urethral warming catheter prevents urethral sloughing. Helium heating elements allow more precise control of the freeze zone.

○ **After radiation therapy, if a reoccurrence is biopsied, how does the recurrent prostate cancer compare to the original cancer?**

There is frequently an increase in the Gleason score.

○ **Is obesity an independent predictor of biochemical failure after radical prostatectomy?**

Yes. Obese patients were found to have a higher rate of biochemical failure after their radical prostatectomy surgery than normal weight patients. Obesity has also been associated with higher-grade tumors and a higher risk of positive surgical margins.

○ **True or False: Following definitive therapy, a PSA doubling time of 1 year or less is associated with a high risk of dying from prostate cancer.**

True. If the PSA doubling time is over 1 year, they are unlikely to die from prostate cancer within the next 10 years.

○ **True or False: Men older than age 70 are more likely to have an upgraded Gleason score on final pathological examination after radical prostatectomy than men younger than 70.**

True. A large study of 4000 men who had all received radical prostatectomy found a substantially higher incidence of Gleason score upgrading in the older age cohort.

○ **Is bladder neck invasion an independent predictor of PSA recurrence after radical prostatectomy?**

While some of the data is conflicting, the more recent studies suggest that bladder neck invasion by prostate cancer is associated with a higher preoperative PSA level, a higher incidence of extraprostatic extension in areas other than the bladder neck, a larger overall tumor volume, and a higher incidence of positive surgical margins and a higher rate of PSA recurrence.

CHAPTER 47

Treatment of Locally Advanced or Recurrent Prostate Cancer

Badar M. Mian, MD, FACS and
Bilal Chughtai, MD

○ **What is the incidence of locally advanced prostate cancer?**

The incidence of clinical stage T3-4 has decreased from 11.8% to 3.5% over the last 10 to 15 years. Similarly, there has been a decrease in the high-risk prostate cancer group (high Gleason grade and PSA) from 32.3% to 21.9%.

○ **What is the incidence of pathological T3 disease in patients who are initially treated with radical prostatectomy?**

The incidence of pathological extraprostatic disease has decreased from 39% (1983–1991) to 31% (1992–2003). In more contemporary series, the incidence may be lower, depending upon patient selection criteria.

○ **Does PSA level reliably predict pathological stage?**

Up to 70% of patients with locally advanced prostate cancer may have a serum PSA level of >10 ng/mL, but serum PSA level alone cannot reliably predict pathological stage.

○ **What is the survival of patients with locally advanced disease for 5, 10, and 15 years without early treatment?**

Overall survival is reported from 25% to 92% at 5 years and 14% to 78% at 10 years for patients who harbor cancers of high grade or stage who are treated only when disease progression is noted. The 15-year cancer-specific mortality in men with Gleason sum 6 was 18% to 30%, compared with the 25% to 59% risk of death from other causes. The chances of death from prostate cancer increased with Gleason score 7 (42%–70%) and 8 to 10 (60%–87%).

○ **What is the incidence of seminal vesicle invasion (SVI) when performing radical retropubic prostatectomy in patients with clinical T3a disease?**

Approximately 5% to 15% of patients will have SVI after radical prostatectomy.

○   **What are the pitfalls of seminal vesicle biopsies to assess local tumor extent in patients with locally advanced prostate cancer?**

A significant number of *false-negative* biopsy results can occur due to sampling error in the presence of focal SVI. Even when SVI is suspected clinically and biopsies are performed, only 50% of patients will have positive biopsy results. *False-positive* results can occur because of a drag-through artifact where the needle goes through the base of the prostate. Lipofuscin staining can identify seminal vesicle tissue and help minimize the *false-positive* results.

○   **What is the extent of clinical staging error for locally advanced prostate cancer?**

Clinical overstaging occurs in up to 20% of patients who are actually found to have organ-confined disease. Understaging has been reported in 20% to 35% of patients who are found to have T3-4 lesions or microscopic nodal metastases.

○   **What percentage of patients with locally advanced prostate cancer will require surgical or medical intervention for disease progression if initially placed on watchful waiting?**

Approximately 70% will require some form of intervention secondary to local or distant disease progression. Depending upon the extent of disease progression, most patients are treated with hormonal ablation therapy or with radiation therapy plus hormonal ablation therapy. Up to 50% of patients may need a transurethral resection of the prostate (TURP) for obstruction or hematuria or nephrostomy tube placement for ureteral obstruction.

○   **What are the long-term results following radical prostatectomy for clinical T3 disease without adjuvant therapy?**

Cancer-specific survival rates are 85% to 92% and 79% to 82% at 5 and 10 years, respectively, regardless of adjuvant therapy. Without the use of secondary treatment, 5-year biochemical (PSA) relapse is noted in 50% to 60% of men.

○   **What effect does local failure have on quality of life after external beam radiation therapy (EBRT)?**

A significant decrease in quality of life is noted secondary to pelvic pain, hematuria, bladder outlet obstruction, and ureteral obstruction requiring nephrostomy tube placement. There is a significantly higher incidence of metastatic progression with bone pain and pathological progression.

○   **A patient with recurrent prostate cancer after radiation therapy does not want to undergo salvage radical prostatectomy but does desire further local therapy. Other than salvage radical prostatectomy, what other salvage local therapies are available?**

Salvage cryotherapy and salvage brachytherapy are alternate salvage local therapies. Approximately 50% of patients undergoing salvage cryotherapy will have a durable biochemical response. The 5-year biochemical disease-free survival rate following salvage brachytherapy is only 34%, which appears lower than the biochemical disease-free survival rates reported for salvage prostatectomy or cryotherapy.

○   **What percentage of patients with local disease progression following external beam radiation therapy may require surgical procedures?**

Local recurrence rates after EBRT for cT3 range from 24% to 74%. It is reported that 36% of patients required transurethral resection of the prostate because of urinary obstruction after RT alone, without hormonal ablation therapy. Other morbidities included hydronephrosis (20%) and incontinence (13%). Due to the technological advances in radiation therapy and more frequent use of hormonal ablation, these complications have become less frequent in contemporary series of patients.

○   **What is the percentage of patients who will become incontinent if they have a TURP after external beam radiation therapy?**

Approximately 30% to 50%. The incidence is higher if the TURP is done less than 1 year after the radiation therapy.

○   **What strategies have been used to improve local control and the disease-free survival rate following EBRT?**

Combination therapy with androgen ablation appears to improve the rate of disease control following XRT. The duration of androgen ablation may be 4 to 6 months in the moderate-risk, localized prostate cancer group. For the high-risk, locally advanced prostate cancer, 3 years of androgen ablation has demonstrated a significant overall survival advantage. Hormonal ablation for less than 3 years was not tested in this clinical setting.

○   **What are the results of cryotherapy for patients with clinical stage T3 prostate cancer?**

For men with high-risk features, those with PSA ≥10 ng/mL or Gleason score ≥8, 6-year biochemical disease-free rates of 35% can be achieved. Reported recurrences are more common in cancers located at the apex (9.5%) and the seminal vesicles (43.8%), in contrast to those located in the midgland (4.1%), and base (0%).

○   **What are the most common complications following cryotherapy?**

The most common complication is erectile dysfunction, as with other treatments for prostate cancer. Other complications include tissue sloughing, perineal ecchymosis, incontinence, strictures, and pelvic or rectal pain. Rectal fistulas are possible but rare with modern equipment and monitoring. Incontinence is more common in patients undergoing salvage cryotherapy who had received radiation therapy previously. Hydronephrosis may be noted in those with extensive damage to the trigone or bladder neck area.

○   **A patient presents with Gleason score 9, clinical stage T2b, N0, M0 prostate cancer. After a lengthy discussion of treatment options, the patient decides to pursue initial observation. What are the disease-specific and metastasis-free survival rates at 10 years for patients with high-grade, clinically localized prostate cancer that has been observed?**

Patients with clinically localized (clinical stage ≤T2) high-grade prostate cancer who are treated conservatively, will have a disease-specific survival rate of only 34% at 10 years, and only 26% of these patients will be free of metastasis at 10 years. Patients with high-grade prostate cancers are over six times more likely to die of prostate cancer than are patients with low-grade tumors.

○   **A patient with initial clinical stage T3 prostate cancer undergoes external beam radiation therapy and is noted to have a rising PSA level. The patient elects to be initially observed for his rising PSA. What is the time interval from the rise in the PSA level to development of clinically detectable prostate cancer?**

A rising PSA level after initial radiation therapy precedes clinically detectable disease (i.e., on digital rectal examination or radiographic metastasis) relapse by 3 to 5 years on average. In the absence of salvage therapy, up to three quarters of men will have clinical evidence of recurrent disease 5 years after PSA elevation is detected.

○   **A 55-year-old man with Gleason score 7, clinical stage T2a prostate cancer elects to receive initial external beam radiation therapy. His pretreatment PSA value is 7.5 ng/mL and falls to a nadir level of 1.2 ng/mL. It then rises to 3.5 ng/mL. The patient is now 60 years old. What staging studies should be considered prior to salvage radical prostatectomy?**

Restaging for patients with rising PSA levels after radiation therapy should include a bone scan and a computerized tomography of the abdomen and pelvis to rule out metastatic disease. The role of a ProstaScint scan is not entirely clear. Although it is well established that bone scans rarely detect metastasis in untreated patients with a PSA value below 20 ng/mL, this has not been established for patients with rising PSA levels after previous therapy. For patients who are candidates for salvage radical prostatectomy, cystoscopic examination is helpful to rule out bladder neck involvement.

○   **For the patient described above, what is the role for prostate biopsies and what is the likelihood that prostate biopsies will be positive in this clinical setting?**

A biopsy is indicated only in those patients who are considering further aggressive local therapy, namely salvage prostatectomy or cryotherapy. Performing a prostate biopsy under transrectal ultrasound (TRUS) guidance is important, as 50% to 80% of patients with a rising PSA after initial radiation therapy are reported to have positive biopsies, depending upon the PSA level at the time of biopsy. Gleason scores usually are increased compared to the original untreated tumor; however, this may be due in part to the therapy-related tissue architectural changes.

○   **The above-described patient elects to undergo a salvage radical prostatectomy. What are his chances of having an undetectable serum PSA 5 years later?**

The 5-year biochemical disease-free survival rate is 60% to 70% for patients undergoing salvage prostatectomy with a presalvage PSA <5 ng/mL compared with 25% to 40% for patients with a presalvage PSA >10 ng/mL.

○   **In salvage prostatectomy series performed in the PSA era, what are the rates of capsular penetration, positive margins, and seminal vesicle involvement?**

Many patients with recurrent prostate cancer after radiation therapy have larger cancers with more advanced pathological stage than anticipated from the preoperative clinical staging. Adverse pathologic features are commonly present. Series that include patients diagnosed in the PSA era have shown a 26% to 43% rate of capsular penetration, a 32% to 36% rate of positive surgical margins, and a 28% to 49% rate of seminal vesicle involvement. The biochemical outcome after salvage prostatectomy appears superior to the biochemical outcome after salvage cryotherapy or brachytherapy. Salvage radical prostatectomy may cure approximately 50% of well-selected patients.

○   **A patient undergoes a salvage radical prostatectomy following radiation therapy. The final pathologic evaluation shows Gleason score 9 adenocarcinoma with extracapsular extension and a positive surgical margin. The seminal vesicles and lymph nodes are negative. Is a positive surgical margin in a patient undergoing salvage radical prostatectomy biologically significant?**

A positive surgical margin in a previously irradiated patient is biologically significant, and patients with positive margins have a worse cancer-specific survival rate than do those with negative surgical margins. In previously irradiated patients, there are no curative treatments to fall back on should the surgery fail to remove all the cancer.

○   **What is the risk of urinary incontinence following salvage radical prostatectomy?**

Incontinence in recent salvage prostatectomy series remains high at almost 50%, despite improvements in operative technique.

○ **What is the biochemical disease-free survival rate for patients with high-risk prostate cancer who undergo external beam radiation therapy alone?**

Overall survival after RT alone for stage III cancer is approximately 60% to 70% at 5 years and less than 50% at 10 years. In high-risk patients, defined by individual parameters alone or in combination, the 5-year progression-free survival rates after RT are typically less than 50%. Because the results of external beam radiation therapy alone for locally advanced prostate cancer have been disappointing, there has been a dramatic shift toward treating patients with combined androgen ablation and radiation therapy.

○ **What are the biochemical disease-free survival rates and complications of these alternate salvage local therapies?**

The main complications of salvage cryotherapy are urinary incontinence, obstructive symptoms, impotence, and severe perineal pain. There is a 37% incidence of serious gastrointestinal or genitourinary complications following salvage brachytherapy. Obstructive symptoms are common, and up to 14% of patients undergo a transurethral resection for relief of obstructive symptoms following salvage brachytherapy. Four percent of patients develop significant rectal ulceration, and there are reports of patients undergoing colostomy for rectal bleeding.

○ **Pathological features are extremely important in establishing risk for local versus distant recurrence after radical prostatectomy. For patients with a rising PSA level after radical prostatectomy, which pathological features of the radical prostatectomy specimen support the presence of distant metastasis?**

Patients with a radical prostatectomy specimen Gleason score of ≥8, seminal vesicle invasion, or positive pelvic lymph nodes are at higher risk for distant metastasis. Patients with a specimen Gleason score ≤7, positive surgical margins, no seminal vesicle invasion, and negative pelvic lymph nodes may be at higher risk for local recurrence rather than distant mets.

○ **Does the presence of negative surgical margins in a radical prostatectomy specimen preclude the development of a local recurrence?**

Previous reports indicate that patients with negative surgical margins may still be at risk for local recurrence. Of patients with an elevated PSA level and negative bone scan following radical prostatectomy, the chances of a biopsy-proven local recurrence have been reported to be 10% to 30%. This rate depends entirely upon the degree and speed of PSA rise (i.e., PSA kinetics). Patients with negative surgical margins should, therefore, not be excluded from salvage radiation therapy. With the current practice patterns, the patients are often treated early and the PSA is not allowed to rise to a substantial level. Thus, a biopsy of the prostatic fossa is not helpful and is uncommonly utilized in the contemporary era.

○ **What are the PSA kinetics of local versus distant disease recurrence following radical prostatectomy?**

Short interval from surgery to detectable PSA is often indicative of distant metastasis. The development of a detectable PSA ≤1 year following radical prostatectomy and a PSA doubling time of ≤6 months have all been associated with significant risk for distant metastasis in patients with a rising PSA level after radical prostatectomy. By comparison, patients who develop a detectable PSA >1 year following radical prostatectomy, or have a PSA doubling time of >6 to 12 months are more likely to harbor local recurrence. It should be noted that there can be a significant overlap in the PSA kinetics which define local versus distant disease.

○ **A 70-year-old man develops a rising PSA value after radical prostatectomy. This patient elects to undergo observation. What is the median actuarial time from postsurgical PSA elevation to the development of clinically evident metastasis?**

It may take an average of 8 years from the initial PSA elevation to the development of clinically detectable recurrence as noted on a CT scan or bone scan or with the development of symptoms. This interval would be shorter in the presence of adverse pathological features such as capsular penetration or positive surgical margins.

○ **A 60-year-old patient has a rising PSA value of 1.2 ng/mL 4 years after radical prostatectomy. The patient is concerned about the possibility of metastasis, and staging studies including a bone scan and CT scan are ordered. What is the likelihood that a bone scan, ProstaScint, or CT scan will be positive in this patient?**

Although bone scans and CT scans of the pelvis are often recommended for patients with a rising PSA value after surgery, results of these studies are initially negative in the vast majority of patients, particularly in those with lower PSA values (<10 ng/mL). There have been anecdotal cases of patients who had positive bone scans but undetectable PSA levels, although this is extremely rare. The literature supports the low likelihood of a positive bone scan (<5%) in this setting until the PSA increased to over 20 ng/mL. Furthermore, CT scans of the pelvis are often inaccurate for assessing lymph node metastasis. A ProstaScint scan may be helpful in select situations, but this is still controversial due to the associated false-negative rates and some false-positive results.

○ **What proportion of patients with a detectable PSA level after radical prostatectomy will experience a decrease in their PSA level following salvage radiation therapy?**

Approximately 35% to 75% of patients with rising PSA who receive postoperative radiation therapy to the prostatic bed experience a decrease in their serum PSA. This depends upon whether the PSA ever declined to undetectable or if it began to rise at some interval from the surgery. As mentioned above PSA kinetics (timing and rate of rise) are also very important in determining the usefulness of salvage XRT for presumed local recurrence. This fact objectively demonstrates that at least some cancer cells persisted in the local field after radical prostatectomy.

○ **In what proportion of patients who undergo salvage radiation therapy for a detectable PSA level does the PSA level become undetectable and stay undetectable?**

The PSA becomes undetectable and stays undetectable in approximately 10% to 59% of patients following salvage radiation therapy. This widely divergent outcome in terms of a persistently undetectable PSA level is related to substantial differences in patient selection, dose of radiation, and timing of radiation therapy from the initial PSA rise.

○ **Five years after radical prostatectomy, a patient has a PSA value of 0.8 ng/mL. What is his likelihood of having a durable biochemical response to salvage radiation? What would his chance of having a durable biochemical response be if his PSA value was 3.5 ng/mL?**

The preradiation PSA value has a profound effect on outcome following salvage radiation therapy. It is clear that the lower the preradiation PSA value, the greater the likelihood of achieving a durable biochemical response. If the preradiation PSA is <2 ng/mL, then 83% of such patients will have biochemical control at 4 years compared with only 33% of patients with a PSA >2 ng/mL. For this reason, patients who have a rising PSA value after surgery, and who have pathologic features favorable for salvage radiation therapy, should have the radiation therapy administered early (PSA <2 ng/mL or even lower). Observing these patients and allowing the PSA to rise above 2 ng/mL may significantly compromise their chances for a cure.

○   **What pathologic features of radical prostatectomy specimens have been shown to have prognostic value for patients undergoing salvage radiation therapy?**

Several studies have shown that patients with pathological evidence of seminal vesicle or lymph node involvement are unlikely to have a durable response to salvage radiation therapy. The risk of treatment failure is several times higher if patients have pathological evidence of lymph node or seminal vesicle involvement. Some reports have shown that patients with higher-grade cancer (Gleason score of 8–10) in the radical prostatectomy specimen are at much higher risk for biochemical failure following salvage radiation therapy.

○   **What are the complications of salvage radiation therapy for a detectable PSA level following radical prostatectomy? If a patient has normal continence, is he likely to develop incontinence?**

In general, salvage radiation therapy is extremely well tolerated with few serious side effects. The most common side effects are related to radiation-induced cystitis and proctitis, which is often mild, and may cause irritative voiding symptoms and diarrhea. The irritative voiding symptoms and diarrhea typically resolve within 3 months of therapy. A worsening of incontinence has been noted in approximately 4% to 8% of patients undergoing salvage radiation therapy. In general, however, most patients who have good urinary control following radical prostatectomy continue to maintain urinary control after salvage radiation therapy. The salvage radiation therapy also has an adverse effect on the erectile function in men who may have regained their potency following surgery.

○   **Is there convincing evidence to indicate that the combined use of hormonal therapy along with radiation therapy is superior to radiation therapy alone?**

Based on randomized control trials, a limited period of hormonal ablation (4–6 months) appears to be appropriate for those men with intermediate-risk cancers. More prolonged hormonal ablation (up to 3 years) is beneficial for those with high-risk disease characteristics, including locally advanced cancers or very high pretreatment serum PSA values.

○   **A 60-year-old man presents with palpable extracapsular extension with Gleason score 7 adenocarcinoma and a PSA value of 15 ng/mL. He is considering 3 months of neoadjuvant hormonal therapy prior to radical prostatectomy. Is there any evidence that neoadjuvant hormonal therapy results in downstaging of clinical stage T3 prostate cancer?**

There have been many studies of neoadjuvant hormonal therapy in patients with clinical stage T3 disease. These studies showed a drop in PSA level in more than 90% of cases, with a 30% to 50% decrease in prostate volume after neoadjuvant hormonal therapy. However, only about 21% of these patients had organ-confined disease, which is not substantially different from the frequency of organ-confined disease noted in patients undergoing surgery without neoadjuvant hormonal therapy for stage T3 disease. Thus, there is no evidence that neoadjuvant hormonal therapy results in downstaging of T3 prostate cancer.

○   **The use of neoadjuvant hormonal therapy prior to radical prostatectomy has been shown to reduce the risk of positive surgical margins in which patients?**

In clinically localized (T2) cancers, there was decrease in the rate of positive surgical margins. For locally advanced tumors (specifically cT3), current data, both retrospective and prospective, do not support a significant benefit of neoadjuvant androgen ablation before surgery.

○ **Is there any proven reduction in the rate of biochemical failure for patients treated with 3 months of neoadjuvant hormonal therapy prior to radical prostatectomy?**

There is no overall benefit of short-term neoadjuvant therapy as measured by biochemical recurrence (34%–38%), regardless of the clinical stage or any reduction in the positive margin rate.

○ **What is the value of the ProstaScint scan?**

It is approved for the evaluation of soft tissue metastases in high-risk patients and for patients with rising PSA levels after definitive therapy. Fusing the Prostascint scan with CT and particularly MRI increases its usefulness. It may be useful in locally advanced cancers to detect extraprostatic disease, or when clinical parameters suggest a high likelihood of advanced disease despite negative conventional imaging.

CHAPTER 48

Testicular and Paratesticular Tumors

John D. Seigne, MB, and
Brian F. Kowal, MD

○ The following are the number of new cancer cases for several urinary cancers in men in 2007. Match the number of cases to the tumor type

Number of Cases	Tumor Type
1280	Bladder
7920	Penis
31,590	Prostate
50,040	Renal
218,890	Testis

Number of Cases	Tumor Type
50,040	Bladder
1280	Penis
218,890	Prostate
31,590	Renal
7,920	Testis

○ **What are the most common genetic alterations found in testis cancer?**

An isochromosome of the short arm of chromosome 12, i (12p), is a relatively frequent finding in germ cell tumors. Tumors not containing i (12p) generally have additional genetic material located on the short arm of chromosome 12. Isochromosome 12p is found in up to 80% of germ cell tumors. Interestingly, neither gain nor amplification of 12p material is commonly seen in CIS (although many other germ cell genomic changes are already present) suggesting that gain of genetic material from 12p is associated with the progression from CIS to invasive disease.

○ **A 2-year-old child undergoes a right orchiopexy for a high inguinal undescended testicle. What is his risk of developing testis cancer in that testicle at some point in the future?**

Patients with cryptorchidism have a 3 to 14 times increased risk of developing testicular cancer. The lifetime probability of developing testis cancer is therefore between 0.6% and 2.8%.

○   **A 2-year old child with a high inguinal undescended testicle has an orchiopexy. To what degree will the orchiopexy affect his future risk of developing testis cancer?**

There is controversy about the degree to which orchiopexy decreases the risk of testis cancer. Orchiopexy certainly allows for easier examination of the affected testicle and potentially earlier detection. A large population-based study showed children who had an orchiopexy prior to age 13 had an increased relative risk of testis cancer of 2.2, whereas those who had an orchiopexy after age 13 had an increased relative risk of 5.4 when compared to the general population.

○   **A 2-year-old child undergoes a right orchiopexy for a high inguinal undescended testicle. He is at increased risk of developing testis cancer in the right testicle. Is he at greater risk than the general population of developing a tumor in his left testicle?**

Yes. Patients with an undescended testicle have an increased risk of developing testis cancer in the contralateral normally descended testicle. The exact level of the risk is uncertain. However, 2% to 4% of patients who have had testis cancer develop a contralateral testis tumor and approximately half of these patients have a history of having an undescended testicle.

○   **What is the peak age group for Leydig cell tumors and how do they present?**

Usually ages 4 to 5. They present most often as gynecomastia, precocious puberty, or breast tenderness.

○   **β-hCG is a tumor marker that is commonly measured in patients with testis cancer. What cells produce β-hCG? What percentage of patients will demonstrate an elevated β-hCG with pure seminoma and NSGCT?**

β-hCG is produced by syncytiotrophoblastic cells. β-hCG is elevated in approximately 15% of patients with pure seminoma and 40% to 60% of those with a nonseminomatous germ cell tumor (NSGCT).

○   **Alpha feto protein (AFP) is a tumor marker that is commonly measured in patients with testis cancer. What percentage of patients with pure seminoma have an elevated AFP and what percentage of patients with NSGCT have elevated AFP levels?**

AFP is not elevated in patients with pure seminoma. AFP is elevated in 50% to 70% of patients with NSGCT.

○   **A 25-year-old has a right orchiectomy for a NSGCT. Prior to orchiectomy, his AFP was 124 and his β-hCG was 88. What is the half-life of AFP and β-hCG? Assuming that he has no metastatic disease, when should his AFP and β-hCG return to normal?**

The metabolic half-life of AFP is 5 to 7 days. Thus, using conservative estimates, the AFP should be normal (<9) in about 4 weeks. The serum half-life of β-hCG is 24 to 36 hours. Thus, using conservative estimates, the β-hCG should be normal (<2) in about 11 days.

○   **A family practitioner refers a 3-month-old boy to you for evaluation of a left testis mass. He was concerned about a testis tumor and sent tumor markers. AFP was 57 and β-hCG was <2. On examination, the infant has a swollen left testis that is twice the size of the right testis. The epididymis cannot readily be distinguished from the testis. What is the next step in the evaluation and how likely is this child to have testicular cancer?**

The next step in evaluation is a testicular ultrasound. The child is very unlikely to have testis cancer. The physical examination is much more suggestive of epididymitis or a missed torsion. Testicular cancer is unusual in infants. The most common testicular cancer would be a yolk sac tumor where the peak incidence is 2 years of age. AFP is produced by the fetus and is measurable at very high levels from the 12th week of gestation. The level gradually falls thereafter and reaches normal levels by the end of the first year of life.

○   **A 22-year-old college student was playing a vigorous game of touch football. He does not specifically remember being hit in the genital area but following the game he has an aching pain in his right testicle. He performs a testicular self-examination and feels a testicular mass. Your examination confirms that the right testicle is larger than the left with some thickening at the lower pole. What is the most likely diagnosis and how should the testicle be evaluated?**

Scrotal ultrasound should be the next step in the evaluation. Many testis tumors are noticed after only minor trauma, but in this case, the diagnosis is uncertain. Therefore, the initial evaluation should be the inexpensive, noninvasive, and sensitive screening study of a scrotal ultrasound.

○   **A 24-year-old has a testicular ultrasound for evaluation of a dragging sensation in his right testicle. He is referred to see you as the ultrasound showed "bilateral microlithiasis." The patient has no other complaints or problems. His discomfort is improving and has been attributed to a sports injury. His physical examination is normal with no testicular masses. The ultrasound is a good-quality study and shows approximately 15 to 20 small (<2 mm) microcalcifications distributed throughout the body of both testes. What is the risk of testicular cancer and what should be the next step in his evaluation? What is the recommended follow-up?**

Instruct the patient to perform regular testis self-examination and seek prompt evaluation if he notices a mass. Large studies of army recruits have demonstrated that testicular microlithiasis is not associated with a substantially increased risk of subsequent testis cancer development. Thus, no further evaluation is necessary, short of teaching the patient to perform testicular self-examination.

○   **A 62-year-old man has gradual painless swelling of his left testicle. Physical examination is noticeable for diffuse enlargement and firmness of the left testicle. The right testis is normal. The remainder of his physical examination is normal. A left radical orchiectomy is performed. A low-power photomicrograph is shown below. What is the diagnosis?**

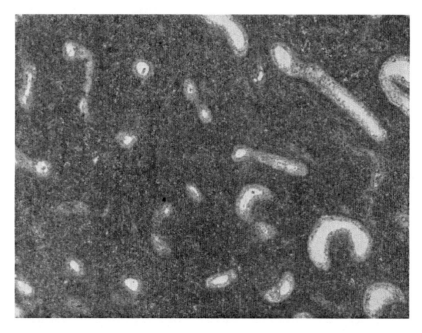

Lymphoma. It is the most common testicular tumor in men older than 60 years. The photomicrograph shows tubules surrounded by monotonous blue staining cells, an appearance that is characteristic for testicular infiltration by lymphoma.

○ A 59-year-old man noticed a mass at the upper pole of the right testicle. He is otherwise healthy and asymptomatic. β-hCG is 110 (normal <2). Alpha feto protein is 256 (normal < 9). His ultrasound is shown below. He undergoes a right radical orchiectomy. What is the most likely diagnosis?

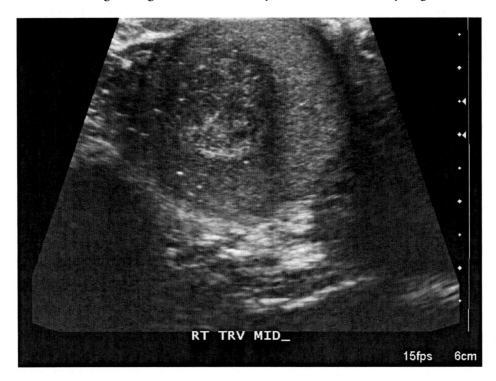

Mixed germ cell tumor. A seminoma would be a more common tumor in this age group. However, the presence of an elevated alpha feto protein excludes this diagnosis. The presence of elevated tumor markers essentially rules out a lymphoma and a Leydig cell tumor.

○ A 35-year-old man has a right testis biopsy as part of an evaluation for infertility and is found to have carcinoma in situ (CIS) (or intratubular germ cell neoplasia). Prior to the testis biopsy, he had a small right testis but no masses were palpable. A right testis U/S showed a decrease in testicular volume with normal echo texture throughout. As a child, he had a left undescended testicle that was removed at age 8. He is otherwise healthy. His physical examination is normal. He is azoospermic. His FSH is elevated at three times normal. Serum testosterone is normal. What are the treatment options and what is his best option to both minimize his risk of developing testis cancer and maintain as much physiological function as possible?

Options include immediate radical orchiectomy, observation, radiation to the testicle, and chemotherapy. The best option to minimize testis cancer risk and preserve as much physiological function as possible is low-dose radiation to the testicle (14 Gy). The patient is almost certainly infertile given his elevated FSH and azoospermia. Therefore, preservation of endocrine function and eradication of CIS are the primary goals of therapy; 14 Gy of irradiation has been shown to effectively achieve this goal in European studies. Chemotherapy can also eradicate CIS. However, the optimal schedule is not known and it is less reliable than radiation. Observation is an option but the patient is quite likely to develop a germ cell tumor at a future date. Radical orchiectomy will cure the cancer but not help his physiological functioning.

○ **A 32-year-old man undergoes a right orchiectomy for a stage I nonseminomatous germ cell tumor and enters a surveillance protocol. At the end of 1 year, he is asymptomatic, all radiologic and laboratory studies are negative. He asks you what are his chances of developing a tumor in the opposite testicle?**

Approximately 2% to 4% of patients develop a contralateral germ cell tumor which is a 20- to 40-fold increased risk compared to the general population. For this reason, it is important to teach patients with testicular tumors to perform regular contralateral testicular self-examination.

○ **A 28-year-old man, treated by a left radical orchiectomy with adjuvant chemotherapy for a stage II nonseminomatous germ cell tumor presents with a 2-cm right lower pole testicular mass. Tumor markers are negative. An ultrasound demonstrates a solid mass located on the anterior surface of the lower pole of the right testis. The remainder of the testis is normal. The patient is recently married and is interested in having children in the future. What are the management options?**

There are three management options:

1. Radical orchiectomy, which is associated with significant permanent endocrine abnormalities and sterility but assures local control.

2. Partial orchiectomy followed by low-dose radiation (20 Gy), which is associated with sterility but preserves endocrine function and is associated with a low incidence of local recurrence.

3. Partial orchiectomy alone, which preserves endocrine function and may preserve fertility but is associated with a higher risk of local failure. As this patient has a favorably located tumor, partial orchiectomy with negative margins preceded by sperm banking would be a good therapeutic choice.

○ **A 28-year-old man, 4 years following orchiectomy and adjuvant chemotherapy (three cycles of BEP) for a left stage II nonseminomatous germ cell tumor, presents with a 2 cm right lower pole testicular mass. Tumor markers are negative. An ultrasound demonstrates a solid mass. What is the likely histology and why did the systemic chemotherapy not prevent the formation of this tumor?**

Patients less than 30 years of age, who are diagnosed with germ cell tumors, are at higher risk of developing recurrent tumors. If the tumor is diagnosed within 5 years of the prior tumor it is more likely to be of similar histology. There is some controversy as to whether prior chemotherapy is protective in preventing subsequent germ cell tumor formation. The likely reason for the absence of full protection is poor diffusion of chemotherapy across the blood testis barrier. Additionally, 5% of patients with unilateral testis cancer have contralateral CIS and studies have shown that the cumulative incidence of recurrent CIS after chemotherapy in this subgroup is approximately 40%.

○ **A 22-year-old man has a right orchiectomy for a pT2 mixed germ cell tumor. Prior to orchiectomy, his β-hCG was 256, alpha feto protein (AFP) was 58, and lactic dehydrogenase (LDH) was normal. He is asymptomatic and his physical examination is unremarkable. All of the following are imaging options chest x-ray, CT of chest and abdomen, PET/CT fusion imaging of chest and abdomen. Which is the most appropriate choice?**

CT of the chest and abdomen: The most common sites of disease in a patient with a newly diagnosed NSGCT are the retroperitoneal lymph nodes and the lungs. These areas should be routinely imaged. In the past, investigators have argued that a chest x-ray is sufficient for lung imaging in the absence of disease in the retroperitoneum. However, a chest CT has a much higher sensitivity than a chest x-ray and is almost certainly a better choice. A PET CT fusion study is much more expensive and in a prospective study has not been shown to provide reliable additional information in patients with NSGCT.

○   **A 19-year-old has a right orchiectomy for a pT2 NSGCT. His tumor markers, which were previously elevated, have returned to normal as predicted by their half-lives. His CT scan of the chest and abdomen are normal. He has seen a medical oncologist, who, after reviewing the pathology report, told him that if he had an RPLND the chances that microscopic disease would be found in his lymph nodes was approximately 60%. What additional information in the pathology report allowed the medical oncologist to draw this conclusion?**

The presence of vascular invasion and the percentage of embryonal cancer. The combination of vascular invasion and a high percentage (>40%) of embryonal cancer in the primary tumor is associated with an elevated risk of finding disease in the retroperitoneum at RPLND.

○   **A 22-year-old single student has a newly diagnosed IGCCC (international germ cell cancer consensus) low risk metastatic testis cancer. He has seen a medical oncologist and is fit for and understands the risks of chemotherapy. However, prior to initiating chemotherapy, he should consider what additional precautionary procedure?**

Sperm Banking. Treatment of testis cancer has the potential to lead to azoospermia. Therefore, all patients should be encouraged to consider sperm banking prior to initiating therapy. Between 40% and 60% of patients with testicular cancer are hypofertile at diagnosis with sperm counts returning to normal in 75% of patients following orchiectomy. With newer reproductive technologies, fertility is likely to be possible for more than 80% of patients. Sperm banking is a sensible precaution as the sperm can be discarded after 2 to 3 years if the patient remains disease-free and the sperm count reverts to normal.

○   **A 30-year-old man presents with a left testicular mass. He undergoes a left orchiectomy. Pathology shows a 4-cm embryonal cancer invading the tunica albuginea. Vascular invasion is noted. Metastatic workup consists of an abdominal MRI scan. (A representative slice is shown below.) Chest CT scan shows five 0.5-cm to 2-cm lung nodules. LDH is three times normal. β-hCG is 3000. AFP is 1500. What stage is the patient according to the 6th Edition (c.2002) of the Manual of American Joint Commission on Cancer TNM staging system?**

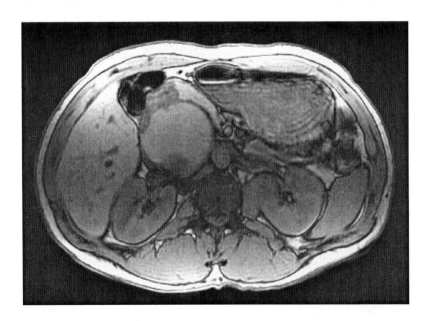

MRI shows a 9-cm intra-aortocaval nodal mass. The patient has a T2N3S2M1a, stage IIIB tumor.

○ **A 35-year-old man is diagnosed with a T1N0M0S1 pure seminoma. His β-hCG was 56 at diagnosis and 14 days later is <2. A CT scan of the chest, abdomen, and pelvis are normal. What is his risk of recurrence if he has no further treatment? How does this risk change if he elects to receive 20 to 25 Gy of radiation therapy to the standard retroperitoneal field?**

The risk of recurrence for a patient with a stage I seminoma on surveillance is approximately 15%. In large studies, the risk of recurrence with adjuvant radiation for stage I seminoma is 2% to 4%.

○ **The same patient of the previous question is considering either adjuvant radiation or a single dose of carboplatin as adjuvant therapy for his stage I seminoma. What are the advantages, if any, of single dose of carboplatin when compared to radiation therapy?**

A large, randomized study demonstrated equivalence of 20 Gy of retroperitoneal irradiation to a single dose of carboplatin. Subjects in the carboplatin arm had less of a decrease in their quality of life scores and more recent data suggests that they also had a decrease in the frequency of secondary contralateral testis tumors.

○ **A 28-year-old man is diagnosed with an anaplastic seminoma after a left radical orchiectomy. Tumor markers are normal. A CT scan of the chest is normal. A CT scan of the abdomen demonstrated a 2-cm left para-aortic lymph node just below the left renal vein. The patient is asymptomatic and otherwise healthy. What is the recommended treatment? How would this be different if the patient had a pure seminoma as compared to an anaplastic seminoma?**

The recommended treatment is 35 to 40 Gy of retroperitoneal radiation to a retro peritoneal and ipsilateral iliac field. There is no evidence that anaplastic seminomas should be treated differently to standard seminomas stage for stage. There is some evidence that seminomas with an anaplastic histology present at a more advanced stage. Standard therapy for a low-volume stage II seminoma is retroperitoneal irradiation.

○ **A 63-year-old man is diagnosed with a spermatocytic seminoma after a left radical orchiectomy. Tumor markers are normal. A CT scan of the chest, abdomen, and pelvis are normal. What is the recommended treatment? How would this be different if the patient had a pure seminoma as compared to a spermatocytic seminoma?**

The risk of metastatic disease associated with spermatocytic seminoma is extremely low. Thus, surveillance is the recommended course of action. If the patient had a pure seminoma, the risk of recurrence is approximately 15%, thus a discussion of adjuvant radiation or single dose of carboplatin (AUC = 7) is appropriate.

○   A 44-year-old man has a right orchiectomy for a 4-cm testis tumor. A representative high power micrograph is shown below. Preoperative tumor markers were notable for a β-hCG of 200. AFP is four and LDH is one and a half times normal. A CT scan of the chest is normal. A CT scan of the abdomen and pelvis shows a large 7-cm mass surrounding the aorta and inferior vena cava, just below the renal vessels. The patient is otherwise healthy and asymptomatic. One week after his orchiectomy, his β-hCG is 108. What is the diagnosis, tumor stage, and recommended therapy?

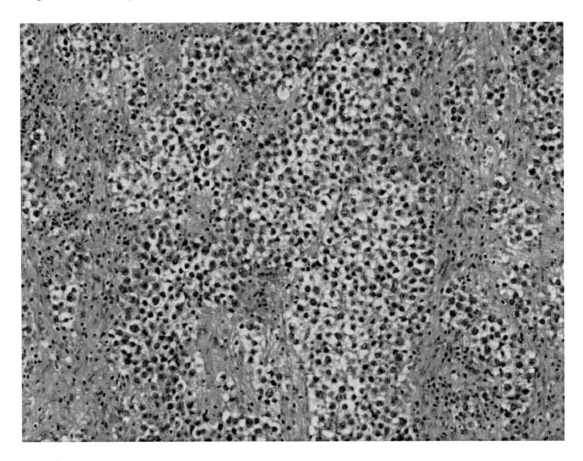

The slides show a pure seminoma, thus the patient has bulky stage II seminoma (T1N3M0S1). In the past, treatment would have consisted of retroperitoneal irradiation (35–40 Gy). Now, most centers recommend chemotherapy (three cycles BEP or four cycles EP). Results with retroperitoneal irradiation are variable with recurrence-free survival rates ranging between 45% and 100%. Most patients who fail radiation are salvaged with subsequent chemotherapy. Initial chemotherapy in patients with bulky (>5 cm) disease avoids the necessity for dual treatment in 20% to 50% of patients.

○   A 38-year-old man has a right orchiectomy for a 5-cm pure seminoma. Preoperative tumor markers were notable for a β-hCG of 200. AFP is four and LDH is one and a half times normal. A CT scan of the chest shows three separate 1-cm lung nodules. A CT scan of the abdomen and pelvis shows a large 9.8-cm mass surrounding the aorta and inferior vena cava just below the renal vessels. The patient is otherwise healthy and asymptomatic. He completes three cycles of BEP chemotherapy. Restaging CT scans show resolution of the lung nodules. The mass in the abdomen has shrunk to 3.4 cm in maximum diameter 2 weeks after completing chemotherapy. Tumor markers are normal. What additional testing should be performed and how will this be used in decision making regarding further therapy?

There is considerable controversy about the best management of a residual mass after chemotherapy for a pure seminoma with some groups suggesting resection of residual masses >3 cm in size and others recommending observation or irradiation. A PET/CT scan can help assess the risk that the mass contains residual active germ cell tumor. Recent reports indicate that a PET scan has an 80% sensitivity and 100% specificity for the detection of viable germ cell tumor in a retroperitoneal mass following chemotherapy for pure seminoma.

In general, surgery should be confined to resecting residual masses. A bilateral retroperitoneal lymph node dissection is not recommended after the chemotherapy for seminoma because of the increased risk of complications due to the extensive fibrosis and desmoplastic reaction.

○ **A 37-year-old patient has an orchiectomy for a 6-cm pure seminoma. He refuses additional therapy and is lost to follow-up. Two years later he is admitted to the hospital with extensive metastatic seminoma with bone and liver metastases. AFP is <6, β-hCG is normal, and LDH is 13 times normal. Liver biopsy confirms metastatic seminoma. What is his international germ cell consensus classification (IGCCC) risk level? What is the recommended therapy and what is the patient's likelihood of cure?**

The patient has intermediate risk disease by the international germ cell consensus classification (IGCCC). Although the patient has what would be considered to be high-risk disease if he had a NSGCT, no seminoma is considered high risk. The recommended therapy for intermediate risk disease is four cycles of BEP, which is likely to achieve about an 80% cure rate.

○ **A 19-year-old man has a right orchiectomy for a mixed NSGCT (40% embryonal, 20% teratoma, 30% seminoma, 10% yolk sac). Vascular invasion is noted on pathology. Prior to orchiectomy, β-hCG was 4 and AFP was 52. A CT scan of the chest, abdomen, and pelvis show no evidence of disease. He decides to proceed with a right template nerve sparing RPLND. He comes for his preoperative visit 3 weeks after his orchiectomy and 1 week prior to surgery. He feels well and his examination is completely normal. His β-hCG is <2 his and AFP is 40. On the morning of surgery his AFP is 56. How should you proceed?**

Cancel the surgery and proceed with three cycles of bleomycin, etoposide, and cis-Platinum chemotherapy or four cycles of etoposide and cis-platinum. Patients with clinical stage I NSGCT who have persistently elevated markers prior to RPLND have a higher incidence of microscopic metastatic disease outside the retroperitoneum, therefore, primary chemotherapy is the preferred alternative.

○ **A 27-year-old has a left orchiectomy for a mixed NSGCT (10% embryonal, 50% teratoma, 20% seminoma, 20% yolk sac). Vascular invasion is not noted on pathology (T1N0M0). AFP was 200 and β-hCG was 60 prior to orchiectomy. Both tumor markers are now normal. The patient is otherwise healthy. What is the likelihood of finding retroperitoneal disease if he has an RPLND.**

Approximately 15%. The patient has a low percentage of embryonal cancer and no vascular invasion, thus is at lower risk of retroperitoneal disease and a candidate for surveillance.

○ **A 27-year-old has a left orchiectomy for a mixed NSGCT (10% embryonal, 50% teratoma, 20% seminoma, 20% yolk sac). Vascular invasion is not noted on pathology (T1N0M0). AFP was 200 and β-hCG was 60 prior to orchiectomy. Both tumor markers are now normal. The patient is otherwise healthy. He elects surveillance. If he has a normal physical examination, tumor markers, and CT scan of the chest abdomen and pelvis at 1 year, what is his likelihood of having a recurrence now?**

The patient has low risk NSGCT with only a 15% chance of relapse in total. Of those on surveillance 85% will relapse within the first year. Thus, with no evidence of relapse at 12 months, his risk of relapse in the future is <3%.

○   A 36-year-old homeless alcoholic undergoes a left orchiectomy for a pathological stage T1 nonseminomatous germ cell tumor (20% embryonal, 40% seminoma, 40% yolk sac). Tumor markers prior to orchiectomy were β-hCG 30 and AFP 45. An abdominal CT scan and chest x-ray show no evidence of disease. He is lost to follow-up. Five-years later he returns to your office and wants follow-up. He has recently married and is currently working. He has no complaints and physical examination is normal. Tumor markers are notable for an AFP of 20 (normal <9). β-hCG is normal. Chest X-ray and abdominal CT scans are normal. What is the cause of his AFP elevation and what further management is necessary?

Elevated AFP can be seen in patients with hepatocellular, pancreatic, gastric, and lung carcinomas as well as benign conditions such as cirrhosis and hepatitis. This patient had a low-risk tumor at diagnosis (T1, low percentage of embryonal cell) and has negative evaluation 5-years after diagnosis. He is unlikely to have recurrent testicular cancer and should be evaluated for liver disease due to his history of alcohol abuse.

○   A 25-year-old male receives four cycles of chemotherapy for a stage III nonseminomatous germ cell tumor. At diagnosis, both β-hCG and AFP were markedly elevated. He is now 1 month after completing chemotherapy and his β-hCG has been stable for 2 months but slightly elevated at four (normal <2). He has no complaints. Physical examination is notable only for an absent right testicle and a small soft left testicle. An extensive radiologic evaluation demonstrates a complete response. What is the next step in this patient's management?

Low-level β-hCG elevations following treatment of germ cell tumors have been divided into three categories: (1) false-positive (phantom hCG), (2) quiescent germ cell tumor, and (3) unexplained increase in hCG. In general, false-positive assays can be diagnosed by demonstrating that hCG cannot be measured by (a) a different assay or (b) cannot be measured simultaneously in the urine. Differentiating between quiescent germ cell tumors and an unexplained increase can be more difficult. The diagnosis often only becomes clear by either resolution of the elevation (unexplained increase) or successive increases (quiescent germ cell tumor).

○   A 29-year-old has a left orchiectomy for a mixed germ cell tumor (70% embryonal, 30% yolk sac). Tumor markers are negative. Laboratory tests and chest x-ray are normal. CT scan of the abdomen and pelvis is shown below. What is the likelihood that the patient will be found to have metastatic germ cell tumor at the time of RPLND?

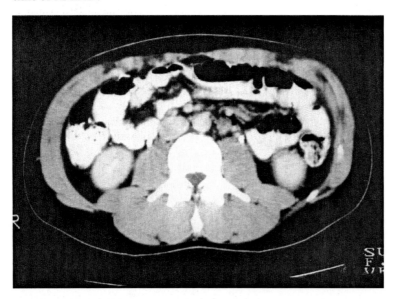

The CT scan shows a 1.5-cm node in the primary landing site of the left testicle. The likelihood that this contains tumor is approximately 75%.

○ **A 27-year-old man undergoes a left orchiectomy. Pathology shows a T1 nonseminomatous germ cell tumor (50% teratoma, 40% embryonal cell carcinoma, and 10% seminoma. Vascular invasion is noted). Within the teratomatous component, foci of dedifferentiation to squamous cell carcinoma are noted. Metastatic evaluation including chest x-ray, abdominal CT scan, and tumor markers are all normal. How does the presence of the squamous cell carcinoma effect the management of this patient?**

The presence of dedifferentiation into another malignant tumor type within a teratoma is found in approximately 2% of patients. If the patient has stage I disease the current recommendation is to treat these patients as you would a patient with a standard NSGCT. Thus, the recommendation would be for the patient to undergo a modified left template nerve sparing RPLND. In the presence of metastatic disease, most patients do not respond to primary cisplatin-based chemotherapy. In these cases, the treatment needs to be tailored to the stage and histologic subtype of the tumor.

○ **A 28-year-old man with an embryonal carcinoma of the left testicle, normal tumor markers, and negative metastatic evaluation undergoes a modified template RPLND. What are the chances that he will have normal antegrade ejaculation? If the surgeon prospectively preserves the sympathetic nerves at the time of the template RPLND, how much will that improve the rate of antegrade ejaculation?**

A template RPLND will result in approximately 75% of patients ejaculating normally. If prospective nerve sparing is performed, this will increase up to approximately 98%.

○ **RPLND can be performed in either an open or laparoscopic fashion. What is the major criticism that open surgeons have of a laparoscopic RPLND?**

Although many criticisms have been leveled at laparoscopic surgery, the main concern is that the completeness of the laparoscopic dissection is less than that of an open procedure, thus the recurrence rates in the retroperitoneum may turn out to be higher. Open surgeons claim that the low recurrence rates reported in laparoscopic RPLND series are a reflection of the increased use of chemotherapy for patients found to have pN1 disease. The validity of these claims is uncertain and this is an area of continuing controversy.

○ **A 25-year-old man is undergoing a right modified template RPLND for a clinical stage I testis cancer. On abdominal exploration, you note he has a 4 cm healthy appendix. Should an appendectomy be performed at the time of RPLND?**

An incidental appendectomy performed at the time of RPLND increases the risk of an infectious complication from 2% to approximately 10%. Therefore, incidental appendectomy at the time of RPLND is not recommended.

○ **You are planning a left nerve-sparing template RPLND for a T2N0M0 NSGCT in a 24-year-old, newly married man who desires four children. What are your boundaries of the dissection?**

The boundaries of dissection are superiorly the renal artery and vein, inferiorly the bifurcation of the common iliac artery, laterally the ureter, and medially the medial boarder of the aorta to the level of the inferior mesenteric artery. Below the inferior mesenteric artery, the boundaries are the lateral aspect of the aorta and the common iliac artery. Additional inter aortocaval nodes should be removed below the right renal artery.

○ **A 25-year-old man with an embryonal carcinoma of the right testicle, normal tumor markers, and negative metastatic evaluation undergoes a modified right nerve sparing RPLND. What are the boundaries of dissection?**

The boundaries of dissection are superiorly the right renal artery and vein, inferiorly the bifurcation of the common iliac artery, laterally the ureter, and medially the midpoint of the aorta to the level of the inferior mesenteric artery. Below the inferior mesenteric artery, the boundaries are the lateral aspect of the aorta and the common iliac artery.

○   **What are the anatomical/physiological types of the nerves that control emission and ejaculation that are preserved at the time of a nerve sparing RPLND?**

Postganglionic sympathetic fibers originating from the T12 through L4 vertebral levels.

○   **A 23-year-old man with a stage I NSGCT undergoes a template RPLND for a final T1N0M0 NSGCT. A total of 26 nodes are resected and all are negative. What is his risk of relapse? If a relapse were to occur, what anatomical site would be the most likely?**

His risk of relapse within 2 years is between 5% and 10% and the likely site of relapse is the lungs. Approximately 75% of these patients relapsed in the lungs and approximately 15% of patients developed a marker-only recurrence. A properly performed negative RPLND makes patient follow-up substantially easier as it makes relapse in the retroperitoneum unlikely. Thus follow-up can be focused with tumor markers and chest x-rays.

○   **A 25-year-old man with an embryonal carcinoma of the left testicle, normal tumor markers, and negative metastatic evaluation undergoes a modified left template nerve sparing RPLND. At the time of RPLND, gross nodal disease is unexpectedly discovered in the interaortocaval area. What is the appropriate course of action?**

The surgeon should abandon the plan to perform a modified left template operation and proceed with a full bilateral node dissection (nerve sparing if possible).

○   **Two cycles of BEP chemotherapy is an option for adjuvant therapy in a patient with a stage I nonseminomatous germ cell tumor with high-risk features in the primary tumor. What are the primary advantages of adjuvant BEP as compared to RPLND?**

The primary advantage of chemotherapy, especially for high-risk patients (>40% embryonal cancer and vascular invasion) is the avoidance of surgery and the decreased risk of systemic relapse.

○   **A 32-year-old is referred to you after undergoing a transscrotal exploration followed by an inguinal orchiectomy for an unsuspected nonseminomatous germ cell tumor. After orchiectomy, his tumor markers remain persistently elevated and he receives three cycles of BEP chemotherapy. Clinical, laboratory, and radiological examination show no evidence of disease 1 month after completion of his chemotherapy. He is referred to you for a hemiscrotectomy. What is your recommendation?**

Reports indicate that scrotal violation at the time of orchiectomy demonstrated no evidence of local recurrence in those patients who had received subsequent chemotherapy. Therefore, no surgery is indicated and the patient should be observed.

○   **A 24-year-old man has a right orchiectomy for a T1 NSGCT (40% embryonal, 40% teratoma, and 20% yolk sac). Tumor markers prior to orchiectomy were AFP 78 and a β-hCG of <2. Following orchiectomy, his tumor markers return to normal. A CT scan of the chest is normal. A CT of the abdomen demonstrates a single 1.3-cm lymph node in the intra aortocaval area at the level of the inferior mesenteric artery. He undergoes an RPLND. He has 3/18 lymph nodes that demonstrate <1 cm of embryonal cancer. What is the recommended adjuvant therapy and what are the chances of a relapse without it? What is the likelihood of a relapse following adjuvant therapy? What is the overall difference in survival for such patients treated with immediate adjuvant therapy or surveillance and definitive therapy if relapse occurs?**

In several series, RPLND has been shown to cure 85% to 90% of patients with low-volume N1 testis cancer. However, in a large randomized trial, about 48% of patients with N1-3 disease relapsed following RPLND. Two cycles of adjuvant BEP chemotherapy prevented relapse in 98% of pN1-3 patients. Both an initial observation (followed by chemotherapy on relapse) and an immediate adjuvant approach cured a similar proportion (>97%) of patients.

○ **A 28-year-old, newly married patient is diagnosed with a low-risk metastatic nonseminomatous germ cell tumor. He has fathered a child in a previous relationship. His wife wants to know what are his chances of future fertility and how long will it take his sperm count to recover from chemotherapy. She also wants to know if future children will be at increased risk of developing congenital abnormalities.**

Combination chemotherapy for testis cancer is toxic to both spermatogenesis and Leydig cell function. Almost all patients become azoospermic during chemotherapy. The toxicity is usually reversible with approximately 50% of patients having normal sperm counts at 2 years. Approximately 25% of patients have persistent azoospermia. The couple should be advised to delay conception for at least 6 months after completing chemotherapy as there is a risk of congenital malformations during this period. Children conceived after 6 months of patients been treated for testis cancer do not appear to be at increased risk of congenital malformations.

○ **A patient with intermediate risk nonseminomatous germ cell tumor is about to start BEP chemotherapy. He requests that you inform him of the major long-term risks of this treatment.**

There are six major long-term risks:

(1) Infertility—Combination chemotherapy for testis cancer is toxic to spermatogenesis. Almost all patients become azoospermic during chemotherapy. The toxicity is usually reversible with approximately 50% of patients having normal sperm counts at 2 years. Approximately 25% of patients have persistent azoospermia.

(2) Nephrotoxicity—Most patients have an irreversible decline in renal function after cisplatin chemotherapy. However, in general, this is subclinical.

(3) Raynaud's phenomenon, which occurs in 20% to 50% of patients following cisplatin and bleomycin chemotherapy.

(4) Neurotoxicity—Clinically relevant peripheral neuropathy occurs in 10% to 40% of patients. Injury to the 8th cranial nerve from cisplatin causes tinnitus in up to 30% of patients. However, major hearing loss is rare.

(5) Pulmonary toxicity—Bleomycin-induced pulmonary fibrosis occurs when the dose exceeds 450 to 500 units (four cycles of standard BEP contains 360 units of bleomycin). Bleomycin pulmonary toxicity is fatal in 1% to 2% of patients and clinically significant fibrosis occurs in an additional 2% to 3%.

(6) Cardiovascular toxicity—Cisplatinum-based chemotherapy is associated with a relatively small risk of short-term cardiovascular toxicity (MI, thromboembolic disease). However, more concerning is the apparent long-term increased risk of hypertension, hyperlipidemia, and the metabolic syndrome with a consequent increased risk of early cardiovascular morbidity and mortality in patients receiving a total dose of greater than 400 mg/m^2 of cisplatinum.

○ **A 29-year-old man has a left orchiectomy for a T2 NSGCT. His AFP prior to orchiectomy is 3517, β-hCG is 286, and LDH 3.5 times normal. The chest CT shows multiple lung metastases. His abdominal CT scan shows a 6-cm mass surrounding the aorta. He has moderate back pain but is otherwise asymptomatic and healthy. What is his IGCCC risk class? What is recommended therapy? What is his chance of being disease free in 5 years?**

Intermediate risk. The IGCCC risk category is useful to stage patients with metastatic testis cancer. The patient has an IGCCC intermediate risk category based on his AFP being between 1000 and 10,000 and LDH that is between 1.5 and 10 times normal and no extrapulmonary metastatic disease. The patient should receive four cycles of BEP chemotherapy. Progression free survival at 5 years is about 80%.

○   **A 29-year-old man has a left orchiectomy for a T2 NSGCT. His AFP prior to orchiectomy is 3517, β-hCG is 286, LDH three and a half times normal. The chest CT shows multiple lung metastases. His abdominal CT scan shows a 6-cm mass surrounding the aorta. He receives four cycles of BEP chemotherapy. Tumor markers are normal and repeat CT scans show a residual 2-cm left lung nodule and a 4-cm intra-aortocaval residual mass. What is the next step in management?**

The next step in management is resection of the residual retroperitoneal mass and bilateral RPLND followed by lung resection. In general, following chemotherapy for metastatic NSGCT, all significant residual masses should be surgically removed. The general recommendation is to resect the retroperitoneal mass prior to proceeding to resection of the lung masses. The reason is that the residual retroperitoneal tissue is more likely to represent viable germ cell cancer. In patients with a NSGCT, it is recommended that a bilateral RPLND be performed in the postchemotherapy setting rather than a modified dissection, as lymphatic channel obstruction by the tumor can result in changes of the lymphatic drainage pattern thus resulting in microscopic residual disease outside the primary lymphatic drainage area of the effected testicle.

○   **In the same patient as above, the retroperitoneal mass is resected followed by a bilateral RPLND and wedge resection of the lung mass. The retroperitoneal mass is resected followed by a bilateral RPLND and then the lung mass is removed by a wedge resection. Pathology reveals necrosis and benign teratoma. What is the next step in management and what is the patient's risk of recurrence at 5 years?**

The next best step in management is follow-up with tumor markers and a chest x-ray every 2 to 3 months with an abdomen/pelvis CT scan in 6 months. The final pathology does not show active germ cell tumor; therefore, additional therapy is not necessary. The patient's risk of recurrence at 5 years is <10%.

○   **A 22-year-old man is scheduled for a postchemotherapy retroperitoneal node dissection. On reviewing the records, it is apparent that he has received a total of 550 units of bleomycin over the course of his chemotherapy. He reports that he noticed a dry cough during the last cycle of chemotherapy, but currently has no respiratory symptoms. What perioperative testing and precautions may aid in the management of this patient?**

A series of five deaths after bleomycin chemotherapy in the 1970s drew attention to the problem of postoperative pulmonary problems. The causes of bleomycin pulmonary toxicity are not entirely clear but an increased incidence occurs once the cumulative dose is greater than 400 to 450 units. Preoperative pulmonary function tests (CO diffusion and forced vital capacity) maybe useful in identifying patients at higher risk. Careful management (restriction) of perioperative fluids and transfusions as well as minimizing the operative time are important interventions that may decrease the risk of this complication. More recent studies have questioned the need to maintain low levels of inspired (28%) oxygen during the perioperative period.

○   **A 25-year-old man with an embryonal carcinoma of the left testicle, normal tumor markers, and negative metastatic evaluation undergoes a modified left nerve sparing RPLND. At the time of RPLND, gross nodal disease is unexpectedly discovered in the inter aortocaval area. The surgeon performs a bilateral non-nerve-sparing dissection. How likely is the patient to ejaculate normally?**

Reports indicate that 18% of patients undergoing a bilateral infra hilar node dissection had antegrade ejaculation. If an extended suprahilar dissection was performed, the rate decreases to 9%.

○   **A 30-year-old with a clinical stage I nonseminomatous germ cell tumor is considering having an RPLND and asks that aside from ejaculatory problems, what are the most common short- and long-term complications of the procedure. What would you tell him?**

In a report from the Testicular Inter Group Study, 3.4% of patients undergoing RPLND had a prolonged ileus for greater than 7 days, 3.3% developed pneumonia, and 2% a UTI. Long-term complications included a 2.3% incidence of small bowel obstruction for an overall significant complication rate of 13.8%. Rarer complications included intraoperative hemorrhage, enterotomy, unplanned nephrectomy, thromboembolism, chylous fistula, lymphocele, and pancreatitis.

○ **Resection of residual masses after chemotherapy for seminoma is controversial. However, resection of residual masses after chemotherapy for a NSGCT is not. What is the reason for this controversy?**

The reasons for controversy are twofold and related. First, surgery after chemotherapy for seminoma is more difficult and with increased risk due to an extensive fibrotic reaction. Secondly, surgery is less likely to be beneficial to the patient with seminoma as just scar/necrotic tissue is identified in approximately 70% to 80% of patients; therefore, these patients will not benefit from the surgery. In patients with NSGCT, approximately 60% to 70% benefit as benign teratoma or active germ cell tumor is identified and removed.

○ **In patients with NSGCT, three things are commonly found in residual masses following chemotherapy: in approximately 20% active germ cell tumor, in about 40% benign teratoma, and in about 40% necrosis. What possible complications can result from failing to resect residual masses that just contain benign teratoma following chemotherapy for testis cancer?**

Benign teratoma can undergo secondary malignant degeneration within one of its elements leading to a carcinoma or sarcoma that, in general, is poorly responsive to chemotherapy. Benign teratomas grow slowly in size and eventually cause symptoms because of a local mass effect. These are the two primary rationales for resection of benign teratoma.

○ **An 18-year-old has a T2N3M0 S1 NSGCT. He undergoes a right orchiectomy followed by three cycles of BEP. Tumor markers are now normal and a 10-cm retroperitoneal mass has decreased in size to 5.8 cm. He undergoes resection of the mass. Final pathology shows necrosis and benign teratoma with several nodes containing multiple small foci of embryonal cancer. All margins are negative. What is the risk that this patient will have a recurrence of testis cancer following his surgery and what is the next step in his management?**

The patient should receive two further cycles of chemotherapy. Studies indicate that 100% of patients with this clinical scenario who do not receive adjuvant therapy relapse compared to less than 70% receiving chemotherapy. There is controversy as to the best choice of chemotherapy with some authors recommending BEP and others a change in drug choice given the incomplete response in the primary tumor.

○ **A patient has an RPLND for a nonseminomatous germ cell tumor. At RPLND he is found to have 4/12 nodes containing 1 cm³ of tumor each. Two cycles of BEP chemotherapy are recommended to the patient. He is reluctant to undergo the treatment as he has heard that chemotherapy can give you cancer. What information can you give him to support or refute this assertion?**

Large databases have suggested that patients treated for testicular cancer incur slightly increased risk of secondary malignancies. Etoposide treatment is associated with an increased risk of developing a secondary leukemia. However, the rate is less than 0.5% and would probably not occur unless additional cycles of etoposide-based chemotherapy are required.

○   A 35-year-old man presents with back pain. Physical examination is notable for a palpable abdominal mass. External genitalia is notable for bilaterally small testes but no palpable testis mass. Testis U/S is normal. A CT scan shows a 12-cm left para-aortic mass (see "A" below). β-hCG is 55 and AFP is 187. A CT biopsy of the retroperitoneal mass is consistent with a germ cell tumor, embryonal type. He attempts sperm banking but insufficient sperm are identified on semen analysis. He receives three cycles of BEP. Tumor markers normalize and his mass shrinks to 6 cm (see "B" below). Testis U/S continues to be normal. What is the next best step in management? If he has a left orchiectomy, what is the chance evidence of a prior germ cell tumor will be found in his testicle on pathological assessment?

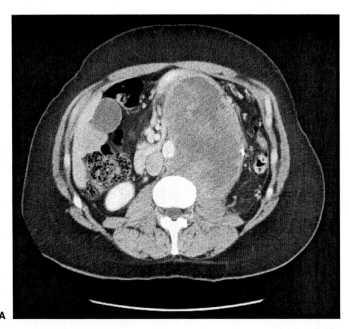

A

Prechemotherapy

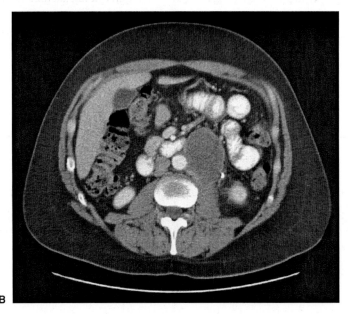

B

Postchemotherapy

It is unclear if the patient has a primary germ cell tumor of the retroperitoneum or a testis cancer that arose in the left testicle and has since undergone regression at the primary site. In small series, in which there is a clinical suspicion that the tumor arose in one particular testicle based on the pattern of the retroperitoneal nodal disease and no primary can be seen on testis U/S, a simultaneous orchiectomy identifies germ cell tumor or prior evidence of germ cell tumor in >70% of the resected testicles.

○ **A 26-year-old man has a right orchiectomy for a nonseminomatous germ cell tumor. Metastatic workup reveals a 10-cm interaortocaval mass and multiple 1-cm pulmonary nodules. β-hCG is 25,000, AFP is 2000 and LDH is six times normal. He receives four cycles of BEP with shrinkage of pulmonary metastases and the retroperitoneal mass. However, the β-hCG, which had been falling at the appropriate rate, is now noted to be increasing significantly. How should this patient be treated and what is his chance of a complete response?**

The patient is showing signs of progression upon completion of chemotherapy. The optimum treatment would be high-dose therapy with carboplatin and etoposide combined with peripheral blood stem cell or autologous bone marrow transplantation. Such regimens have reported long term survival rates of up to 70%.

○ **A 50-year-old man with a 3-year history of gynecomastia discovers a left testicular mass. A radical orchiectomy is performed. On bisecting the testicle, a 2-cm homogeneous brown tumor is seen in the upper pole. Pathology shows closely packed uniform cells with eosinophilic cytoplasm and Reinke crystals. What is the diagnosis and malignant potential of this tumor?**

The patient has a Leydig cell tumor. Approximately 10% of Leydig cell tumors are malignant. The malignant potential of these tumors is difficult to predict based on histology. However, in the absence of a histological suspicion of malignancy (no hemorrhage, uniform cells, few mitoses), observation is the preferred form of management.

○ **A 30-year-old man is referred to you by his family physician for a 1.5-cm epididymal mass. The patient has no complaints and did not notice anything unusual himself. Physical examination reveals a 1.5-cm mass in the epididymis that does not transilluminate. Ultrasound confirms a 1.5-cm homogeneous, solid, intraepididymal mass. What is the differential diagnoses and which is most likely?**

The most likely diagnosis is an adenomatoid tumor since it is the most common solid epididymal tumor. The differential diagnoses are paratesticular sarcoma, atypical spermatocele, or epididymal cyst. The mass is probably growing very slowly as the patient has not noticed a change. Therefore, it is likely a benign process and transscrotal excision is appropriate. If there is any suspicion of malignancy, an inguinal exploration is indicated.

○ **A 40-year-old man notices a mass in his right groin that has doubled in size in the last 2 months. He otherwise feels well. A radical orchiectomy is performed. Final pathology demonstrates a rhabdomyosarcoma. What are the major determinants of prognosis in patients with sarcomas?**

The main prognostic determinants of sarcomas are tumor grade, tumor size (greater or less than 5 cm), and the presence of metastases. Complete surgical resection with wide margins holds the best prospect for cure.

○ **What are epidermoid cysts of the testicle?**

Testicular epidermoid cysts are round, hard, well-circumscribed, and encapsulated intratesticular masses. They account for about 1% of all testicular tumors. They have a claylike, yellow center on cut section and are thought to be a monolayer form of teratoma. They are generally considered to be benign, although they may be associated with germ cell elements. Treatment is usually by radical orchiectomy because of the germ cell elements that may be present. However, local excision is possible and appropriate in select cases.

○ **How is teratoma in children different from teratoma in adults?**

In the pediatric age group, teratoma is always benign.

○ **What are the most common mesenchymal tumors of the testis?**

Fibromas, angiomas, leiomyomas, and neurofibromas. They are important mainly because they need to be distinguished from germ cell tumors.

○ **Sertoli cell tumor of the testis in prepubertal boys is associated with what genetic disorder?**

Peutz–Jeghers syndrome.

CHAPTER 49 Penile Cancer

Michael B. Williams, MD, MS,
John W. Davis, MD, and
Donald F. Lynch, Jr. MD, FACS

○ **True or False: Bowenoid papulosis of the penis is a premalignant condition with the natural history of progression to invasive disease.**

False. Bowenoid papulosis has the histologic criteria of carcinoma in situ, but usually has a benign course. Malignant transformation occurs only in 2.6%.

○ **What causes Bowenoid papulosis?**

It's caused by human papilloma virus, most often type 16.

○ **What is the best palliative treatment for a patient with AIDS and Kaposi's sarcoma of the glans penis causing obstruction?**

Radiation therapy.

○ **Which forms of Kaposi's sarcoma (KS) are associated with acquired immunodeficiency syndrome?**

Classic KS, immunosuppressive treatment-related KS, African KS, and epidemic KS.

○ **True or False: Verrucous carcinoma is a well-differentiated variant of squamous cell carcinoma with similar metastatic potential.**

False. Verrucous carcinoma of the penis invades locally and can cause local tissue destruction; metastasis does not occur unless invasive SCC coexists.

○ **True or False: Both verrucous carcinoma and condyloma acuminatum typically remain superficial lesions.**

False. Verrucous carcinoma can invade locally causing unrestrained local growth.

○ **Which of the following local treatments is not recommended for verrucous carcinoma and which is the standard recommended therapy: partial or total penectomy, Mohs surgery, radiation therapy, topical podophyllin, 5-fluorouracil, or Nd:YAG laser?**

Radiation therapy has been associated with malignant degeneration and is ineffective. Partial or total penectomy is standard therapy.

○ **What differentiates condyloma acuminata from Buschke–Lowenstein tumors?**

Condyloma never invade adjacent normal tissues and always remain superficial. Buschke–Lowenstein tumors displace and invade adjacent tissues destroying them.

○ **What other terms are used for penile carcinoma in situ?**

Penile carcinoma in situ is also known as erythroplasia of Queyrat when it involves the glans penis or prepuce, and Bowen's disease if it involves the penile shaft.

○ **A 55-year-old uncircumcised male presents with a 0.5-cm reddish, well-defined, barely raised plaque on the glans. The biopsy diagnosis is erythroplasia of Queyrat (CIS). What is the chance of progression to invasive disease and how is the lesion best managed?**

The relative risks of progression to an invasive lesion and development of metastases is 10% and 2%, respectively. Superficial premalignant lesions may be treated with local excision, topical 5-fluorouracil, or laser therapy. Sexual partners should be counseled and examined for CIS.

○ **For the lesion described in the previous question, what is the clinical differential diagnosis?**

Chronic circumscribed balanitis, inflammatory process, drug eruption, psoriasis, and lichen planus among others.

○ **True or False: The diagnosis of erythroplasia of Queyrat requires a biopsy.**

True.

○ **What is the importance in differentiating Bowenoid papulosis from Bowen's disease in the clinical setting?**

Bowenoid papulosis is a dysplastic lesion of the epithelium involving the penile shaft in younger men. The histopathologic appearance may be similar to other forms of CIS. The lesions are light brown to gray papules that may coalesce to form plaques. These lesions generally have an indolent course, respond well to excision or podophyllin, may spontaneously regress, and do not usually progress to invasive cancer. Bowenoid papulosis is similar to multifocal vulvovaginal dysplasia in young women.

○ **How does the incidence of squamous cell carcinoma of the penis (SCC) differ in the United States and Europe versus African and South American countries?**

In the United States and Europe, SCC of the penis accounts for only 0.4% to 0.6% of all male malignances. In some African and South American countries, SCC accounts for up to 10% of all diagnosed malignancies in men.

○ **In the United States, what is the ethnic population with the highest age-adjusted incidence of penile cancer per million?**

Hispanics are the highest at nearly seven patients per million. This is followed by blacks, whites, American Indians, and Asian Pacific islanders.

○ **Which age range has the highest incidence of penile cancer?**

If broken down by age, males older than 85 years of age have the highest incidence.

○ **Over the past three decades, is the incidence of penile carcinoma in the United States increasing, decreasing, or remaining constant?**

Based on SEER data, penile carcinoma rates are decreasing.

○ **Describe the relationship between penile cancer and circumcision.**

Chronic exposure to smegma in the prepubertal period is thought to contribute to the development of penile cancer. Phimosis may accentuate this effect, as it is a finding in up to 50% of cases of penile cancer. Neonatal circumcision virtually eliminates the risk of penile cancer, whereas adolescent or adult circumcision has no protective effect.

○ **True or False: In populations that practice good hygiene but are uncircumcised, the incidence of penile carcinoma is similar to that of circumcised populations.**

True.

○ **Name the risk factors for penile carcinoma.**

Sexually transmitted human papilloma virus (HPV), phimosis (smegma accumulation), lack of childhood circumcision, and smoking have been associated.

○ **What is human papilloma virus (HPV), approximately how many HPV subtypes are known, and which are well know to be benign versus malignant?**

HPV is a double-stranded, supercoiled DNA virus with more than 65 subtypes identified. "Low risk" strands HPV-6 and HPV-11 are associated with benign condylomata of the anogenital area. "High risk" types such as HPV-16, -18, -31, -33, -35, and -39 are associated with premalignant lesions of the cervix and penis.

○ **HPV has been identified in what percentage of penile cancers?**

HPV has been demonstrated in 50% of penile SCC cases.

○ **True or False: Penile carcinoma secondary to HPV infection causes p53 and retinoblastoma (Rb) dysregulation.**

True. Cells that are infected with high-risk HPV (i.e., 16, 18, 31, 33, 35, and 39) continue to make viral genes known as E6 and E7. These genes have products that act to disrupt apoptotic pathways and proliferation pathways via Rb and p53 tumor suppressors.

○ **How are penile cancer and cervical cancer related?**

Both cancers have HPV as a potential etiology. In some studies, female sexual partners of men with SCC of the penis have a threefold increased risk of invasive cervical carcinoma. However, there are key differences as cervical carcinoma is much more common and affects younger women whereas penile cancer is rare and affects older men.

○ **Describe the lymphatic spread of penile cancer.**

Lymphatics from the glans and shaft drain to the superficial inguinal, deep inguinal, and pelvic lymph nodes. Drainage is bilateral, and crossover may occur.

○   **What is the natural history of untreated penile cancer.**

Untreated penile cancer progresses to death in the majority of patients within 2 years. Local and regional nodal enlargement and complications predominate over distant metastases to lung, liver, bone, or brain. Death may occur by erosion into the femoral vessels with subsequent hemorrhage. Spontaneous remission has not been reported.

○   **List the sites of the primary tumor in penile cancer in order of frequency.**

Glans (48%), prepuce (21%), glans and prepuce (9%), coronal sulcus (6%), and shaft (<2%).

○   **What precautions should be taken to prevent dissemination of tumor during biopsy of a penile lesion?**

None. Tumor dissemination due to a biopsy has not been reported.

○   **True or False: The most important factors in determining prognosis in penile cancer are stage and presence of lymph node metastasis.**

True. Of the two, the presence or absence of nodal metastases is the strongest predictive factor for survival. Additionally, the histologic characteristics of the primary tumor provide further valuable prognostic information.

○   **How does the appearance of well-differentiated (grade 1) SCC differ from poorly differentiated (grade 3)?**

Grade 1 SCC shows downward finger-like projections of atypical squamous cells from the papillomatous epidermis. Keratin pearls are present, and there is limited cellular atypia and mitotic figures. Grade 3 SCC shows little to no keratin pearls and marked cellular nuclear pleomorphism, mitoses, necrosis, and deep invasion.

○   **Compare the 5-year survival for the following groups of patients with SCC of the penis: all patients, negative nodes, positive inguinal nodes, and positive pelvic nodes.**

All patients = 50%, negative lymph nodes = 66%, positive inguinal nodes = 27%, positive pelvic lymph nodes = rare.

○   **What radiologic studies have proven useful in staging penile cancer?**

Lymphangiography has been replaced by CT and MRI due to their technical ease and ability to image the hypogastric and presacral nodes. Ultrasound and MRI can stage the depth of invasion of the primary lesion. Ultrasound and CT scan image the inguinal nodal regions, where physical examination is hindered by obesity or prior surgery. However, do not forget that lymph nodes can undergo reactive changes yielding higher false-positive rates with these modalities.

○   **What is the utility for PET in the assessment of patients with penile cancer?**

Several small studies have demonstrated that F^{18}-FDG uptake is found in lymph nodes with metastatic deposits of squamous cell carcinomas.

○   **Describe the utilization of lymphotrophic nanoparticle-enhanced MRI with Ferumoxtran-10 in the evaluation of lymph nodes.**

This new method of MRI utilizes iron particle injection with subsequent imaging 24 hours later. The goal is to limit the number of individuals that undergo lymph node dissection that do not require such a treatment.

In lymph nodes that are metastatic, an area of hypointensity will be seen, whereas normal lymph nodes take up the iron particle. One case series demonstrated a negative predictive value of 100% with high sensitivities. Further research is ongoing and appears promising.

○   **Assessment of the primary tumor is important in deciding whether to perform inguinal lymph node dissections. List the TNM staging system for penile cancer (UICC, 1994).**

- Primary tumor:

    Tx = primary tumor not assessed.

    T0 = no primary tumor.

    Tis = carcinoma in situ.

    Ta = verrucous carcinoma.

    T1 = tumor invades subepithelial connective tissue.

    T2 = tumor invades corpus spongiosum or cavernosum.

    T3 = tumor invades urethra or prostate.

    T4 = tumor invades other adjacent structures.

- Regional lymph nodes:

    Nx = nodes not assessed.

    N0 = no regional nodes.

    N1 = metastasis in a single, superficial inguinal lymph node.

    N2 = metastasis in multiple or bilateral superficial nodes.

    N3 = metastasis in deep inguinal or pelvic lymph nodes, unilateral or bilateral.

- Distant metastases:

    MX = distant metastasis not assessed.

    M0 = no distant metastases.

    M1 = distant metastases.

○   **Review the Jackson staging and how it equates to the TNM system above. What is the disadvantage of the Jackson staging system?**

Jackson staging system:

- Stage I = limited to the glans or prepuce.
- Stage II = involving the shaft.
- Stage III = palpable nodes.
- Stage IV = invades adjacent structures or distant metastases.

The Jackson system roughly equates to TNM as follows:

- Stage 0 = Tis-Ta N0M0.
- Stage I = T1N0M0.
- Stage II = T1-2N1M0 or T2N0M0.
- Stage III = T1-3N2M0 or T3N0-1M0.
- Stage IV = T4anyNM0 or AnyTN3M0 or AnyTAnyNM1.

The Jackson system has the disadvantage of conveying less information about the tumor and makes interpretation of studies using different staging systems difficult.

○   **What is the gold standard treatment for the primary tumor in penile cancer?**

The gold standard is resection of the primary tumor with a 2-cm margin to ensure complete resection of microscopic finger-like projections of tumor that may extend from the grossly evident tumor. This goal can be accomplished with a partial penectomy if the residual stump is serviceable for upright voiding and/or sexual function. Otherwise, total penectomy is indicated.

○ **What surgical margin is required when performing tumor excision for localized penile cancer?**

Historically, teaching has emphasized a 2-cm margin at the time of excision. However, this has recently come into question with new studies demonstrating a more conservative approach to radical disfiguring surgery. Although a definitive margin has not yet been established, it appears a 1-cm margin with close oncologic follow-up can be implemented safely in localized penile cancer with low grades (1–2).

○ **When is circumcision appropriate treatment for penile cancer and what are the risks/benefits?**

Circumcision is less disfiguring than partial penectomy and may be appropriate for small lesions of the prepuce. However recurrence rates are as high as 50%. Close patient follow-up and low threshold for biopsy and additional surgery is necessary for this approach to the primary tumor.

○ **What is the best management for a primary tumor located on the proximal penile shaft?**

In rare circumstances when the tumor invades only the epidermis, excision of skin only is appropriate. In cases of a deeply invasive tumor of the shaft where a 2-cm margin is not possible, or if the residual stump would not allow upright voiding, then total penectomy with perineal urethrostomy is the best management.

○ **A 70-year-old male underwent a partial penectomy 1 year ago for a T1 N0M0 grade I SCC of the glans penis. He presents with increasing lower urinary tract symptoms. What operative complications apply to this scenario?**

Stricture of the neomeatus is a common complication of partial penectomy and can be avoided by widely spatulating the urethra, performing a tension-free anastomosis, and adequate vascularization of the urethral stump. Strictures are initially managed by dilation or meatotomy. Recurrent local disease must be ruled out.

○ **What are the risks and benefits of Mohs micrographic surgery (MMS) for penile cancer?**

MMS for small, distal lesions in the hands of an experienced Mohs surgeon can provide cure rates equivalent to partial penectomy with a decrease in the amount of tissue that is sacrificed. MMS is less successful for larger (>3 cm) lesions because large resections can create defects in the glans that are difficult to reconstruct. Excessive resections can create significant glans defects and meatal stenosis that is difficult to reconstruct.

○ **What are the risks and benefits of radiation therapy for penile cancer?**

Many patients undergoing radiation therapy (external beam or brachytherapy) refused surgery. Organ preservation is accomplished with cancer control rates for minimally invasive T1-2 lesions that are comparable to conventional surgery. Radiation therapy for larger lesions is less successful and carries higher morbidity. Potential complications include urethral fistula, stricture, penile necrosis requiring penectomy, lengthy treatment schedule, and difficulty distinguishing postirradiation scar from tumor recurrence.

○ **What are the indications for lasers in penile cancer?**

Both CO_2 and Nd:YAG lasers are effective in treating CIS. Select patients with low stage invasive SCC can be treated as long as they are followed carefully for local recurrence.

○ **What is the major drawback to laser surgery for small squamous cell carcinomas of the penis?**

No histologic specimen to assess stage and grade.

○ **A 40-year-old healthy man presents with a large fungating lesion of the glans penis with erosion into the penile shaft and extensive fungating bilateral inguinal lymphadenopathy. The patient delayed seeing a doctor for a considerable amount of time but now requests maximal therapy. Describe the treatment options.**

In such extreme cases, the anatomy will dictate treatment possibilities. Fixed lymph nodes may require neoadjuvant chemotherapy followed by treatment of the primary lesion and lymphadenectomy. Aggressive approaches for these extreme cases include total emasculation, scrotectomy, resection of the lower abdominal wall and pubic symphysis, and hemipelvectomy.

○ **What is the most common reconstructive option for a patient following partial or total penectomy?**

Free flap reconstruction of the penis with a ulnar forearm flap is the procedure of choice at many centers. Subsequently, a prosthesis can be placed for erectile function.

○ **What is the efficacy of inguinal lymphadenectomy in terms of cure and palliation?**

Inguinal lymphadenectomy is curative in approximately 80% of cases and palliates possible complications of inguinal disease such as ulceration, infection, and vascular compromise.

○ **At the time of diagnosis of an invasive penile cancer, a patient has palpable inguinal lymph nodes. Following 4 to 6 weeks of oral antibiotics therapy, the lymphadenopathy persists. What is the likelihood that the lymph nodes are pathologic?**

Initially: 50%; after 4 to 6 weeks of antibiotics: 70% to 85%.

○ **What are the disadvantages of routine inguinal lymphadenectomy?**

Early complications include phlebitis, pulmonary embolism, wound infection, and flap necrosis. Long-term complications include severe lymphedema from the scrotum to the lower extremities.

○ **Define the terms "early" or "immediate" inguinal lymphadenectomy (LND), and "delayed" LND as they relate to the management of cancer of the penis.**

Early/immediate LND is carried out following 4 to 6 weeks of antibiotic therapy even though the inguinal nodes are not palpably abnormal. Delayed LND is performed when an abnormal inguinal node examination demonstrates lymphadenopathy sometime after penectomy is performed.

○ **True or False: Penectomy and lymphadenectomy should be performed concurrently to maximize staging information.**

False. Mortality from sepsis can occur when a combined procedure is performed. Additionally, the histology of the nodes is often difficult to assess in the presence of severe inflammation.

○ **What is the incidence of subclinical metastasis (negative groin examinations) and what factors increase the likelihood of metastatic nodal disease?**

The reported incidence of subclinical metastasis ranges from 2% to 25% in most reports. Primary tumor stage (tumor invading the basement membrane of the penile skin) and higher tumor grade increase the likelihood of nodal disease.

○ **What is the major drawback to the sentinel node concept of penile cancer metastasis?**

Some series have shown metastatic spread to the inguinal nodes without involvement of the sentinel node. Hence sentinel node biopsy alone can miss the diagnosis of inguinal metastasis.

○ **What is the key advantage of prophylactic groin dissections of clinically negative nodes versus delayed dissection if they become palpable?**

Recent studies have pooled results and indicate a potential survival advantage for patients with positive inguinal nodes who underwent prophylactic versus delayed groin dissection. The survival benefit of prophylactic LND if the nodes are positive must be weighed against the risk of morbidity in the 75% of patients who will have negative dissections.

○ **What are the key elements of the modified inguinal lymph node dissection?**

Shorter skin incision, skin flaps elevated deep to Scarpa's fascia, narrower field of dissection—exclude dissection lateral to the femoral artery and caudal to the fossa ovalis, preservation of the saphenous vein, and elimination of sartorius muscle transposition (unless subsequent deep nodes dissected).

○ **When and why is sartorius muscle transposition performed?**

When standard inguinal lymphadenectomy is performed, the deep nodes and fascia lata over the femoral vessels are resected. In the event of erosion from wound infection or major flap necrosis, a sartorius muscle transposition protects the femoral vessels.

○ **What are the boundaries of the femoral (Scarpa's) triangle?**

Base—inguinal ligament; laterally—sartorius muscle, medially—adductor longus muscle; floor—(lateral to medial) the iliacus, psoas major, pectineus, and adductor brevis muscles; roof—fascia lata with small opening (fossa ovalis) through which the greater saphenous vein enters the underlying femoral vein.

○ **What three small branches of the femoral artery and vein are usually encountered in inguinal lymph node dissection?**

Circumflex iliac, superficial epigastric, and superficial external pudendal.

○ **Name the six subtypes of squamous cell carcinoma of the penis. Which are the most aggressive?**

They are as follows: usual type, papillary, basaloid, warty, verrucous, and sarcomatoid. The basaloid and sarcomatoid variants are the most aggressive with the verrucous being the least. Additionally, the basaloid variant has a strong association with HPV expression (approximately 80%).

○ **A 65-year-old male with SCC of the penis s/p penectomy has bulky eroded groin metastases that would necessitate excision of a large portion of overlying skin. What are treatment approaches?**

Palliative or neoadjuvant chemo/radiation therapy may be given for inoperable nodes. Lymph node dissection is preferred and with the assistance of a reconstructive surgeon to rotate a myocutaneous skin flap such as the tensor fascia lata, gracilis, or rectus abdominis flap, the large defect can be covered.

○ **A 60-year-old male presents with a biopsy-proven SCC of the glans penis and is found to have T1 grade I SCC at partial penectomy. Clinical examination reveals palpable lymphadenopathy on the right and a negative left groin. Describe the management of the lymph nodes.**

Following treatment of the primary tumor, 4 to 6 weeks of oral antibiotics should be administered. If the unilateral lymphadenopathy resolves, then the patient can be carefully followed for recurrence. If the unilateral adenopathy does not resolve, then bilateral superficial inguinal LND should be performed as anatomic crossover of penile lymphatics is well established. If either superficial dissection is positive for malignancy, then a deep inguinal dissection is performed. If any deep dissection is positive, then complete ilioinguinal/pelvic lymph node dissections may be indicated.

○ **How does pelvic lymphadenectomy for penile cancer differ from prostate and bladder cancer?**

Pelvic lymphadenectomy for penile cancer should extend more distally removing all lymph nodes tissue between the deep inguinal node group and the iliac group.

○ **A patient with clinically negative inguinal nodes undergoes resection of a TI grade III penile tumor. During follow-up, he develops unilateral inguinal adenopathy. What is the appropriate management?**

In this setting, unilateral dissection of the palpable lymph nodes is appropriate. The elapsed time has increased the likelihood that the clinically negative side is free of metastasis.

○ **Describe the optimal strategy for surveillance of low stage SCC of the penis and clinically negative inguinal nodes.**

Most inguinal metastases occur within 2 to 3 years of the diagnosis of the primary tumor. Patients must be closely examined during these 2 to 3 years at 2- to 3-month intervals, as well as taught self-examination. Follow-up should continue indefinitely.

○ **A 60-year-old male undergoes partial penectomy for a T2 grade II glanular SCC (corporeal tissue invasion); inguinal nodes are nonpalpable. Appropriate management of the lymph nodes includes:**

T2-3, N0M0 patients have a higher incidence of metastases and should undergo 6 weeks of oral antibiotics followed by bilateral inguinal lymph node dissection even if the nodes remain negative. The extent of dissection varies, but it is common to start with a superficial dissection and only perform a deep dissection if positive nodes are encountered; "skip" metastases are rare.

○ **What role does chemotherapy have in penile cancer?**

Multiagent regimens have yielded partial responses of short duration in most patients (approximately 65%) with advanced disease. Complete responses are unfortunately uncommon (approximately 10%–15%). Various regimens have been utilized to include methotrexate, bleomycin, cisplatin, vinblastine, and ifosfamide. All clinical trials utilize multimodal consolidative approaches with regard to chemotherapy plus either surgery or radiotherapy due to shortened overall responses.

○ **What percentage of patients with metastatic penile cancer exhibit hypercalcemia and what is the mechanism?**

Approximately 20%. The cause is unknown, but systemic release of paraneoplastic hormonal substances is suspected.

○ **How does the incidence of SCC compare with other types of penile cancer?**

SCC accounts for more than 95% of penile cancers. The remaining cancers are rare and include sarcomas, melanomas, basal cell carcinomas, and metastases.

○ **How does malignant melanoma of the penis differ from SCC?**

Malignant melanoma of the penis is rare with <100 cases reported. The glans and prepuce are most common sites. The Breslow thickness scale provides important prognostic information. Most cases of penile melanoma present at an advanced stage with early metastases and poor survival. Hematogenous metastases are more common than lymphatic spread.

○ **How does sarcoma of the penis differ from SCC?**

Sarcomas of the penis are usually locally invasive, low grade, and respond well to local excision. Local recurrence is characteristic, but metastases are rare.

○ **Where do penile metastatic lesions usually originate?**

While rare, metastases to the penis may come from the bladder, prostate, and rectum. The primary disease is usually very advanced when the penis is involved and survival is <1 year.

○ **What is the most common presenting sign of involvement of the penis with metastatic tumor?**

Priapism.

○ **For advanced penile cancer, which chemotherapy agents have shown the most activity?**

Bleomycin, cisplatin, and methotrexate have demonstrated the most activity.

○ **What percentage of patients who ultimately develop squamous cell carcinoma of the penis had a preexisting premalignant penile lesion?**

Approximately 30% to 40%.

○ **What is a cutaneous horn and how should it be treated?**

It's a hyperkeratotic growth on the penis that is usually related to a preexisting lesion such as a wart, scratch, or laceration. Due to its malignant potential, local excision is recommended.

CHAPTER 50 Pediatric Oncology

Fernando Ferrer, MD, FAAP, FACS

○ **The Wilms' tumor suppressor gene WT-1 is located on which chromosome?**

The Wilms' tumor suppressor gene (WT-1) is located on the distal portion of the short arm of chromosome 11, in the 11p13 location. A second putative Wilms' tumor gene has been found at 11p15. Abnormalities here are associated with overgrowth syndrome and Beckwith–Weidemann syndrome.

○ **What congenital anomalies are associated with Wilms' tumor and what chromosomal abnormalities are associated with these anomalies?**

Congenital anomalies are seen in approximately 15% of patients with Wilms' tumor. These include the following:
- WT-1

  Aniridia

  WAGR syndrome (**W**ilms', **A**niridia, **G**enitourinary anomalies, and **R**etardation)
- Hemihypertrophy

  Denys–Drash syndrome (Wilms', pseudohermaphroditism, glomerulopathy, retardation)
- WT-2

  Beckwith–Wiedemann syndrome (macroglossia, gigantism, organomegaly)

○ **What is the significance of loss of heterozygosity at sites 16 q and 1 p in Wilms tumor?**

LOH at 16q (seen in 20% of all tumors) and 1p (seen in 10% of all tumors) have been identified as biomarkers of worse outcome. When occurring together they represent an indication for more aggressive therapy.

○ **The histologic picture of Wilms' tumor is described as "triphasic." What are these three components?**

The classic microscopic appearance of Wilms' tumor includes blastemal, epithelial, and stromal components.

○ **A patient with Wilms' tumor undergoes nephrectomy. The tumor penetrates the surface of the capsule. At the time of nephrectomy there is tumor spillage, which is confined to the flank. Lymph nodes are negative. Contralateral kidney is negative. Chest x-ray is negative. What stage is this tumor?**

This is a stage III Wilms' tumor. The staging system is as follows:

Stage I—Tumor limited to kidney, completely resected. The renal capsule is intact. The tumor was not ruptured or biopsied prior to removal. The vessels of the renal sinus are not involved. There is no evidence of tumor at or beyond the margins of resection.

Note: For a tumor to quality for certain therapeutic protocols as stage I, regional lymph nodes must be examined microscopically.

Stage II—The tumor is completely resected and there is no evidence of tumor at or beyond the margins of resection. The tumor extends beyond kidney, as is evidenced by any one of the following criteria:

- There is regional extension of the tumor (i.e., penetration of the renal capsule, or extensive invasion of the soft tissue of the renal sinus, as discussed below).
- Blood vessels within the nephrectomy specimen outside the renal parenchyma, including those of the renal sinus, contain tumor.

Note: Rupture of spillage confined to the flank, including biopsy of the tumor, is no longer included in stage II and is now included in stage III.

Stage III—Residual nonhematogenous tumor present following surgery and confined to abdomen. Any one of the following may occur:

- Lymph nodes within the abdomen or pelvis are involved by tumor. (Lymph node involvement in the thorax, or other extra-abdominal sites is a criterion for stage IV.)
- The tumor has penetrated through the peritoneal surface.
- Tumor implants are found on the peritoneal surface.
- Gross or microscopic tumor remains postoperatively (e.g., tumor cells are found at the margin of surgical resection on microscopic examination).
- The tumor is not completely resectable because of local infiltration into vital structures.
- Tumor spillage occurring either before or during surgery.
- The tumor was biopsied (whether, tru-cut, open or fine needle aspiration) before removal.
- Tumor is removed in greater than one piece (e.g., tumor cells are found in a separately excised adrenal gland; a tumor thrombus within the renal vein is removed separately from the nephrectomy specimen).

Stage IV—Hematogenous metastases (lung, liver, bone, brain, etc.), or lymph node metastases outside the abdomino-pelvic region are present. (The presence of tumor within the adrenal gland is not interpreted as metastasis and staging depends on all other staging parameters present).

Stage V—Bilateral renal involvement by tumor is present at diagnosis. An attempt should be made to stage each side according to the above criteria on the basis of the extent of disease.

○ **What is the most important factor in the prognosis of patients with Wilms' tumor?**

The most important aspect of Wilms' tumor is the histology. Unfavorable histology (anaplasia) at any stage is associated with a worse prognosis. Anaplasia is seen in approximately 10% of all Wilms' tumors. Anaplasia is defined by the presence of gigantic polyploid nuclei within the tumor sample. It is rare in the first 2 years of life, but the incidence increases to 13% in children older than 5 years old. Anaplasia is further divided into focal and diffuse forms, with diffuse anaplasia carrying a worse prognosis that focal. Anaplasia is believed to be a marker of chemoresistance.

○ **What are the chemotherapeutic agents used to treat patients with Wilms' tumor?**

Patients with Wilms tumor are treated according to a risk schema. Current COG protocols divide patients into very low-, low-, standard-, and higher-risk groups. Patients with bilateral tumors are treated under a separate protocol.

Patients with standard-risk tumors (stage III, favorable histology) are treated with vincristine, dactinomycin + doxorubicin + radiation. Patients with higher stage disease and/or anaplasia may also receive cyclophosphamide/ carboplatin/etoposide and cyclophosphamide.

○ **What is the current survival in Wilm's tumor?**

Data from NWTS IV indicated that for patients with favorable histology unilateral tumors stages I–IV 10-year overall survival ranged from 96% to 81%, respectively. For patients with anaplastic tumors stage II to III survival was 49%, stage IV patients with anaplasia had a survival rate of 18% at 10 years.

○ **What is the most common renal tumor of infancy and which renal tumor is most common during childhood?**

Congenital mesoblastic nephroma is the most common tumor in infants, while Wilms' is the most common tumor in children. After the age of 10, renal tumors in children are just as likely to represent a Wilms tumor or a pediatric renal cell carcinoma.

○ **What is the most common extracranial solid tumor of childhood?**

Neuroblastoma is the most common extracranial solid tumor in children. It accounts for 6% to 10% of all childhood malignancies.

○ **An 18-month-old male presents with malaise, weight loss, and diffuse pain. An abdominal mass is palpable. What is the most likely diagnosis?**

Neuroblastoma. At the time of presentation of neuroblastoma, approximately 70% of patients have disseminated disease versus less than 10% to 15% with Wilms'. Patients with Wilms' tumor generally appear in good health, in contrast to patients with neuroblastoma in whom the tumor may be widespread at presentation and systemic symptoms are very often present.

○ **When does the peak incidence of neuroblastoma occur?**

The peak incidence of neuroblastoma is seen in the first year of life. The incidence decreases progressively with age, and is rarely diagnosed in patients older than 6 to 7 years.

○ **Neuroblastoma is a malignant neuroendocrine tumor. There is a spectrum from this to benign tumors. What are these other tumors, and what are their characteristics?**

Ganglioneuroma is the benign counterpart to neuroblastoma. It does not metastasize, but can envelop adjacent structures and even extend into intervertebral foramina. Histologically, they contain mature ganglion cells in a collagen-rich background.

Ganglioneuroblastoma is intermediate between neuroblastoma and ganglioneuroma. There is a histologic spectrum between these; the outcome for ganglioneuroblastoma is varied.

○ **What is the most common site of occurrence of neuroblastomas?**

Seventy-five percent originate in the abdomen (retroperitoneum) and two-thirds of these are in the adrenal gland.

○ **Is age a significant determinant of outcome in neuroblastoma?**

Yes, age less than 1 year is an indicator of better outcome when compared to older children, likely due to more favorable biology in tumors occurring at a younger age. Other predictive factors include site of origin; survival is better for nonadrenal tumors. Stage of disease is also an important predictor as stage I and II patients have excellent survival statistics.

○ **When is a bone marrow aspirate and/or biopsy indicated in the evaluation of patients with confirmed or suspected neuroblastoma?**

All patients with neuroblastoma should undergo bone marrow aspirate and/or biopsy. As many as 70% of bone marrow aspirates have been reported to be positive in patients with neuroblastoma.

○ **What molecular markers have been shown to carry prognostic significance in patients with neuroblastoma?**

N-*myc* amplification is associated with a poor prognosis and is found in about 30% to 40% of patients with advanced disease.

Hyperdiploid tumors (those that contain more than the normal amount of DNA material found in somatic cells) have demonstrated a favorable outcome.

○ **What are the characteristics of stage IV-S neuroblastoma?**

The definition of stage IV-S is patients who would otherwise be classified with stage I (tumor confined to the organ of origin) or stage II (tumor extending in continuity beyond the organ of origin, but not crossing the midline; ipsilateral regional nodes may be involved) but who have remote spread of tumor confined to one or more of the following: liver, skin, or bone marrow (without evidence of bony involvement). This stage disease is limited to patients younger than 1 year. This group typically has an excellent prognosis with survival rate in excess of 80%.

○ **What diagnostic tests can be useful for making the diagnosis of neuroblastoma?**

Urinary metabolites of catecholamines. Vanillymandelic acid and homovanillic acid are found to be elevated in 90% to 95% of patients.

Anemia is associated with diffuse bone marrow involvement.

In addition to standard radiologic imaging tests, MIBG scintigraphy can be useful in identifying primary and metastatic lesions.

○ **What are the histologic types of rhabdomyosarcoma, and which is most common in childhood?**

The types of rhabdomyosarcoma are embryonal, alveolar, and pleomorphic. Mixed rhabdomyosarcomas also occur, and in about 10% to 20% of cases, the tumor is so undifferentiated that it does not fit into the standard classification.

Embryonal rhabdomyosarcoma is the most common type seen in childhood, accounting for two-thirds of GU rhabdomyosarcomas, and 50% to 70% of all rhabdomyosarcomas in children.

Sarcoma botryoides is a descriptive term for an exophytic embryonal tumor that looks grossly like a cluster of grapes. It tends to arise in hollow organs (bladder, vagina).

Another histologic variant of the embryonal type is the "spindle cell sarcoma." It often arises in a paratesticular location and is associated with an especially favorable outcome.

○ **What are the most common GU sites?**

Prostate, bladder, paratesticular appendages, followed by the vagina and uterus.

○ **If a patient has a posttreatment biopsy indicating mature rhabdomyoblasts, should the patient have exonerative surgery to remove these elements?**

No, current evidence suggests that rhabdomyoblasts alone on biopsy after treatment does not require aggressive surgical treatment. Observation alone is needed.

○ **Besides histologic type, what are some adverse prognostic factors in patients with rhabdomyosarcoma?**

Tumors arising in the prostate, children younger than 1 year, and tumors in adults and older children generally have a poorer prognosis.

○ **A 4-year-old male has a rhabdomyosarcoma of the bladder. At the time of surgery the tumor appears grossly removed. However, pathological analysis reveals positive margins. Lymph nodes are negative. According to the International Rhabdomyosarcoma Study (IRS) staging system, what stage disease is this?**

This patient is in group IIA. The staging system is as follows:

Intergroup Rhabdomyosarcoma Study Group Clinical Grouping Classification

Group I	Localized disease completely resected
	Confined to the organ of origin
	Contiguous involvement
Group II	Total gross resection with evidence of regional spread
	Microscopic residual
	Positive nodes but no microscopic residual
	Positive nodes but microscopic residual in nodes or margins
Group III	Incomplete resection with gross residual disease
	After biopsy only
	After gross or major resection of the primary (>50%)
Group IV	Distant metastasis at diagnosis (lung, liver, bones, bone marrow, brain, and nonregional nodes)
	Positive cytology in cerebrospinal, pleural, or peritoneal fluid or implants on pleural or peritoneal surfaces are regarded as stage IV

○ **What is the primary mode of therapy for patients with stage T2a rhabdomyosarcoma of the bladder?**

Multiagent chemotherapy is the primary mode of treatment for patients with rhabdomyosarcoma. The combination of agents is often determined based on randomized trials but often includes one or more of the following: vincristine, actinomycin D, ifosfamide, etoposide, and/or cyclophosphamide. Radiation therapy may be added, and patients who do not have complete response to these treatments undergo surgical excision. The current trend, however, is toward organ preservation.

○ **What is the most common testicular tumor in a prepubertal boy?**

Yolk sac tumors are the most prevalent in prepubertal boys, accounting for nearly half of all testicular tumors in this age group.

○ **What is the histologic hallmark of a testicular teratoma?**

Teratomas contain elements derived from more than one of the three germ tissues: ectoderm, endoderm, and mesoderm.

○ **A 14-month-old male presents with a testicular mass. Tumor markers are negative. Radical orchiectomy is performed, and the pathology reveals a teratoma. What is the next step in management of this patient?**

Observation. Teratomas in prepubertal boys are consistently benign. Either orchiectomy or enucleation of the tumor with preservation of the remaining testicular tissue is curative. An older, postpubertal patient with teratocarcinoma, however, is managed the same as an adult with a nonseminomatous germ cell tumor.

○ **What testicular tumor must be ruled out in boys who present with precocious puberty?**

Leydig cell tumors can produce high levels of testosterone resulting in increased somatic growth, deepening of the voice, phallic growth, and secondary sexual characteristics. Serum levels of testosterone and gonadotropins must be checked, along with testicular ultrasonography.

○ **What disease can mimic a Leydig cell tumor?**

Congenital adrenal hyperplasia (non-salt-wasting) can present similar to a Leydig cell tumor. This is particularly true if a hypertrophic adrenal rest is present in the scrotum. These patients will exhibit elevated 17-ketosteroids as well as testosterone; gonadotropin levels will be low. Treatment with corticosteroids usually results in prompt resolution of the scrotal mass (adrenal rest).

○ **What condition or conditions are associated with the development of gonadoblastoma?**

Gonadoblastoma is a tumor that contains both germ cells and germinal stromal cells (although often the germ cells predominate and the tumor resembles a seminoma). This tumor develops almost exclusively in patients with abnormal gonads. The karyotype of these children contains either a Y chromosome or a translocation, which includes a portion of the Y chromosome, most commonly 46XY or 45XO/46XY. All of these children have genital/sexual abnormalities. Eighty percent are phenotypic females with intra-abdominal testes (or streak gonads); 20% occur in patients with predominantly male phenotype, often with ambiguity. The risk of tumor development increases at puberty, and the preferred treatment is gonadectomy prior to tumor development.

○ **True or False: The younger the patient is at the time of diagnosis of a sacrococcygeal teratoma the worse the prognosis.**

False. The prognosis for malignant sacrococcygeal teratomas is much worse than that for benign lesions. Malignancy is seen in 7% of girls and 10% of boys diagnosed at less than 2 months of age. In contrast, malignancy was seen in 48% of girls and 67% of boys diagnosed after 2 months of age.

○ **What structure must be excised along with a sacrococcygeal teratoma?**

Resection of the coccyx is an extremely important part of the surgical management of sacrococcygeal teratoma. Failure to resect the coccyx has been associated with a recurrence rate of up to 35%.

○ **What is the primary mode of treatment for a sacrococcygeal teratoma?**

Surgical excision is the mainstay in the management of patients with sacrococcygeal teratoma. Patients with benign tumors need to be followed with imaging to detect any recurrence. Patients with malignant tumors have a poor long-term prognosis despite the multiagent chemotherapy that is required following surgical resection.

CHAPTER 51 Radiology: CT/Ultrasound

Stephen Haltom, MD, and
Anthony Smith, MD

○ **What is the role of renal CT and MR angiography?**

CT and MR renal angiography are used to diagnose renal artery stenosis (RAS), the most common cause of secondary hypertension. Etiologies include atherosclerosis and fibromuscular dysplasia. Atherosclerotic lesions typically occur at the ostium or within the proximal 2 cm of the renal artery. They present as a focal/segmental stenosis. It typically affects men older than 50 years.

Fibromuscular dysplasia is the second most common cause of RAS and the most common cause in children and young adults. It is bilateral in two-thirds of cases and affects the mid-to-distal renal artery. The renal artery classically has a "string of beads" pattern with stenosis involving a long segment in fibromuscular dysplasia.

CT angiography is also useful in the evaluation of living renal donors prior to surgery to define the anatomy. MR angiography has traditionally also been used to evaluate the vena cava for renal masses where a suspicion of vena caval thrombus exists.

The scan below is a normal CT angiogram showing arterial and venous anatomy of the left kidney. The appearance of the vena cava is dark due to incomplete mixing with the contrast. The aorta is still bright white indicating an arterial phase picture.

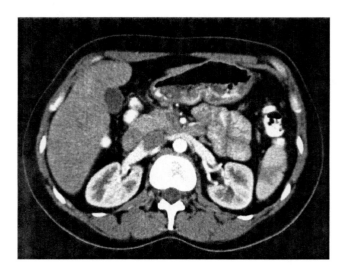

○ **What are the ultrasound findings in renal artery stenosis?**

Direct signs of RAS include increased peak systolic velocity and poststenotic turbulent flow (spectral broadening). Indirect signs or distal manifestations of RAS include a dampened systolic waveform (tardus et parvus waveform) and decreased renal resistive index.

○ **What is the renal resistive index and how is it used?**

The renal resistive index is calculated from Doppler ultrasound studies of the renal vasculature. It is defined as the peak systolic velocity minus the end-diastolic velocity divided by the peak systolic velocity. Resistive index can be elevated in acute obstruction, acute tubular necrosis, allograft rejection, and cyclosporin toxicity. Resistive index may be decreased in renal artery stenosis due to decreased peak systolic flow.

○ **How does a nuclear medicine study evaluate for renovascular hypertension (RVH)?**

Technetium 99m-DTPA and MAG3 are radionuclide agents cleared by the kidneys. Patients with RVH may show a unilateral reduction in flow, while function is preserved. This study may be performed in conjunction with an ACE inhibitor, such as captopril. The ACE inhibitor blocks efferent arterial vasoconstriction, resulting in a decrease in the GFR and ERPF. The study is considered suggestive of RAS if one of the kidneys GFR drops by 30% after captopril is administered.

○ **What is the role of a renal captopril study in suspected RVH?**

The renal captopril study is a good screening test for those suspected of renal artery stenosis. However, patients with positive studies should undergo additional imaging, such as magnetic resonance angiography or renal angiography.

○ **Which urinary tract stones are radiolucent on CT?**

Indinavir stones can only be seen by secondary findings and usually require an IVP. Matrix stones are soft tissue attenuation density. Uric acid and cystine stones range from 100 to 300 Hounsfield units (HU), while calcium stones are typically 400 to 600 HU.

Before the widespread use of CT, it was assumed that most calcium stones are visible on plain films. In reality, plain KUB radiography misses many calculi due to their small size and overlying abdominal or bony structures.

○ **What is the advantage of assessing hematuria with CT urogram versus an intravenous pyelogram (IVP)?**

CT urogram (contrast study) affords improved detection of calculi, better bladder visualization, and demonstrates vascular pathology. Renal masses will be evident on the intermediate contrasted phase where both cortex and medulla are opacified (nephrographic phase). Advances in CT technology have enabled fast acquisition of thin slices that allows improved visualization of the urothelial surfaces.

○ **In the region of the renal medulla, multiple, bilateral calcifications are present. What are the top three diagnoses?**

1. Renal tubular acidosis.
2. Medullary sponge kidney.
3. Hyperparathyroidism.

The scan below shows medullary nephrocalcinosis.

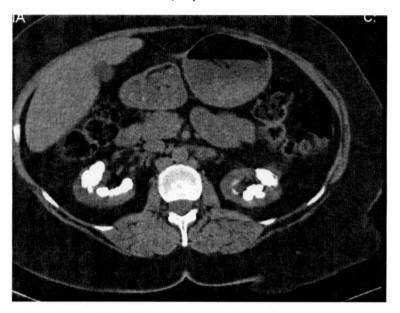

○ **What are the ultrasound characteristics of renal stones?**

Calculi are seen as crescent-shaped echogenic foci with posterior acoustic shadowing. Posterior shadowing distinguishes small stones from other echogenic structures in the central sinus. Ureteral stones are frequently not seen because of the overlying bowel gas.

Color Doppler is used to visualize ureteric jets of urine into the bladder that excludes high-grade ureteric obstruction. Twinkling artifact or rapid color change posterior to a stone is a useful ancillary finding to confirm a urinary tract stone.

○ **What are the secondary signs of acute obstruction from ureteral calculi on CT scan?**

Typical findings are renal enlargement, striated cortex, perinephric stranding, and ureteral dilation with hydronephrosis (right image), and a tissue rim sign (left image) around the ureter where the stone is located.

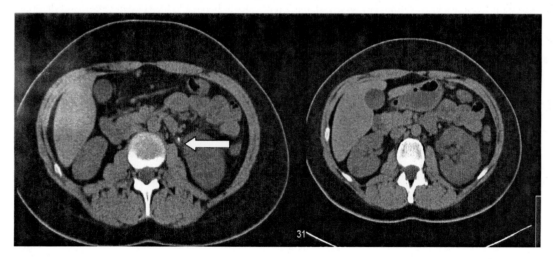

○   **What are the CT characteristic of xanthogranulomatous pyelonephritis (XGP)?**

Lipid-laden macrophages create multiple focal low attenuation masses. There is contrast enhancement of parenchyma surrounding the collections. Cortical involvement is often diffuse but can be focal. The kidney is nonfunctioning or poorly functioning. The process can extend beyond renal capsule. Renal cutaneous and renal enteric fistulas are a complication. XGP can mimic renal cell carcinoma, transitional cell carcinoma, lymphoma, metastases, abscess, and pyonephrosis (The scan below shows xanthogranulomatous pyelonephritis with concomitant psoas abscess).

Staghorn calculi are associated with xanthogranulomatous pyelonephritis. Staghorn calculi fill the collecting system, forming a cast of the pelvis and calyces. Most are composed of struvite and associated with chronic renal infection.

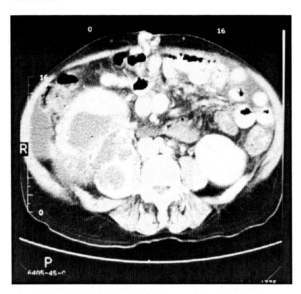

○   **An adult patient presents with hematuria, hypertension, and an elevated serum creatinine. An ultrasound shows multiple, bilateral large cysts. A representative CT scan is shown as well as a typical renal ultrasound. What is the diagnosis and recommended treatment?**

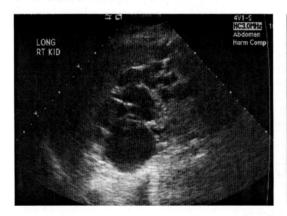
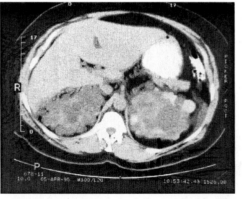

Autosomal dominant polycystic kidney disease (ADPCKD) is the diagnosis. The ultrasound/CT findings are pathognomonic with bilaterally large kidneys containing multiple cysts. The mean age at diagnosis is 43 years. ADPCKD is associated with cysts in the liver and pancreas and saccular berry aneurysms of the cerebral arteries. Renal insufficiency gradually develops. Treatment is a renal transplant.

○ **What other entities present with renal parenchymal cysts?**

Acquired cystic disease from long-term dialysis, multiple simple cysts, von Hippel–Lindau disease, tuberous sclerosis, and medullary cystic disease all cause renal cysts.

○ **What are the characteristics of a simple cyst on renal ultrasound?**

A simple cyst appears as a round or oval anechoic structure, with an imperceptible wall and smooth margins. There is increased through transmission and no internal echoes.

○ **How can one characterize a simple renal cyst on CT?**

Simple cysts are round, low attenuation structures without complexity of the wall. Hounsfield units are less than 20.

○ **What are the typical CT and US findings of renal lymphoma?**

CT demonstrates a homogeneous mass with minimal contrast enhancement. On ultrasound, lymphoma is hypoechoic and may show posterior acoustic enhancement. Diffuse infiltration is characterized by renal enlargement. Primary renal lymphoma is rare. It is most often secondary to hematogenous spread from extra renal lymphoma.

○ **How are renal cystic lesions characterized on CT?**

The Bosniak classification:

- Class I—Benign cysts (well-defined, round, homogeneous, lucent (<HU 20), avascular, thin-walled).
- Class II—Minimally complicated cysts; benign (well-marginated, mildly irregular, calcified, septated, avascular, hyperdense, usually ≤3 cm).
- Class IIF—Possibly benign (hyperdense, thick or nodular calcifications in wall or septa, vaguely enhanced, may be ≥3 cm) (see figure below).
- Class III—Indeterminate.
- Class IV—Malignant lesions with large cystic or necrotic components (irregular wall thickening or an enhancing mass).

The CT scan shows right renal cyst with dense calcification centrally and multiple septations (Bosniak IIF–III). This proved to be a cystic renal cell carcinoma. Contrast in this case makes identification of calcification difficult to prove conclusively.

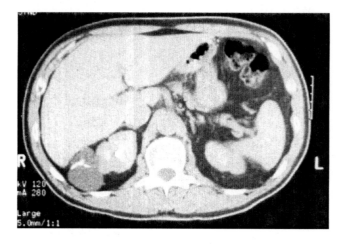

○   **What is the characteristic appearance of renal cell carcinoma on imaging?**

It most often presents as a solid, expansile, hyperenhancing renal lesion: 10% have calcifications and 20% are at least partially cystic. There is often tumor extension into the renal vein and IVC. Lymphatic metastases present as retroperitoneal adenopathy. However, necrotic tumors can illicit reactive hyperplasia in regional nodes.

   Patients with acquired cystic renal disease (long-term dialysis), tuberous sclerosis, and von Hippel–Lindau syndrome are predisposed to renal cell carcinoma.

○   **What is the pattern most often seen on CT of distant metastasis in renal cell carcinoma (RCC)?**

Metastases to the lungs can be solitary or demonstrate a miliary pattern. Bone metastases are lytic, aggressive, and can be solitary or multiple. Hepatic metastases are usually hypervascular.

○   **What is the best imaging test to evaluate for vascular invasion of renal cell carcinoma?**

Both multiphasic contrast-enhanced CT and MRI yield 90% to 95% accuracy in identifying renal vein thrombus. Multislice CT adds the capability of coronal and sagittal reconstructions, which are desirable for surgical planning.

   CT scan (below) showing vena caval thrombus and renal cell carcinoma and another typical CT appearance of a renal cell cancer.

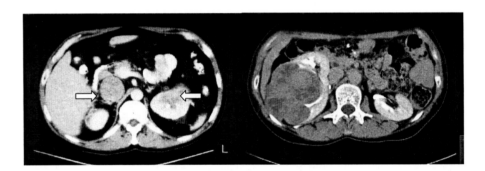

○   **An echogenic, 2-cm renal mass is found on ultrasound. What imaging study should be performed next?**

If fat is found in the mass on CT, the diagnosis of an angiomyolipoma is confirmed. Fat is hypodense on CT and the Hounsfield units should measure less than zero. Angiomyolipomas are benign lesions consisting of fat, smooth muscle, and blood vessels. If they reach a large size they may hemorrhage, therefore, they may be resected.

   Ultrasound (below) showing a subtle upper pole hyperechoic angiomyolipoma and a CT scan from a patient with tuberous sclerosis showing multiple bilateral angiomyolipomas.

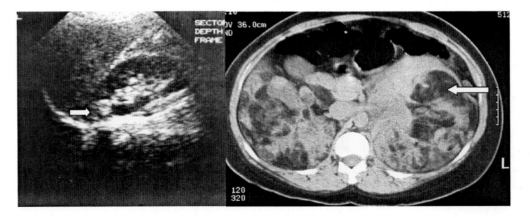

○ **What renal transplant complications may occur immediately postoperatively and what are their characteristics?**

- Acute tubular necrosis (ATN)—Transient renal enlargement and increased renal resistive index.
- Acute rejection—Similar to ATN but does not resolve.
- Renal artery stenosis—Tardus et parvus waveform distal to stenosis, peak systolic velocity >250 cm/s.
- Renal vein thrombosis—Reversal of diastolic flow on Doppler ultrasound.
- Urine leak—Anechoic collection (urinoma) without septations.

○ **Acute tubular necrosis (ATN) is suspected in a renal transplant patient. What findings would you expect on the nuclear medicine renal scan?**

The classic findings of ATN are blood flow is preserved; however, poor concentration and excretion is present resulting in an increasingly dense nephrogram. Rejection and dehydration can have a similar appearance.

○ **How can one tell the difference on nuclear renal scans between ATN and rejection?**

Subsequent renal scans show improvement in flow and function in the setting of ATN, whereas flow and function continue to decrease with rejection. Serial examinations to differentiate ATN from rejection should be performed with ultrasound, monitoring resistive indices.

○ **What factors are evaluated on a renal transplant ultrasound?**

The kidney is identified, measured, and the flow in the kidney is examined. The flow is evaluated with color and power Doppler imaging. The main renal artery and vein blood flows are evaluated. The resistive index should typically not exceed 0.80. Remember, the resistive index is the peak systolic velocity (PSV) minus the end-diastolic velocity (EDV) divided by the peak systolic velocity or (PSV − EDV)/PSV.

○ **Fluid collections may accumulate around the transplanted kidney. Name the differential for the fluid collections immediately postop, 3 months, and 6 months from surgery.**

- Urinoma—1 to 2 weeks posttransplant.
- Hematoma—1 to 3 weeks posttransplant.
- Lymphocele—a few weeks to several months posttransplant.
- Abscess—4 to 5 weeks posttransplant.

○ **What ultrasound findings are suggestive of obstruction of the transplanted kidney?**

Either increasing dilatation of the renal collecting system on subsequent ultrasounds or significant dilatation of the collecting system may represent obstruction (ureteral stenosis or a blood clot). However, mild dilatation is often seen in normal transplants.

○ **What is the normal appearance of the adrenal glands on CT/MRI?**

Each limb of the adrenal gland has straight or slightly convex borders, may measure up to 4 cm in length, and should measure less than 10 mm in thickness. T1 signal on MRI is homogeneous and slightly less intense than that of a normal liver and renal cortex.

○ **Which imaging study is best to differentiate adrenal masses from upper pole renal masses?**

Historically, multiplanar MRI (coronal, sagittal) has made this modality the best choice in evaluating a renal versus adrenal mass. Newer multislice CT scanners can easily reconstruct axial sequences into coronal and sagittal planes. Subtle fat planes between the renal mass and adrenal gland may be distinguished on a coronal or other planar imaging sequence.

○ **What is the CT imaging characteristic of an adrenal adenoma?**

Adrenal adenomas are typically 3 cm or less and appear as focal low densities with a smooth round margin. Hounsfield units that are less than 10 on noncontrast CT is 95% specific for adrenal adenoma. Adenomas, unlike metastases, demonstrate rapid washout of intravenous contrast. Thus, indeterminate lesions can be evaluated with contrast CT scans. A lesion that demonstrates 60% or greater washout of contrast on the 15 minutes delayed scan compared with the portal venous phase scan will be an adenoma 98% of the time.

○ **What is the MRI imaging characteristic of an adrenal adenoma?**

Chemical shift imaging with in and out of phase sequences is 95% to 100% specific for a diagnosis of adrenal adenoma. False negatives may be encountered in lipid poor adenomas.

○ **What are the CT and MRI imaging characteristic of an adrenal hemorrhage?**

CT demonstrates a round mass with increased attenuation (50–90 HU). The mass does not enhance and will decrease in size over a 6-month period of time.

MRI characteristically demonstrates a ring pattern of high T1 low T2 signal peripherally caused by methemoglobin and hemosiderin.

○ **What are the clinical entities associated with adrenal hemorrhage?**

Adrenal hemorrhage is associated with trauma, anticoagulation, septicemia, burns, recent surgery, and metastatic melanoma. It is more common in the right adrenal gland.

○ **Describe the imaging characteristics of an adrenal pheochromocytoma on CT and MRI.**

Pheochromocytomas are usually greater than 2 cm at presentation. They are indistinguishable from metastases. Larger tumors will have areas of central necrosis. Correlation with blood tests is required to establish the diagnosis. The use of intravenous contrast in patients with pheochromocytoma is controversial in the setting of a history of hypertensive episodes or if the patient has not had adequate adrenergic blockade.

MRI may not be as useful as previously thought secondary to cost, time, and increased artifacts. Furthermore, the classic description of "light bulb" appearance on T2 sequences is seen in less than half of adrenal pheochromocytomas. Other tumors with cystic components will also have a high T2 signal.

A whole body Iodine 131-labeled metaiodobenzylguanidine (MIBG) is used when looking for an extra-adrenal tumor. The scan below is an MRI of adrenal pheochromocytoma showing bright signal on T2-weighted imaging. Note compression of the underlying kidney.

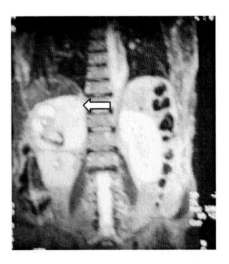

○ **If a single kidney were seen in the abdomen on ultrasound, what differential would one consider?**

- Congenital absence of a kidney.
- Renal hypoplasia or atrophy.
- An ectopic location, such as the pelvis.
- Prior resection.
- Nonfunctioning kidney (trauma or obstruction).

○ **What are the imaging findings in renal trauma?**

Intrarenal hematoma presents as an area of decreased enhancement on nephrographic (parenchymal) phase of contrast CT. Infarct has a similar appearance but is classically a peripheral wedge-shaped defect. Subcapsular hematomas are elliptical or round and have 40 to 70 HU. Lacerations are linear low attenuation areas that can extend into the collecting system and result in contrast extravasation of urine. Delayed phase images should be performed to evaluate collecting system injury when lacerations are present. Extensive areas of devascularization are common in higher-grade lesions.

CT scan (below) demonstrating a classic right-sided "rim sign," where the external kidney cortex is perfused by cortical perforators. This is a classic sign of an intimal disruption and significant renovascular trauma.

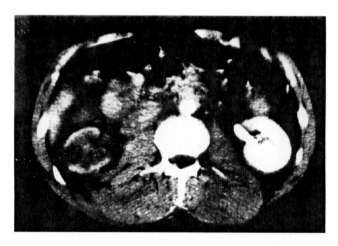

○ **What are the imaging characteristics of a horseshoe kidney?**

The lower poles of the kidneys fuse, creating a single band of tissue crossing the midline. The orientation of the kidneys is altered with the lower poles directed more medial and the collecting systems directed anterior. This condition is associated with an increased incidence of UPJ obstruction, recurrent urinary infections, Wilms' tumor in children, and is more predisposed to injury in trauma.

○ **What are the characteristics of adrenal myelolipoma on CT?**

Adrenal myelolipoma is a rare benign lesion containing myeloid, fat, and hematopoietic tissue. Size is usually 2 to 10 cm. They demonstrate heterogeneous attenuation and are very rarely bilateral. Large tumors can hemorrhage. Fat content creates increased echogenicity on ultrasound and negative Hounsfield units on CT. It can mimic retroperitoneal lipoma or liposarcoma. They are T1 hyperintense on MRI. Signal drops out on fat suppression sequences.

The scan (below) shows classic right adrenal myelolipoma with fat density.

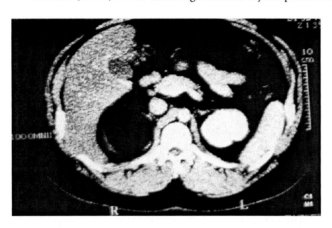

○ **What are the most common causes of adrenal hemorrhage in pediatric and adult patients?**

In neonates, the most common cause of adrenal hemorrhage is birth trauma, hypoxia, or septicemia. Most cases are bilateral. In neonates, ultrasound is the imaging study of choice. In adults, trauma, anticoagulation, and infection are the most common causes of hemorrhage. Typically, unilateral hemorrhage involving the right adrenal gland occurs in adults. CT is performed in adult patients being evaluating for adrenal hemorrhage.

○ **What are the imaging characteristics of adrenal hemorrhage on ultrasound?**

Ultrasound initially images acute hemorrhage as hyperechoic. Over time, the blood becomes more hypoechoic and smaller.

○ **What are the CT findings of pyelonephritis?**

Imaging studies, including CT, is normal in 75% of cases. However, a contrast-enhanced CT study may show wedge-shaped areas of decreased density (striated nephrogram) or renal enlargement. CT can rule out potential complications of pyelonephritis, such as abscess, hydronephrosis, stones, or scarring. Differential diagnosis for a striated nephrogram includes contusion, infarct, and radiation.

○ **What are the ultrasound and CT findings in emphysematous pyelonephritis?**

Ultrasound demonstrates echogenic foci in the renal sinus and parenchyma with dirty posterior shadowing. Ring down artifacts from trapped air bubbles can be seen. Perinephric gas may obscure visualization of the kidney.

CT demonstrates gas radiating from the medulla to the parenchyma. There is often a crescentic subcapsular gas collection. Gas can extend into the ipsilateral and contralateral anterior pararenal space.

The scan (below) depicts bilateral emphysematous pyelonephritis showing gas in the parenchyma.

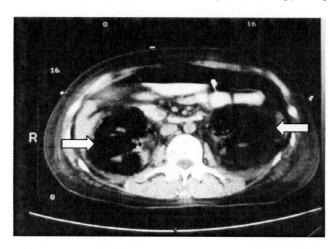

○ **What are the imaging findings of medullary sponge kidney?**

CT urogram and IVP: Retained contrast in dilated tubules in renal pyramids. Medullary nephrocalcinosis and urolithiasis may be present. These patients have an increased incidence of urinary tract infections and nephrolithiasis due to renal leak type hypercalciuria and hypocitraturia.

○ **What are the imaging findings of papillary necrosis?**

- Ultrasound shows echogenic foci in renal papillae progressing to cystic cavities in the pyramids.
- CT urogram/IVP demonstrates contrast-filled clefts in the renal parenchyma, sloughed papillae (renal pelvis filling defect), and ring-shaped medullary calcifications.
- Papillary necrosis is associated with analgesic abuse. Diabetic and sickle cell patients are also susceptible.

○ **Unilateral hydronephrosis and hydroureter is identified on an ultrasound. The patient has no history of compromised renal function. Which imaging study should be ordered next?**

A CT urogram with contrast is best to evaluate for the cause of obstruction, such as an obstructing bladder stone or a bladder cancer obstructing the UVJ. If there is a reasonable suspicion for nephrolithiasis, a single phase CT without contrast may be sufficient for diagnosis and save the patient considerable radiation exposure. If there is compromised renal function, consider an MR urogram.

Causes of obstruction include ureteral stricture, sloughed papilla, prior stone, prior infection, pelvic neoplasm, retroperitoneal fibrosis, ureterocele, or prior instrumentation.

○   **What are the ultrasound and CT imaging findings of a ureterocele?**

A ureterocele is a cystic dilatation of the distal ureter with prolapse into the bladder. Orthotopic ureteroceles insert normally at the trigone. Ectopic ureteroceles insert below the trigone and are associated with duplicated collecting systems in 80% of the time.

CT demonstrates an intravesicular mass at the UVJ. CT urogram findings can be similar to the IVP. Orthotopic ureteroceles present as a dilated distal ureter projecting into the bladder. Ectopic variety is often best demonstrated by ancillary findings of duplication.

On ultrasound, an orthotopic ureterocele presents as a round, thin walled sac, continuous with the distal ureter. Size fluctuates with ureteral peristalsis. A full bladder can occasionally cause a ureterocele to invert, giving the appearance of a bladder diverticulum.

Ultrasound (below) showing ureterocele in the base of the bladder.

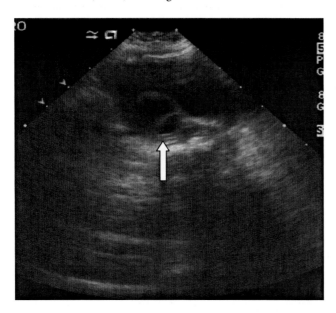

○   **What are the imaging findings of a collecting system duplication?**

CT demonstrates a duplex kidney. Absence of a renal sinus at the junction of upper and lower pole creates "faceless kidney" appearance. There are two ureters. The upper pole is most often obstructed. It can insert medial and caudal to the insertion of the lower pole ureter (Meyer–Weigert rule) or ectopically.

Ultrasound shows two renal sinus echo complexes and intervening renal parenchyma as well as upper pole hydronephrosis.

○   **In a duplicated collecting system, hydronephrosis of the upper pole moiety is due to what entity?**

The upper pole ureter inserts ectopically. An ectopic ureter inserting into the bladder (not at the trigone) is usually stenotic at its orifice and may end in an ectopic ureterocele. Extravesicular insertion in males is most common at the prostatic urethra. In females, insertion is most commonly at the urethra or vestibule. Males, unlike females, do not experience incontinence because the ectopic orifice is always above the external sphincter.

○   **What is the preferred imaging modality for suspected urolithiasis?**

The noncontrast CT of the abdomen and pelvis is now the preferred imaging study. A plain x-ray of the abdomen (KUB) is recommended when the CT scan is positive for stones. The KUB is useful to establish the radiopacity or radiolucency of the stone as well as to characterize its shape and surgical orientation. It also provides a simple and inexpensive way to track the progress of the stone.

○   **What is the role of the CT urogram in the evaluation of the patient with microhematuria?**

CT urogram of the abdomen and pelvis is gaining favor over the IVP. The study consists of a noncontrasted scan to look for urolithiasis. If stones are present, the study may be terminated to spare the patient unnecessary radiation exposure. After administration of contrast, the nephrographic phase (maximum cortical enhancement) and excretory phase images are performed. A series of excretory scans are often performed to ensure complete visualization of contrast throughout the renal collecting systems, ureters, and bladder. The nephrographic phase is most sensitive for evaluation of cortical lesions.

   The bladder should be carefully evaluated with contrast opacifying the majority of the structure. If contrast is especially dense, bone windows help "see through" the contrast in the bladder so no masses are missed.

   CT urogram (below) showing transitional cell carcinoma of the right renal pelvis seen as multiple filling defects in the collecting system.

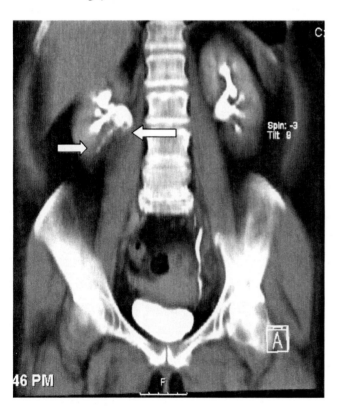

○   **How is transitional cell carcinoma (TCC) distinguished from a blood clot on ultrasound?**

TCC will have color flow on ultrasound and is immobile. Blood clots are immobile and will move as patient changes position. TCC can involve any part of the urothelium but is most common in the bladder. Lesions can be low-grade papillary or high-grade nonpapillary (nodular or flat). Echogenic polypoid tumor can mimic fungus ball or bladder stone.

○   **What are the CT/MRI characteristics of transitional cell carcinoma (TCC)?**

TCC is a hypovascular, infiltrative tumor. In the renal pelvis, it can present as urothelial thickening or as a polypoid or sessile mass. There may be invasion of the renal cortex and sinus fat. Look for thin rims of contrast filling caliceal spaces around the periphery of the tumor. In the ureter, it presents as circumferential or eccentric wall thickening. Hydronephrosis is often present.

Bladder TCC may enhance and protrude into the bladder lumen. MRI is the study of choice to assess invasion of the bladder wall and adjacent organs. Lesions are hyperintense on T2 sequences compared with normal bladder wall and perivesical tissues. Bladder TCC mildly enhances with gadolinium.

○   **How is transitional cell carcinoma distinguished from tuberculosis on CT urogram?**

Strictures are the earliest finding and can result in an amputated infundibulum and irregular caliceal contour. Papillary necrosis results in irregular cavities. Calcifications are common.

○   **What imaging modality is best for evaluation of prostatic cysts? Can you name any of the types of cysts?**

Transrectal ultrasound or MRI with endorectal coil are the best studies for evaluating prostatic cysts.

Utricle and Müllerian cysts are derived from the paramesonephric duct. Utricle cyst will fill on retrograde urethrogram via connection with the posterior urethra. A Müllerian cyst can be larger extending cephalad to the prostate and does not communicate with the urethra.

Cysts associated with benign prostatic hypertrophy and ejaculatory duct cysts are usually paramedian in location. Congenital and retention cyst are usually more lateral.

○   **What neoplasm is associated with a urachal remnant? What are the imaging features?**

Urachal remnants result from persistence of the embryonic connection between the bladder dome and allantoic duct. This can result in a patent urachus, urachal cyst, urachal sinus, or urachal diverticulum. CT demonstrates a midline cystic lesion above the bladder dome. It may have rim calcifications. Urachal carcinoma (adenocarcinoma is most common) presents as a mass in this region and often invades the bladder dome.

The scan (below) shows urachal adenocarcinoma presenting as a mass in the dome of the bladder and space of Retzius.

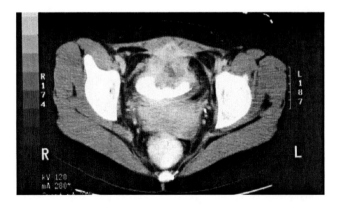

○   **Which zone of the prostate is the site of benign prostatic hypertrophy?**

The transitional zone is the site of origin (greater than 95%) of benign prostatic hypertrophy.

○ **What is the percentage of prostate cancer arising from each zone?**

- Peripheral zone 70%.
- Central zone 10%.
- Transitional zone 20%.

○ **Which imaging modality is used to evaluate acute scrotal pain?**

Ultrasound.

○ **What are the ultrasound findings of testicular torsion?**

Early torsion (less than 4 hours) may be normal on gray scale images. However, color imaging shows an absence of flow to the affected testis. By 24 hours, the testicle may be hyper- or hypovascular on color images and enlarged with a heterogeneous echotexture on gray scale imaging.

○ **What are the ultrasound findings in epididymitis?**

The epididymis is enlarged and hypervascular. If the testis is involved, increased blood flow will be present. A reactive hydrocele and skin thickening may also be present.

○ **What is the importance of differentiating an extra/intratesticular mass?**

The majority of intratesticular masses are malignant. Most extratesticular masses are benign.

Primary and metastatic malignancies can involve the testicles. The vast majority of testicular neoplasms are primary. The most common germ cell tumors include seminoma, embryonal carcinoma, choriocarcinoma, and teratocarcinomas. Common primaries that may metastasize to the testicles are lymphoma (the most common in patients older than 60), prostate, leukemia, and kidney.

Testicular ultrasound (below) showing an intraparenchymal neoplasm suspicious for a germ cell tumor.

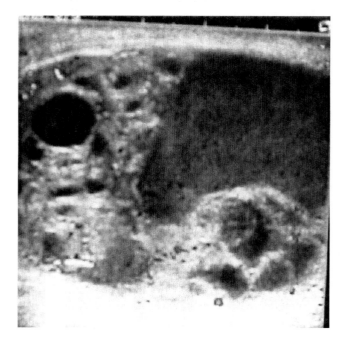

○ **Ultrasound appearance of an epidermoid cyst.**

Layers of keratin and desquamated squamous cells create an "onion skin" appearance.
　Other nonmalignant mass-like testicular lesions seen on ultrasound include the following:

- Hematoma—Hypoechoic and avascular.
- Segmental infarct—Focal hypoechoic, avascular area; painful. No palpable abnormality.
- Focal orchitis—Increased vascularity, reactive hydrocele/epididymitis, and scrotal wall thickening.

○ **What is the ultrasound appearance of Fournier's gangrene?**

Gas in the scrotum and perineum is echogenic with dirty posterior shadowing. Ring down artifact can also be seen. There is thickening of the scrotum.

○ **An infant's renal ultrasound shows the right kidney to have multiple cysts of varying sizes, which do not communicate. A right renal pelvis is not identified. What is the diagnosis?**

Multicystic dysplastic kidney (MCDK) is the result of atresia of the renal pelvis. If the disorder is bilateral, it is incompatible with life. MCDK is associated with contralateral renal abnormalities, most commonly ureteropelvic junction obstruction and vesicoureteral reflux.
　It is one of the most common causes of abdominal mass in an infant.

○ **Prenatal ultrasound demonstrates oligohydramnios and large echogenic kidneys. What is the diagnosis?**

Autosomal recessive polycystic kidney disease. Microcystic dilatation of the renal tubules causes an echogenic appearance without visible cysts (macrocysts).

○ **What is nephroblastomosis and what is its significance?**

Nephroblastomatosis presents in young patients with multiple renal masses and renal enlargement. Nephroblastomosis are persistent embryonal remnants (metanephric blastoma) in the kidney. Although not malignant itself, nephroblastomosis is considered a precursor to Wilms' tumor. The involved kidney is enlarged with a lobulated contour. Lesions are hypovascular, with little to no enhancement on contrast CT.

○ **What is mesoblastic nephroma and what is its significance?**

It is the most common neonatal renal neoplasm. It is a hamartoma of the kidney. Most are nonfunctioning. It can mimic Wilms' tumor. Most are diagnosed pathologically.

○ **What is the typical age range for diagnosing Wilms' tumor?**

Wilms' tumor is diagnosed between the first and fifth years of life. They are uncommon in the first year of life.

○ **Describe the typical imaging findings of a Wilms' tumor.**

Wilms' tumor commonly presents as a large (mean 12 cm) mass arising from the renal cortex, displacing and distorting the pelvocaliceal system, with less contrast enhancement than the surrounding parenchyma. There is frequent invasion of the renal vein and IVC. They are poorly enhancing and heterogeneous on CT and usually have well-defined margins.

A large left-sided Wilms' tumor (2) on CT (see below) with a vena caval thrombus (3).

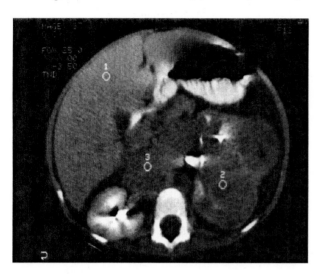

○   **What is the sequence of imaging tests for hydronephrosis found on prenatal ultrasound?**

• Postnatal ultrasound performed 4 to 7 days after birth to avoid false-negatives from physiologic postnatal dehydration.
• VCUG should be ordered in severe cases to evaluate for vesicoureteral reflux and posterior urethral valves.
• If obstruction is suspected, nuclear medicine renogram with diuretics will evaluate the degree of obstruction and differential renal function.

○   **What is the normal appearance of infant kidneys on ultrasound?**

They can have an undulating contour. Renal pyramids are hypoechoic compared with the cortex. This finding can be mistaken for hydronephrosis.

The scan (below) is the ultrasound appearance of a normal infant kidney showing fetal lobulation and hypoechoic renal pyramids. This is due to impaired concentrating ability of these kidneys with a relatively dilute medullary interstitium.

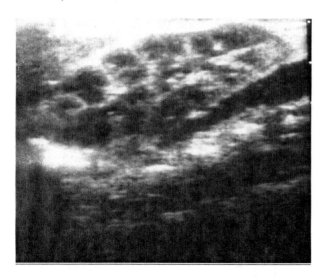

○   A 74-year-old man is admitted to the hospital for treatment of a foot infection. He has noted increasing abdominal distension over the last 3 months but no pain. He thinks he is just been gaining weight. His voiding is unchanged from his usual habit of small amounts and moderate frequency. Urology is consulted because of hydronephrosis and kidney stones. What is the correct diagnosis?

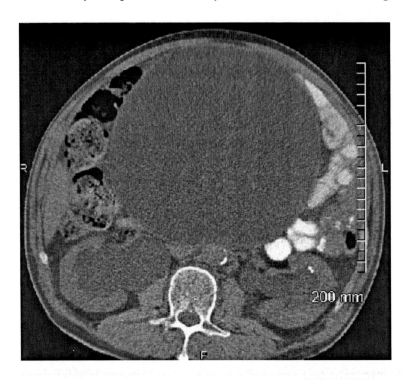

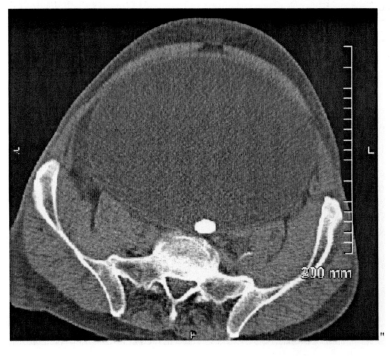

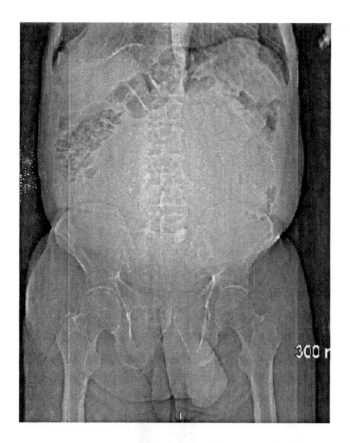

The images show significant hydronephrosis, renal calculi, a large bladder stone, and an enormous cystic structure extending from the pelvis to the kidneys and beyond. This cystic structure extended beyond the kidneys to the diaphragm. This is his bladder, which has become decompensated and stretched out to an enormous degree. He was catheterized for 9,350 cc of urine and developed postobstructive diuresis that lasted another 24 hours. His PSA was 54 and he was diagnosed with prostate cancer as the underlying cause of his prostatic obstruction. He was treated with a suprapubic tube and IMRT for his localized prostate cancer.

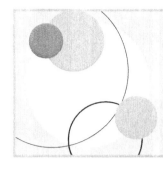

Urological Grab Bag Challenge

Stephen W. Leslie, MD, FACS

○ **What is the most common cause of urinary retention in pregnancy and at what gestational age is it most likely to occur?**

An impacted retroverted uterus is the most common cause of urinary retention in pregnancy. Most of these cases will present at approximately 16-week gestational age.

○ **The bladder may become palpable if it holds what minimum amount of urine?**

Usually, the bladder is palpable if it contains at least 200 mL of urine. It can be percussed if it is holding at least 150 mL of urine.

○ **True or False: Acute urinary retention can raise PSA levels.**

True, so do not bother checking the PSA level in situations of acute urinary retention.

○ **What is the clinical significance of "atypical small acinar proliferation" on a prostate biopsy and how often is it found?**

It represents approximately 2% of cases and has a 60% chance of developing into prostate cancer.

○ **What percentage of low-risk prostate cancer patients with focal or localized disease who undergo saturation prostatic biopsies are ultimately found to have significantly higher Gleason scores or previously undetected contralateral cancer?**

Nineteen percent would have their Gleason scores upgraded and approximately thirty percent will have contralateral disease.

○ **True or False: The bladder should always be emptied rapidly and completely, without clamping the Foley catheter, in cases of acute urinary retention even when the volume is well over 1000 mL.**

True. There is no benefit and possibly some harm if the catheter is clamped.

○ **α-Adrenergic blockers are often started immediately after placing a catheter for acute urinary retention. What is the recommended optimal duration of α-blocker therapy before removing the catheter for a voiding trial after an episode of acute retention?**

Three days appears to be the reasonable minimum time period to wait for the α-blocker therapy to be effective before catheter removal in most cases of acute retention.

○ **Is mumps orchitis more common in prepubertal or postpubertal boys and what percentage of boys with mumps will get mumps orchitis?**

Mumps orchitis is rare in prepubertal boys. Approximately 30% (20%–40%) of boys with mumps will get mumps orchitis.

○ **What cardiac drug at what dosage can cause a chemical epididymitis, what portion of the epididymis is involved most often and how should it be treated?**

Amiodarone at dosages more than 200 mg/d can cause a chemical epididymitis in 3% to 11% of patients on the medication. This type of chemical epididymitis typically involves the head of the epididymis. Treatment is discontinuation of the drug.

○ **Pyuria is present in roughly what percentage of patients with acute epididymitis?**

Only approximately 25%.

○ **What exactly is the function of fructose in the semen and what is the significance of its absence?**

Fructose nourishes the sperm. Absence of fructose in the semen suggests the absence of the seminal vesicles.

○ **What three medical diseases or disorders can cause calcification of the vas deferens?**

Tuberculosis, diabetes, and gonorrhea.

○ **Which kidney is affected most often with angiomyolipomas and with what other disease is it closely associated?**

The right kidney is affected 80% of the time. Approximately 20% of renal angiomyolipomas are associated with tuberous sclerosis and 80% of patients with tuberous sclerosis have angiomyolipomas.

○ **What percentage of patients with renal tuberculosis present with hematuria?**

Approximately 30%.

○ **What is the normal volume of the renal pelvis?**

The normal value is 5 to 8 cm^3.

○ **What are the most common benign and malignant tumors of the spermatic cord?**

The most common benign tumors are adenomatoid tumors and lipomas. Malignancies are uncommon in the spermatic cord, but the most frequent malignant tumor is a liposarcoma.

○ **Painful ejaculation is caused by what problems?**

Ejaculatory duct obstruction, prostatitis, BPH, and chronic pelvic pain syndrome.

○ **Are adult men with cystic fibrosis sterile and, if so, why?**

Adult cystic fibrosis men are sterile because of the absence of the vas deferens.

○ **A patient getting a TURP under spinal anesthetic develops epigastric and/or chest pain radiating to the left shoulder. What has probably happened?**

While a cardiac event is possible, it is far more likely that there has been an intraperitoneal bladder rupture.

○ **What is Dietl's crisis?**

Recurrent renal colic pain caused by intermittent kinking or twisting of the ureter, associated with nephroptosis.

○ **Fanconi syndrome is sometimes associated with what other disorder sometimes in kidney stone disease?**

Cystinuria.

○ **How does vaginal atresia differ from vaginal agenesis?**

Vaginal atresia involves only the distal vagina. The Mullerian structures are not affected. The uterus, cervix, and proximal vagina are all normal and intact.

  Vaginal agenesis is the absence of a proximal vagina in a normal 46 XX female with normal hormones. A hymenal fringe and a small distal vaginal pouch are usually present.

○ **What is Mayer-Rokitansky-Kuster-Hauser (MRKH) syndrome?**

Another name for vaginal agenesis.

○ **What urological problems are most commonly associated with vaginal agenesis?**

Unilateral renal agenesis or ectopia of one or both kidneys occurs in 74% of patients.

○ **What are Fordyce's spots and how are they treated?**

Fordyce's spots are the small, 1- to 3-mm painless fleshy bumps commonly found on the shaft of the penis. They are a form of ectopic sebaceous gland and are not considered pathologic so no treatment is necessary or recommended. A CO_2 laser can be used to remove them for cosmetic reasons if desired.

○ **True or False: The ascending loop of Henle contains active sodium transport and is impermeable to water.**

True.

○ **What are Tyson's glands?**

These are identical to Fordyce's spots, except that they are located on the glans.

○ **Gadolinium can cause what potentially serious complication when used in patients with renal failure?**

Nephrogenic systemic fibrosis.

○ **What is NAION, what causes it, and how is it treated?**

NonArteric Ischemic Optic Neuropathy, a type of blindness, has been associated extremely rarely with PDE5 inhibitors. There is no effective treatment.

○ **What is Stauffer syndrome?**

Stauffer syndrome is a paraneoplastic liver disorder associated with renal cell carcinoma.

○ **What are the four major effects of angiotensin II?**

Arteriolar vasoconstriction, decreased renal blood flow, sodium retention, and stimulation of aldosterone synthesis.

○ **What is Balkan nephropathy and why is it important urologically?**

Balkan nephropathy is a rare degenerative interstitial nephritis found typically in rural areas of the Balkans. It is urologically significant because of its associated 100- to 200-fold increase in the risk of upper tract transitional cell carcinoma.

○ **What type of renal tumor is associated with staghorn calculi?**

Squamous cell carcinoma.

○ **Describe the mechanism of action of thiazides.**

Thiazide diuretics inhibit NaCl reabsorption from the luminal side of the early segments of the distal convoluted tubule, resulting in a diuresis. This causes a compensatory increase in the proximal tubular reabsorption of calcium and NaCl, which explains the hypocalciuric effect of thiazides and why it is blunted by excess NaCl.

○ **What is the ipsilateral recurrence rate of transitional cell cancer when a segmental ureterectomy is done for distal ureteral disease?**

Approximately 25%.

○ **What is the most common site of ureteral TB?**

At the UVJ.

○ **What is the most common tumor metastatic to the kidneys?**

Lymphoma.

○ **Eighty percent of angiomyolipomas are associated with what other disorder?**

Tuberous sclerosis.

○ **What is the nephrectomy rate in major renal trauma cases that are surgically explored?**

Approximately 18%.

○ **Identify the most common location for iatrogenic injury to the ureter.**

At the pelvic brim, where the ureter crosses the iliac artery and courses posterior to the broad ligament and ovarian vessels in women.

○ **A retrocaval ureter develops due to the persistence of what vein?**

The subcardinal vein.

○ **What percentage of chronic dialysis patients developed renal failure due to polycystic kidney disease?**

Approximately 10%.

○ **Explain the underlying pathophysiology of polycystic kidney disease and how it causes renal cysts expansion and growth.**

Excessive expansion of renal cysts is due to a heightened sensitivity to the proliferative stimulation of epidermal growth factor.

○ **Explain the underlying etiology of hypertension in polycystic kidney disease, and is it renin mediated?**

As the renal cysts enlarge, they stretch the renal tubules that causes ischemia to the distal portions of the renal parenchyma resulting in renin release and hypertension.

○ **Name at least four other disorders besides hypertension and renal failure that are associated with polycystic kidney disease.**

Circle of Willis and Berry aneurysms, subarachnoid bleeds, colonic diverticula, and mitral valve prolapse.

○ **A simple renal cortical cyst will have what kind of T2-weighed image on an MRI?**

Homogenous hyperdense image.

○ **Name nine separate treatments to help control bleeding in hemorrhagic cystitis.**

1) Continuous bladder irrigation.
2) Intravesical therapy with alum, formalin, or silver nitrate.
3) Systemic therapy with Elmiron and Amicar.
4) Electrocautery.
5) Laser coagulation therapy.
6) Hydrodistension.
7) Hyperbaric oxygen.
8) Urinary diversion.
9) Hypogastric artery embolization.

○ **"Moth-eaten" calices on IVP are typical of what disease and how is it treated?**

Renal tuberculosis. Treatment is with INH, rifampin, and pyrazinamide.

○ **Physiologic hydronephrosis of pregnancy affects which side most often and why?**

The right side is affected approximately three times more often than the left. The left ureter is partially protected from compression by the sigmoid colon.

○ **Which antibiotics are preferred during pregnancy for UTI's?**

Penicillins and cephalosporins are preferred. Nitrofurantoin is acceptable but may be more likely to cause GI upset. Sulfa can be used except near term. Avoid quinolones and tetracyclines.

○ **Can aminoglycosides be used during pregnancy?**

Yes, but only when other agents are not suitable in patients with normal renal function.

○ **What is the average number of sperm that ultimately reach the site of fertilization in the fallopian tube?**

Only approximately 300.

○ **When is INH therapy useful in urology?**

INH can be used in TB but is most useful as the primary antibiotic for severe side effects of BCG therapy.

○ **What complication of INH therapy can be prevented with pyridoxine therapy?**

Peripheral neuropathy.

○ **What is the significance of poor endothelial cell functional testing in men with ED?**

Poor endothelial cell function would suggest a higher risk of cardiovascular disease.

○ **After a vasectomy, what percentage of men develop antisperm antibodies?**

Approximately 60%.

○ **What is the most common epididymal tumor?**

A benign adenomatoid tumor.

○ **Incomplete dissolution of Chwalla's membrane will cause what?**

A ureterocele.

○ **What is the most common renal tumor in infants?**

Congenital mesoblastic nephroma.

○ **Which is more sensitive in the detection of vesicoureteral reflux: a radionuclide cystogram or a VCUG, and which delivers less radiation to the patient?**

The radionuclide cystogram is more sensitive and more specific than a VCUG in the detection of vesicoureteral reflux. It also delivers considerably less radiation exposure to the patient.

○ **Explain the differences among detrusor overactivity, overactive bladder, detrusor hyperreflexia, and detrusor instability. (Warning: this could be the toughest single question in the whole book!)**

Detrusor overactivity describes the urodynamic observation of involuntary detrusor contractions during bladder filling which may be spontaneous or provoked. It requires urodynamic testing.

Overactive bladder is a symptomatic diagnosis secondary to detrusor overactivity usually defined as urgency with or without incontinence usually associated with frequency and nocturia.

Detrusor hyperreflexia is defined as bladder overactivity or increased bladder contractile activity caused by a disturbance in the nervous control mechanism. It requires identification of a relevant, underlying neurologic disorder. If no neurologic disorder is identified, then the term idiopathic detrusor hyperreflexia should be used.

Detrusor instability has previously been used to describe uninhabitable bladder contractions typically occurring at bladder volumes below capacity. Idiopathic detrusor hyperreflexia describes the same situation although the term idiopathic detrusor overactivity is now preferred.

○ **Angiomyolipomas are associated with what disease?**

Tuberous sclerosis.

○ **Calcification of the vas occurs in association with what three disorders?**

Diabetes, TB, and gonorrhea.

○ **The majority of the calcium ultimately excreted in the urine is determined where in the nephron?**

The distal convoluted tubule and proximal collecting tubule. No significant changes in calcium occur anywhere else in the nephron.

○ **Tuberous sclerosis is an inheritable autosomal dominant disorder associated with angiomyolipomas and what other renal problems?**

Cysts and renal cell carcinoma.

○ **What tumors are associated with von Hippel-Lindau disease?**

Renal cell carcinomas, pheochromocytomas, and hemangioblastomas of the central nervous system.

○ **Topamax (topiramate), a drug used for migraine and epilepsy, causes what specific GU problem and how?**

Calcium phosphate nephrolithiasis. It is a carbonic anhydrase inhibitor that causes metabolic acidosis resulting in hypocitraturia and increased urinary alkalinity. This results in calcium phosphate stones. The increase in risk is roughly 2 to 4 times normal.

○ **True or False: Measuring bone mineral density is recommended before long-term, androgen-deprivation therapy?**

True.

○ **Name three oral drugs that can be used specifically for prostatic bleeding.**

Dutasteride (Avodart), finasteride (Proscar), and epsilon aminocaproic acid (Amicar).

○ **What is the treatment for stuttering (intermittent) priapism?**

Intermittent intracorporal self-injection with a diluted α-agonist solution. LHRH therapy can also be used in resistant or persistent cases.

○ **In which gender and racial group is nocturia most common?**

It is most common in non-white females.

○ **True or False: Diuretics increase nocturia by approximately 40%.**

True.

○ **Nocturia is associated with what chronic conditions? (Name 10.)**

Diabetes, cardiac disease, hypertension, sleep disorders such as sleep apnea, overactive bladder, neurogenic bladder, urinary retention, interstitial cystitis, radiation cystitis, renal disease, diabetes insipidus, and depression.

○ **True or False: Evening fluid restriction is a reasonably effective initial treatment for nocturnal polyuria.**

False. It is reasonable but usually ineffective.

○ **Differentiate between nocturnal polyuria and global polyuria.**

Nocturnal polyuria is a relative increase in nocturnal urinary volume but with a normal 24-hour urine total volume. Global polyuria has an abnormally high 24-hour urine volume, usually >40 mg/kg/24 h.

○ **What does a "beehive in the bladder" on cystogram or cystoscopy typically indicate?**

A colovesical fistula.

○ **Colovesical fistulas are typically located in what part of the bladder?**

The dome.

○ **Is there any clinical significance to a colovesical fistula that involves the right side versus the left side of the bladder?**

Lesions on the right side (dome or posterior wall) are most likely due to Crohn's disease, while left-sided lesions are typically due to diverticular disease.

○ **An acute left varicocele suggests what underlying pathology?**

Testicular vein occlusion from a renal cell tumor thrombus extending into the left renal vein.

○ **What common urologic anomaly can mimic a sacral metastasis on a bone scan?**

A pelvic horseshoe kidney.

○ **Patients treated with sorafenib for renal cell carcinoma have a significant higher risk of what common medical disorder?**

Hypertension.

○ **Is testicular cancer more common on one side?**

The right side is involved more often.

○ **What is a Quackel shunt and what is it used for?**

It is a cavernosal–spongiosum shunt used for priapism performed through a perineal approach.

○ **What is the preferred intracavernosal injection agent for reversal of low-flow priapism and why?**

Diluted phenylephrine solution is preferred due to its pure α-agonist activity with minimal β effects.

○ **True or False: Cranberry juice and tablets are recommended for both recurrent UTIs and nephrolithiasis patients.**

False. Cranberry juice has a relatively high oxalate content and therefore is not recommended for kidney stone patients. It may be of some use in UTIs.

○ **True or False: A 24-hour urine for metabolic kidney stone risk factors is required in renal transplant patients.**

True.

○ **True or False: Tetracycline lowers testosterone levels by approximately 20% and nitrofurantoin depresses spermatogenesis.**

True.

○ **What is the mortality rate associated with urinary retention?**

12.5% without comorbidities and 28.8% with comorbidities.

○ **Define and differentiate the following terms: microhematuria, dipstick hematuria, dipstick pseudohematuria, and significant microhematuria.**

Microhematuria is the presence of red blood cells in the urine.

Dipstick hematuria means a positive dipstick test for urinary blood with or without any actual RBCs on microscopic examination.

Dipstick pseudohematuria is defined as a positive dipstick test for urinary blood with no RBCs actually present on microscopic examination.

Significant microhematuria, according to the Official AUA Panel Definition, means an average of three or more RBCs /HPF in two of three properly collected urine specimens.

○ **Is the incidence of penile cancer in the world increasing, decreasing, or stable and what is the incidence in the United States?**

Decreasing in the world. Approximately 1200 cases are reported yearly in the United States.

○ **Name seven risk factors for penile cancer.**

Age (incidence increases significantly after age 60), smoking, poor personal hygiene, phimosis, increased number of sexual partners, BXO, HPV infection, lichen sclerosis, giant condyloma, bowenoid papulosis, and penile intraepithelial neoplasia.

○   **What is the overall mortality rate from penile cancer?**

The National Cancer Institute's Surveillance, Epidemiology and End Results program found a mortality rate of 22.4%, while the National Cancer Database (2007) reported a 5-year mortality rate of 25%.

○   **True or False: Circumcision offers almost complete protection from penile cancer.**

False. Adult circumcisions offer no significant protection. To be effective as a prophylactic measure, circumcision must be done during the neonatal period. When circumcision is done at puberty, the risk is reduced but if done while the patient is a neonate, penile cancer almost never develops.

○   **What is the difference between erythroplasia of Queryat and Bowen's disease?**

Both are histologically carcinoma-in-situ intraepithelial neoplasms. Erythroplasia of Queryat involves the foreskin and glans, while Bowen's disease affects the penile shaft and the remainder of the male genitalia and perineum.

○   **Most (95%) of penile cancers are squamous cell cancers. What other primary cell type tumors can occur in the penis?**

Carcinoma-in-situ (Queryat, Bowen's), adenocarcinoma (from sweat glands), melanoma, basal cell, and sarcomas (from blood vessels, smooth muscle, and connective tissue).

○   **Does circumcision reduce the risk of HIV transmission and, if so, by how much?**

Circumcision reduces HIV transmission by approximately 50% to 60%.

○   **Rate the risk of chemotherapy-induced nausea and vomiting from highest to lowest for the following chemotherapy agents: cisplatin, cyclophosphamide, adriamycin, docetaxel, mitomycin, mitoxantrone, bleomycin, vincristin, and vinblastin.**

They are in correct descending order with cisplatin having the highest risk. The risk is low to minimal from docetaxel on.

○   **What is a Page kidney, what is its most common cause, how is it diagnosed, and how should it be treated?**

A Page kidney is a kidney exposed to external compression of the renal parenchyma resulting in renin-mediated hypertension and renal ischemia. The most common example would be a subcapsular hematoma following a trauma, but it can also be caused by a needle biopsy. Compression by a cyst or tumor is also possible but less common. Doppler ultrasound typically shows no or diminished diastolic renal blood flow. Treatment is surgical decompression. It was named after Dr. Irvine Page (1901–1989) who demonstrated in 1939 that wrapping cellophane tightly around an animal kidney would cause hypertension.

○   **What is the ipsilateral recurrent rate for ureteral cancers treated by segmental or partial ureterectomy?**

The recurrent rate is 45% to 50%.

○   **True or False: Statins are harmful to patients receiving BCG therapy for superficial bladder cancer.**

True. Studies suggest that the use of statins is associated with a threefold increased risk of tumor progression and subsequent need for radical cystectomy.

○   **True or False: Epirubicin intravesical chemotherapy has recently been shown to have comparable recurrence rates to BCG therapy for superficial bladder cancer and CIS.**

False. BCG remains superior.

○   **Describe the "trigger and maintenance" theory of hyperoxaluric nephrolithiasis and what causes the "trigger." (For extra credit, who first suggested this theory and when?)**

Vermeulen CW et al. (1967) first suggested that many calcium oxalate stone formers would have mild or borderline hyperoxaluria with transient spikes in urinary oxalate excretion caused by "dietary indiscretions."

○   **True or False: According to the Stress Incontinence Surgical Treatment Efficacy Trial (SISTER), overall success from the Burch colposuspension and the pubovaginal sling are roughly comparable.**

False. The sling procedure had significantly better success rates for controlling stress incontinence than the Burch.

○   **Male slings are most useful and effective for men with what severity level of incontinence?**

Male slings are best suited for men with mild-to-moderate incontinence. Artificial urinary sphincters are the preferred treatment for more severe male incontinence.

○   **Does the percentage of smooth muscle and α-adrenergic receptors in the prostate change with age and, if so, how?**

The percentage increases with age.

○   **True or False: A slower ESWL rate of 60 shocks per minute achieves better stone fragmentation and higher stone-free rates than 120 shocks per minute.**

True. An 18% improvement in stone-free rate has been reported with the slower shock wave frequency.

○   **True or False: Osteopenia is more prevalent in infertile, oligospermic men than in normal men.**

True. Low total sperm counts and low FSH levels have been reported to correlate to decreased bone mineral density.

○   **True or False: Co Q_{10} (Coenzyme Q_{10}) can increase sperm motility in idiopathic asthenozoospermia.**

True.

○   **What infertility treatments, if any, are available to a man with nonmosaic Klinefelter's syndrome?**

Microdissection testicular sperm extraction (Micro-TESE) and intracytoplasmic sperm injection (ICSI) have demonstrated success.

○   **Which of the following have been found to be good predictors of sperm detection during microscopic sperm extraction surgery: serum inhibin, spermatogenic cells in semen, Y chromosome microdeletions, testicular size, FSH level, and positive testicular histopathology.**

Only the first three listed.

○   **What is the significance of Yq11.23 (interval 6)?**

This is the designated area on the long arm of the Y chromosome considered critical for male fertility.

○ **Which is more common: ED or premature ejaculation?**

ED is more common in the older age group, but overall premature ejaculation is the most common male sexual disorder.

○ **Premature ejaculation is often associated with ED and what other urologic problem?**

Chronic prostatitis is present in more than 55% of men with premature ejaculation.

○ **Daily use of what drug appears to yield the longest ejaculatory delay when used for premature ejaculation?**

Paroxetine (Paxil).

○ **What is the major contraindication for daily SSRI medication?**

The presence or reported history of bipolar depression.

○ **True or False: Oxytocin analogues may be possible future treatments for premature ejaculation.**

False. Oxytocin analogues may prove useful for stimulating ejaculation in patients with delayed ejaculation, while oxytocin inhibitors may play a future role in premature ejaculation treatment.

○ **In postobstructive diuresis, what IV fluid should be used for fluid replacement and how should the rate be calculated?**

The recommended replacement fluid in postobstructive diuresis is half-normal saline. The suggested rate of fluid replacement is 50% of the hourly urinary output up to 1000 mL less than the 24-hour total urine output. Check electrolytes at least every 6 to 8 hours.

○ **How long does postobstructive diuresis typically last?**

24 to 72 hours.

○ **What relationship, if any, has been established between FSH, LH, inhibin, testosterone, free T4, and abnormal semen parameters in infertile men?**

No clear association has been found.

○ **Which vasopressin subtype affects the renal collecting duct cells causing increased free-water reabsorption?**

Type V_2. (A type V_2 antagonist is now available as conivaptan (Vaprisol) to treat persistent or refractory hyponatremia but only in hospitalized patients with hypervolemia or euvolemia without congestive heart failure.) Type 1a increases platelet aggregation and vasoconstriction, while type 1b increases release of ACTH and B-endorphins.

○ **What is the nocturnal polyuria index and what is normal?**

It is the percentage of the 24-hour urinary volume that is produced during sleep. Normal is 35% or less. A higher percentage would be diagnostic of nocturnal polyuria.

○ **Compared to normal controls, do patients with nocturnal polyuria demonstrate different patterns of water intake or body water distribution?**

No difference in water intake is found, but patients with nocturnal polyuria generally demonstrate increased water volume in the lower extremities compared to controls. This process usually begins at about noon and gradually increases through the afternoon and evening until bedtime. This may explain the observed benefits noted with lower extremity elevation and evening walks in patients with nocturnal polyuria.

○ **Which condition tends to lose urinary and rectal continence earlier and why: Shy–Drager syndrome or amyotrophic lateral sclerosis (ALS)?**

ALS tends to preserve urinary and rectal continence until very advanced stages of the disease. Shy–Drager syndrome patients lose continence early in the course of the disease. The difference is due to preservation/ destruction, respectively, of Onuf's nucleus in the sacral spinal cord. The nucleus is preserved in ALS but destroyed early in Shy–Drager syndrome.

○ **Which of the following is NOT a treatment for nocturia:**
1) **Vasopressin (DDAVP) therapy.**
2) **Decreased oral fluid intake before bedtime.**
3) **Elevation of the lower extremities before bedtime.**
4) **Taking an afternoon nap.**
5) **Changing the timing of daily furosemide from early morning to midafternoon.**
6) **Use of anticholinergics or imipramine.**
7) **Use of sleeping pills/aids.**

None of the above. All are possible therapies for nocturia.

○ **What is the recommended number of ejaculations needed to achieve azoospermia after a bilateral vasectomy?**

Approximately 32.

○ **What is cabergoline (Dostinex) and what urologic problem does it address?**

Cabergoline is an ergot-derived dopamine receptor agonist that is used primarily in the United States as a second-line oral agent for hyperprolactinemia when bromocriptine alone is insufficient. It has also been used in Parkinson's. There is also some evidence that it may be reasonably effective in the treatment of ED in PDE5 inhibitor failures.

○ **What is the specific medical risk for cabergoline (Dostinex)?**

It has been associated with an increased risk of heart valve disease, although this usually occurs only at the higher dosages.

○ **What is the most common cause of male infertility and what is its frequency in infertile men?**

Varicocele, which is found in approximately 40% of all male infertility cases.

○ **Renal colic from intractable stone disease can be treated with what last resort surgical procedure?**

Renal autotransplantation with a pyelovesicostomy.

○   **Intracorporeal laser lithotripsy of cystine and uric acid stones produces what chemicals?**

Laser treatment of cystine stones produces hydrogen sulfide, while treatment of uric acid stones can make cyanide.

○   **MUSE is contraindicated in what conditions?**

Abnormal penile anatomy, allergy to alprostadil, multiple myeloma, sickle cell anemia or trait, thrombocythemia, and polycythemia.

○   **What is the "poppy seed" test?**

Visual inspection of the urine after oral ingestion of poppy seeds. It is a simple, cost-effective screening test for colovesical fistula.

○   **True or False: Renal cell cancer patients with a positive family history for renal cell carcinoma have a greater risk of dying from that cancer than renal cell cancer patients without a positive family history.**

False. However, those with a positive family history are more likely to develop bilateral disease.

○   **What factors are associated with the degree or severity of the penile deformity/curvature in Peyronie's disease?**

Age, lateral location of the plaque, and ED.

○   **Balanitis xerotica obliterans (BXO) has been linked to what other urological disorder?**

Hypogonadism that may play a significant role in the development, progression, and recurrence of BXO. Application of 2% testosterone cream and testosterone-replacement therapy has shown normalization of tissue in BXO cases who are hypogonadal.

○   **Children with nocturnal enuresis have a higher incidence of what other disorders?**

Obesity and sleep apnea.

○   **What percentage of patients with gross hematuria and a totally negative initial urological workup will eventually be diagnosed with a urological cancer?**

Approximately 3.4%.

○   **Which has shown, so far, better rates of suppressing local tumor progression and metastases in renal tumors: cryoablation or radiofrequency ablation?**

Cryoablation appears to be significantly better in reducing tumor progression according to most studies.

○   **Capsular invasion in renal cell cancer has what impact on tumor recurrence and survival? How does it change the staging?**

Capsular invasion does not change the staging, but it tends to indicate more aggressive disease.

○   **Obstructive azoospermia due to ejaculatory duct obstruction should be suspected in azoospermic men with what clinical findings?**

At least one palpable vas, low semen volume, acidic semen pH, and low or absent semen fructose.

○ **What is the expected pregnancy rate after ejaculatory duct resection in men with ejaculatory duct obstruction?**

Only approximately 20% to 30%.

○ **You are called by a patient on a PDE5 inhibitor such as sildenafil (Viagra) about sudden blindness or hearing loss. According to the pharmaceutical's manufacturer, what advice should you give the patient?**

Stop taking the medication. They offer no other advice. However, referral to an appropriate specialist (ENT or ophthalmology) would seem reasonable, as there might be other treatable causes of the patient's problem.

○ **During a long laparoscopic procedure, the patient's blood pressure starts to drop slowly and ventilation is becoming more difficult according to the anesthesiologist. New cardiac arrhythmias have been detected. You have encountered no obvious problems with the surgery and no significant bleeding. What is the diagnosis, pathophysiology, and treatment for this condition?**

Most likely, the patient is developing a tension pneumoperitoneum due to the persistently elevated intra-abdominal pressure. High intraperitoneal pressures over time lead to vena caval compression that decreases the venous return, resulting in hypotension as well as direct pressure on the diaphragm making ventilation more difficult. Higher amounts of carbon dioxide are absorbed into the blood eventually causing acidosis, hypoxia, and arrhythmias. Cardiovascular collapse will ultimately develop if recognized and treated promptly. Treatment involves immediate desufflation, correcting any Trendelenburg position, IV fluids, and hyperventilation with 100% oxygen.

○ **What is the "eggplant sign" and what problem does it indicate?**

This is the typical appearance of the penis immediately after a penile fracture with extensive hematoma formation and extravasation of blood.

○ **What is tumor necrosis factor-α, what does it normally do, and why is it important urologically?**

Tumor necrosis factor-α (TNF-α) is a cytokine that is involved with homeostasis of the immune system, inflammation, and host defense as well as malignant disease. TNF is secreted by a number of tumor cells including renal cell carcinoma where it appears to act as an autocrine growth factor. The presence of TNF in tumors is associated with cachexia, hormone resistance, and more aggressive disease with a poorer prognosis. Tumor necrosis factor-α is one of the targets of renal cell cancer chemotherapy along with vascular endothelial growth factor and mammalian target of rapamycin (mTOR).

○ **True or False: Tumor necrosis factor-α is elevated in prostate cancer patients with advanced or extensive disease.**

True.

○ **What is the most common site of malignant melanoma in the urinary tract?**

The urethra. In men, it is most often in the fossa navicularis.

○ **What is the overall incidence and significance of testicular microcalcifications on testicular ultrasound examinations? How should it be treated and followed?**

Testicular microcalcifications are not rare and occur in approximately 0.6% to 9% of men. There is an increased risk of testicular cancer associated with these microcalcifications. α-Fetoprotein and β-HCG tumor markers along with yearly follow-ups are suggested.

○   **What is the medication and recommended dilution formula for intracorporeal injection therapy of priapism?**

The most commonly used medication is phenylephrine. Typically, the standard ampule is 10 mg/mL, which is too concentrated to use directly. One-half a milliliter of the drug in 9.5 mL of NS provides sufficient dilution to use safely. 0.5 to 1 mL is injected directly into the corpora every 15 minutes until the priapism is resolved, up to a maximum of three injections. If this fails, then a shunt will be needed. Vital signs should be checked regularly during this process because of the risk of hypertension when injecting an α-agonist.

○   **What is the modality of choice for evaluating the nodal status of penile cancer patients with impalpable nodes?**

Dynamic sentinel node biopsy.

○   **True or False: α-Blocker therapy reduces the incidence of ureteral colic after ureteroscopy and improves the stone-free rate after both ESWL and ureteroscopy.**

True.

○   **True or False: Shockwave therapy has shown slight benefits when used for Peyronie's disease.**

False. No benefit has been demonstrated from shockwave therapy in Peyronie's.

○   **True or False: Testosterone does not influence PSA levels in older men.**

True. For men older than 50 years, testosterone does not appear to affect PSA levels.

○   **What is the cause of nephrogenic systemic fibrosis?**

Use of gadolinium-contrast in patients with azotemia or renal failure. First recognized in 1997, the typical patient is already on dialysis. It begins with subacute swelling of the distal extremities and progresses to severe skin induration, which can spread to internal organs. Transmetallation from prolonged exposure to gadolinium-contrast media is thought to be the underlying cause.

○   **Can nephrogenic systemic fibrosis occur in patients without significant renal failure?**

Apparently not, since no confirmed cases have been reported without severe azotemia or end-stage renal disease.

○   **True or False: C-reactive protein is an independent prognostic variable for outcomes in renal cell carcinoma and can be used to monitor response to chemotherapy in metastatic disease.**

True.

○   **True or False: Cryoablation of small renal tumors has similar outcomes to radiofrequency ablation.**

False. Cryoablation appears to have better outcomes according to meta-analysis.

○   **When performing a partial nephrectomy, what is the maximum recommended warm ischemia time?**

No more than 36 to 40 minutes are recommended.

○ **What is elastography, how does it work, and what is its urological application?**

Elastrography is thought to be potentially helpful in identifying prostate cancer. It is performed by compressing prostate tissue, then measuring its tissue strain and degree of elasticity. It is thought that areas of increased stiffness would indicate prostate cancer due to the increased cell density present in cancer tissue.

○ **True or False: Penile ultrasonography can be useful in categorizing and following Peyronie's disease.**

True. The density of echogenic areas and acoustic shadows can be easily followed.

○ **What are the contraindications for laparoscopic radical nephrectomy?**

Need for nephron-sparing surgery, locally advanced (T4) disease with tumor invasion of surrounding tissues, and significant vena caval tumor thrombus or vena caval wall invasion. Tumor size is a relative contraindication if more than 20 cm in size.

○ **What are the characteristics and differential diagnosis of inflammatory myofibroblastic tumors of the bladder?**

These are rare, benign tumors that typically occur in younger patients. The most common bladder location is the posterior lateral wall. The etiology is thought to be inflammatory but there is evidence of a neoplastic process as well. The main differential diagnosis is sarcoma where the treatment is more surgically aggressive. The correct diagnosis of inflammatory myofibroblastic tumor of the bladder often requires a final histologic confirmation, so this entity must be considered when dealing with bladder masses of undetermined etiology to avoid overtreatment if benign, and potentially dangerous undertreatment if it is ultimately determined to be a malignant sarcoma.

○ **Micturition syncope is classically caused by what disorder?**

Pheochromocytoma involving the bladder.

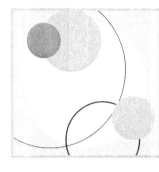

Just for Fun: Urology Trivia

Stephen W. Leslie, MD, FACS

○ **Who first coined the name "nephrostomy" and was the first to actually do this as a planned surgical procedure? For extra credit, what is this urologist's full name, his nationality, when did this happen, and what is he better known for?**

The first nephrostomy was done by Joaquin Albarran Maria y Dominguez in 1896. He was a prominent French urologist born in Cuba. He is better known for inventing the deflecting cystoscope lever or bridge.

○ **What is Gerota's full name and nationality?**

Dimitrie Gerota was Romanian.

○ **What is another name for Highmore's body?**

The hilum of the testis.

○ **What is the Fick principle and what is its urological application?**

Developed by Adolf Eugen Fick. It is the basic principle and formula used to measure blood flow to an organ. Originally used for cardiac output, a modified form of Fick's formula is currently used to calculate the creatinine clearance.

○ **What is pilimiction and how does it happen?**

Pilimiction means hair passing in the urine. It is most commonly caused by a pelvic dermoid cyst that breaks through into the bladder.

○ **"Suprasegmental reflex mechanisms becoming integrated with the spinal reflex arc" describes what urological milestone event?**

Toilet training.

○ **Annual amount of money spent on urology-related medical care in the United States is?**

$11 billion.

○   **Harrison Ford came up with the idea for the famous scene in "Raiders of the Lost Ark" where Indiana Jones shoots the big swordsman. What was his inspiration?**

He urgently needed a bathroom break.

○   **The first episode of "Joanie Loves Chachi" was the highest rated American program ever in the history of Korean television. How come?**

Chachi is Korean for "penis."

○   **True or False: Dutch researchers have found a way to measure the resistance of the urethra using sound via a microphone placed behind the scrotum.**

True. Apparently, the sound's frequency varies according to the degree of urethral narrowing.

○   **Birt-Hogg-Dube syndrome, a type of small papular skin lesion on the scalp, forehead, face, and neck, is associated with what two urological conditions?**

Multiple or bilateral renal cell carcinomas and renal oncocytomas.

○   **Lo Prado, Chile, a suburb of Santiago, was the first city in the world to do what?**

Give all its senior male residents free Viagra.

○   **What does "cock-throppled" mean?**

That your Adam's apple is larger than normal.

○   **Who first placed the eyes or openings on a catheter on opposite sides instead of just using a terminal opening? (Hint: He was also the first to use a catheter introducer and a stylet.)**

Rhazes, an Arab physician who lived 850–923 AD.

○   **What is the origin of the word penis? (Hint: It is Latin.)**

It is Latin for "tail."

○   **How far would the seminiferous tubules reach if fully stretched out?**

Approximately one-fourth mile.

○   **What is the total lifetime male semen production volume?**

Approximately 18 quarts.

○   **What is the average speed of a sperm and how far can a sperm swim in an hour?**

Approximately 1/8 in/min or approximately 7 in/h.

○   **Who performed the first successful artificial insemination in a human and when?**

Scottish surgeon John Hunter in the 1780s.

○ **Where did the term "missionary position" come from?**

It came from Trobriand Islanders, who were urged by missionaries to adopt the "man on top" position as the only morally acceptable way to have intercourse.

○ **What is a spermologer? (Hint: The editor of this book is one.)**

A person who collects trivia.

○ **What is the most common neoplastic condition affecting males?**

BPH.

○ **Hypospadius is associated with how many other syndromes, anomalies, and congenital malformations?**

49.

○ **What is "Tire Pump syndrome," how does it happen, who gets it, and when?**

It refers to abdominal and shoulder pain after sexual activity, which improves quickly on its own without further treatment. It occurs only in females, usually after hysterectomy. The abdominal and shoulder pain is caused by pneumoperitoneum produced by the sexual intercourse in the presence of a salpingovaginal fistula. It is quite rare but reported.

○ **Living, laboratory-grown skin for skin grafts has been successfully developed using what original source for the cellular material?**

Neonatal foreskin.

○ **What age group is affected most often by acute urinary retention?**

From 75 to 84 years.

○ **What is the world's largest recorded human urinary bladder volume from retention?**

So far, the largest documented human bladder capacity was 9350 cm^3. The patient never went to the physician and thought his increasing abdominal distension was just gaining weight. He might have gone on for several more months except he got a severe foot infection that required hospitalization. The underlying cause of his retention was found to be prostate cancer. If anyone has found a larger bladder, please inform the editor!

○ **What noted urologist was able to achieve a BA, MA, and an MD degree from the University of Virginia in only 4 years?**

High Hampton Young.

○ **What is "Soot Wart," what causes it, and why did it affect people in England more than in other countries? (For extra credit, who discovered it and when?)**

Soot wart was the original name for squamous cell carcinoma of the scrotum. It was associated with chimney sweeps in England in the 18th century and was the first proven occupational cancer. Soot from the chimneys would easily penetrate their clothes and reach the scrotum, ultimately causing cancer. English chimney sweeps, unlike those in other countries, were notoriously averse to washing and therefore had much higher scrotal cancer rates. First reported by Sir Percival Pott in 1775.

○ **Name five predisposing factors to squamous cell carcinoma of the scrotum.**

Compromised immune system, scrotal trauma, UV and x-ray radiation exposure, chemical exposure, and arsenic.

○ **What is the most common malignancy in men in Uganda? (Hint: It is a urological malignancy.)**

Penile cancer.

○ **Phimosis comes from the Greek word for what?**

Muzzling.

○ **The foreskin represents approximately what percentage of the total skin of the penis?**

Approximately 50%.

○ **Buschke-Lowenstein tumor is another name for what urological neoplasm?**

Verrucous carcinoma of the penis.

○ **Name the two urologists who have won the Nobel Prize and describe their contributions.**

Dr. Charles Huggins was a Canadian-born urologist who discovered that male sex hormones stimulate prostate growth in dogs while estrogens inhibit it. This finding rapidly became the basis for hormonal therapy for the treatment of prostate cancer. Dr. Huggins won the Nobel Prize in 1966.

Dr. Werner Forssmann was a general surgery resident during the depression in 1929. He passed a ureteral catheter through his antecubital vein into the right atrium. He then ran to the radiology department to take a picture. Up until that time, it was widely believed that passage of a tube into the heart would be instantly fatal. His goal was to find a better way to deliver drugs directly to the heart for cardiac resuscitation. For this momentous discovery, Dr. Forssman was immediately fired from the hospital and general surgery residency program. He eventually became a urologist (no other surgical field would take him). He later received the Nobel Prize in 1956 for his role in the discovery of cardiac catheterization.

○ **Several decades ago, then AUA President Dr. Logan Holtgrewe surveyed practicing urologists approximately the minimum number of TURP cases necessary to achieve minimal proficiency. What was the consensus conclusion?**

A minimum of 80 TURP cases.

○ **What is the average total number of TURP procedures currently done by urology residents in a 4-year urology residency training program?**

Approximately 60 and decreasing.

○ **Claudius Galen, the famous Roman physician from 200 AD, died from what urological disorder?**

Hydrocele. His hydrocele was so large that he had to drain it periodically. Eventually, it got infected and he succumbed to sepsis.

○ **What animals have a urogenital diaphragm similar to humans?**

None.

○ **Which medical specialty is the least likely to refer a patient with hematuria to urology or order any imaging studies?**

Ob-Gyn. Their usual treatment is to repeat the urinalysis or send a urine culture.

○ **How did syphilis contribute to modern urography and who was responsible?**

In 1923, a dermatology resident named Earl Osborne was experimenting with intravenous sodium iodide as a possible treatment for syphilis. He discovered that the x-rays he obtained on patients given the sodium iodide showed clearly opacified urinary tracts.

○ **Who first correctly described Gerota's fascia? (Hint: It was not Gerota!)**

Emil and Otto Zuckerkandl in 1883. Dimitrie Gerota's description of the same entity was not published until 1895.

○ **What famous and momentous urological event occurred on Monday, April 18, 1983 at exactly 7 PM in Las Vegas, NV; who did it, and what medication was involved?**

That was when British neurophysiologist Dr. Giles Brindley injected his own penis with phenoxybenzamine and then showed the entire AUA meeting delegates his induced erection!

○ **What is the precise, formal chemical descriptive name for conivaptan hydrochloride (Vaprisol), what is it, and what is it used for?**

[1,1′-biphenyl]-2-carboxamide, N-[4-[[(4,5-dihydro-2-methylimidazo[4,5-d][1]benzazepin-6(1H)-yl)carbonyl] phenyl]-monohydrochloride is the chemical formula. It is a type V_2 vasopressin antagonist that is approved for the treatment of hyponatremia. It increases free-water excretion while retaining sodium.

○ **Who was the first Board certified female urologist?**

Dr. Elisabeth Pauline Pickett was the first female certified in urology in 1962.

○ **As of 2008, how many Board certified women urologists are there in the United States?**

324, not counting the 237 who are Board eligible and another 229 still in urology residency.

○ **What is the association between snoring and male sexual function?**

Heavy snoring is associated with decreased ejaculatory function and overall sexual satisfaction. There does not appear to be a relationship between snoring and libido or erectile function.

○ **What is the Nutcracker syndrome, how is it diagnosed and what is the treatment?**

It is left renal venous hypertension caused by compression of the left renal vein between the aorta and superior mesenteric artery. This causes left-sided hematuria, left gonadal vein varices, varicoceles in men, and possibly pain. Diagnosis is difficult but may be picked up with CT or MR angiography. Current treatment is with stents as a minimally invasive option, but embolization and vascular repositioning are acceptable alternatives.

○ **What is the most commonly litigated procedure that involves urologists, how many are done annually, and how many does the average urologist do a year?**

Vasectomy is the most commonly litigated procedure routinely performed by urologists. Approximately 527,000 are done yearly in the United States with the average urologist doing approximately 70 annually.

○ **What is infibulation?**

The placement of a ring or stick through the foreskin, presumably to prevent masturbation, sexual activity, and the spread of STDs by the ancient Greeks and Romans. It was done permanently in slaves and entertainers, but was removable for soldiers at age 25.

○ **Was infibulation ever accepted medical practice in the United States?**

It was commonly practiced starting in the 1860s and was not totally abandoned until 1929.

○ **What is an escutcheonectomy and what is its urological application?**

Excision of excessive suprapubic fat. It is one of several procedures to treat adult acquired buried penis. (The other procedures are scrotoplasty, split-thickness skin grafts, Y-V plasty, and panniculectomy.)

○ **Name the Roman god for lust and the god for marriage.**

Priapus for lust and Hymen for marriage.

○ **The early Christian church allowed sex in marriage only on what days?**

Tuesdays and Wednesdays.

○ **According to the Urologic Diseases in America Project by the NIDDK, what are the five most expensive urological conditions (in order) that accounted for more than $9 billion in 2007?**

In order, UTIs, kidney stones, prostate cancer, bladder cancer, and BPH.

○ **What are the estimated total yearly expenditures for overactive bladder in the United States?**

Approximately $16.4 billion.

○ **What percentage of patients can accurately and reliably fill out their AUA symptom scores by themselves without help?**

Sixteen percent.

○ **What is Zoon's balanitis, is it dangerous, and how is it treated?**

Also called plasma cell balanitis, Zoon's balanitis is a rare, idiopathic, benign penile dermatocytis. It causes a bright red skin in the glans under the foreskin. Microscopically, it shows significant plasma cell infiltration. The lesion does not respond to steroids. Recommended treatment is a circumcision.

○ **Achille Boari first described his successful method for ureteral extension in dogs in 1894. When was the first human trial of this technique and who did it? (Hint: It was not Boari and it was done somewhere in the United States.)**

The first human case was in 1936 by Ockerblad of Yale.

○ **Describe in detail the unique connection between urine and matches.**

German alchemist Hennig Brand was looking for the "philosopher's stone." In 1669, he distilled a small amount of a glowing chemical that burned brilliantly by boiling a large amount of urine. This new chemical was noticed by Robert Boyle who added it to sulfur-tipped wooden splinters to facilitate ignition—the first matches. (Fortunately, early commercial matches used crushed bone treated with acid instead of urine as a source of this chemical.) Today we call Brand's chemical "phosphorus."

○ **Define "Koro" and "Dhat" and where they are most prevalent.**

"Koro" syndrome is the pathologic fear that the penis is shrinking. "Dhat" is a significant decrease in vitality from excessive loss of semen. Koro is found mostly in Southeast Asia while Dhat is typical of India.

○ **What is a Candiru?**

It is the name of the small catfish of the Amazon that reportedly can swim up the human male urethra.

○ **Premature ejaculation, as defined by the International Society for Sexual Medicine includes what general time limit for ejaculation after vaginal penetration?**

One minute.

BIBLIOGRAPHY

Akerlund S, Campanello M, Kaijser B, et al. Bacteriuria in patients with a continent ileal reservoir for urinary diversion does not regularly require antibiotic treatment. *Br J Urol*. 1994;74:177–181.

Aparicio AM, Elkhouiery AB, Quinn DI: The current and future application of adjuvant systemic chemotherapy in patients with bladder cancer following cystectomy. *Urol Clin North Am*. 2005;32:217–230.

AUA Guidelines: Guidelines for the Management of Nonmuscle Invasive Bladder Cancer (Stage Ta, T1, and Tis), 2007.

Barzon L, Boscaro M. Diagnosis and management of adrenal incidentalomas. *J Urol*. 2000;163:398–407.

Baseman AG, Young RR Jr, Young AK, et al. Conservative management of spontaneous rupture of Kock orthotopic ileal reservoir. *Urology*. 1997;49:629–631.

Bauer SB. Anomalies of the kidney and ureteropelvic junction. In: Walsh PC, Retik AB, Vaughan ED, Wein AJ, eds. *Campbell's Urology*. 7th ed. Philadelphia, PA: W.B. Saunders; 1998.

Bearhs OH, Hanson DR, Hutter RVP, Kenedy BJ. *Manual for Staging of Cancer*. 4th ed. Philadelphia, PA: J.B. Lippincott; 1992:181.

Beilby JA, Keogh EJ. Spinal cord injuries and anejaculation. *Paraplegia*. 1989;27:152.

Benson MC, Olsson CA. Continent urinary diversion. In: Walsh PC, Retik AB, Vaughan ED, Wein AJ, eds. *Campbell's Urology*. 7th ed. Philadelphia, PA: W.B. Saunders; 1998:3190.

Benson MC, Olsson CA. Continent urinary diversion. *Urol Clin North Am*. 1999;26:125–147.

Bihrle R. The Indiana pouch continent urinary reservoir. *Urol Clin North Am*. 1997;24:773–779.

Bloch MJ, Trost DW, Pickering TG, Sos TA, August P. Prevention of recurrent pulmonary edema is patients with bilateral renovascular disease through renal artery stent replacement. *Am J Hypertens*. 1999;12(1, pt 1):1–7.

Blyth B, Snyder HM. Ureteropelvic junction obstruction in children. In: Krane RJ, Siroky MB, Fitzpatrick JM, eds. *Clinical Urology*. Philadelphia, PA: J.B. Lippincott; 1994.

Bosi GJ, Motzer RJ. Testicular germ-cell cancer. *N Engl J Med*. 1997;337(4):242–253.

Breneman JC, Donaldson SS, Hays DM. The management of pediatric genitourinary rhabdomyosarcoma. In: Vogelzang NJ, Scardino PT, Shipley WU, Coffey DS, eds. *Comprehensive Textbook of Genitourinary Oncology*. Baltimore, MD: Williams and Wilkins; 1996.

Bricker EM. Bladder substitution after pelvic evisceration. *Surg Clin North Am*. 1950;30:1511–1521.

Brossner C, Bayer G, Madersbacher S, Kuber W, Klinger C, Pycha A. Twelve prostate biopsies detect significant cancer volumes (>0.5 mL). *Br J Urol*. 2000;85(6):705.

Bukowski RM, Klein EA. Management of adrenal neoplasms. In: Vogelzang NJ, Scardino PT, Shipley WU, Coffey DS, eds. *Comprehensive Textbook of Genitourinary Oncology*. Baltimore, MD: Williams and Wilkins; 1996;125–153.

Buvat J, Lemaire A. Endocrine screening in 1022 men with erectile dysfunction: clinical significance and cost-effective strategy. *J Urol*. 1997;158:1764–1767.

Caldamone AA, Woodard JR. Prune Belly syndrome. In: Wein AJ, Kavoussi LR, Novick AC, Partin AW, Peters CA, eds. *Campbell-Walsh Urology*, 9th ed. Philadelphia, PA: W.B. Saunders; 2007.

Campbell-Walsh Urology (9th edition) Saunders-Elsevier Inc. Philadelphia, PA 2007.

Campbell MF, Wein AJ, Kavoussi LR. In: Wein AJ, Kavoussi LR, Novick AC, Partin AW, Peters CA, eds. *Campbell-Walsh Urology*. 9th ed. Philadelphia, PA: W.B. Saunders; 2007.

Carroll P, ed. Testis cancer. *Urol Clin North Am*. 1998;23(3).

Carson CC. Management of penile prosthesis infection. *Probi Urol*. 1993;7:368–380.

Cassady JR, Hutter JJ Jr, Whitesell LJ. Neuroblastoma: natural history and current therapeutic approaches. In: Vogelzang NJ, Scardino PT, Shipley WU, Coffey DS, eds. *Comprehensive Textbook of Genitourinary Oncology*. Baltimore, MD: Williams and Wilkins; 1996.

Catalona WJ. Urothelial tumors of the urinary tract. In: Walsh PC, Retik AB, Stamey TA, Vaughan ED Jr, eds. *Campbell's Urology*. Philadelphia, PA: W.B. Saunders; 1992:1094–1158.

CDC Surveillance Reports. Reported Tuberculosis in the United States, www.cdc.gov.

Cendron M, Elder JS, Duckett JW. Perinatal urology. In: Gillenwater JY, Grayhack JT, Howards SS, Duckett JW, eds. *Adult and Pediatric Urology*. Vol III. 3rd ed. St. Louis, MO: Mosby-Year Book, Inc.; 1996:2075–2169.

Cesaro S, Facchin C, Tridello G, et al. A prospective study of BK-virus-associated hemorrhagic cystitis in pediatric patients undergoing allogenic hematopoietic stem cell transplantation. *Bone Marrow Transplant*. 2008;41:363.

Cheville JC. Classification and pathology of testicular germ cell and sex cord-stromal tumors. *Urol Clin North Am*. 1999;26(3):595–609.

Chodak GW, Keller P, Scheonberg HW. Assessment of screening for prostate cancer using digital rectal examination. *J Urol*. 1989; 141:1136.

Choong SK, Gleeson M. Conservative management of a spontaneous rupture of a continent cutaneous urinary diversion. *Br J Urol*. 1998;82:592–593.

Clayman RV, McDougal EM, Figenshau RS. Endourology of the upper urinary noncalculous applications. In: Gillenwater JY, Grayhack JT, Howards SH, Duckett JW, eds. *Adult and Pediatric Urology*. 3rd ed. St. Louis, MO: Mosby; 1996.

Cohen and Resnik. Reoperative Urology. 1995.

Colding-Jorgensen M, Poulsen AL, Steven K. Mechanical characteristics of tubular and detubularized bowel for bladder substitution: theory, urodynamics and clinical results. *Br J Urol*. 1993;72:586–593.

Connolly JA, Peppas DS, Jeffs RD, Gearhart JP. Prevalence and repair of inguinal hernias in children with bladder exstrophy. *J Urol*. 1995;154(5):1900–1901.

Coplen DE, Snow BW, Duckett JW. Prune Belly syndrome. In: Gillenwater JY, Grayhack JT, Howards SS, Duckett JW, eds. *Adult and Pediatric Urology*. 3rd ed. St. Louis, MO: Mosby; 1996:2297.

Cruz DN, Huot SJ. Metabolic complications of urinary diversions: an overview. *Am J Med*. 1997;102:477–484.

Dahl DM, McDougal WS. Use of intestinal segments in urinary diversion. In: Wein AJ, Kavoussi LR, Novick AC, Partin AW, Peters CA, eds. *Campbell-Walsh Urology*, 9th ed. Philadelphia, PA: W.B. Saunders; 2007.

Davidson AJ, Hartman DS, eds. *Radiology of the Kidney and Genitourinary Tract*. 3rd ed. Philadelphia, PA: W.B. Saunders; 1999.

Davidsson T, Akerlund S, Forssell-Aronsson E, et al. Absorption of sodium and chloride in continent reservoirs for urine: comparison of ileal and colonic reservoirs. *J Urol*. 1994;151:335–337.

deKernion JB, Trapasso JG. Urinary diversion and continent reservoir. In: Gillenwater JY, Grayhack JT, Howards SS, Duckett JW, eds. *Adult and Pediatric Urology*. 3rd ed. St. Louis, MO: Mosby; 1996:1465.

Diamond M. Pediatric management of ambiguous and traumatized genitalia. *J Urol*. 1999;162(2):1021–1028.

Diamond DA, Gosalbez R. Neonatal urologic emergencies. In: Walsh PC, Retik AB, Vaughn ED, Wein AJ, eds. *Campbell's Urology*. Vol II. 7th ed. Philadelphia, PA: W.B. Saunders; 1998:1629–1654.

Dunnick NR, McCallum RW, Snadler CM. *Textbook of Uroradiology*. 2nd ed. Baltimore, MD: Williams and Wilkins; 1997.

Einhorn LH, Donohue JP. Advanced testicular cancer: update for urologists. *J Urol*. 1998;160(6, pt 1):1964–1969.

Eisenberger CF, Schoenberg M, Fitter D, Marshall FF. Orthotopic ileocolic neobladder reconstruction following radical cystectomy: history, technique and results of the Johns Hopkins experience, 1986–1998. *Urol Clin North Am*. 1999;26:149–156.

El Bahnasawy MS, Osman Y, Gomha MA, et al. Nocturnal enuresis in men with an orthotopic ileal reservoir: urodynamic evaluation. *J Urol*. 2000;164:10–13.

Elder JR, Hladky D, Selzmann AA. Outpatient nephrectomy for non-functioning kidneys. *J Urol*. 1993;154:712–715.

Endogenous Hormones and Prostate Cancer Collaborative Group. *J Natl Cancer Inst*. 2008;100:158.

Feldman HA, Goldstein I, Hatzichristou DG, Krane RJ, McKinlay JB. Impotence and its medical and psychosocial correlates. Results of the Massachusetts Male Aging Study. *J Urol*. 1994;151:54–46.

Fitzgerald J, Malone MJ, Gaertner RA, Zinman LN. Stomal construction, complications, and reconstruction. *Urol Clin North Am*. 1997;24:729–733.

Fowler JE, Koshy M, Strub M. Priapism associated with the sickle cell hemaglobinopathies: prevalence, natural history, and sequelae. *J Urol*. 1991;145:65–68.

Furness PD, Cheng EY, Franco I, Firlit CF. The Prune-Belly syndrome: a new and simplified technique of abdominal wall reconstruction. *J Urol*. 1998;160:1195.

Garovic V, Textor SC. Renovascular hypertension: current concepts. *Semin Nephrol*. 2005;25(4):261–271.

Gburek BM, Lieber MM, Blute ML. Comparison of Studer ileal neobladder and ileal conduit urinary diversion with respect to perioperative outcome and late complications. *J Urol*. 1998;160:721–723.

Gillenwater JY, Grayhack JT, Howards SS, Duckett JW, eds. *Adult and Pediatric Urology*. 3rd ed. St. Louis, MO: Mosby; 1996:2061–2758.

Goldfarb DS, Modersitzki F, Asplin JR. A randomized controlled trial of lactic acid bacteria for idopathic hyperoxaluria. *Clin J Am Soc Nephrol*. 2007;2(4):745–749.

Goldstein I, Lue TF, Padma-Nathan H, Rosen RC, Steers WD, Wicker PA. Oral Sildenafil in the treatment of erectile dysfunction. *N Engl J Med*. 1998;338:1397–1404.

Gonzales ET Jr. Anomalies of the renal pelvis and ureter. In: Kelalis PP, King LR, Belman AB, eds. *Clinical Pediatric Urology*. 3rd ed. Philadelphia, PA: W.B. Saunders; 1992.

Gordon I. Ultrasonography in uronephrology. In: O'Donnell B, Koff SA, eds. *Pediatric Urology*. 3rd ed. Oxford: Butterworth-Heinemann; 1997:41–64.

Gorelick JI, Goldstein M. Loss of fertility in men with varicocele. *Fertil Steril*. 1993;59:613.

Gow JG. The current management of patients with genitourinary tuberculosis. AUA Update Series, Lesson 26, Vol. XI, 1992.

Graves FT. The anatomy of the intrarenal arteries and its application to segmental resection of the kidney. *Br J Surg*. 1955;2:132.

Gray H. *Gray's Anatomy, the Anatomical Basis of Medicine and Surgery*. 38th ed. New York: Churchill Livingstone; 1995.

Gray H, Carter HV, Pick TP, Howden R. *Gray's Anatomy*. London: Senate; 2003.

Gray SW, Skandalakis JE. *Embryology for Surgeons*. Philadelphia, PA: W.B. Saunders; 1972.

Greskovich FJ, Nyberg LM. The prune belly syndrome: a review of its etiology, defects, treatment and prognosis. *J Urol*. 1988;140: 707.

Grossman HB, Natale RB, Tangen CM, et al.: Neoadjuvant chemotherapy plus cystectomy compared with cystectomy alone for locally advanced bladder cancer. *N Engl J Med*. 2003;349:859–866.

Guiney EJ. Emergency room problems. In: O'Donnell B, Koff SA, eds. *Pediatric Urology*. 3rd ed. Oxford: Butterworth-Heinemann; 1997:281–285.

Gulml FA, Felsen D, Vaughan ED. Pathophysiology of urinary tract obstruction. In: Walsh PC, Retik AB, Vaughan ED, Wein AJ, eds. *Campbell's Urology*. 7th ed. Philadelphia, PA: W.B. Saunders; 1998.

Guyton AC. *Textbook of Medical Physiology*. 8th ed. Philadelphia, PA: W.B. Saunders; 1991.

Haas GP, Triest J, Pontes E, Trump DL. Nonsurgical treatment of adrenocortical cancer. In: Raghavan D, Scher HI, Leibel SA, Lange P, eds. *Principles and Practice of Genitourinary Oncology*. Philadelphia, PA: Lippincott-Raven; 1997:1001–1006.

Hanno PM. Diagnosis of interstitial cystitis. *Urol Clin North Am*. 1994;21(1):1, 63.

Hautmann RE. The ileal neobladder to the female urethra. *Urol Clin North Am*. 1997;24:827–835.

Hautmann RE, Simon J. Ileal neobladder and local recurrence of bladder cancer: patterns of failure and impact on function in men. *J Urol*. 1999;162:1963–1966.

Hedge GA, Colby HD, Goodman RL. *Clinical Endocrine Physiology*. Philadelphia, PA: W.B. Saunders; 1987.

Hendren WH. Historical perspective of the use of bowel in urology. *Urol Clin North Am*. 1997;24:703–713.

Hendren WH. Urinary undiversion: refunctionalization of the previously diverted urinary tract. In: Walsh PC, Retik AB, Vaughan ED, Wein AJ, eds. *Campbell's Urology*. 7th ed. Philadelphia, PA: W.B. Saunders; 1998:3247.

Henly DR, Farrow GM, Zincke H. Urachal Carcinoma: Role of conservative surgery. *Urology*. 1993;42:635–639.

Hensle TW, Bingham JB, Reiley EA, et al. The urologic care and outcome of pregnancy after urinary tract reconstruction. *BJU Int*. 2004;93:588–590.

Herr HW: Superiority of ratio based lymph node staging for bladder cancer. *J Urol*. 2003;169:943–945.

Herr HW: Restaging transurethral resection of high risk superficial bladder cancer improves the initial response to bacillus Calmette-Guérin therapy. *J Urol*. 2005;174:2134–2137.

Hinman F. *Atlas of Urosurgical Anatomy*. Philadelphia, PA: W.B. Saunders; 1993.

Hinman F Jr. *Atlas of Urologic Surgery*. 2nd ed. Philadelphia, PA: W.B. Saunders; 1998.

Hoffman DM, Resnick MI. Return of perineal prostatectomy, *MediGuide Urol*. 1993;6(3).

Hogan JD, Smith AD. Endopyelotomy and pyeloplasty. In: Krane RJ, Siroky MB, Fitzpatrick JM, eds. *Clinical Urology*. Philadelphia, PA: J.B. Lippincott; 1994.

Husmann DA, Levy JB, Cain MP, et al. Micropenis: Current Concepts and Controversies. In: AUA Update Series. Lesson 10, Vol. XVII. Houston, TX: American Urological Association; 1998:74–79.

Ibarra F, Casanova JL, Solsona E. Tolerance of external urinary diversion (Bricker) followed for more than 10 years. *Eur Urol*. 2001;39(suppl 5):146–147.

Inman BA, Harel F, Tiguert R, et al. Routine nasogastric tubes are not required following cystectomy with urinary diversion: a comparative analysis of 430 patients. *J Urol*. 2003;170:1888–1891.

Johnson DE, Hodges GB, Abdul-Karim FW, et al. Urachal carcinoma. *Urology*. 1985;26:218–221.

Kabalin JN. In: Walsh PC, Retik AB, Vaughan ED Jr, Wein AJ, eds. *Campbell's Urology*. Vol I. 7th ed. Philadelphia, PA: W.B. Saunders; 1998.

Kaefer M, Retik AB. The Mitrofanoff principle in continent urinary reconstruction. *Urol Clin North Am*. 1997;24:795–811.

Kass EJ. Megaureter. In: Kelalis PP, King LR, Belman AB, eds. *Clinical Pediatric Urology*. 3rd ed. Philadelphia, PA: W.B. Saunders; 1992.

Katz MD, Imperato-McGinley J. Adrenal cancer: endocrinology, diagnosis and clinical staging. In: Raghavan D, Scher HI, Leibel SA, Lange P, eds. *Principles and Practice of Genitourinary Oncology*. Philadelphia, PA: Lippincott-Raven; 1997:981–992.

Kelalis PP, King LR, Belman AB, eds. *Clinical Pediatric Urology*. Vol. 2, 3rd ed. Philadelphia, PA: W.B. Saunders; 1992.

Kim J-H, et al. Contemporary management of renovascular hypertension. *AUA Update Series*. 2007;26:Lesson 14.

King LR. Vesicoureteral reflux, megaureter and ureteral reimplantation. In: Walsh PC, Retik AB, Vaughan ED Jr, Wein AJ, eds. *Campbell's Urology*. 6th ed. Philadelphia, PA: W.B. Saunders; 2007.

Koch MO, Gurevitch E, Hill DE, et al. Urinary solute transport by intestinal segments: a comparative study of ileum and colon in rats. *J Urol*. 1990;143:1275–1279.

Koch MO, McDougal WS. Chlorpromazine: adjuvant therapy for the metabolic derangements created by urinary diversion through intestinal segments. *J Urol*. 1985;134(1):165–169.

Koch MO, Smith JA. Surgical management of adrenal tumors. In: Raghavan D, Scher HI, Leibel SA, Lange P, eds. *Principles and Practice of Genitourinary Oncology*. Philadelphia, PA: Lippincott-Raven; 1997:993–1000.

Kogan BA. Disorders of the ureter and ureteropelvic junction. In: Tanango EA, McAnich JW, eds. *Smith's General Urology*. 14th ed. Norwalk, CT: Appleton and Lange; 1995.

Kogan S, Hadziselimovic F, Howards SS, Snyder HM, Huff D. Pediatric andrology. In: Gillenwater JY, Grayhack JT, Howards SS, Duckett JW, eds. *Adult and Pediatric Urology*. 3rd ed. St. Louis, MO: Mosby; 1996:2623–2674.

Koo HP, Bloom DA. Laparoscopy for the nonpalpable testis. *Semin Laparosc Surg*. 1998;5:40–46.

Korman HJ: Monographs in Urology. 1996: 17:83–95.

Korman HJ, Watson RB, Soloway MS. Bladder cancer: clinical aspects and management, 1996. In: Stamey TS, ed. *Monographs in Urology*. Vol 17. 1996:6, 81–110.

Koziol JA. Epidemiology of interstitial cystitis. *Urol Clin North Am*. 1994;21(1):1, 7.

Kramer SA. Vesicoureteral reflux. In: Kelalis PP, King LR, Belman AB, eds *Clinical Pediatric Urology*. 3rd ed. Philadelphia, PA: W.B. Saunders; 1992.

Krane RJ et al., eds. *Clinical Urology*. Philadelphia, PA: J.B. Lippincott; 1994.

Kristjansson A, Bajc M, Wallin L, et al. Renal function up to 16 years after conduit (refluxing or anti-reflux anastomosis) or continent urinary diversion. 2. Renal scarring and location of bacteriuria. *Br J Urol*. 1995b;76:546–550.

Kristjansson A, Wallin L, Mansson W. Renal function up to 16 years after conduit (refluxing or anti-reflux anastomosis) or continent urinary diversion. 1. Glomerular filtration rate and patency of uretero-intestinal anastomosis. *Br J Urol*. 1995a;76:539–545.

Lee PA. Fertility in cryptorchidism: does treatment make a difference? *Endocrinol Metab Clin North Am*. 1993;22:479.

Lecouvet FE et al. *J. Clin. Oncol*. 2007;25:3281–3287.

Leissner J, Black P, Fisch M, et al. Colon pouch (Mainz Pouch III) for continent urinary diversion after pelvic irradiation. *Urology*. 2000; 56:798–802.

Levy DA, Resnick MI. Laparoscopic pelvic lymphadenectomy and radical perineal prostatectomy: a viable alternative to radical retropubic prostatectomy. *J Urol*. 1994;151:905.

Licht MR, Lewis RW, Wollan PC, Harris CD. Comparison of RigiScan and sleep laboratory nocturnal penile tumescence in the diagnosis of organic impotence. *J Urol*. 1995;154:1740–1743.

Madersbacher S, Mohrle K, Burkhard F, et al. Long-term voiding pattern of patients with ileal orthotopic bladder substitutes. *J Urol*. 2002;167:2052–2057.

Malone MJ, Izes JK, Hurley LJ. Carcinogenesis: the fate of intestinal segments used in urinary reconstruction. *Urol Clin North Am*. 1997;24:723–728.

Mansson W, Colleen S, Mardh PA. The microbial flora of the continent cecal urinary reservoir, its stoma and the peristomal skin. *J Urol*. 1986;135:247–250.

Mansson W, Davidsson T, Konyves J, et al. Continent urinary tract reconstruction—The Lund experience. *BJU Int*. 2003;92: 271–276.

Manyak MJ, Hinkle GH, Olsen JO, et al. Immunoscintigraphy with indium-111-capromed pendetide: evaluation before definitive therapy in patients with prostate cancer. *Urology*. 1999;54(6):1058.

Matzkin H, Moinuddin SM, Soloway MS. Value of urine cytology versus bladder washing in bladder cancer. *Urology*. 1992;39:201–203.

McDougal WS. Metabolic complications of urinary intestinal diversion. *J Urol*. 1992;147:1199–1208.

McDougal WS. Use of intestinal segments and urinary diversion. In: Walsh PC, Retik AB, Vaughan ED, Wein AJ, eds. *Campbell's Urology*. 7th ed. Philadelphia, PA: W.B. Saunders; 1998:3121.

McDougal WS, Koch MO. Effect of sulfate on calcium and magnesium homeostasis following urinary diversion. *Kidney Int*. 1989;35: 105–115.

Meyers RP. Practical pelvic anatomy pertinent to radical retropubic prostatectomy. AUA Update Series XIII, Lesson 4, 1994.

Mills RD, Studer UE. Metabolic consequences of continent urinary diversion. *J Urol.* 1999;161:1057–1066.

Morris PJ ed. *Kidney Transplantation: Principles and Practice.* 4th ed. 1994.

Muruve NA. E-medicine: radiation cystitis. Feb 7, 2008.

Narayan P, Konety BR. Surgical treatment of female urethral carcinoma. *Urol Clin North Am.* 1992;19(2):373–382.

Nieh PT. The Kock pouch urinary reservoir. *Urol Clin North Am.* 24:755–772.

Nippgen JB, Hakenberg OW, Manseck A, et al. Spontaneous late rupture of orthotopic detubularized ileal neobladders: report of five cases. *Urology.* 2001;58:43–46.

Noh PH, Cooper CS, Winkler AC, et al. Prognostic factors for long-term renal function in boys with prune-belly syndrome. *J Urol.* 1999;162:1399.

Norman and Suki, eds. Primer on Transplantation. 1998.

Novick AC, Howards SS. The adrenals. In: Gillenwater JY, Grayhack JT, Howards SS, Duckett JW, eds. *Adult and Pediatric Urology.* 3rd ed. Mosby; 1996:587–616.

Novick AC, Streem SB. Surgery of the kidney. In: Walsh PC, Retik AB, Vaughan ED, Wein AJ, eds. *Campbell's Urology.* 7th ed. Philadelphia, PA: W.B. Saunders; 1998.

Oates RD, Lipshultz LI. Fertility and testicular function in patients after chemotherapy and radiotherapy. *Adv Urol.* 1989;10:52.

O'Donnell B, Koff SA, eds. *Pediatric Urology.* 3rd ed. Oxford: Butterworth Heinemann; 1997.

Parekh DJ, Gilbert WB, Koch MO, et al. Continent urinary reconstruction versus ileal conduit: a contemporary single-institution comparison of perioperative morbidity and mortality. *Urology.* 2000;55:852–855.

Parsons CL, Parsons JK. Interstitial cystitis. In: Shlomo Raz, ed. *Female Urology.* 2nd ed. Saunders; 1996.

Partin AW, Yoo J, Carter HB, et al. The use of prostatic specific antigen, clinical stage and gleason's score to predict pathological stage in men with localized prostate cancer. *J Urol.* 1993;150:110.

Partin AW, Yoo J, Carter HB, et al. Letter to the Editor. *J Urol.* 1994;152:172.

Penn I. Renal transplantation in patients with pre-existing malignancies. *Transplant Proc.* 1983;15:1079.

Peters P. "Ball Peen Hammer" appearance of the duplicated collecting system. Personal communication.

Pisansky T et al. An enhanced prognostic system for clinically localized carcinoma of the prostate. *Cancer.* 1997;79:2154–2161.

Presti JC, Chang JJ, Bhargava V, Shinohara K. The optimal systematic prostate biopsy scheme should include 8 rather than 6 biopsies: results of a prospective clinical trial. *J Urol.* 2000;163(1):163.

Pryor JP, Hendry WF. Ejaculatory duct obstruction in subfertile males: analysis of 87 patients. *Fertil Steril.* 1991;56:725.

Racioppi M, D'Addessi A, Fanasca A, et al. Acid-base and electrolyte balance in urinary intestinal orthotopic reservoir: ileocecal neobladder compared with ileal neobladder. *Urology.* 1999;54:629–635.

Ramos CG, Carvalhal GF, Smith DS, Mager DE, Catalona WJ. Retrospective comparison of radical retropubic prostatectomy and 125-iodine brachytherapy for a localized prostate cancer. *J Urol.* 1999;161(4):1212–1215.

Ravi R, Dewan AK, Pandey KK. Transverse colon conduit urinary diversion in patients treated with very high dose pelvic irradiation. *Br J Urol.* 1994;73:51–54.

Redman JF. In: Raghavan D, Scher HI, Leibel SA, Lange P, eds. *Principles and Practice of Genitourinary Oncology.* Philadelphia, PA: Lippincott-Raven; 1997.

Resnik MI, Kursh ED. Extrinsic obstruction of the ureter. In: Walsh PC, Retik AB, Vaughan ED, Wein AJ, eds. *Campbell's Urology.* 7th ed. Philadelphia, PA: W.B. Saunders; 1998.

Retik AB, Peters CA. Ectopic Ureter and Ureterocele. In: Walsh PC, Retik AB, Vaughan ED Jr, Wein AJ, eds. *Campbell's Urology.* 6th ed. Philadelphia, PA: W.B. Saunders; 1992.

Ritchie JP. Testicular neoplasms. In: Walsh P, Retik A, Vaughan E, Wein A, eds. *Campbell's Urology.* 7th ed. Philidelphia, PA: W.B. Saunders; 1998:2411.

Rob DH, Blascoe JC, Grim PD, et al. Interstitial iodine—125 radiation without adjuvant therapy, the treatment of clinically localized prostate. *Cancer.* 1997;80:442.

Sadler TW. *Langman's Medical Embryology.* 6th ed. Baltimore, MD: Williams & Wilkins; 1990:260–296.

Sarosdy MF. Immunotherapy of superficial bladder carcinoma, AUA Update Series, Lesson 29, Volume XIV, 1995:234–239.

Schaeffer AJ. Urinary tract infections. In: Gillenwater JY, Grayhack JT, Howards SH, Duckett JW, eds. *Adult and Pediatric Urology.* 3rd ed. Mosby, MO: St. Louis; 1996.

Schaeffer AJ. Infections and Inflammations of the Genitourinary Tract. In: Walsh PC, Retik AB, Vaughan ED, Wein AJ, eds. *Campbell's Urology.* Philadelphia, PA: W.B. Saunders; 1998.

Shokeir AA. The diagnosis of upper urinary tract obstruction. European Urology Update Series 1999:3. *BJU*. 1999;83:893.

Singh G, Wilkinson JM, Thomas DG. Supravesical diversion for incontinence: a long-term follow-up. *BJU Int*. 1997;79:348–353.

Siroky MB, Edelstein RA, Krane RJ, eds. *Manual of Urology*. 2nd ed. Philadelphia, PA: Lippincott Williams & Wilkins; 1999.

Smith RB, Ehrlich RM, eds. *Complications or Urologic Surgery, Prevention and Management*. 2nd ed. Philadephia, PA: W.B. Saunders; 1990:386–411.

Snyder HM III, D'Angio GJ, Evans AE, Raney RB. Pediatric oncology. In: Walsh PC, Retik AB, Vaughan ED, Wein AJ, eds. *Campbell's Urology*. 7th ed. Philadelphia, PA: W.B. Saunders; 1998.

Sobin LH, Wittekind CH, eds; International Union Against Cancer. *TNM Classification of Malignant Tumours*. New York: Wiley-Liss, 1997:187–190.

Soloway MS. Expectant treatment of small, recurrent, low-grade, noninvasive tumors of the urinary bladder. *Urol Oncol*. 2006;24:58–61.

Splinter TA, Scher HI. Adjuvant and neoadjuvant chemotherapy for invasive (T3-T4) bladder cancer. In: Vogelzang NJ, Scardino PT, Shipley WU, Cofffey DS, Miles BJ, eds. *Comprehensive Textbook of Genitourinary Oncology*. Baltimore, MD: Williams and Wilkins; 1996:464–471.

Stamey TA, Yang N, Hay AR, McNeal JE, Freiha FS, Redwine E. Prostate-specific antigen as a serum marker for adenocarcinoma of the prostate. *N Engl J Med*. 1987;317:909.

Stamm WE. Treatment of acute uncomplicated urinary tract infection. In: Bergan T, ed. *Urinary Tract Infections*. Basel, Switzerland: Karger; 1997.

Stampfer DS, McDougal WS, McGovern FJ. Metabolic and nutritional complications. *Urol Clin North Am*. 1997;24:715–722.

Stein R, Fisch M, Beetz R. Urinary diversion in children and young adults using the Mainz Pouch I technique. *Br J Urol*. 1997;79:354–361.

Stein JP, Cai J, Groshen S, Skinner DG. Risk factors for patients with pelvic lymph node metastases following radical cystectomy with en bloc pelvic lymphadenectomy: Concept of lymph node density. *J Urol*. 2003;170:35.

Stein JP, Clark P, Miranda G, Cai J, Groshen S, Skinner DG. Urethral tumor recurrence following cystectomy and urinary diversion: Clinical and pathological characteristics in 768 male patients. *J Urol*. 2005;173:1163–1168.

Stephens FD. *Congenital Malformations of the Urinary Tract*. New York: Praeger; 1983.

Studer UE, Hautmann RE, Hohenfellner M, et al. Indications for continent diversion after cystectomy and factors affecting long-term results. *Urol Oncol*. 1998;4:172–176.

Studer UE, Zingg EJ. Ileal orthotopic bladder substitutes: what we have learned from 12 years experience with 200 patients. *Urol Clin North Am*. 1997;24:781–793.

Tanagho EA, McAninch JW, eds. *Smith's General Urology*. 14th ed. Norwalk, CT: Appleton & Lange; 1995.

Tchetgen MB, Sanda MG, Montie JE, et al. Collagen injection for the treatment of incontinence after cystectomy and orthotopic neobladder reconstruction in women. *J Urol*. 2000;163:212–214.

Tolkoff-Rubin NE, Rubin RH. Urinary tract infection in the renal transplant recipient. In: Bergan T, ed. *Urinary Tract Infections*. Basel, Switzerland: Karger; 1997.

Turek PJ, Lipshultz LI. Immunologic infertility. *Urol Clin North Am*. 1994;21:447.

Valicenti RK et al. Effect of higher radiation dose on biochemical control after radical prostatectomy for pT3N0 prostate cancer. *Int J Rad Oncol Biol Phys*. 1998;42(3):501–506.

Varol C, Studer UE. Managing patients after an ileal orthotopic bladder substitution. *BJU Int*. 2004;93:266–270.

Vates TS, Steinberg GD. Testicular, sacrococcygeal, and other tumors. In: Vogelzang NJ, Scardino PT, Shipley WU, Coffey DS, eds. *Comprehensive Textbook of Genitourinary Oncology*. Baltimore, MD: Williams and Wilkins; 1996.

Vaughan ED, Blumenfeld JD. The adrenals. In: Walsh PC, Retik AB, Vaughan ED, Wein AJ, eds. *Campbell's Urology*. 7th ed. Philadelphia, PA: W.B. Saunders; 1998.

Vermeulen CW et al. *J Urol*. 1967;97(7):573–582.

Vogelzang NJ et al., eds. *Comprehensive Textbook of Genitourinary Oncology*. 2nd ed. Philadelphia, PA: Lippincott Williams & Wilkins; 1999.

Vogelzang NJ, Scardino P, Shipley WU, Coffey DS, eds. *Comprehensive Textbook of Genitourinary Oncology*. Baltimore, MD: Williams & Wilkins Press; 1996.

Walsh PC, Retick AB, Vaughn ED Jr, Wein AJ. *Cambell's Urology*. 6th ed. Philadelphia, PA: W.B. Saunders; 1992:1194–1221.

Walsh PC, Retik AB, Darracott Vaughan E Jr, Wein AJ, eds. *Campbell's Urology*. 7th ed. Philadelphia, PA: W.B. Saunders; 1998.

Wein AJ, Broderick GA. Interstitial cystitis: current and future approaches to diagnosis and treatment. 1994;21(1):1, 153.

Weiss RE, Fair WR. Urachal anomalies and urachal carcinoma. In: AUA Update Series, Vol. XVII, Lesson 38, 1998, American Urological Association.

Wilimas JA, Greenwald CA, Rao BK. Wilms' tumor. In: Vogelzang NJ, Scardino PT, Shipley WU, Coffey DS, eds. *Comprehensive Textbook of Genitourinary Oncology*. Baltimore, MD: Williams and Wilkins; 1996.

Williams O, Vereb MJ, Libertino JA. Noncontinent urinary diversion. *Urol Clin North Am*. 1997;24:735–744.

Williamson MR, Smith AY. *Fundamentals of Uroradiology*. Philadelphia, PA: W.B. Saunders; 2000.

Woodard JR, Smith EA. Prune-Belly syndrome. In: Walsh PC, Retick AB, Vaughan ED, Wein AJ, eds. *Campbell's Urology*. 7th ed. Philadelphia, PA: W.B. Saunders; 1998:1917.

Woodard JR, Zucker I. Current management of the dilated urinary tract in prune belly syndrome. *Urol Clin North Am*. 1990;17: 407.

World Health Organization. A double-blind trial of clomiphene citrate for the treatment of idiopathic male infertility. *Int J Androl*. 1992;15:299.

World Health Organization (WHO) Consensus Conference on Bladder Cancer; Hautmann RE, Abol-Enein H, Hafez K, Mansson W, Mills RD, Montie JD, Sagalowsky AI, Stein JP, Stenzl A, Studer UE, Volkmer BG. Urinary diversion. *Urology*. 2007;69(1 suppl): 17–49.

Yeung CK, Jennifer DY Sihoe. In: Wein AJ, Kavoussi LR, Novick AC, Partin AW, Peters CA, eds. *Campbell-Walsh Urology*. 9th ed. Philadelphia, PA: W.B. Saunders; 2007:3605–3624.

Young RH. Pathology of carcinomas of the urinary bladder. In: Vogelzang NJ, Scardino PT, Shipley WU, Coffey DS, eds. *Comprehensive Textbook of Genitourinary Oncology*. Philadelphia, PA: Lippincott Williams & Wilkins; 2000.